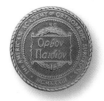
American Academy of Orthopaedic Surgeons

OKU

Orthopaedic Knowledge Update:

Pediatrics

2

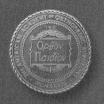

American Academy of Orthopaedic Surgeons

OKU

Orthopaedic Knowledge Update:

Pediatrics

2

Edited by
Paul D. Sponseller, MD, MBA
Professor and Head, Division of Pediatric Orthopedics
Johns Hopkins Medical Institutions
Baltimore, Maryland

Developed by the
Pediatric Orthopaedic Society of North America

Published 2002
by the American Academy of Orthopaedic Surgeons
6300 North River Road
Rosemont, IL 60018
1-800-626-6726

The material presented in *Orthopaedic Knowledge Update: Pediatrics 2* has been made available by the American Academy of Orthopaedic Surgeons for educational purposes only. This material is not intended to present the only, or necessarily best, methods or procedures for the medical situations discussed, but rather is intended to represent an approach, view, statement, or opinion of the author(s) or producer(s), which may be helpful to others who face similar situations.

Some drugs or medical devices demonstrated in Academy courses or described in Academy print or electronic publications have not been cleared by the Food and Drug Administration (FDA) or have been cleared for specific uses only. The FDA has stated that it is the responsibility of the physician to determine the FDA clearance status of each drug or device he or she wishes to use in clinical practice.

The U.S. FDA has expressed concern about potential serious patient care issues involved with the use of polymethylmethacrylate (PMMA) bone cement in the spine. A physician might insert the PMMA bone cement into vertebrae by various procedures, including vertebroplasty and kyphoplasty. Orthopaedic surgeons should be alert to possible complications.

PMMA bone cement is considered a device for FDA purposes. In October 1999, the FDA reclassified PMMA bone cement as a Class II device for its intended use "in arthroplastic procedures of the hip, knee, and other joints for the fixation of polymer or metallic prosthetic implants to living bone." The use of a device for other than its FDA-cleared indication is an off-label use. Physicians may use a device off-label if they believe, in their best medical judgment, that its use is appropriate for a particular patient (eg, tumors).

The use of PMMA bone cement in the spine is described in Academy educational courses, videotapes, and publications for educational purposes only. As is the Academy's policy regarding all of its educational offerings, the fact that the use of PMMA bone cement in the spine is discussed does not constitute an Academy endorsement of this use.

Furthermore, any statements about commercial products are solely the opinion(s) of the author(s) and do not represent an Academy endorsement or evaluation of these products. These statements may not be used in advertising or for any commercial purpose.

First Edition
Copyright © 2002 by the
American Academy of Orthopaedic Surgeons

ISBN 0-89203-238-3

Acknowledgments

Contributors

Mark F. Abel, MD
Associate Professor
Department of Orthopaedic Surgery
and Pediatrics
University of Virginia
Charlottesville, Virginia

Stephen A. Albanese, MD
Professor
Department of Orthopedic Surgery
SUNY Upstate Medical University
Syracuse, New York

R. Tracy Ballock, MD
Associate Professor of Orthopaedics
and Pediatrics
Department of Orthopaedics
Case Western Reserve University
University Hospitals of Cleveland
Rainbow Babies and Children's
Hospital
Cleveland, Ohio

J. Sybil Biermann, MD
Assistant Professor
Department of Orthopaedic Surgery
University of Michigan
Ann Arbor, Michigan

Brian E. Black, MD
Medical Director, Spinal Performance
Center of St. Francis Hospital
Department of Pediatric Orthopedic
Surgery
Sports Medicine and Orthopedic
Center, S.C.
Milwaukee, Wisconsin

John S. Blanco, MD
Associate Professor of Orthopedic
Surgery and Pediatrics
Department of Orthopedic Surgery
University of Virginia
Charlottesville, Virginia

R. Dale Blasier, MD, FRCSC
Professor of Orthopaedic Surgery
University of Arkansas for Medical
Science
Arkansas Children's Hospital
Little Rock, Arkansas

Steven L. Buckley, MD
Children's Orthopedics
Huntsville, Alabama

Alvin H. Crawford, MD
Director of Orthopaedic Surgery
Cincinnati Children's Hospital Medical
Center
Department of Pediatric Orthopaedic
Surgery
Cincinnati Children's Hospital
Cincinnati, Ohio

Diane L. Damiano, PhD, PT
Associate Professor
Department of Neurological Surgery
Washington University
St. Louis, Missouri

Richard S. Davidson, MD
Associate Clinical Professor
Department of Orthopaedic Surgery
Children's Hospital of Philadelphia
Shriners Hospital of Philadelphia
Philadelphia, Pennsylvania

Peter A. DeLuca, MD
Pediatric Orthopaedic Surgeon
Connecticut Orthopaedic Specialists
New Haven, Connecticut

Luciano Dias, MD
Professor of Orthopedic Surgery
Northwestern University
Department of Orthopedic Surgery
Children's Memorial Hospital
Chicago, Illinois

Atiq Durrani, MD
Resident
Department of Orthopedic Surgery
University of Cincinnati
Cincinnati, Ohio

John C. Eldridge, MD
Assistant Clinical Professor of
Orthopaedics and Pediatrics
Children's Orthopaedics of Louisville
Louisville, Kentucky

David W. Gray, MD
Medical Director
Department of Orthopaedics
Cook Children's Hospital
Fort Worth, Texas

John J. Grayhack, MD, MS
Assistant Professor of Orthopedic
Surgery
The Children's Memorial Medical
Center
Northwestern University Medical
School
Chicago, Illinois

Lori A. Karol, MD
Associate Professor
University of Texas, Southwestern
Department of Orthopaedic Surgery
Texas Scottish Rite Hospital
Dallas, Texas

Erik C. King, MD
Attending Physician, Division of
Pediatric Orthopaedic Surgery
Children's Memorial Hospital
Instructor, Department of Orthopaedic
Surgery
Northwestern University Medical
School
Chicago, Illinois

Steven E. Koop, MD
Medical Director
Associate Professor of Orthopedics
Gillette Children's Specialty Healthcare
St. Paul, Minnesota

Shobha Malviya, MD
Associate Professor of Anesthesiology
Section of Pediatric Anesthesiology
University of Michigan Hospital and
Health Center
Ann Arbor, Michigan

Gregory A. Mencio, MD
Associate Professor
Department of Orthopaedics and
Rehabilitation
Vanderbilt University
Nashville, Tennessee

Sandra I. Merkel, MS, RN
Clinical Nurse Specialist
Pediatric Pain Service
C.S. Mott Children's Hospital
University of Michigan Health System
Ann Arbor, Michigan

Vincent S. Mosca, MD
Associate Professor and Chief of
    Pediatric Orthopedics
Children's Hospital and Regional
    Medical Center
University of Washington School of
    Medicine
Seattle, Washington

Charles Paidas, MD
Director, Pediatric Trauma
Department of General Pediatric
    Surgery
Johns Hopkins Hospital
Baltimore, Maryland

B. Stephens Richards, MD
Assistant Chief of Staff
Associate Professor
Department of Orthopaedic Surgery
Texas Scottish Rite Hospital for
    Children
Dallas, Texas

John F. Sarwark, MD
Interim Division Head
Department of Pediatric Orthopaedic
    Surgery
Children's Memorial Hospital
Associate Professor
Department of Orthopaedic Surgery
Northwestern University Medical
    School
Chicago, Illinois

William J. Shaughnessy, MD
Chair, Division of Pediatric
    Orthopedics
Assistant Professor of Orthopedic
    Surgery
Department of Orthopedics
Mayo Clinic
Rochester, Minnesota

Stephen R. Skinner, MD
Chief of Staff, Orthopaedics
Shriners Hospitals for Children
Sacramento, California

Brian G. Smith, MD
Associate Professor
Newington Department of
    Orthopaedics
Connecticut Children's Medical Center
Hartford, Connecticut

Paul D. Sponseller, MD, MBA
Professor and Head, Division of
    Pediatric Orthopedics
Johns Hopkins Medical Institutions
Baltimore, Maryland

Carl L. Stanitski, MD
Professor of Orthopaedic Surgery
Medical University of South Carolina
Charleston, South Carolina

Deborah F. Stanitski, MD
Professor
Department of Orthopaedic Surgery
Medical University of South Carolina
Charleston, South Carolina

John G. Thometz, MD
Professor
Department of Orthopaedic Surgery
    (Pediatric)
Medical College of Wisconsin
Milwaukee, Wisconsin

Laura L. Tosi, MD
Chair, Department of Orthopaedics
Children's National Medical Center
Washington, District of Columbia

Peter M. Waters, MD
Associate Professor, Orthopedic
    Surgery
Clinical Director, Hand and Upper
    Extremity Surgery
Children's Hospital
Harvard Medical School
Boston, Massachusetts

Table of Contents

American Academy of Orthopaedic Surgeons

Section 3: Lower Extremity
Section Editor: Steven L. Buckley, MD

Section 4: Neuromuscular Disorders
Section Editor: Mark F. Abel, MD

Section V: Spine
Section Editor: Stephen A. Albanese, MD

Preface

The second edition of *Orthopaedic Knowledge Update: Pediatrics* builds upon the success of the first edition, fulfilling a need for a text written for the general orthopaedic surgeon that provides a concise review and update on recent developments in the field. In addition to sections on general pediatric orthopaedics, trauma, disorders of the lower extremity, and disorders of the spine, we have added a new section on neuromuscular disorders. The principles we have used throughout the book include concise style, practical modern focus, use of summary tables, and an annotated bibliography that summarizes recent literature. Most chapters also include a classic bibliography noting literature that was published before 1995.

The high quality of this book is due in large part to the efforts of the section editors—William Shaughnessy, Steven Buckley, Mark Abel, and Stephen Albanese—each a leader in the field and an experienced author. They have chosen a panel of expert chapter authors who have volunteered their efforts on behalf of the American Academy of Orthopaedic Surgeons. Great credit and thanks also goes to the publications staff at the Academy, particularly Susan Baim, Lynne Shindoll, Lisa Moore, Sophie Tosta, and Marilyn Fox. We hope that the readers find this a useful resource in caring for children with musculoskeletal disorders. We welcome suggestions to make future editions as helpful as possible.

Paul D. Sponseller, MD
Editor

Section 1

General Pediatric Orthopaedics

Section Editor:
William J. Shaughnessy, MD

Section 1

General Pediatric Orthopaedics

Overview

This section updates the reader on a variety of subjects of interest in pediatric orthopaedics. The limping child is discussed, specifically options for differential diagnoses and timely updates on several conditions, including transient synovitis, diskitis, and a variety of inflammatory, neoplastic, and developmental disorders. The chapter on evaluation of back pain emphasizes the importance of appropriate imaging studies and lists the differential diagnoses. The chapter on rotational and angular deformities of the lower extremities reviews such disorders as intoeing and outtoeing, as well as less common conditions such as focal fibrocartilaginous dysplasia. Osteomyelitis, septic arthritis, and the changing nature of musculoskeletal infections in children resulting from widespread vaccination for *Haemophilus influenzae B* are updated in the chapter on pediatric orthopaedic infections. HIV, resistance to antibiotics, and relatively uncommon conditions such as SAPHO and tuberculosis are discussed as well. In the chapter on pain management, physiologic measurement and self-reporting of pain are presented as tools available to the physician. The genetic basis for many neoplasms in children is the focus of the chapter on musculoskeletal neoplasms. Finally, substantial new information regarding osteogenesis imperfecta is presented, specifically the molecular genetic basis of the condition and treatments with bisphosphonates. Even among the long-standing topics covered in this section, new material is presented that will allow the orthopaedic surgeon to better understand the underlying condition and more effectively treat the pediatric patient.

William J. Shaughnessy, MD
Section Editor

Chapter 1

The Limping Child

B. Stephens Richards, MD

Introduction

A new episode of limping is often the reason for a child's visit to a physician in the emergency department. Ultimately, the responsibility to correctly identify the source of the limp falls on the orthopaedic surgeon. Some causes of a limp, such as septic arthritis, osteomyelitis, or slipped capital femoral epiphysis, require urgent treatment. Other causes, such as transient synovitis, require minimal management of the symptoms. This chapter is intended to provide information that will allow the orthopaedic surgeon to systematically evaluate a child with a limp.

Many of the conditions that lead to painless or painful limping in childhood will also be discussed in other chapters; therefore, only a brief mention will be found here. Rather, an organized approach to the cause of the limp and any urgent treatment programs will be described (Table 1).

The importance of a thorough history of the child's limp cannot be overemphasized. The time of onset, presence of antecedent trauma or infection, treatment provided before the initial evaluation, and pertinent perinatal history all are useful pieces of information that may lead to a provisional diagnosis. A meticulous physical examination should identify the site responsible for the limp. Further work-up consisting of laboratory evaluation and necessary imaging studies nearly always results in a definitive diagnosis. If the cause of the child's limp remains uncertain following completion of this evaluation, the family often can be reassured that a serious disorder is not likely and observation may be all that is needed.

The Limping Toddler (Ages 1 to 3 Years)

The cause of a toddler's limp can be an enigma. Undoubtedly, the most common concern facing the health care provider is to determine whether or not the child has an infection. Frequently, the orthopaedic surgeon must determine whether an irritable joint in a toddler's lower extremity is caused by a mild self-limited disorder, such as transient synovitis, or a condition that requires urgent care, such as septic arthritis or osteomyelitis. In this instance, the patient's medical history may provide little useful information to differentiate between the two. A physical examination and appropriate laboratory and imaging studies are necessary to determine the proper diagnosis. Because this clinical picture can occur frequently in the toddler, the differences between infection and transient synovitis will be described here in depth.

Septic Arthritis and Osteomyelitis

In the irritable toddler whose painful joint of the lower extremity is due to infection, the history may reveal mild antecedent trauma to the extremity or a coexisting illness. Fever is common. The onset of joint pain is rapidly followed by the toddler's refusal to use the affected extremity. Symptoms are usually localized to one particular area or joint and are accompanied by swelling and tenderness. The toddler often resists any attempts to examine range of motion of the joint.

Laboratory studies reveal notable elevation of the C-reactive protein (CRP) and erythrocyte sedimentation rate (ESR). Because the CRP shows a quicker response to treatment, it appears to be the more useful investigation. However, it is the more expensive of the two tests. The white blood cell (WBC) count and differential may be unremarkable or slightly abnormal. In reality, a clear distinction between infection and transient synovitis is not always evident, particularly when the CRP and ESR are only mildly abnormal.

Imaging studies can be extremely useful. Ultrasonography can clearly demonstrate an effusion in the hip joint when the affected hip is compared with the normal side. Ultrasonography does not differentiate pus from normal synovial joint fluid; however, if no joint effusion is noted, the presence of septic arthritis is unlikely. Plain radiographs may be normal early in the

TABLE 1 | Common Causes of a Limp

Age Group	Signs and Symptoms
Toddler (Age 1 to 3 Years)	
Septic arthritis, osteomyelitis	Fever
	Pain
	Refusal to use extremity
	Localized swelling and tenderness
Transient synovitis	Acute onset of joint pain
	Restricted range of motion
Diskitis	Painful walk (limp or refusal to walk)
	Back "stiffness"
Toddler's fracture	Refusal to bear weight
Neuromuscular disorders (cerebral palsy, muscular dystrophy)	Abnormal gait patterns
DDH	Painless limp (Trendelenburg gait)
Inflammatory disorders (juvenile rheumatoid arthritis, Lyme disease, rheumatic fever)	Mild painful limp
	Localized swelling and warmth of the knee, ankle, or subtalar joint
	Restricted range of motion
Neoplasms (leukemia, neuroblastoma, osteoid osteoma)	Variable intensity and duration of pain
	Irritable hip or knee
	Mild to moderate fever
	Lymphadenopathy
Older Child (Age 4 to 10 Years)	
Transient synovitis	Acute onset of joint pain
	Restricted range of motion
LCPD	Pain
	Restricted range of motion
Discoid lateral meniscus	Clicking in the knee
	Discomfort
	± Bulge at joint line
	Tenderness
LLD	Asymmetrical gait
Adolescent (Age 11 to 15 Years)	
Overuse syndromes (Osgood-Schlatter disease, jumper's knee)	Activity-related tenderness
SCFE	Recent onset of hip, groin, thigh, or knee pain (usually in overweight preadolescent or adolescent)
Hip dysplasia	Pain (related to activity)
	Trendelenburg gait
Chondrolysis	Pain
	Restricted range of motion
Osteochondritis dissecans	Pain
Tarsal coalition	Midfoot and hindfoot discomfort
	Loss of normal motion

course of infection. When the affected and unaffected extremities are compared, a widened joint space in the affected hip strongly suggests that a joint is distended with fluid. This finding may be confirmed with ultrasonography. However, many infected hips do not show a widened joint space. Bone destruction from osteomyelitis usually becomes evident only after 7 to 10 days.

In patients with septic arthritis or transient synovitis, skeletal scintigraphy may reveal increased periarticular localization on any or all phases of a three-phase study. In patients with hip involvement, the opposite may be found. Diminished or absent tracer in the femoral capital epiphysis may be noted if tamponade of the intracapsular vessels by the effusion has occurred. If so, scintigraphy findings may be normal following an arthrocentesis. A localized area of increased uptake in the bone is generally consistent with an accompanying osteomyelitis and is a finding that essentially excludes the diagnosis of transient synovitis. Less extensive scintigraphic findings do not conclusively distinguish septic arthritis from transient synovitis.

In the future, MRI may become useful in differentiating transient synovitis from septic arthritis. Results of a recent study on the differential MRI findings between these two entities have been reported. Although signal intensity alterations consisting of juxta-articular changes in the bone marrow were seen in patients with septic arthritis but not in patients with transient synovitis, it is too early for this information to be used routinely for differentiation.

A diagnosis of septic arthritis is likely in a patient with a fever, a very irritable joint, notably elevated CRP and ESR, and effusion noted on ultrasound. The diagnosis is confirmed and the bacterial organism identified with aspiration of the joint. Cloudy fluid that reveals a WBC count between 80,000 and 200,000/mm^3, with more than 75% polymorphs, indicates infection. Gram stains may be helpful in the preliminary antibiotic selection. *Staphylococcus aureus* remains the most common organism responsible for septic arthritis. A significant reduction in instances of septic arthritis or osteomyelitis caused by *Haemophilus influenza* has occurred following the introduction of the *H influenza* type B vaccination in the late 1980s. At present, if *S aureus* is not responsible for the infection, group B streptococcus and *Kingella kingae* are likely causes. One recent study suggests that cultures of suspected infected joint fluid may be negative for bacterial growth in nearly 70% of patients. Despite this negative result, treatment should be aggressive in patients in whom other findings are consistent with infection.

The standard treatment of septic arthritis remains incision and drainage of the joint, followed by administration of antibiotics. If aspiration of the joint is unremarkable for purulence, but skeletal scintigraphy or MRI indicates the possibility of osteomyelitis, parenteral antibiotics followed by oral antibiotics may be appropriate without the need for surgery. Clinical response to treatment is best determined by noting symptoms and obtaining serial CRP measurements.

Transient Synovitis

Fortunately, transient (toxic) synovitis of a joint is far more common than infection, particularly in patients between ages 3 and 8 years. Transient synovitis has an uncertain etiology and remains a diagnosis of exclusion. As with septic arthritis, transient synovitis can be present in a patient with an acute onset of joint pain, limping, and restriction in the joint range of motion. Features that help to differentiate transient synovitis from septic arthritis include absence of significant fever or systemic illness, near-normal laboratory values (WBC, CRP, and ESR), and normal radiograph findings. Gentle hip range of motion usually reveals a greater arc in transient synovitis than in septic arthritis. An ultrasound of the hip may demonstrate an effusion with transient synovitis, which generally resolves over a period of several days. Usually, joint aspiration is performed only if an accompanying septic arthritis is strongly suspected. The joint aspirate count is usually between 5,000 and 15,000 cells/mL, with fewer than 25% polymorphs.

Clinical symptoms gradually resolve over the course of 7 to 10 days. Treatment consists of nonsteroidal anti-inflammatory drugs (NSAIDs) and activity restriction. Occasionally, bed rest may hasten recovery for patients with transient synovitis.

Diskitis

Diskitis usually affects children between ages 6 months and 4 years, most commonly at the L2-3 and L3-4 disk spaces. Toddlers will find that walking causes pain, and they may limp or actually refuse to walk. When picking up an object from the floor, the toddler keeps the spine straight and bends at the knees and hips only.

Laboratory investigation reveals elevation in the CRP and ESR. Early radiographs are normal. Narrowing of the disk space with erosion of the adjacent end plates may not be apparent for 2 to 7 weeks following the onset of symptoms. A bone scan, which generally is abnormal after symptoms have been present for a week, provides an earlier diagnosis than radiographs. MRI generally is not needed; however, if obtained, it may show signs consistent with an accompanying osteomyelitis.

The cause of diskitis usually is *S aureus*. Although needle biopsies into the disk space can confirm this, they generally are not necessary. Results of blood cultures frequently are positive for *S aureus*. Current treatment recommendations include short-term parenteral antibiotics followed by oral antibiotics. Parenteral antibiotics lead to more rapid resolution of symptoms than do oral or no antibiotics. External immobilization generally is not necessary.

Toddler's Fracture

Toddler's fracture is a well-recognized cause of limping. The history frequently is unremarkable for any particular traumatic event. Toddler's fracture typically is a hairline, oblique fracture at the diaphysis of the tibia. In some patients, the fracture can be so subtle that bone scan, or radiographs obtained 7 to 10 days later, may be required to confirm the suspected diagnosis. A variety of other difficult-to-detect fractures can also occur elsewhere in the tibia and foot, including plastic bowing or buckle-type fractures of the fibula, calcaneal and cuboid fractures, and metatarsal fractures. Children with any of these injuries usually refuse to bear weight on the affected extremity. Bone scan is quite helpful in diagnosing any of these other subtle fractures. Recently, it has been proposed that the term toddler's fracture be expanded to include all of these subtle lower extremity traumatic injuries. For treatment, short-term immobilization is all that is necessary for relief of symptoms.

Neuromuscular Disorders

With neuromuscular disorders, abnormal gait patterns (often described by parents as a limp) usually are present from the time the toddler begins walking. If so, the medical history, including the child's prenatal, perinatal, and postnatal condition, should be thoroughly explored. The most common example of a subtle neuromuscular limp occurs in a patient with mild static encephalopathy (cerebral palsy), specifically with a hemiplegic pattern.

Physical examination reveals increased muscle tone (particularly of the gastrocnemius-soleus complex), hyperreflexia, and an exaggeration of the limp when the child runs. If there also is a history of premature birth, difficult pregnancy or delivery, low birth weight, ventilator requirements, or postnatal infections, the diagnosis of mild cerebral palsy is readily confirmed. If there is no consistent history with an underlying static encephalopathy, the patient should be referred to a pediatric neurologist.

Developmental Dysplasia of the Hip

Developmental dysplasia of the hip (DDH) should always be suspected in the ambulatory toddler who has a painless limp. This abnormal walking pattern, known as a Trendelenburg gait, results from functionally weakened hip abductor muscles. Although the muscles are normal, the dislocated hip puts the muscles at a mechanical disadvantage. As a result, during the stance phase of gait, the hip abductors function ineffectively and the pelvis tilts away from the affected side. In an attempt to lessen this effect, the toddler will compensate by leaning over the affected hip, which gives the appearance of a limp. Increased lumbar lordosis, apparent shortening of the extremity, asymmetric thigh skin folds, and limited hip abduction usually accompany DDH. If DDH is suspected, an AP radiograph of the pelvis is mandatory. This imaging test always confirms the diagnosis, making further imaging studies unnecessary.

Congenital coxa vara will mimic the limp that is seen in patients with DDH. As with DDH, this painless limp is caused by an insufficient abductor mechanism. Congenital coxa vara is clearly differentiated from DDH upon review of an AP radiograph of the pelvis.

Inflammatory Disorders

The initial visit to the physician of a child with pauciarticular juvenile arthritis often occurs at approximately age 2 years. The child usually has a mild painful limp that is accompanied by localized swelling and warmth in the knee, ankle, or subtalar joint. Several joints may be involved simultaneously, and range of motion often is restricted. This condition affects girls four times more often than boys. Laboratory evaluation of the inflammatory indices is often normal. If swelling is localized and arthritis is suspected, the patient should be referred to a pediatric rheumatologist. Most patients do well without orthopaedic intervention and will return to normal with the proper management.

If the patient has pain in one or more joints associated with swelling, erythema, skin rash, and systemic symptoms, other inflammatory disorders should also be suspected. These disorders include acute rheumatic fever, Lyme disease, lupus erythematosus, and Guillain-Barré syndrome. Appropriate inflammatory indices, lumbar puncture, and electromyographic tests may be required to confirm these diagnoses.

Neoplasms

Leukemia

Acute lymphoblastic leukemia is the most common form of leukemia. Its peak incidence is in children between ages 2 and 6 years. Boys are most commonly affected. In 20% of patients, musculoskeletal complaints are the presenting feature. In a recent study, 12% of children with leukemia had a chief complaint of a limp. The physician should suspect leukemia if the patient has an antalgic gait and reports pain of variable intensity and duration, an irritable hip or knee, a mild to moderate elevation of body temperature, lymphadenopathy, hepatosplenomegaly, elevated ESR, thrombocytopenia, anemia, decreased neutrophils, increased lymphocytes, or blast cells on the peripheral smear. A bone marrow biopsy confirms the diagnosis. Although radiographs are generally nonspecific in patients with leukemia, metaphyseal bands (if present) are one of the earliest findings.

Osteoid Osteoma

Osteoid osteoma is a benign neoplasm that is uncommon in children younger than age 5 years. However, because it is a source of an occult limp throughout the childhood years, it should always be considered in the differential diagnosis. Radiographs may be unremarkable, but a bone scan almost always identifies the abnormality. Follow-up CT provides a clear delineation of the lesion.

The Limping Child (Ages 4 to 10 Years)
Transient Synovitis

As mentioned earlier, transient synovitis occurs most commonly in children between ages 3 and 8 years. In the toddler, transient synovitis must be differentiated from septic arthritis; in the child older than age 4 years, it must be differentiated from the early onset of Legg-Calvé-Perthes disease (LCPD).

Legg-Calvé-Perthes Disease

Idiopathic osteonecrosis of the femoral head occurs more commonly in children between ages 4 and 8 years. Initially, the child has a limp but no reports of pain. As the condition worsens, pain accompanies the limp. Range of motion of the hip becomes increasingly restricted. Radiographs may appear normal early in the disorder, which makes the differentiation between transient synovitis and early LCPD difficult. If clinical suspicion is high, either bone scintigraphy or MRI will demonstrate changes of the femoral head earlier than plain radiographs.

With the passing of time, radiographs reveal a subchondral lucency (crescent sign) that is followed later by collapse and fragmentation of the femoral epiphysis.

The cause of LCPD remains uncertain. Results of recent studies that suggest deficiencies in antithrombotic factor C or S, elevated levels of lipoprotein(a), hypofibrinolysis, or the presence of factor V Leiden require further confirmation to determine their role in the etiology of LCPD.

Discoid Lateral Meniscus

A discoid lateral meniscus is an infrequent cause of childhood limping. The child experiences clicking in the knee that is accompanied by discomfort, occasional swelling, and tenderness along the lateral joint space. Symptoms are usually exacerbated by increased activity. Discoid lateral menisci typically present in children between ages 3 and 12 years. MRI confirms the diagnosis.

Treatment consists of partial excision (saucerization) of the discoid meniscus. Occasionally, total excision is required to relieve the symptoms. Long-term results of total meniscectomy are controversial. Results of one recent study indicated that total meniscectomy provided a long-term symptom-free knee in patients younger than age 16 years. Conversely, results of another recent study indicated that clinical symptoms of osteoarthrosis were present in most of the knees that had undergone total meniscectomy. At present, saucerization of the discoid meniscus is the optimal treatment, assuming that it allows for full range of motion without persistent residual clicking.

Limb-Length Discrepancy

Very mild limb-length discrepancies (LLD) in children may go unnoticed. As discrepancies increase, gait asymmetry becomes evident. Causes of LLD are numerous and include idiopathic hemiatrophy or hemihypertrophy, trauma (overgrowth that is secondary to physeal stimulation or shortening that is secondary to fracture alignment or physeal injury), prior infection, neoplasm, metabolic disorders, and congenital anomalies. Some of these causes may be subtle and do not become evident until the child is between ages 4 and 10 years. Once the discrepancy is clinically recognized, an AP radiograph of the lower extremities should be obtained to clearly discern the abnormal area. Follow-up with periodic scanograms monitors changes over time. Results of a recent study have shown that limping as a result of significant LLD can be corrected following equalization procedures.

The Limping Adolescent (Ages 11 to 15 Years)
Overuse Syndromes

The combination of rapid growth in early adolescence and increased participation in athletic sporting events often leads to lower extremity overuse syndromes and, subsequently, the presence of a limp. The site most frequently affected is the knee, with inflammation involving the tibial tubercle (Osgood-Schlatter disease), patellar tendon (jumper's knee), and peripatellar region. These abnormalities are usually readily identified during the physical examination. Treatment consists of short-term rest and NSAIDs. Long-term activity modification may be needed to avoid persistent discomfort.

Slipped Capital Femoral Epiphysis

Slipped capital femoral epiphysis (SCFE) is considered to be the most common hip problem in adolescents. Although SCFE is frequently reported on in orthopaedic and pediatric journals, it remains a poorly recognized entity outside of pediatric orthopaedics. Anytime an overweight limping adolescent describes pain of recent onset involving the hip, groin, thigh, or knee, the physician should consider a diagnosis of SCFE. With SCFE, a thorough hip examination clearly reveals abnormal motion and discomfort. When the hip joint is flexed, it externally rotates automatically because of displacement of the femoral head on the femoral neck. Internal rotation is severely limited for the same reason. To exclude a diagnosis of SCFE, radiographs of the hip, particularly a lateral view, must be obtained; however, further imaging studies usually are not necessary. Once SCFE is recognized, it is considered an urgent surgical matter that requires the orthopaedic surgeon's immediate attention.

Hip Dysplasia

Primary dysplasia of the hip may not become clinically apparent until the patient has reached adolescence. Generally, the symptoms, pain and limping, are related to activity and relieved with rest or NSAIDs. An AP radiograph of the pelvis confirms the diagnosis. Once hip dysplasia becomes symptomatic in an adolescent, surgical intervention is necessary to improve the acetabular coverage of the femoral head.

Idiopathic Chondrolysis of the Hip

Idiopathic chondrolysis is a rare cause of limping in the adolescent. Pain and restricted range of motion accompany the radiographic appearance of joint space narrowing, subchondral lucencies, and juxta-articular osteopenia. Once idiopathic chondrolysis of the hip is identified, treatment includes using NSAIDs for the synovitis and range of motion exercises. Some improvement in the joint range of motion and restoration of some joint space may occur when the synovitis is resolved; however, ultimately, this condition remains very unpredictable.

Osteochondritis Dissecans

Osteochondritis dissecans occurs most commonly in the adolescent. Typically the patient experiences pain

and limping. The lateral aspect of the medial femoral condyle of the knee is affected most commonly, followed by the ankle and hip. Once identified, treatment depends on the condition of the overlying cartilage of the defect. Options include joint immobilization in patients with open physes with nondisplaced fragments, arthroscopic drilling of small nondisplaced fragments in older adolescents, internal fixation of larger nondisplaced fragments, or excision of displaced fragments followed by débridement of the remaining defect.

Tarsal Coalitions

Tarsal coalitions occur in fewer than 1% of adolescents. The two most common sites are the calcaneonavicular joint and middle facet of the talocalcaneal joint. Midfoot and hindfoot discomfort is associated with loss of normal motion of the subtalar joint. Radiographically, the calcaneonavicular coalition can be identified on the oblique view of the foot. If a talocalcaneal coalition is suspected, it will be clearly defined on the CT scan. Initial treatment includes immobilization and NSAIDs. Calcaneonavicular coalitions have better long-term surgical results following excision than do subtalar coalitions.

Annotated Bibliography

Introduction

Renshaw TS: The child who has a limp. *Pediatr Rev* 1995;16:458-465.

In a review article intended for pediatricians, but applicable for every orthopaedist, numerous causes of limping are briefly discussed. Appropriate clinical assessment, diagnostic work-up, and treatment programs are presented. All of the causes that are discussed can be classified into one or more of three categories: pain, weakness, and structural abnormalities.

The Limping Toddler

Connolly LP, Treves ST: Assessing the limping child with skeletal scintigraphy. *J Nucl Med* 1998;39: 1056-1061.

Skeletal scintigraphy is frequently used in the clinical investigation of children who limp. This review article presents techniques used for pediatric skeletal scintigraphy, skeletal tracer distribution in the immature skeleton, and scintigraphic manifestations of relatively common conditions that can produce limping in children ages 1 to 6 years. Acute osteomyelitis, vertebral infections, transient synovitis, septic arthritis, LCPD, lower extremity injuries in toddlers, and osteoid osteoma are discussed.

Howard AW, Viskontas D, Sabbagh C: Reduction in osteomyelitis and septic arthritis related to Haemophilus influenzae type b vaccination. *J Pediatr Orthop* 1999;19:705-709.

Before vaccinations against *H influenzae* became routine, this organism was responsible for 5% of culture-positive osteomyelitis and 41% of culture-positive septic arthritis. Since administration of the vaccine began in 1992, *H influenzae* type b has been eliminated as an infective agent in hematogenous septic arthritis and osteomyelitis.

John SD, Moorthy CS, Swischuk LE: Expanding the concept of the toddler's fracture. *Radiographics* 1997; 17:367-376.

The toddler's fracture, a hairline oblique tibial shaft fracture, may require bone scintigraphy or follow-up radiographs to confirm its presence. This article describes other fractures in the tibia (compression, impaction, stress) or foot (tarsal or metatarsal) in which the clinical picture is similar to that of the classic toddler's fracture. The authors propose that the term "toddler's fracture" be expanded to include all of these fractures.

Lawrence LL: The limping child. *Emerg Med Clin North Am* 1998;16:911-929.

This review article, which is written from the perspective of an emergency department physician, examines the child with a limp. Pertinent history and physical examination, appropriate diagnostic tests, and proper emergency department disposition are presented. Common disorders leading to a limp are summarized, with emphasis on urgent and emergent conditions such as septic arthritis, osteomyelitis, diskitis, SCFE, and child abuse.

Lee SK, Suh KJ, Kim YW, et al: Septic arthritis versus transient synovitis at MR imaging: Preliminary assessment with signal intensity alterations in bone marrow. *Radiology* 1999;211:459-465.

This is a report on the differential MRI findings between septic arthritis and transient synovitis in children. The authors state that signal intensity alterations, consisting of juxta-articular changes in the bone marrow, were seen in patients with septic arthritis but not in those with transient synovitis. In the future, this noninvasive method may help differentiate between the two disorders; however, at this time, these results should be considered preliminary.

Lundy DW, Kehl DK: Increasing prevalence of Kingella kingae in osteoarticular infections in young children. *J Pediatr Orthop* 1998;18:262-267.

K kingae was found in 10 of 60 patients with culture-positive hematogenous septic arthritis and osteomyelitis. *H influenzae* was found in only one patient. *H influenzae* has become less prominent since immunizations have become routine.

Lyon RM, Evanich JD: Culture-negative septic arthritis in children. *J Pediatr Orthop* 1999;19:655-659.

Seventy-six children with joint infection underwent aspiration of the joint with synovial fluid analysis, including culture. Results indicated that all patients had a synovial WBC count of greater than 50,000 or the presence of purulent material. Culture-negative septic arthritis was seen in 70% of patients, a figure that is much higher than previous reports. Aggressive treatment should be undertaken in those patients with negative cultures if their clinical presentation is consistent with infection.

Myers MT, Thompson GH: Imaging the child with a limp. *Pediatr Clin North Am* 1997;44:637-658.

This review article is intended to guide pediatricians in selecting and interpreting appropriate imaging tests for various disorders that result in a limp. The expected findings of infection, trauma, acquired disorders, and tumors are described for each radiographic modality (plain radiographs, bone scintigraphy, ultrasound, MRI, and CT scan).

Ring D, Johnston CE II, Wenger DR: Pyogenic infectious spondylitis in children: The convergence of discitis and vertebral osteomyelitis. *J Pediatr Orthop* 1995;15:652-660.

Forty-seven patients with pyogenic infectious spondylitis (diskitis) were reviewed to determine the spectrum of disease. MRI scans were obtained in nine patients and found to be identical to MRI findings in adult vertebral osteomyelitis, which provides strong evidence for an infectious process in diskitis. The investigation confirmed the usually benign course of spine infections in children but also emphasized the potential for serious sequelae. Symptoms were resolved more rapidly with intravenous antibiotics than they were with oral or no antibiotics.

Tuten HR, Gabos PG, Kumar SJ, et al: The limping child: A manifestation of acute leukemia. *J Pediatr Orthop* 1998;18:625-629.

Nine children, who were ultimately diagnosed with acute leukemia, presented initially with antalgic limps. When a painful limp of variable intensity and duration is accompanied by an irritable joint, slight increase in body temperature, lymphadenopathy, hepatosplenomegaly, increased ESR, abnormal complete blood count (anemia, thrombocytopenia, neutropenia, increased lymphocytes), and blast cells on the peripheral smear, there should be a high index of suspicion for leukemia. Bone marrow biopsy will confirm the diagnosis.

The Limping Child

Bhave A, Paley D, Herzenberg JE: Improvement in gait parameters after lengthening for the treatment of limb-length discrepancy. *J Bone Joint Surg Am* 1999;81: 529-534.

Eighteen patients with lower limb-length discrepancies underwent equalization to within 1 cm. Gait analysis before lengthening was compared to that after lengthening. Both the stance time and the second peak of the vertical ground-reaction-force vector were normalized. The authors concluded from the data that equalization can improve gait patterns and eliminate limps that are due to limb-length discrepancies.

Raber DA, Friederich NF, Hefti F: Discoid lateral meniscus in children: Long-term follow-up after total meniscectomy. *J Bone Joint Surg Am* 1998;80: 1579-1586.

Fourteen patients who underwent a total of 17 meniscectomies for discoid menisci in childhood were reviewed as young adults (average 19.8 years follow-up). Ten of 17 knees had clinical symptoms of osteoarthrosis. In distinct contrast to Washington and associates' study, the authors recommended that total meniscectomy for the treatment of a discoid meniscus in children should be avoided whenever possible.

Washington ER, Root L, Liener UC: Discoid lateral meniscus in children: Long-term follow-up after excision. *J Bone Joint Surg Am* 1995;77:1357-1361.

Fifteen patients who underwent a total of 18 meniscectomies for discoid menisci in childhood were reviewed as young adults (average 17 years follow-up). Ten excellent, three good, and five fair results were achieved. The authors concluded that for children younger than age 16 years with symptomatic discoid menisci, a total meniscectomy may still offer the best prognosis for a symptom-free knee.

The Limping Adolescent

Vincent KA: Tarsal coalition and painful flatfoot. *J Am Acad Orthop Surg* 1998;6:274-281.

A review article of tarsal coalitions describes a 1% incidence. Two sites are commonly affected: calcaneonavicular joint and middle facet of the talocalcaneal joint. Surgical intervention consisting of bar excision and fat-graft (or muscle) interposition is warranted in most patients. Long-term results following bar excision are moderately successful in relieving symptoms in calcaneonavicular coalitions, but less so in talocalcaneal coalitions.

Classic Bibliography

Royle SG: Investigation of the irritable hip. *J Pediatr Orthop* 1992;12:396-397.

Terjesen T, Osthus P: Ultrasound in the diagnosis and follow-up of transient synovitis of the hip. *J Pediatr Orthop* 1991;11:608-613.

Chapter 2

Evaluation of Back Pain

Lori A. Karol, MD

Introduction

Although back pain in the pediatric population is believed to rarely occur, recent studies show that more than half of adolescents report back pain by age 15 years, but few seek medical evaluation. In one study of 225 children who went to the emergency department for treatment of back pain, trauma and muscle strain were found to be the most common diagnoses given and 13% of the patients were left with an "idiopathic" diagnosis. Yet in an earlier study, an identifiable cause was found in 84% of children with reports of back pain. The goal of this chapter is to help orthopaedic surgeons decide which of their patients with back pain are likely to have a musculoskeletal pathologic process that requires a comprehensive evaluation and then to direct that evaluation efficiently.

History

The most important information in the evaluation of the child with back pain is the history (Table 1). The patient's age is critical. Children age 4 years and younger are most likely to have infections and tumors and therefore require immediate extensive evaluations. Adolescents are more likely to have developmental problems such as spondylolysis or Scheuermann's kyphosis.

The character of the back pain is important. Constant and worsening pain or pain that awakens the patient from sleep are associated with tumors. Constitutional symptoms such as fever and weight loss are warning signs that infection or a malignancy such as leukemia may exist. Intermittent pain that worsens with activities and is relieved by rest is more likely secondary to spondylolysis. The physician should question the patient regarding participation in athletic activities and the intensity of participation. Sports in which there is repetitive hyperextension of the lumbar spine, most commonly gymnastics and football, may predispose a patient toward spondylolysis.

Both the patient and parents should be questioned about symptoms of neurologic compromise. Gait disturbances such as increased clumsiness, decreased endurance, and inability to climb stairs may be due to motor weakness. Some patients may be reluctant to admit to bowel and bladder control changes, so questions should be directed to these issues.

The location of the pain directs the radiographic examination. Certain conditions have anatomic predilections. For example, spondylolysis and spondylolisthesis produce lumbar symptoms, thoracic pain occurs in patients with Scheuermann's kyphosis, and pain radiating to the buttocks and legs results most commonly from a herniated disk or avulsed vertebral apophysis.

Physical Examination

The physical examination should be performed with the patient disrobed. Examination of the spine begins with inspection for midline skin abnormalities that may represent occult spinal dysraphism or tethered cord. The patient should be assessed for scoliosis using the Adams forward bend test. Trunk lean or decompensation is often seen in patients with irritative lesions such as herniated disks or tumors. Spinal mobility is disturbed in the presence of pathology, and reversal of normal lumbar lordosis with forward bending may be absent. The child with back pain often has hamstring tightness, which leaves the child unable to bend and touch the floor and produces a diminished straight leg raise. A young child with diskitis will bend the knees rather than bend over from the spine to retrieve a toy from the floor. If spondylolysis is present, the child's lumbar pain may be exacerbated when the spine is hyperextended and twisted simultaneously. Palpation for areas of tenderness is important.

A thorough neurologic examination is necessary when evaluating the child with back pain. Motor strength, sensation, deep tendon reflexes, and abdomi-

TABLE 1 | History of Back Pain

Description	Importance
Duration	Long duration suggests developmental process
Frequency	Infrequent pain suggests a condition of a less serious nature than that with frequent pain
Location	Location of pain suggests the region that should be imaged
	Pain may not be in the midline or lumbar regions
Timing	Shorter duration of pain episode may be less serious than a longer duration
Night pain	Night pain suggests an inflammatory or a tumor source
Interference with activities or sports	Interference with activities is the most important gauge of the severity of the condition
Changes in gait and movement	A "stiff back" suggests diskitis or disk protrusion
Bladder or bowel changes	Bladder or bowel changes are rare but may indicate neurologic impairment
Use of analgesics	Use of pain relievers helps gauge the severity of the condition and the patient's response

nal reflexes should be tested. The presence of clonus or an abnormal Babinski reflex may indicate cord abnormalities or compression. Atrophy of the lower extremity and cavus foot deformity may result from spinal cord abnormalities. Loss of strength or hamstring tightness may result in gait disturbances.

Radiographic Examination

Plain radiographs are the most helpful imaging studies to obtain in a child with back pain. AP and lateral plain radiographs that have excellent bony detail should be examined for lesions and deformity. Methodical inspection of the radiographs for disk space narrowing, lytic or blastic lesions, presence of the pedicles, alignment, and vertebral scalloping is required. If a specific area of the spine is painful, or if a lesion is suspected on screening radiographs, a coned-down view taken with the patient supine yields better bone detail. In the lumbar spine, oblique radiographs are helpful to identify spondylolysis. Because patients with back pain may have pelvic tumors or sacroiliac joint disease, the pelvis should always be included in the radiographic examination. Gonadal shields can obscure lumbosacral lesions and should not be used in female patients with back pain.

If plain radiographs are nondiagnostic and further studies are indicated based on the results of the history and physical examination, a technetium bone scan is recommended in children who have normal neurologic examinations. The bone scan is a sensitive, although not specific, study that will show increased uptake in areas of increased bone turnover, such as in infection, fracture, and most tumors. Although a bone scan can

localize the abnormality, it is usually inadequate to definitively diagnose the disease process. CT scans define bony involvement best. Single photon emission computed tomography (SPECT) combines the physiology of a bone scan with the localization of tomography. SPECT shows bright uptake in areas of increased bony turnover and allows precise anatomic localization of the lesion and has been used to identify occult spondylolysis when the lysis was questionable on plain radiographs. If physical examination reveals a neurologic abnormality, MRI is indicated for visualization of the entire spinal cord. If MRI reveals concomitant bony pathology, CT also should be obtained to map out geographically the extent of bony abnormality and its encroachment on the spinal canal.

Laboratory Evaluation

All children with a history of fever, weight loss, or night pain, and those children who appear acutely ill, should be evaluated with laboratory studies. A complete blood count with differential, platelet count, peripheral smear, erythrocyte sedimentation rate (ESR), C-reactive protein (CRP), and urinalysis should be obtained for children age 4 years or younger at the initial visit.

Causes of Back Pain
Diskitis

Diskitis is the most common cause of back pain in the young child (Table 2). The distinction between diskitis and osteomyelitis in children is unclear because of the common blood supply of the intervertebral disk and

TABLE 2 | Causes of Back Pain

Condition	Characteristics of Pain
Spondylolysis/Spondylolisthesis	Pain with activity and hyperextension in young children and adolescents Patient may have flattened lordosis and short stride
Scheuermann's kyphosis	Pain in the region of the curve
Scoliosis	Children usually experience no pain or occasional mild to moderate pain (other causes of pain must first be ruled out)
Herniated disk	Stiffness and low lumbar pain that may radiate down the legs
Slipped vertebral apophysis	Sudden onset of low lumbar pain and stiffness that may radiate down the legs, usually in teenagers
Diskitis	Symptoms of infection and back stiffness
Tuberculosis	Mild to moderate pain that may involve any region
Inflammatory spondyloarthropathy	Low back pain and stiffness that may be associated with inflammatory bowel disease or ankylosing spondylitis
Juvenile osteoporosis	Pain in any region that increases when standing or active (rare cause of pain)
Sickle cell anemia	Severe, constant localized pain that occurs as part of a crisis
Eosinophilic granuloma	Localized pain in a younger patient "Vertebra plana" appearance
Osteoid osteoma/osteoblastoma	Localized pain and night pain that improves with use of NSAIDs
Aneurysmal bone cyst	Pain often occurs in the upper lumbar or thoracic regions
Leukemia	Pain is associated with fatigue, malaise, bruising
Spinal cord tumor	Night pain and neurologic changes
Osteosarcoma	Constant localized pain that stays the same or worsens at night
Ewing's sarcoma	Constant localized pain that stays the same or worsens at night and a low-grade fever
Chordoma	Pain in the sacrum with bowel or bladder changes
Neuroblastoma	Pain, stiffness, or weakness in infants

the vertebral body in the young child. The term pyogenic spondylitis describes this spectrum aptly. The patient may report a range of symptoms that includes back pain, abdominal pain, a limp, or refusal to walk. A history of fever is common. The patient often will appear ill; patients with diskitis commonly visit the emergency department for evaluation. Physical examination reveals stiffness in the spine and a reluctance to bend over to touch the floor. The neurologic examination is nearly always normal.

Early in the disease, radiographs are normal. Mild disk space narrowing is the first sign to appear and can be quite subtle. Careful inspection sometimes reveals paravertebral soft-tissue swelling. End plate irregularities follow. Because initial radiographs usually are normal, the diagnosis frequently is made from the bone scan, which shows increased uptake on both sides of

the involved disk. Although MRI generally is unnecessary for initial diagnosis, gadolinium-enhanced MRI is helpful when an abscess is suspected in patients who do not respond to empiric antibiotic treatment.

In the past, the treatment of diskitis was controversial. Some authors advocated orthotic management and rest without antibiotics. However, recent reports all describe improved outcomes with antibiotic therapy and cite fewer refractory cases and recurrences. Disk cultures are not necessary and are positive only 60% of the time. Blood cultures are obtained easily and therefore should be ordered routinely.

Because most culture results yield *Staphylococcus aureus* when positive, antibiotic treatment is recommended empirically. Many strains of *S aureus* are now penicillinase-producing, so second-generation cephalosporin may be indicated. A 3-week course of antibiotic

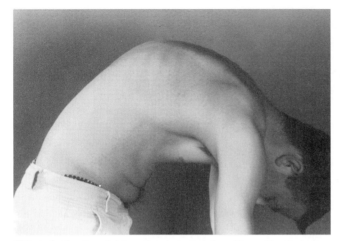

Figure 1 Sharply angled lower thoracic kyphosis in a 17-year-old patient with Scheuermann's kyphosis.

administration has been proposed. Clinical response and the normalization of the white blood cell (WBC) count and CRP should determine the change from intravenous to oral antibiotics.

Tuberculous osteomyelitis is becoming more prevalent; however, it is usually seen in immunosuppressed children and patients from undeveloped countries. Radiographic destruction of the vertebral body is more obvious in patients with tuberculosis. Drug regimens change frequently, and resistant strains of tuberculosis are emerging.

Scoliosis

Although orthopaedic teaching has traditionally deemed that idiopathic scoliosis does not result in back pain, 33% of girls with presumed idiopathic scoliosis do report a history of pain. When pain is caused by a concomitant bony abnormality, plain radiographs are most likely to identify the pathology in the apex of the concavity of the curve or at the lumbosacral junction. Results of a recent study indicated that if a thorough neurologic examination was normal, then the MRI results were also normal, and further imaging studies of the spinal cord are unnecessary in those patients with normal neurologic examinations. However, painful left thoracic curves are particularly predisposed to pathology and have been linked with syringomyelia and other intraspinal abnormalities; therefore, obtaining an MRI in these patients appears to be justified.

Scheuermann's Kyphosis

Scheuermann's kyphosis is a common cause of thoracic back pain in adolescents. The peak age of incidence is the midteens, and there is a slight male predominance. Pain is typically located over the apex of the kyphosis and/or in the hyperlordotic lumbar spine. Although

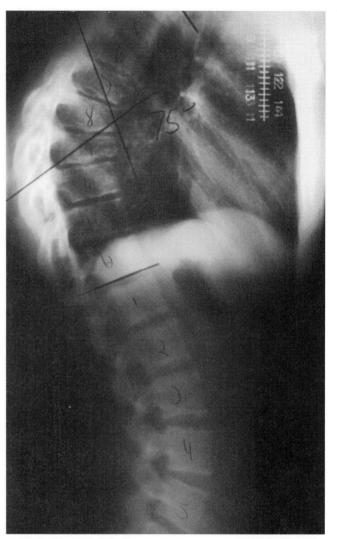

Figure 2 Lateral radiograph of the patient seen in Figure 1. Kyphosis is increased, measuring 75°, and there is apical wedging of the T8, T9, and T10 vertebral bodies.

Scheuermann's kyphosis can be painful, the chief complaint in many of these adolescents is a painless cosmetic deformity noted by the parents.

Physical examination reveals a stiff increased thoracic kyphosis, differentiating the condition from the more common and flexible postural round back of adolescence. The kyphosis appears sharply angled when viewed from the side (Fig. 1), in comparison to the more gently rounded appearance in patients with postural kyphosis. Results of the neurologic examination should be normal. Although present, increased lumbar lordosis is less obvious. Hamstring tightness may limit the child's ability to touch the toes.

Normal thoracic kyphosis is defined as between 20° and 40°. Classic radiographic findings of Scheuermann's kyphosis include increased thoracic kyphosis on a standing lateral view of the spine and wedging of the anterior vertebral body of three contiguous vertebrae

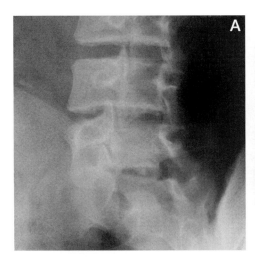
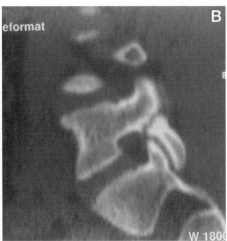

Figure 3 **A,** Oblique radiograph of the lumbar spine in a 16-year-old football player that reveals possible spondylolysis of L5. **B,** Three-dimensional CT scan confirms the diagnosis of spondylolysis.

in excess of 5° each (Fig. 2). Associated findings are end plate irregularities known as Schmorl's nodes. These radiographic changes are usually appreciable by age 12 or 13 years.

Treatment begins with a home program of exercises to stretch the tight hamstrings and improve thoracic hyperextension with the goal of relieving pain. Nonsteroidal anti-inflammatory drugs (NSAIDs) also can lessen symptoms. Patients with a kyphosis of 60° or greater and remaining spinal growth may be candidates for bracing. The Milwaukee brace, which includes a neck ring and posterior pads placed over the apex of the kyphotic deformity, is used most commonly. However, compliance with bracing is generally poor. If the kyphosis is severe and rigid, Risser casting prior to brace application may improve the flexibility of the deformity. Surgical indications are controversial. Patients with kyphosis greater than 75°, progressive deformity, persistent pain, or significant dislike for their kyphotic appearance may benefit from surgical correction.

Scheuermann's kyphosis infrequently involves the thoracolumbar and lumbar spine, causing mechanical back pain in older teens. Boys are affected more frequently than girls. Radiographs reveal Schmorl's nodes, end plate irregularities, and anterior wedging with loss of lordosis or frank kyphosis. Symptoms often improve with the use of an orthosis and restriction of heavy activities. Spinal fusion is rarely needed for persistent pain.

Spondylolysis and Spondylolisthesis

Spondylolysis is the most common cause of lumbar back pain in the teen athlete. In one pediatric sports medicine clinic, 47% of teens with back pain had either spondylolysis or spondylolisthesis. Repetitive hyperextension of the spine stresses the pars interarticularis, predisposing this area to stress fracture. The main symptom is low back pain with occasional

radiation into the legs. The pain is activity related and improves when the patient stops participation in sports. Hyperextension and twisting exacerbate the pain. If spondylolisthesis has occurred, physical examination may reveal reduced lumbar lordosis and flattened buttocks. Hamstring tightness is usually present.

A lateral radiograph may reveal a lytic defect in the pars, but oblique radiographs may identify spondylolysis in less obvious cases (Fig. 3). Patients with spondylolisthesis may have lysis through the pars interarticularis or elongation of the pars without fracture in the dysplastic variant. Scintigraphy has been useful because SPECT scans show increased uptake in the prefracture and acute stages. As the lysis becomes chronic, increased uptake is no longer seen. Scoliosis can coexist with spondylolysis and

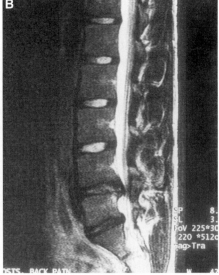
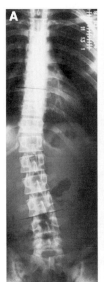

Figure 4 **A,** Atypical scoliosis seen in a 15-year-old boy with a herniated disk. **B,** Herniation of the L4-5 disk is confirmed by MRI.

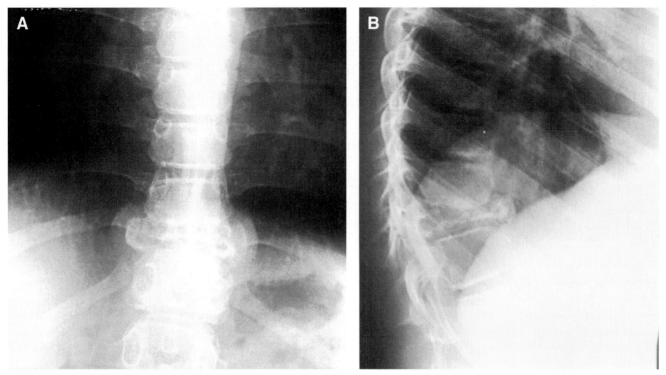

Figure 5 **A,** The AP radiograph of a 12-year-old boy with an eosinophilic granuloma of T11. **B,** The lateral view reveals complete collapse of the vertebral body with vertebra plana.

spondylolisthesis, but the curves are usually mild and appear atypical.

Treatment begins with stopping the aggravating activity. Patients may gradually return to their sport after the pain resolves; however, changes in training should be recommended to avoid repetitive hyperextension and repeat injury. If the fracture is acute on bone scan, a low-profile thoracolumbosacral orthosis can limit motion, relieve symptoms, and promote healing. Surgery is indicated if pain persists following 6 to 12 weeks of bracing, rest, hamstring stretching, and abdominal and paraspinal musculature strengthening. Repair of the spondylolytic defect is an alternative to posterolateral fusion in spondylolysis at L4 and higher. Treatment of spondylolisthesis varies with the severity of the slip. Surgery is indicated in patients with slips with greater than 50% translation and in milder slips that remain painful despite conservative treatment.

Traumatic Etiologies

Herniated Disk

Herniated nucleus pulposus is seen infrequently in the pediatric population, and young children in particular do not sustain herniated disks. Disk herniations are first seen generally in the second decade of life. The patient reports back pain that radiates down one or both legs. A history of trauma is often present. A positive straight leg raise sign is revealed most frequently on examination. Neurologic findings such as absent reflexes and weakness are less common in this age group than in the adult population. Symptoms that mimic a herniated disk in a young child should be considered secondary to a spinal tumor until proven otherwise.

Plain radiographs may show atypical scoliosis or listing, or they can be normal. A herniated disk is most clearly demonstrated on MRI (Fig. 4). False-positive findings such as bulging or degenerative changes in the disk do occur in teenagers, so clinical correlation with the physical examination is important to prevent over-diagnosis and inappropriate treatment.

Initial treatment of a herniated disk is conservative and includes pain control and rest. If pain persists following an adequate trial of decreased activity and physical therapy, surgical diskectomy leads to better results than prolonged conservative management. Following surgical diskectomy, 90% of pediatric patients experience short-term pain relief. However, results of long-term studies are now indicating that many patients who undergo surgical diskectomy as teenagers have further degeneration of additional disks and recurrent symptoms of back pain years later, possibly as a result of an inherent predisposition to disk disease. The role of percutaneous diskectomy in the pediatric population is currently undefined.

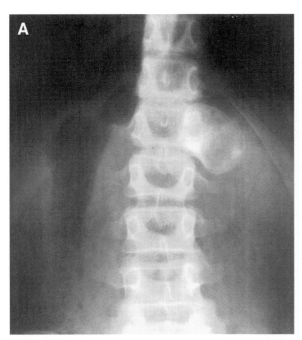

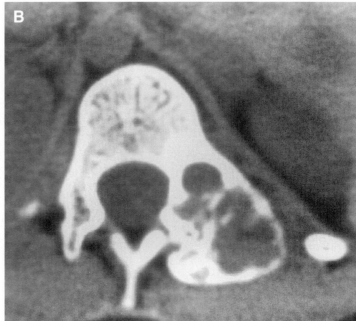

Figure 6 A, Aneurysmal bone cyst of L1 in an adolescent girl. **B**, The anterior extent of the lesion into the pedicle is best appreciated on CT scan.

Slipped Vertebral Apophysis

An uncommon condition that is unique to the skeletally immature patient is the slipped vertebral apophysis. This condition occurs in adolescents in whom the posterior inferior apophysis fractures away from the lumbar vertebral body, avulsing posteriorly into the spinal canal. Male weight lifters are most commonly affected. The mechanism of injury is rapid flexion with axial compression. The patient experiences a sudden onset of pain in the back that radiates down the legs. The pain resembles the pain that occurs with an acute disk herniation. CT is the best modality to visualize the bony fragment in the canal. Excision of the avulsed fragment is necessary.

Inflammatory Etiologies

Back pain in children is attributable only rarely to juvenile arthritis. Ankylosing spondylitis, which is more common in boys, can first be seen in adolescence and is linked with a positive HLA-B27 blood test result. Physical examination reveals loss of spinal flexibility. Plain radiographs may show irregularity or sclerosis in the sacroiliac joint. When radiographic results are questionable, MRI best identifies the inflamed sacroiliac joint.

Sickle Cell Anemia

Two recent studies have emphasized the association of sickle cell anemia with back pain. In one recent study, up to 26% of vascular-occlusive crises in children with sickle cell anemia involved the spine. In another study, 13% of visits to an urban emergency department for back pain were for treatment of sickle cell crises. Phy-

sician awareness of sickle cell disease as a possible etiology for back pain in black children should be raised.

Psychologic Etiologies

In some patients, a musculoskeletal cause of back pain cannot be identified. Psychosomatic pain and conversion reactions occur most commonly in the older teenager and are diagnoses of exclusion. An aggressive multidisciplinary approach using psychology and physical therapy can be successful in treating patients with this difficult problem.

Neoplasms
Eosinophilic Granuloma

Children between age 5 and 10 years with back pain might have eosinophilic granuloma, also known as Langerhans' cell histiocytosis or histiocytosis X. Spinal involvement is seen in 7% to 15% of children with eosinophilic granuloma. Lesions can be multiple or single, and patients can have systemic manifestations such as in Hand-Schüller-Christian disease or Letterer-Siwe disease.

Radiographs typically reveal lytic lesions in the anterior vertebral body or the classic coin-on-end appearance of vertebra plana (Fig. 5). Posterior element involvement is less common. Differential diagnosis includes leukemia, neuroblastoma, and infection. Bone scintigraphy may show increased uptake in multifocal disease, but also can be normal if the lesions have poor radioisotope uptake. A bone scan is helpful if it yields a positive result, but is not helpful if the result is neg-

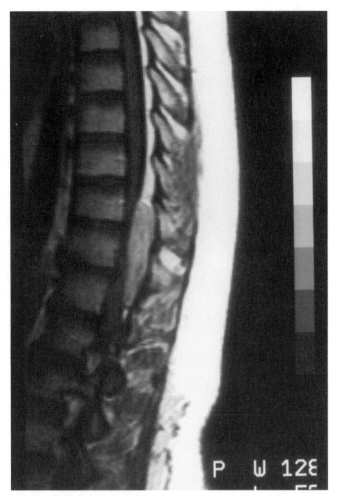

Figure 7 An MRI study of a 12-year-old boy with progressive weakness of the lower extremities reveals spinal cord compression by a ganglioneuroma.

ative. A skeletal survey is recommended to identify other lesions and can help establish the diagnosis.

Treatment consists of observation and bracing. Orthoses are used to decrease pain and encourage restoration of vertebral body height and therefore decrease kyphosis. Surgery is reserved for the minority of patients who have either neurologic compromise or questionable diagnoses. Biopsy is indicated for atypical lesions, but the presence of multiple lesions can either confirm the diagnosis or may provide a less invasive biopsy site if necessary. The roles of chemotherapy and low dose radiation are controversial.

Osteoid Osteoma and Osteoblastoma
Osteoid osteomas may develop within the posterior elements of the spine in children older than age 5 years. Characteristic symptoms are night pain that is relieved by aspirin. Physical examination may reveal loss of flexibility and painful scoliosis. Plain radiographs are usually nondiagnostic, but increased uptake is seen on bone scans. The radiolucent nidus surrounded by sclerosis is identified most easily by CT.

The lesion is nearly always located near the apex in the concavity when scoliosis is present. Treatment usually consists of surgery, but NSAIDs may provide symptomatic relief in rare cases.

Osteoblastoma may occur in the posterior elements of the spine, but can extend into the vertebral body as a result of its larger size. Forty percent of osteoblastomas occur in the spine. Whereas osteoid osteomas do not cause neurologic symptoms, osteoblastomas commonly do cause symptoms, based on the size of the lesions. Scoliosis occurs in 40% of children with osteoblastomas. The lesions are best characterized by CT. MRI can overestimate the extent of the mass and may misrepresent soft-tissue involvement because of surrounding edema. Treatment is surgical excision, with a local recurrence rate of 10%.

Aneurysmal Bone Cysts
Aneurysmal bone cysts (ABC) appear most commonly in the second decade of life. They usually originate in the posterior elements of the spine, but if large, they may extend into the vertebral body. Radiographs reveal an expansile lytic lesion with an eggshell-thin blown-out appearance. The extent of the cyst, the many communicating cavities, and the thin rim of surrounding bone can be further documented by CT (Fig. 6). Multiple fluid-fluid levels characteristic of ABC may be seen on T2-weighted MRI.

The expansile nature of the vertebral ABC leads to neurologic deficits in up to two thirds of patients. The ABC also can involve contiguous vertebrae, but does not involve the intervertebral disk. Because of the expansion and destruction of the vertebrae and the ABC's ability to involve multiple vertebrae, it can be confused with a malignancy.

Treatment usually consists of surgical curettage and bone grafting, with a recurrence rate of approximately 10%. If the ABC invades the vertebral body, an anterior approach to the spine should be performed to decrease the risk of recurrence. Spinal fusion should be performed at the time of curettage if the stability of the spine has been compromised by the extent of the lesion or surgical excision. Preoperative selective arterial embolization can decrease the intraoperative blood loss; however, caution should be taken to prevent cord ischemia. Definitive treatment of ABC of the spine with repeated embolization has been reported.

Malignancies
Leukemia is the most common malignancy that produces back pain. Back pain is reported in 6% of children with acute lymphocytic leukemia. Symptoms of fatigue, increased bruising, and fever should prompt the physician to suspect leukemia. Radiographic findings in the spine include diffuse osteopenia, vertebral

body compression fractures, and breaks along the vertebral cortical margins with translucent areas. Until proven otherwise, any child with vertebral compression fractures should be suspected of having leukemia. A complete blood count (CBC) may reveal deviations in any of the blood cell lines, such as an elevated WBC count, anemia, or decreased platelet count. The CBC and differential are normal at presentation in 5% to 10% of patients, so inspection of the peripheral smear is required to definitively rule out leukemia. An elevated ESR and WBC count also can indicate infection, resulting in confusion about the diagnosis. Because laboratory abnormalities can be subtle, the diagnosis may not be obvious. The diagnosis is confirmed by bone marrow aspiration that reveals lymphoblasts.

Constant worsening back pain, night pain, and pain in young children may indicate malignant tumors of the spine and spinal cord. Neurologic signs such as weakness and impaired reflexes are frequently present. The extent of the lesion and involvement of the spinal cord are best demonstrated by MRI (Fig. 7). Primary malignant tumors that arise in the spine include osteosarcoma, Ewing's sarcoma, and chordoma. Neuroblastoma metastasizes to the spine. The most common cord tumor is astrocytoma. Very rarely has malignant degeneration of neurofibromata into neurofibrosarcoma been reported in children with neurofibromatosis.

Annotated Bibliography

Introduction

Burton AK, Clarke RD, McClune TD, Tillotson KM: The natural history of low back pain in adolescents. *Spine* 1996;21:2323-2328.

Back pain occurs in more than half of children by age 15 years, but an orthopaedic evaluation is rarely sought.

King HA: Back pain in children. *Orthop Clin North Am* 1999;30:467-474.

Richards BS, McCarthy RE, Akbarnia BA: Back pain in childhood and adolescence. *Instr Course Lect* 1999; 48:525-542.

Both of these articles provide a comprehensive review of back pain in children.

Selbst SM, Lavelle JM, Soyupak SK, Markowitz RI: Back pain in children who present to the emergency department. *Clin Pediatr (Phila)* 1999;38:401-406.

Diagnoses of trauma and muscle strain were given in half of the children who were taken to the emergency department for evaluation of their back pain. Infections were more rare than sickle-cell crises.

Causes of Back Pain

de Kleuver M, van der Heul RO, Veraart BE: Aneurysmal bone cyst of the spine: 31 cases and the importance of the surgical approach. *J Pediatr Orthop Br* 1998;7: 286-292.

This large series advocates an anterior approach for resection of the lesion when the vertebral body is involved and adjuvant preoperative embolization.

Floman Y, Bar-On E, Mosheiff R, Mirovsky Y, Robin GC, Ramu N: Eosinophilic granuloma of the spine. *J Pediatr Orthop Br* 1997;6:260-265.

Radiographic vertebra plana was present in 40% of 20 children. The remaining children had lytic lesions in the vertebral body or posterior elements.

Glazer PA, Hu SS: Pediatric spinal infections. *Orthop Clin North Am* 1996;27:111-123.

This article is a comprehensive review of diskitis and other spinal infections. The authors recommend 3 weeks of a second-generation cephalosporin for the treatment of diskitis.

Kayser R, Mahlfeld K, Nebelung W, Grasshoff H: Vertebral collapse and normal peripheral blood cell count at the onset of acute lymphatic leukemia in childhood. *J Pediatr Orthop Br* 2000;9:55-57.

Automated cell counts in acute lymphocytic leukemia are normal in 5% to 10% of children. Suspicion should be high in children with vertebral compression fractures and osteopenia.

Lowe TG: Scheuermann's disease. *Orthop Clin North Am* 1999;30:475-487.

In this article, the author notes that the mode of inheritance of Scheuermann's kyphosis is likely autosomal dominant and the etiology is largely unknown. Brace treatment is effective with an early diagnosis, and surgery is rarely indicated for severe kyphosis.

Luukkonen M, Partanen K, Vapalahti M: Lumbar disc herniations in children: A long-term clinical and magnetic resonance imaging follow-up study. *Br J Neurosurg* 1997;11:280-285.

A 6-year follow-up of 12 patients who underwent diskectomy prior to age 16 years revealed persistent or recurrent symptoms in 60%. Persistent stenosing changes at the surgery site in 60% of patients and adjacent disk degeneration in 65% of patients were demonstrated on MRI. The outcome was graded as good or moderate in 90% of patients.

Mammano S, Candiotto S, Balsano M: Cast and brace treatment of eosinophilic granuloma of the spine: Long-term follow-up. *J Pediatr Orthop* 1997;17:821-827.

This article reveals that nonsurgical treatment in all patients was prolonged but successful.

Martinez-Lage JF, Martinez Robledo A, Lopez F, Poza M: Disc protrusion in the child: Particular features and comparison with neoplasms. *Childs Nerv Syst* 1997;13: 201-207.

Patients with herniated disks were all older than age 11 years; most of the children with tumors were younger. Neurologic findings of weakness and sensory loss were more frequently present in the patients with tumors.

Micheli LJ, Wood R: Back pain in young athletes: Significant differences from adults in causes and patterns. *Arch Pediatr Adolesc Med* 1995;149:15-18.

Spondylolysis was present in 47% of pediatric athletes seen for treatment of back pain. Disk herniations were uncommon.

Papagelopoulos PJ, Currier BL, Shaughnessy WJ, et al: Aneurysmal bone cyst of the spine: Management and outcome. *Spine* 1998;23:621-628.

The current treatment recommendation for aneurysmal bone cyst is preoperative selective embolization, intralesional curettage with bone grafting, and fusion in patients who have instability.

Ramirez N, Johnston CE, Browne RH: The prevalence of back pain in children who have idiopathic scoliosis. *J Bone Joint Surg Am* 1997;79:364-368.

Although back pain was noted in 32% of 2,442 patients with presumed idiopathic scoliosis, only 9% of the patients with pain had an underlying pathologic condition. Painful left thoracic curves were associated with pathology. If the neurologic examination was normal and plain radiographs did not reveal lesions, MRI and bone scans were not helpful.

Roger E, Letts M: Sickle cell disease of the spine in children. *Can J Surg* 1999;42:289-292.

Bony pain crises involved the spine in 26% of patients. Anemia was present in 86% of these children. Sickle-cell anemia should be included in the differential diagnosis of back pain in black children.

Saifuddin A, White J, Sherazi Z, Shaikh MI, Natali C, Ransford AO: Osteoid osteoma and osteoblastoma of the spine: Factors associated with the presence of scoliosis. *Spine* 1998;23:47-53.

Sixty-three percent of patients with osteoid osteoma or osteoblastoma had scoliosis. The bony lesions were located in the concavity of the curve in nearly all patients.

Shaikh MI, Saifuddin A, Pringle J, Natali C, Sherazi Z: Spinal osteoblastoma: CT and MR imaging with pathological correlation. *Skeletal Radiol* 1999;28:33-40.

The extent of the mass in osteoblastoma can be overestimated by MRI. The lesions become enhanced with the use of gadolinium, and there may be the erroneous appearance of soft-tissue involvement. The use of CT is more reliable in defining the anatomy of spinal osteoblastomas.

Song KS, Ogden JA, Ganey T, Guidera KJ: Contiguous discitis and osteomyelitis in children. *J Pediatr Orthop* 1997;17:470-477.

Vascular spread of infection between the disk and the vertebral end plate was histologically supported in this article. Disk space narrowing persisted at follow-up. Neurologic deficits are usually absent.

Tribus CB: Scheuermann's kyphosis in adolescents and adults: Diagnosis and management. *J Am Acad Orthop Surg* 1998;6:36-43.

This article provides a review of radiographic criteria and current treatment recommendations for bracing and surgery.

Chapter 3

Rotational and Angular Deformities of the Lower Extremities

John G. Thometz, MD

Metatarsus Adductus

Metatarsus adductus is a common foot problem in which the forefoot is adducted, and the lateral border of the foot is convex. This deformity differs from clubfoot in that the heel is not in the equinovarus position. The natural history of metatarsus adductus tends to be one of spontaneous improvement; 85% or more cases resolve without treatment.

To identify those patients who may need treatment, the flexibility of the foot must be assessed. If the deformity is completely correctable passively, treatment is rarely needed. Parents may perform stretching exercises, and use of a reverse-last shoe can be helpful. If the forefoot deformity is severe and rigid, serial manipulations and weekly casting are indicated until the deformity is fully corrected. Reverse-last shoes will help maintain the correction. Best results are achieved when treatment is begun when the child is younger than age 8 months. Improvement may be seen with casting until the child is age 2 years. When casting, the surgeon must stabilize the hindfoot in the neutral position with one hand, while applying lateral pressure to the first metatarsal head and neck with the other hand. Incorrect casting or splinting techniques may apply valgus force to the hindfoot as well as the forefoot, resulting in a planovalgus foot. If the problem recurs, it usually responds to an additional series of correcting casts.

Metatarsus adductus must be distinguished from the so-called skewfoot, in which there is a combination of forefoot adduction, lateral translation of the midfoot, and hindfoot valgus. Skewfoot is significantly more difficult to treat nonsurgically. It requires a more prolonged period of casting and often requires surgical intervention. In patients for whom nonsurgical management has failed or who are being assessed for the possibility of skewfoot, radiographs of the feet should be taken.

Patients who have a mild to moderate deformity generally are asymptomatic at long-term follow-up.

Surgical intervention rarely is indicated, even in the older child. Older children with deformity associated with pain or shoe-wear problems can be considered for surgical intervention. Surgical procedures for treatment of persistent metatarsus adductus include release of the abductor hallucis, medial capsular release, and extensive tarsometatarsal capsulotomies. Multiple metatarsal osteotomies are an option (with care being taken not to injure the physis of the first metatarsal). However, poor long-term results have been recorded in patients treated with extensive tarsometatarsal capsulotomies. The simplest procedure is a lateral closing wedge osteotomy of the cuboid with an opening wedge osteotomy of the first cuneiform.

Torsional Deformities

Rotational conditions of a child's lower extremities are a common cause for anxiety in parents. Parents, relatives, and neighbors often have a great concern with the child's appearance. Many family members may have been treated in the past with corrective shoes and braces, and therefore, the parents may be convinced of the need for aggressive therapy. Careful explanation of the natural history is important, with emphasis on the fact that unnecessary treatment is not beneficial to the child. Nonsurgical treatment does not help; the need for late surgical intervention is very rare. The orthopaedist can reassure the family by explaining the etiology and natural history of these torsional malalignments. Intrauterine molding is commonly responsible for the rotational appearance. In utero, the hips may be held flexed and laterally rotated. This position may result in a mild flexion and external rotation contracture of the hip, which resolves with time. The in utero molding effect may rotate the feet medially, resulting in medial rotation of the tibia (and also metatarsus adductus). With the passage of time, medial and lateral rotation of the hip becomes more symmetric, and medial rotation of the tibia resolves.

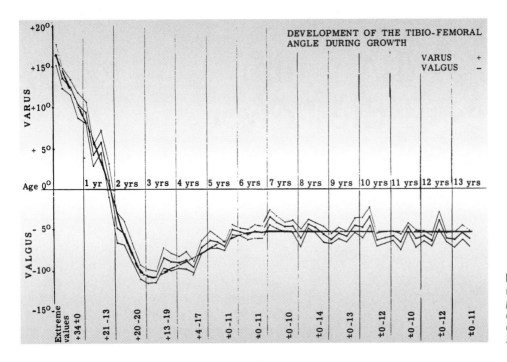

Figure 1 Development of the tibiofemoral angle during growth. (*Reproduced with permission from Salenius P, Vankka E: The development of the tibiofemoral angle in children. J Bone Joint Surg Am 1975;57: 260.*)

TABLE 1 | The Differential Diagnosis of Genu Varum

Problem	Differential Diagnosis
Asymmetric growth	Tibia vara
	Partial physeal arrest
Metabolic causes	Renal disease
	Rickets
Bone dysplasia	Achondroplasia
	Multiple epiphyseal dysplasia
Osteopenia	Juvenile rheumatoid arthritis
	Osteogenesis imperfecta
Physiologic causes	Physiologic genu varum

The rotational profile allows measurement of the severity and location of the rotational problem. The foot-progression angle during gait is noted, followed by evaluation of hip rotation, assessment of the thigh-foot angle, and evaluation of the foot. The magnitude of rotation is quantified in degrees. Hip rotation in the prone position should be symmetric. Medial hip rotation of greater than 70° indicates medial or internal femoral torsion. The thigh-foot angle is the angle between the axis of the foot and the axis of the thigh. Forefoot adduction or abduction should be assessed.

Medial rotation of the hips tends to be greatest in early childhood (after 12 to 18 months) and then declines until adulthood. From middle childhood on, medial rotation of the hip is roughly 50°, and lateral rotation is about 45°. Newborns normally have a slight medial thigh-foot angle, which corrects over time to a lateral thigh-foot angle of 10°. In the older child, an intoeing gait commonly is caused by medial or internal femoral torsion (exhibited by increased medial rotation of the hip) or medial tibial torsion (with a medial thigh-foot angle).

In patients with a persistent deformity, surgical intervention should not be considered before age 10 years. In the older child with significant functional and cosmetic problems, surgical intervention may be warranted. CT can be used preoperatively to assess the degree of rotational deformity of the femur. Generally the child should have at least 80° of medial rotation of the hips clinically, and CT should identify any medial femoral torsion of greater than 50°. For children who have persistent tibial torsion in late childhood and who may have a severe functional abnormality because of this, surgical correction at the supramalleolar level can be considered. The tibial deformities should exceed a medial thigh-foot angle of greater than 10° or a lateral thigh-foot angle of greater than 35°. Very rarely, a patient may have a combination of severe medial femoral torsion and lateral tibial torsion. This combination can complicate the management because patients may have knee discomfort or patellar instability and may require correction of both the femoral and tibial torsion.

Bowlegs and Knock-Knees

Angular deformities in young children also are a common concern of parents, although the natural history of these conditions usually is benign. The orthopaedist must rule out pathologic conditions such as infantile

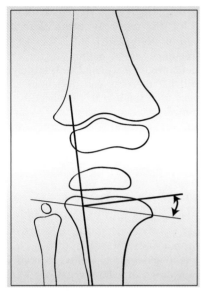

Figure 2 Metaphyseal-diaphyseal angle.

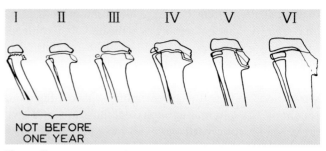

Figure 3 Langenskiöld classification of tibia vara. *(Reproduced with permission from Langenskiöld A, Riska EB: Tibia vara (osteochondrosis deformans tibiae): A survey of seventy-one cases. J Bone Joint Surg Am 1964;46:1405-1420.)*

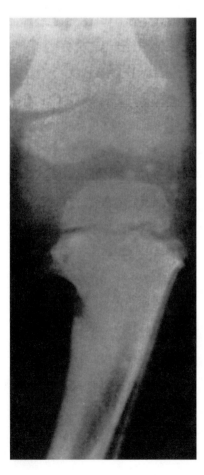

Figure 4 Focal fibrocartilaginous dysplasia. *(Reproduced with permission from Choi IH, Kim CJ, Cho TJ, et al: Focal fibrocartilaginous dysplasia of long bones: Report of eight additional cases and literature review. J Pediatr Orthop 2000: 20:421-427.)*

AP radiographs of the lower extremities should be taken when the patient has a severe angular deformity, significantly short stature, asymmetric involvement, or a positive family history. If varus bowing persists after age 18 to 24 months, the child must be evaluated radiographically for infantile tibia vara (infantile Blount's disease). Usually a metaphyseal-diaphyseal angle of more than 16° predicts the development of infantile Blount's disease (Fig. 2).

Growth inhibition of the medial and posterior aspects of the proximal tibial physis causes infantile tibia vara. Early weight bearing, especially in obese children, may lead to tibia vara, possibly because of excessive compressive forces on the medial aspect of the physis. Over time, the damage in the medial aspect of the physis progresses, usually resulting in severe varus deformity of the proximal tibia. The Langenskiöld radiographic staging classification analyzes the progression of the tibia vara in untreated cases (Fig. 3). For stages I through III, bracing may be effective in correcting the deformity. By stage IV, a proximal tibial valgus osteotomy is required for correction. By stage V or VI, a medial physeal bar is present, and additional procedures such as bar resection, elevation of the medial plateau, and lateral physeal arrest may be necessary.

Bracing works in many cases for tibia vara in patients younger than age 3 years, patients with a metaphyseal-diaphyseal angle of greater than 16° or patients who have Langenskiöld stage I or stage II deformity. Daytime weight-bearing braces are most effective. The orthosis must be a long leg brace with a cuff at the knee providing a valgus force. A single medial upright with locked knee and valgus strap works well. By age 4 years, early tibial valgus osteotomy should be performed. Overcorrection into 5° to 10° valgus angulation (beyond normal) should be the goal.

Tibia vara may also develop in juveniles or adolescents. In the adolescent whose tibial physes are open and who is calculated to have significant remaining growth, a lateral hemiepiphysiodesis will provide cor-

tibia vara, metaphyseal chondrodysplasia, rickets (particularly hypophosphatemic rickets), and focal fibrocartilaginous dysplasia (Table 1).

Mild varus of the knee is normal. Knee alignment is neutral at about age 18 months. Then, slightly increased genu valgum develops, which is most noticeable in the 30- to 36-month old child (Fig. 1). Standing rection. If the patient is near skeletal maturity, a prox-imal tibial valgus osteotomy is indicated. It is difficult to achieve a tibiofemoral angle within 5° of normal in these patients because of their obesity.

The pathology of late-onset tibia vara also shows fis-suring and clefts in the physis along with cartilaginous repair at the physeal-metaphyseal junction and evi-dence of necrotic cartilage. The increased thigh girth associated with obesity causes increased loading of the medial compartment of the knee during the gait cycle. This increased weight damages the physis and leads to the development of adolescent Blount's disease. The mechanical axis is difficult to identify in obese patients. The Ilizarov device has worked well to achieve normal lower extremity alignment.

Focal fibrocartilaginous dysplasia is an unusual con-dition that may be confused with tibia vara. It differs in that radiographs show indentation of the medial aspect of the tibia at the junction of the metaphysis and diaphysis (Fig. 4). Spontaneous improvement is common; therefore, a trial of observation is warranted.

In the older child with excessive genu valgum, under-lying metabolic abnormalities must be ruled out. Per-sistent genu valgum may be corrected either by hemiepiphysiodesis or stapling of the medial physis. If possible, these procedures should be performed after the child reaches age 10 years. However, the successful use of stapling in children younger than age 10 years has been reported, with satisfactory maintenance of growth plate function after staple removal. A horizon-tal knee joint for weight bearing must be maintained.

Even minimally displaced proximal tibial metaphy-seal fractures may develop marked valgus deformity over time. Parents certainly must be informed of this possibility at the time of initial injury. The valgus deformity should be observed for several years, because there is a strong tendency toward spontaneous correction, and corrective osteotomies may be associ-ated with recurrent deformity.

Annotated Bibliography

Choi IH, Kim CJ, Cho TJ, et al: Focal fibrocartilaginous dysplasia of long bones: Report of eight additional cases and literature review. *J Pediatr Orthop* 2000;20:421-427.

The authors reported on eight patients with focal fibrocar-tilaginous dysplasia (FFCD). The deformities were concomi-tantly corrected and lengthened using the Ilizarov method. Results were satisfactory in all but one patient, in whom mild postoperative genu valgum developed. A review of the literature found that tibial FFCD resolves spontaneously in 45% of patients, but femoral and humeral FFCDs rarely resolve spontaneously. Corrective osteotomy is indicated with an increasing or persistent deformity or a severe existing deformity.

Davids JR, Huskamp M, Bagley AM: A dynamic biomechanical analysis of the etiology of adolescent tibia vara. *J Pediatr Orthop* 1996;16:461-468.

The authors used three-dimensional motion analysis to identify the kinematic/kinetic profile associated with fat-thigh gait. The authors believed that dynamic gait deviations are used to compensate for increased thigh girth associated with obesity. Gait deviations noted included dynamic stance limb knee varus with increased stance limb knee rotation and swing-limb circumduction. These gait abnormalities resulted in abnormal compressive forces across the medial aspect of the knee.

Davis CA, Maranji K, Frederick N, Dorey F, Moseley CF: Comparison of crossed pins and external fixation for correction of angular deformities about the knee in children. *J Pediatr Orthop* 1998;18:502-507.

In this study, the preoperative deformity and postoperative correction were similar in both groups; however, there were significantly more complications in the external fixator group—16 complications (62%) compared to five (19%) in the group treated with Steinmann pins and casting. Both groups had a 100% union rate.

Raney EM, Topoleski TA, Yaghoubian R, Guidera KJ, Marshall JG: Orthotic treatment of infantile tibia vara. *J Pediatr Orthop* 1998;18:670-674.

Patients in this study were treated with a brace if they had a metaphyseal-diaphyseal angle of greater than 16°, or an angle between 9° and 16° with a clinical risk factor for progression. Risk factors for progression were ligamentous laxity, obesity, asymmetry, and being female, black, or Hispanic. The success rate with 60 tibiae was 98%. Risk factors for failure were instability, obesity, and delayed bracing. The authors believe that brace treatment favorably altered the natural history of the tibia vara.

Stanitski DF, Dahl M, Louie K, Grayhack J: Manage-ment of late-onset tibia vara in the obese patient by using circular external fixation. *J Pediatr Orthop* 1997; 17:691-694.

A circular external fixator was used to treat 25 tibiae in 17 patients who had exceeded their ideal body weight by greater than 50%. Their late-onset tibia vara was treated with the Ilizarov technique. The treatment time averaged 12 weeks in patients without lengthening, and 17 weeks in those with lengthening. In this study, all patients achieved alignment within 5° of normal.

Stevens PM, Maguire M, Dales MD, Robins AJ: Physeal stapling for idiopathic genu valgum. *J Pediatr Orthop* 1999;19:645-649.

This study reviewed 76 patients (152 knees) who under-went hemiphyseal stapling for idiopathic adolescent genu valgum and had follow-up to skeletal maturity. The authors analyzed the patients' gait, symptoms, and several radiograph-ic parameters. It was noted that adolescent genu valgum may be associated with symptoms such as anterior knee pain. Physeal stapling was effective, and no premature growth arrests were noted.

Zionts LE, Shean CJ: Brace treatment of early infantile tibia vara. *J Pediatr Orthop* 1998;18:102-109.

Brace treatment was initiated for children with a varus deformity that had not improved by age 18 to 24 months or a persistent varus deformity in those older than 24 months. Braces were worn during the day and removed at night. Forty-two extremities in 24 children were treated, and, at follow-up, 29 extremities were rated good, 9 fair, and 4 poor. The authors believe that bracing helped alter the natural history of tibia vara in patients younger than age 3 years and those with Langenskiöld stage I or II deformity.

Classic Bibliography

Farsetti P, Weinstein SL, Ponseti IV: The long-term functional and radiographic outcomes of untreated and non-operatively treated metatarsus adductus. *J Bone Joint Surg Am* 1994;76:257-265.

Feldman MD, Schoenecker PL: Use of the metaphyseal-diaphyseal angle in the evaluation of bowed legs. *J Bone Joint Surg Am* 1993;75:1602-1609.

Heath CH, Staheli LT: Normal limits of knee angle in white children: Genu varum and genu valgum. *J Pediatr Orthop* 1993;13:259-262.

Henderson RC, Kemp GJ Jr, Greene WB: Adolescent tibia vara: Alternatives for operative treatment. *J Bone Joint Surg Am* 1992;74:342-350.

Langenskiöld A, Riska EB: Tibia vara (osteochondrosis deformans tibiae): A survey of seventy-one cases. *J Bone Joint Surg Am* 1964;46:1405-1420.

Langenskiöld A: Tibia vara: A critical review. *Clin Orthop* 1989;246:195-207.

Loder RT, Schaffer JJ, Bardenstein MB: Late-onset tibia vara. *J Pediatr Orthop* 1991;11:162-167.

Salenius P, Vankka E: The development of the tibiofemoral angle in children. *J Bone Joint Surg Am* 1975;57:259-261.

Staheli LT: Rotational problems in children. *Instr Course Lect* 1994;43:199-200.

Steel HH, Sandrow RE, Sullivan PD: Complications of tibial osteotomy in children for genu varum or valgum: Evidence that neurological changes are due to ischemia. *J Bone Joint Surg Am* 1971;53:1629-1635.

Thompson GH, Carter JR: Late-onset tibia vara (Blount's disease): Current concepts. *Clin Orthop* 1990;255:24-35.

Chapter 4

Pediatric Orthopaedic Infections

Laura L. Tosi, MD

Introduction

The differential diagnosis of musculoskeletal infection can be challenging, because a broad range of infectious processes as well as other conditions must be considered. Although many overall approaches to the evaluation and treatment of children with orthopaedic infections have been devised, questions remain regarding the aggressiveness of diagnostic interventions, the value of early surgical intervention, the choice of antimicrobial agents, and the optimal duration and route of antibiotic treatment.

Osteomyelitis

The differential diagnosis of osteomyelitis is quite broad and includes fracture, toxic synovitis, cellulitis, pyogenic arthritis, cellulitis, soft-tissue abscesses, thrombophlebitis, rheumatic fever, bone infarction, Gaucher's disease, and malignancy (osteosarcoma, Ewing's sarcoma, leukemia, neuroblastoma, and Wilms' tumor). Several key considerations can facilitate diagnosis, including consideration of patient age, the causative organism (pyogenic or granulomatous), the nature of onset (acute, subacute, or chronic) and the route of infection (hematogenous direct inoculation or contiguous spread).

Acute Hematogenous Osteomyelitis

Acute hematogenous osteomyelitis (AHO) occurs in one per every 5,000 children younger than age 13 years. One half of these patients are younger than age 5 years, and one third are younger than age 2 years. Boys are affected 1.2 to 3.7 times as often as are girls. The incidence of osteomyelitis is highest in areas that have a warm climate, and the disease demonstrates a peak incidence in late summer and early fall. It has a predilection for the most rapidly growing bones, especially those in the lower extremities. AHO can be difficult to diagnose and typically is confirmed by finding purulence in the bone, positive bone or blood culture results, or positive radiographic, scintigraphic, MRI, or CT findings.

Pathogenesis

The causes of AHO are poorly understood. Infection begins when bloodborne bacteria are deposited in the metaphyseal venous sinusoids. Slow blood flow through the capillary bed allows microorganisms to migrate through fenestrations in the blood vessel walls. The normal ability of endothelial cells to phagocytize particles is deficient in the metaphyseal capillary loops. Thus, during the process of transient bacteremia, organisms may escape into this region of relative phagocytic deficiency and establish infection. As the infection spreads, the medullary vessels become thrombosed and prohibit the inflow of white blood cells (WBCs), causing the WBCs to slowly migrate from the medullary cavity. The early phase in osteomyelitis is called the "cellulitic" phase, because pus has not been produced. In this stage, antibiotic treatment alone may be enough to fight the infection.

Without treatment, pus forms. The purulence typically does not extend into the medullary cavity but exits the bone laterally through the porous metaphyseal cortex, elevating the periosteum and forming a subperiosteal abscess. The elevated periosteum may or may not rupture. As pressure increases under the periosteum, the vascular supply to the denuded cortex and metaphysis is compromised. Necrosis may occur, resulting in the development of a sequestrum, or loosely adherent piece of dead bone. New bone may form over the sequestrum, producing an involucrum. Because of its limited vascular supply, the new bone is relatively inaccessible to antibiotics, and chronic osteomyelitis may result.

In four locations—the proximal femur-hip joint, proximal humerus-shoulder joint, lateral distal tibia-ankle joint, and radial neck in the elbow joint—the metaphysis lies within the adjacent joint capsule. Thus, an infected joint may coexist with infected bone if the infection breaks through the metaphyseal cortex. In addition, infection may rupture into the muscular bed in neonates because they have a relatively thin cortex and loosely applied periosteum. Osteomyelitis is more likely to also involve the epiphysis in the neonate, because nutrient metaphyseal capillaries perforate the epiphyseal growth plate. This also allows infection to spread to the adjacent joint cavity.

Presentation

Initial signs and symptoms of osteomyelitis vary tremendously, ranging from malaise and low-grade fever to severe constitutional symptoms and high-grade fever. Nearly one half of patients have a history of recent or concurrent infection, and most have a history of continuous bone pain for 1 or more days.

In the neonate, the physical examination may be very nonspecific; pseudoparalysis of the limb may be the only clinical finding. In older infants and children, the signs and symptoms tend to localize to the nidus of infection. Pain, usually point tenderness, may be elicited in 50% of toddlers and young children. If the lower extremities are involved, the child may limp or refuse to walk. Joint motion may be limited because of local muscle spasm. Local signs of erythema, swelling, and warmth are absent unless the infection is advanced and has extended from the metaphyseal cortex into the subperiosteal space. A sympathetic joint effusion may occur, which must be differentiated from contiguous septic arthritis. Pain typically is not well localized if the infection is in the spinal or pelvic bones. Adolescents often have more exquisite point tenderness because their bone is more developed and has a thicker metaphyseal cortex with a dense fibrous periosteum. These anatomic features tend to contain the infection; as a result, extension beyond the outer cortical lamellae is limited. For this reason, adolescents may have only minimally restricted movement in the extremity.

Laboratory Tests

A normal WBC count has been reported in as many as 75% of patients and is, therefore, not a reliable indicator of infection. A normal polymorphonuclear cell count has been reported in 35% of patients. The erythrocyte sedimentation rate (ESR), however, is elevated in more than 90% of patients and is believed to be a reliable indicator of infection. Exceptions include the neonate with osteomyelitis, the child with sickle cell disease, and the child who is taking steroids. The ESR is nonspecific and represents the concentration of fibrinogen. It rises slowly and peaks at approximately 3 to 5 days, then it should begin to decline to 1 to 2 weeks after appropriate therapy is initiated. The C-reactive protein (CRP) level rises rapidly and peaks in

2 days, then begins to decline within 6 hours of initiation of appropriate therapy. However, CRP testing is not routinely used in many centers because it is very nonspecific and also will be elevated in the presence of trauma.

Imaging Studies

Plain radiographs may show muscle plane displacement from the adjacent metaphysis within 3 days of infection. Obliteration of normal intermuscular fat planes is evident in 3 to 7 days. These changes are caused by local edema. Actual bony changes do not appear for 7 to 14 days; thus, if the diagnosis remains uncertain, additional studies may be needed. Bone scan is a more sensitive modality for identifying the site of involvement in osteomyelitis when plain radiographs are negative, particularly in difficult areas, such as the pelvis or spine. Bone scans also are helpful in identifying patients with multiple sites of bone involvement, particularly in the neonate or patient with multifocal osteomyelitis or malignancy. However, because of the high incidence of false-negative results in the neonate, plain radiographs are the mainstay for establishing the diagnosis. Bone aspiration will not affect the results of bone scans if the scan is performed within 48 hours of aspiration; therefore, aspiration should not be delayed. Patients with "cold" bone scans appear to have a more aggressive type of infection and typically have a higher temperature, higher pulse rate, elevated ESR, and increased length of hospital stay and rate of surgical intervention than do those with hot bone scans. It is essential to order a whole body bone scan (as opposed to an isolated study of the extremities) because multifocal osteomyelitis and malignancy must be considered in the differential diagnosis. Gallium scans require 24 to 48 hours to complete and much higher doses of radiation, and they rarely add information beyond that provided by a two- or three-phase bone scan; therefore, they rarely are indicated.

CT is quick, easy, and inexpensive, but it does not demonstrate intraosseous changes early in the course of the disease. Late in the course of the disease, CT can provide good definition of cortical destruction, definition of extraosseous abscesses or gas, and evidence of bony sequestration. In recalcitrant infection, CT can provide useful information for surgical planning and also help differentiate osteomyelitis from other lucent lesions, especially chondroblastoma and osteoid osteoma.

MRI is very sensitive, but it is not specific for osteomyelitis. Osteomyelitis can be detected on MRI in the first 3 to 5 days because edema in the bone marrow and soft tissue is revealed, and when MRI is used with gadolinium, the area of necrosis can be defined. However, although cellulitis can be differentiated from osteomyelitis on MRI, a fracture or bone infarction might not be distinguished from an infection. MRI is helpful only if one knows where to look. It is the imaging study of choice when the spinal and/or pelvic area is involved and the diagnosis is uncertain. MRI typically demonstrates a localized area of abnormal bone marrow with decreased signal intensity on T1-weighted images and increased signal intensity on T2-weighted images.

Ultrasound is being used more frequently because of its ability to detect subperiosteal abscesses in the child with diffuse tenderness and swelling of an extremity. Characteristic ultrasound findings include thickening of the periosteum with hypoechogenic zones, both superficial and deep, giving the periosteum the appearance of a "sandwich"; elevation of the periosteum by more than 2 mm; or swelling of the overlying muscle or subcutaneous tissue with altered echogenicity of the tissue, depending on the angle of the scan. When the periosteum is lifted off the bone by 2 mm or more, pus usually can be seen. In children with hip pain who have a normal ultrasound study, extension of the ultrasound examination to include the pelvic muscles may help identify and document the progression of acute pelvic osteomyelitis.

Aspiration

Isolation of the etiologic pathogen is desired; however, blood cultures are positive in only 30% to 50% of patients. Cultures taken from bone have a higher yield of pathogen, but prior antibiotic use decreases the yield; thus, material for culture should be obtained as quickly as possible.

In a recent report, a much higher incidence of adjacent joint involvement was demonstrated in all age groups than previously reported. For this reason, careful evaluation of the adjacent joint in any child with osteomyelitis is necessary.

Management

Many authors believe that empiric antibiotics used to treat *Staphylococcus aureus* in children and adolescents can be initiated without obtaining a bone culture, and aspiration should be reserved for patients whose symptoms do not improve after 36 to 48 hours of appropriate antibiotic treatment. *S aureus* usually is the pathogen, followed by group A streptococcus, *Streptococcus pneumoniae*, and group B β-hemolytic streptococcus. *Haemophilus influenzae B* (Hib), once a common pathogen in childhood, has virtually disappeared with the advent of the Hib vaccine, and coverage for this pathogen is not required in the fully immunized child. The U.S. Food and Drug Administration (FDA) recently approved a conjugate heptavalent pneumococcal vaccine for high-risk children older than age 2 years. This vaccine will be especially helpful to patients with sickle cell disease, asplenia, chronic diseases such as nephrotic syndrome, and compromised immune systems, including patients with human immunodeficiency virus (HIV) infection.

In children with underlying disease, atypical organisms are a concern, and aspiration must be performed. A Gram stain of the aspirate should be obtained. In addition, a routine culture, as well as cultures for anaerobic bacteria, acid-fast bacilli, and fungi should be obtained. Some authors suggest that fine-needle biopsy be performed at the same sitting to obtain material for histologic examination. This procedure requires sedation.

The patient's age and history should be considered when choosing the antibiotic (Table 1). The preferred antibiotic for children and adolescents usually is oxacillin or cefazolin. Cefazolin is used if the patient is allergic to penicillin. If the patient is allergic to both penicillin and cephalosporin, clindamycin or vancomycin is recommended. If methicillin-resistant *S aureus* is suspected, vancomycin should be administered.

Antibiotics always should be administered parenterally, at least initially, for two reasons. First, *S aureus* is prone to dissemination with metastatic abscesses. In the preantibiotic era, the mortality rate of patients with *S aureus* was 20%. Second, concomitant physiologic changes (ie, bacteremia) interfere with absorption of oral agents. The duration of therapy is a subject of great debate and depends on the etiology, extent of infection, and clinical and laboratory response. Patients with acute hematogenous osteomyelitis usually are treated with 3 weeks of parenteral antistaphylococcal antibiotics, followed by 3 weeks of the appropriate oral antibiotic. A shorter course of parenteral antibiotics may be possible if the organism is identified in the laboratory, is known to be very sensitive to the chosen antibiotic, and serum cidal levels are confirmed. Oral agents may be introduced when fever, pain, and signs of inflammation resolve; however, patient compliance with an oral regimen must be considered. If the patient is symptomatic for more than 72 hours before therapy is initiated, responds poorly to 1 week of parenteral therapy, is unable to swallow or retain medications, or if the infection is caused by a microorganism for which no effective oral antibiotic exists, intravenous antibiotics must be continued longer.

The preferred oral agent for treatment of *S aureus* infection is cephalexin. Patients must be monitored for antimicrobial side effects of these drugs. Patients who take cefazolin for more than 2 weeks, especially children younger than age 5 years, are at risk for neutropenia. Use of oxacillin or clindamycin can result in elevated hepatic transaminase levels.

TABLE 1 | Initial Empiric Antibiotic Therapy for Osteomyelitis

Patient Type	Probable Organism	Initial Antibiotic
Neonates*	Group B Streptococci, *S aureus*, or Gram-negative bacilli	Oxacillin 150 mg/kg/24 hours in divided doses q6h plus gentamicin 7.5 mg/kg/24 hours in divided doses q8h; or oxacillin plus cefotaxime 150 mg/kg/24 hours in divided doses q8h
Infants and children	*S aureus*, *S pneumoniae*, group A streptococci	Oxacillin 150 mg/kg/24 hours in divided doses q6h
If allergic to penicillin		Cefazolin 100 mg/kg/24 hours in divided doses q8h
If allergic to penicillin and cephalosporins		Clindamycin 35 to 40 mg/kg/24 hours in divided doses q6h; or vancomycin 40 mg/kg/24 hours in divided doses q6h
Patients with sickle cell disease	*S aureus* or *Salmonella*	Oxacillin and cefotaxime

*Consult neonatologist or infectious disease specialist if the infant is premature

Ultimately, the duration of therapy is determined by the patient's temperature and ESR and evidence of clinical improvement. A decrease in the ESR may lag behind clinical improvement. CRP levels are elevated in 98% of patients with osteomyelitis and decrease rapidly following treatment. However, in most institutions, CRP testing has not replaced ESR testing because CRP levels fall too quickly in patients with osteomyelitis to be a satisfactory criterion for choosing the end point for therapy.

Surgery
Surgery generally is reserved for patients with evidence of a subperiosteal or soft-tissue abscess, intramedullary purulence, sequestra, contiguous focus, or pyogenic arthritis. Although administration of antibiotics decreases mortality, surgery decreases morbidity. At the time of surgery, it is essential to drain the abscess, incise the periosteum, drill the cortex, and remove all dead bone. Specimens should be obtained for bacteriologic and pathologic studies. Persistent fever and pain after surgical drainage strongly suggests inadequate drainage, and repeat drainage should be considered.

Complications
Long-term sequelae of osteomyelitis include recurrent infection, limb-length discrepancy, joint deformity, and gait abnormality.

Special Circumstances
Osteomyelitis in the Neonate
Osteomyelitis in the neonate is a unique disorder for several reasons. First, in infants, small vessels link the metaphysis directly to the cartilaginous anlage of the epiphysis. Thus, an infection that begins in the metaphysis can easily invade and destroy the chondroepiphysis, creating a route for infection to spread into the joint. At age 12 to 18 months, the metaphysis and

epiphysis have matured. The epiphysis develops a separate blood supply, and communication with the metaphyseal vessels ceases. The physis then serves as a mechanical barrier to infection. In addition, the metaphysis of the hip, proximal humerus, proximal radius, and distal lateral tibia are intra-articular. Compared with older children, neonates have a substantially thinner cortex and more loosely adherent periosteum, which are less effective barriers to infection. This allows pus from osteomyelitis to track under the capsule into the joint. The bony architecture of the neonate is also more fragile than that of the older child, and permanent growth arrest may occur if the infection is not appropriately treated.

Second, the organisms responsible for disease in neonates differ from those in older infants and children. Historically, *S aureus* has been the most prevalent organism in the neonate. However, group B streptococcus is now the predominant organism responsible for neonatal sepsis. Invasive procedures such as fetal monitoring, heel punctures, and umbilical catheters are believed to be responsible for many of these infections.

Finally, neonates often are unable to mount a significant inflammatory response to infection. Therefore, the infection spreads rapidly and frequently involves multiple sites. Multiple site involvement has been reported in up to 40% of neonates with acute hematogenous osteomyelitis. At the same time, the clinical presentation may be very subtle. Soft-tissue swelling and pseudoparalysis are hallmarks of neonatal osteomyelitis; however, the infant may demonstrate only minimal symptoms, such as malaise, irritability, poor feeding, or failure to gain weight. The infant may have no fever, and the WBC count and ESR may be normal. Conversely, some neonates may present with fulminant sepsis, specifically with an erythematous, edematous, or discolored limb because of rapid invasion.

The skin overlying the infectious contiguum may have an "orange-peel" appearance caused by local edema. All bones and joints that appear abnormal must be aspirated. Bone scan may help to detect multiple sites of involvement, but should not be relied on to make a diagnosis, because bone scan in the neonate has a high false-negative rate and may not demonstrate all infected sites.

In a recent review of 30 infants younger than age 4 months with osteomyelitis confirmed by radiographic changes, positive bone or blood cultures, and a compatible clinical picture, 17 were premature infants who had received mechanical ventilation and four were full-term infants who had received intensive care. Osteomyelitis was multifocal in 40% of these patients and associated with septic arthritis in 47%. The long bones were affected in 80% of these patients, whereas the flat bones were frequently sites of clinically silent disease. Only 10 patients were febrile.

Because neonates may not absorb oral antibiotics adequately, parenteral therapy for 4 to 6 weeks generally is recommended. In the neonate, the CRP level is believed to be helpful in making the initial diagnosis, because some infants cannot mount an ESR but do have an elevated CRP level. Many authors, however, believe that the CRP level returns to normal too quickly and that it may be misleading to use it to determine the duration of therapy.

Long-term complications of osteomyelitis in the neonate include osteonecrosis of the epiphysis, joint dislocation, and premature physeal arrest. Long-term follow-up is strongly recommended.

Chronic Recurrent Multifocal Osteomyelitis

Chronic recurrent multifocal osteomyelitis (CRMO) is an inflammatory bone disease of unknown etiology that is characterized by an unpredictable course of exacerbations and spontaneous remissions. CRMO occurs primarily during childhood and adolescence and is believed to be a nonpyogenic inflammatory process; no causative agent has been demonstrated. Because CRMO has no clear diagnostic criteria, it is often initially misdiagnosed as acute osteomyelitis or neoplastic disease. However, a number of characteristic features can help differentiate CRMO from other conditions. Whereas hematogenous osteomyelitis is characterized by sudden onset, high fever, and leukocytosis, CRMO generally is characterized by a slow-onset low-grade fever, and normal leukocyte counts. Other typical features of CRMO include (1) local bone pain of gradual onset; (2) multifocal lesions, especially at the long tubular bones, spine, and bones of the foot; (3) inability to culture an infectious agent; and (4) improvement with nonsteroidal anti-inflammatory drugs (NSAIDs).

The WBC count usually is normal; however, the ESR is elevated in most patients.

Plain radiographs reveal nonspecific features suggestive of osteomyelitis, such as osteolysis, sclerosis, and new bone formation, especially in the long tubular bones, spine, and bones of the foot. Areas of lysis and periosteal sclerosis can mimic many primary neoplasms, especially Ewing's sarcoma and Langerhans' cell histiocytosis. Bone scan helps demonstrate the multifocal nature of the disorder and identify initially silent lesions. An open biopsy is not specific, but it will exclude neoplasm.

Because a clear diagnosis of CRMO is frequently impossible at presentation, an initial course of antibiotics with empiric coverage for usual pathogens typically is prescribed. If there is no response to antibiotics, a course of NSAIDs is justified.

Because CRMO is noted to have a good response to NSAIDs, some authors have suggested, but not proved, that this condition is caused by an autoimmune process, particularly a spondyloarthropathy. In the past, this hypothesis has been rejected because no association has been noted between CRMO and HLA-B27 or sacroiliitis, as usually is observed in spondyloarthropathies. Recently, however, in a report on the long-term outcome of eight children and adolescents and seven adults with no family history of rheumatic disease, 80% of these patients satisfied the European Spondyloarthropathy Study Group criteria for spondyloarthropathy. CRMO would, however, appear to be an atypical spondyloarthropathy for several reasons. For example, there is no family history of disease in patients with CRMO, and it affects women more often than men. Anterior thoracic and unilateral sacroiliac involvement are common, and there is no link with the HLA-B27 haplotype. Because CRMO has occurred in association with pustulosis palmaris et plantaris, some authors have suggested that it may be associated with the so-called SAPHO syndrome (synovitis, acne, pustulosis, hyperostosis, and osteitis).

Subacute Hematogenous Osteomyelitis

Subacute hematogenous osteomyelitis develops as a result of increased host resistance and decreased bacterial virulence. Children usually have a history of slow, insidious onset of symptoms such as pain, swelling, and a limp, but with little functional impairment. Laboratory tests usually do not help confirm a diagnosis. The radiologic features can mimic various benign or malignant bone tumors as well as nonpyogenic infections. Most authors believe that histologic confirmation is necessary. However, others believe that a careful radiologic assessment will reveal benign radiologic features and that, in these instances, antibiotics should be the first line of treatment.

Septic Arthritis

Overview

Septic arthritis (SA) requires urgent attention. Three routes of invasion are most common: hematogenous seeding, local spread from a contiguous infection, and traumatic or surgical infection. Duration of symptoms prior to treatment is the most important prognostic factor; therefore, this condition must be quickly identified and treated promptly. Failure to diagnose SA can lead to permanent disability from destruction of the articular cartilage.

The differential diagnosis includes transient synovitis, rheumatic fever, hemarthrosis, juvenile arthritis, cellulitis, osteomyelitis, hemophilia, chondrolysis, Henoch-Schönlein purpura, leukemia, villonodular synovitis, Lyme disease, sickle cell crisis, and reactive arthritis. Reactive arthritis has been documented in a variety of infectious bacterial diseases including *Borrelia burgdorferi*, *Chlamydia*, *Yersinia*, *Salmonella*, *Shigella*, *Mycoplasma*, and *Campylobacter*, as well as some viruses, including hepatitis A and B, rubella, HIV, mumps, parvovirus B19, enterovirus, and herpesvirus. Reactive arthritis may be very difficult to differentiate from septic arthritis by history and physical examination. If the hip is involved, Legg-Calvé-Perthes disease, slipped capital femoral epiphysis, and pelvic, sacroiliac, and vertebral osteomyelitis must be considered.

The initial presentation of an acutely irritable hip warrants particular concern. After Legg-Calvé-Perthes disease, slipped capital femoral epiphysis, and fracture have been ruled out, the differential diagnosis is commonly narrowed to SA and transient synovitis. Differentiation is essential because these two conditions have very different treatments and negative sequelae; however, differentiation can be difficult because the two conditions often have a similar presentation: an irritable, acutely ill child with progressive symptoms and signs of fever, a limp or refusal to bear weight, limited joint motion or effusion, and abnormal laboratory findings. Four clinical predictors that help to differentiate SA from transient synovitis recently have been identified: history of fever, inability to bear weight, an ESR of 40 mm/h or greater, and a serum WBC count of more than 12,000 mm³. If three of these four predictors are present, the probability of SA is 93.1%; if all four predictors are present, the probability is 99.6%.

Presentation

SA is more common in boys than in girls and occurs most commonly in children younger than age 2 years. The patient may have a recent history of upper respiratory tract infection or local soft-tissue infection. Patients with SA generally appear sicker than do those with osteomyelitis. They have a fever of 38° to 40°C and malaise. Physical signs include erythema, restricted joint motion, tenderness, and joint warmth and effusion. Passive joint motion, which stresses the joint capsule, elicits pain. However, in the infant, physical signs may be restricted to limited spontaneous motion or asymmetric posturing of the extremity. The knees, hips, ankles, and elbows account for 90% of affected joints.

Laboratory Tests

With SA, the WBC count is elevated in 30% to 60% of patients, with a left shift in 60% of those with an elevated count. The ESR is a more sensitive test and usually is higher in patients with SA than in those with osteomyelitis; however, the ESR is an unreliable test in the neonate or the patient who has sickle cell disease or is taking steroids. Return of the ESR to normal values is much slower than is clinical improvement; because of this, ESR is of limited use in monitoring resolution of the infection. Monitoring the CRP level may be more useful, particularly in identifying children with osteomyelitis who have concurrent SA.

Imaging Studies

Plain radiographs frequently are normal. Changes are subtle and may include joint space widening, obliteration of the normal fat planes, soft-tissue swelling, and, after 7 to 14 days, bone destruction. Widening of the joint space is an indication of increased joint fluid and pressure that may result in subluxation, dislocation, or ischemic necrosis of the epiphysis. Plain radiographs help to eliminate common differential diagnoses such as fracture or neoplasm. Bone scan is less effective in the treatment of SA than in the treatment of osteomyelitis. The former shows uptake that is focal and less intense than that characteristic of osteomyelitis, especially in the neonate in whom the inflammatory response is limited. A bone scan can be helpful, however, in the pelvis, hip, spine, scapula, shoulder, and swollen foot and ankle, where the exact location of the SA can be difficult to identify. It also may identify multiple sites of infection in the neonate. CT and MRI do not differentiate septic arthritis from nonseptic arthritis.

The role of ultrasound is controversial. Although ultrasound is more sensitive than plain radiography in diagnosing an effusion, it is not specific. Ultrasound is useful in evaluating suspected sepsis in the hips, although neither the quantity nor the echogenicity of the fluid correlates with the severity of the arthritis. In addition, it is not immediately available in most institutions.

TABLE 2 | Initial Empiric Antibiotic Therapy for Septic Arthritis

Patient Age	Probable Organism	Initial Antibiotic
Neonate*	Group B streptococci, S aureus, Gram-negative bacilli	Oxacillin 150 mg/kg/24 hours in divided doses q6h plus cefotaxime 150 mg/kg/24 hours in divided doses q8h
1 month to 6 years	S aureus, S pneumoniae, S pyogenes, H influenzae B	Oxacillin plus cefotaxime or ceftriaxone 75–100 mg/kg/24 hours in divided doses q12h
6 years to adolescence	S aureus, Neisseria gonorrhoeae	Oxacillin (add cefotaxime or ceftriaxone if concerned about gonococcal arthritis)

*Consult neonatologist or infectious disease specialist if the infant is premature

Aspiration

The definitive test for SA is needle aspiration of the joint; therefore, this procedure should not be delayed if SA is suspected. If no fluid is found during aspiration of a hip lesion, an arthrogram is indicated to confirm that the needle has entered the joint. All aspirated fluid should be sent for Gram stain, aerobic and anaerobic bacterial cultures, cell count with a leukocyte differential count, synovial glucose test with a simultaneous serum glucose test, and mucin clot test. Aspirates of infected joints yield positive cultures 54% to 68% of the time. The immunoglobulins in the aspirated fluid may result in a negative synovial fluid culture; therefore, obtaining a Gram stain is essential. Gram stain demonstrates a microorganism in 30% to 40% of patients. If infection is present, the joint fluid usually is cloudy and the WBC count is usually 50,000/mm^3 or greater with a predominance (90%) of polymorphonuclear cells. In addition, the fluid demonstrates a synovial fluid/blood glucose ratio of less than 0.5 and a positive mucin clot test. The mucin clot test assesses the integrity of the hyaluronic acid of the joint fluid and is performed by placing a drop of glacial acetic acid into the fluid while stirring with a glass stirring rod. If bacteria are present, much of the hyaluronic acid is degraded, and the consistency of the fluid resembles that of curdled milk. A positive mucin clot test result is seen with rheumatic fever; however, the results show a fibrous band that resembles a tethered rope forming on the stirring rod.

Microbiology

Prior to the development of an effective vaccine, *H influenzae B* was reported as responsible for 5% of all cases of culture-positive osteomyelitis and more than 40% of cases of culture-positive SA. Since the administration of the conjugated Hib vaccine began in 1992, this pathogen has virtually disappeared; therefore, coverage for this pathogen is not required in the fully immunized child.

S aureus is now the most common causative agent of SA, followed by group A streptococci and *S pneumoniae. Kingella kingae* infections in children are more common than previously recognized and should be actively considered in any child. The recommended empiric therapy is a third-generation cephalosporin until susceptibility to penicillin is confirmed.

Group B β-hemolytic streptococcus is an important cause of SA in the neonate. *Neisseria gonorrhoeae* may be isolated from septic joints in neonates and sexually active adolescents. Adolescents who abuse drugs are at risk for Gram-negative SA. In patients with chronic SA, mycobacteria and fungi must be considered and cultured accordingly. The FDA recently approved a conjugate heptavalent pneumococcal vaccine for high-risk children who are older than age 2 years. This vaccine will be especially helpful to patients with sickle cell disease, asplenia, chronic diseases such as nephrotic syndrome, and immunocompromised children, including those with HIV infection.

Treatment

Treatment of SA should not begin until all of the necessary culture materials have been obtained, because antibiotics diminish the positive yields from blood cultures and aspirations. Aspiration and irrigation of the joint are required to remove the microorganisms, host and bacterial enzymes, and particulate debris in nearly all patients with SA. Open débridement is required for patients with hip involvement, except for those with gonococcal arthritis. In these patients, joint aspiration is sufficient. The role of arthroscopy is unclear.

Treatment with intravenous antimicrobial agents should be initiated as soon as blood, synovial fluid, and other appropriate culture materials have been obtained (Table 2). Results of the synovial fluid Gram stain are the best guide to the selection of an appropriate initial antibiotic. If the Gram stain identifies no microorganisms, the antibiotic should be chosen on the basis of the child's age, immune competency, the joint involved, and local epidemiology. Empiric coverage must include an antistaphylococcal agent, either a β-lactamase–resistant penicillin or a first-generation cephalosporin. These drugs also treat pneumococcus and group B β-hemolytic streptococci. Appropriate Gram-negative coverage should be initiated in all neonates and adolescents to treat gonococcus. Oxacillin and ceftriaxone may be used in immunocompromised patients or in children in whom microorganisms other than traditional Gram-positive organisms, such as *S aureus*, pneumococcus, and group A streptococci, are suspected. Synovial antimicrobial concentrations usually meet or exceed the serum concentrations of parenterally administered antimicrobial agents. Antibiotic therapy is needed for 3 to 4 weeks. Serial laboratory studies should be conducted to detect any adverse drug effects.

Most patients with SA have a normal outcome following appropriate treatment. Factors that contribute to a poor prognosis include delay in treatment, patient age younger than 6 months, prematurity, *Staphyloccus* species infection, and concomitant osteomyelitis.

Other Specific Infections and Conditions
Antibiotic Resistance

The growing number of antibiotic-resistant organisms continues to cause great alarm, particularly in neonatal units. The problem has been attributed both to provider- and patient-related factors. Inappropriate provider practices include imprecise infection diagnoses, "giving in" to patient requests and prescribing an antibiotic when none is needed, limited time spent with patients, fears of liability, and inadequate infection control. Patient-related factors include a lack of knowledge about bacterial versus viral illness, insistence on receiving antibiotics, nonadherence to drug regimens, and exposure to resistant organisms.

The development of new vaccines will help alleviate this problem. In the meantime, two complementary strategies are being encouraged. The first is to avoid use of antibiotics in situations in which they are unlikely to provide benefit, specifically in patients with colds, upper respiratory infections, or bronchitis. The second strategy is to use narrow-spectrum antibiotics as much as possible and thereby minimize selective pressure.

Diskitis and Vertebral Osteomyelitis

Intervertebral disk infection (diskitis) and vertebral osteomyelitis are uncommon entities with many overlapping features. Diskitis generally affects children younger than age 5 years. It occurs almost exclusively in the lumbar region; presenting symptoms that include

refusal to walk or a progressive limp. The child is afebrile or has a low-grade fever. After 2 to 3 weeks, radiographs demonstrate narrowing of the disk space with variable degrees of destruction of adjacent vertebral end plates. A technetium-Tc 99m bone scan demonstrates increased uptake. CT or MRI may demonstrate vertebral disk space involvement with a normal appearance of the nonadjacent vertebrae, but they more commonly demonstrate involvement of two adjacent vertebrae and the intervening disk.

Historically, the word "diskitis" was used to describe a triad of back, abdomen, or lower-extremity pain, fever (or laboratory evidence of an inflammatory process), and radiographic evidence of disk-space narrowing. There was significant debate over whether these findings represented a bacterial infection, viral infection, trauma, or nonspecific osteochondritis. However, recent evidence strongly suggests that the disorder has a pyogenic etiology. Therefore, most authors recommend a course of antibiotics as optimal treatment for this disorder.

Vertebral osteomyelitis is similar to diskitis, but it typically occurs in older children who are febrile and report back pain in the lumbar, thoracic, or cervical region. A pathogen is detected from blood or biopsy specimen, and histopathology demonstrates evidence of osteomyelitis on biopsy. Radiographs first demonstrate a localized rarefaction of one vertebral body; later, destruction of bone, usually of the anterior portion, as well as osteophytic bridging, is evident. Disk space narrowing may or may not occur. MRI is the imaging study of choice and demonstrates edema and purulent material in the marrow or disk space. Vertebral osteomyelitis can be an atypical manifestation of *Bartonella henselae* infection (cat-scratch disease); for this reason, serologic testing should be considered in children with a history of exposure to cats.

Age-dependent differences in the blood supply to the intervertebral disk have been implicated in the pathophysiology of these two conditions. Diskitis is believed to occur as a result of the presence of vascular channels in the cartilaginous region of the disk space during childhood that disappear later in life. Vertebral osteomyelitis, in contrast, is believed to occur when microorganisms lodge in the low-flow, end-organ vasculature adjacent to the subchondral plate region.

Human Immunodeficiency Virus Infection

HIV infection was once largely confined to adolescents with hemophilia. Unfortunately, this disease now affects the general adolescent population. Currently, approximately 25% of individuals who are newly infected with HIV are younger than age 22 years. This trend has been attributed to numerous factors, including unsafe sexual practices, intravenous drug abuse, homelessness, psychiatric disorders, and inadequate psychosocial support.

Efforts to reduce HIV infection in children have focused on discouraging intravenous drug abuse and high-risk sexual activities in women of childbearing age. Zidovudine, or AZT, has been provided to pregnant women to prevent transmission of the disease. Despite these efforts, infants are still being infected perinatally with HIV. Linear growth is stunted in these children, and the severity of delay is correlated with viral load.

Iliopsoas Abscess

Acute pyogenic abscess of the iliopsoas is uncommon in children. The diagnosis is based on clinical, laboratory, and radiologic findings. The clinical presentation varies and may be confused with that of other conditions such as SA of the hip, osteomyelitis, or appendicular abscess. The clinical presentation may include pain or a mass in the iliac fossa or central abdomen, pain and flexion deformity of the hip, a limp, and fever. Passive rotation of the hip in these patients, unlike in those with primary disease of the hip, usually is possible. This condition also differs from primary hip disease in that patients have no posterior hip pain but do report pain on rectal examination. Ultrasound is quick, safe, inexpensive, and readily available, but CT more consistently identifies the iliopsoas muscles and adjacent bony structures.

Historically, iliopsoas abscess was managed with open surgical drainage. In adults, however, image-guided percutaneous drainage currently is used. In children, aspiration (without percutaneous drainage), coupled with intravenous antibiotics, is safe and effective.

Lyme Disease

Lyme disease is a complex, multisystem disease that is caused by the tick-borne spirochete *Borrelia burgdorferi*. The Centers for Disease Control and Prevention (CDC) have reported that the number of reported cases of Lyme disease increased by 70% over a 6-year period, from 9,909 reported cases in 1992 to 16,802 reported cases in 1998. The CDC attributes this rise to an actual increase in the number of cases, as well as improved reporting. Although Lyme disease has been reported in virtually every state in the United States, 92% of all reported cases have been reported in Connecticut, Delaware, Maryland, Massachusetts, New Jersey, New York, Rhode Island, Minnesota, and Wisconsin. Only 2% of infections have been reported in California.

Most cases of Lyme disease occur between May and August. Erythema migrans, a round, red spot at the site of the tick bite that gradually takes on the appearance of a bull's-eye rash is characteristic and appears in approximately 80% of infected patients 3 to 30 days after the bite. Fever, headache, malaise, arthralgias, and multiple secondary skin lesions also may develop. If left untreated, cardiac involvement (usually atrioventricular block), arthralgias, or neurologic disease such as facial nerve palsy or other cranial or peripheral neuropathy may develop. In addition, lymphocytic meningitis, pseudotumor cerebri, or, more rarely, encephalitis may occur. Late manifestations include arthritis, typically of the knee, and various neurologic conditions, including encephalopathy and polyneuropathies.

Transmission of *B burgdorferi* is more likely to occur with tick attachment of more than 24 hours; therefore, prompt removal of the tick can prevent the disease. Because the incidence of infection after a tick bite is low and early treatment of the disease is effective and generally prevents late sequelae, most authors do not recommend prophylactic treatment of tick bites. However, a human recombinant outer-surface-protein vaccine is now available for individuals between age 15 and 70 years who live or work in moderate- to high-risk areas and are exposed frequently to ticks for long periods of time. A preliminary study has found that the vaccine is safe for children, and it currently is being evaluated for approval for use in children.

If treatment is initiated shortly after symptoms first appear, more than 90% of infected individuals are cured with a 21- to 28-day course of oral antibiotics. Oral antibiotics are used to treat erythema migrans and shorten the duration of the rash, and they generally prevent development of late sequelae. Doxycycline is effective but should not be used in children younger than age 8 years or lactating women. Instead, cefuroxime or amoxicillin can be used in these two patient groups. Macrolides are not used as first-line agents because a high rate of clinical failure was found in controlled trials in patients with erythema migrans. Antibody testing does not help confirm diagnosis of early Lyme disease. Serologic testing can help confirm the diagnosis; however, IgG anti-*B burgdorferi* antibodies may not be detectable until 4 to 6 weeks after the initial infection. Serologic testing may help confirm diagnosis if the presence of arthritis, neurologic problems, or cardiac abnormalities cause suspicion of the disease.

Pyomyositis

Pyomyositis is a bacterial infection of muscle caused by *S aureus*. Although pyomyositis initially was described in individuals living in the tropics, it is currently receiving increasing recognition in temperate climates. The differential diagnosis is extensive and includes septic arthritis, cellulitis, osteomyelitis, thrombophlebitis, polymyositis, viral or parasitic myositis, hematoma, contusion, muscle strain, injury, and neoplasm. The natural history includes three stages during which the clinical findings parallel the progression from diffuse inflammation to focal suppuration. The initial invasive stage involves the insidious onset of dull, cramping pain, with or without low-grade fever, that progresses over a period of 10 to 21 days. The suppurative phase of the disease is indicated by an increase in the magnitude of symptoms associated with systemic signs. The late stage includes fluctuance and more profound systemic manifestations. The ESR generally is elevated. MRI is an excellent tool for identifying abscesses.

During the early stages of the disease, antibiotics alone are sufficient treatment; however, once abscesses have formed, open surgical drainage is required. Most patients require surgical débridement, followed by a course of antibiotics. If the patient does not respond quickly, careful evaluation for a second abscess is necessary. The possibility of multiple abscesses always should be considered.

Acute hematogenous peripelvic abscesses commonly occur in tropical climates. However, in a recent article, the authors reported that these infections may occur anywhere and can be overlooked. The most consistent symptom is a hip flexion pseudocontracture in which the hip is held in flexion and in neutral or external rotation. In contrast to patients with SA of the hip, patients with pyomyositis have minimal pain with gentle internal and external rotation of the hip. Although the abscesses may occur in any pelvic muscle, they primarily occur in the psoas. CT is the most helpful imaging modality for both diagnosis and surgical planning.

SAPHO Syndrome

The SAPHO syndrome is a rare constellation of signs and symptoms characterized by synovitis, acne, pustulosis, hyperostosis, and osteitis. It has been primarily reported in Japanese and European children. The most common musculoskeletal complaint is hyperostosis, which causes pain, tenderness, and swelling of the anterior chest wall, although any part of the axial and appendicular skeleton may be affected. The most commonly reported manifestation of this syndrome in adults is osteitis of the sternum, medial clavicle, and anterior portion of the ribs; in children, there is an increased incidence of osteitis of the long bones, which is also characteristic of CRMO. Dermatologic involvement varies and includes pustulosis palmaris et plantaris, pustular psoriasis, and several forms of acne. A combination of clinical, radiographic, and pathologic investigation is required to establish the diagnosis.

Most patients with SAPHO syndrome first report musculoskeletal complaints related to hyperostosis, aseptic osteomyelitis, or synovitis that mimics SA, as in pseudoseptic arthritis. Patients may report a gradual onset of pain, tenderness, and swelling, often before skeletal change is observed. Arthralgias, synovitis, enthesitis, and tenosynovitis may occur.

The etiology and pathophysiology of SAPHO syndrome are unknown, and treatment is difficult and generally ineffective. Because they are ineffective, antibiotics are not recommended. In some patients, NSAIDs have helped alleviate symptoms. Analgesics frequently are required.

Sickle Cell Disease

Although osteomyelitis is uncommon in patients with sickle cell disease, it is still more prevalent in these individuals than in the general population. Bone infarction and microvascular disease probably play a part in the predisposition of these patients to osteomyelitis. Dysfunctional IgG and IgM antibody response, a lack of splenic clearance, defects in alternative pathway fixation of complement, and defects in opsonic activity play a role in the predisposition to invasive infection from polysaccharide encapsulated organisms.

When fever, swelling, erythema, and other signs suggestive of bacterial infection occur in patients with sickle cell disease, it is essential to differentiate between vaso-occlusive pain crisis, caused by bone and/or bone marrow infarction, and osteomyelitis. Making the distinction can be challenging. An elevated ESR and a high WBC count, for example, are common in both conditions. No imaging study reliably differentiates infarction from infection. Bone scans generally are not helpful, although some authors believe that a cold bone scan indicates infarction while normal or increased uptake indicates infection. False-positive and false-negative results have been reported both with gallium scans and MRI. Ultrasound recently has been proven to be quite helpful in patients who have periosteal thickening and elevation and in those who have abscess formation. A positive blood culture is consistent with osteomyelitis, and aspiration of purulent material confirms the diagnosis. Generally, clinical judgment is the primary means of differentiating these two entities. The rare patient with osteomyelitis usually has a high fever, appears toxic with multifocal findings on examination, has a left shift in the peripheral leukocyte count, and has a positive blood and/or bone culture. Infarction is far more common (at least 50-fold in many reports) than is infection. If osteomyelitis does occur, the most common pathogens are *S aureus*, *Salmonella*, and other Gram-negative enteric organisms. *Salmonella* is the most common cause of osteomyelitis in patients with sickle cell disease, in both developed and developing countries. Recent studies have shown that the relative incidence of *Salmonella* is more than twice that of *S aureus*.

If osteomyelitis is suspected, aggressive management is essential. Management should include careful presurgical preparation, which includes exchange transfusion to raise the level of hemoglobin A to 60% and vigorous intravenous hydration to avoid vascular stasis secondary to increased viscosity of the blood; prompt decompression of all abscesses; avoiding the use of tourniquets to prevent vascular stasis and decreased oxygenation; careful collection of culture materials prior to initiation of antibiotics; and administration of parenteral antibiotics for 6 to 8 weeks. A prolonged course of antibiotic treatment is required because of the patient's weakened immune system and the affected bone's compromised vascularity.

Syphilis

The incidence of syphilis has decreased dramatically since 1990. However, focal concentrations of high syphilis prevalence still exist and are predominantly located in inner cities and the southeastern United States. The resurgence of congenital syphilis has been linked to acquired immunodeficiency syndrome, exchange of sex for drugs, teenage pregnancy, limited health care access, and poor prenatal care. In addition, a strong association between maternal illicit drug use, particularly of cocaine, and congenital syphilis has been demonstrated.

Signs and symptoms of active congenital syphilis include temperature instability, mucocutaneous lesions, rhinorrhea, hepatomegaly, splenomegaly, adenopathy, anemia, hydrops fetalis, pathologic jaundice, and pseudoparalysis. In early infancy, the usual radiographic finding is syphilitic metaphysitis (metaphyseal lucent bands, erosions, or a wide zone of provisional calcification), which has been reported in more than 90% of infants with symptomatic congenital syphilis.

Tuberculosis

Physicians must maintain a high index of suspicion for patients with tuberculosis and skeletal tuberculosis. Three related organisms, *Mycobacterium tuberculosis, M africanum,* and *M bovis,* cause tuberculosis. Factors that have contributed to the reappearance of this disease include the rise in the number of individuals with suppressed immune systems, increasingly drug-resistant strains of *Mycobacterium,* an aging population, and an increase in the number of health care workers who are exposed to the disease. HIV remains the leading

known risk factor for the reactivation of latent tuberculous infection, and patients with HIV who are exposed to *M tuberculosis* are more likely to progress to an active disease state than are noninfected patients.

Extrapulmonary tuberculosis is more common in children than in adults, and approximately one third of children who have tuberculosis have extrapulmonary manifestations, most commonly involvement of the superficial lymph nodes (scrofula). Involvement of the cervical spine is rare in children. The clinical presentation of musculoskeletal tuberculosis includes localized pain associated with fever and weight loss. If the spine is involved, truncal rigidity, muscle spasm, and neurologic signs may be present. A cold abscess (swelling without inflammation) strongly suggests musculoskeletal tuberculosis. Any individual who has a skeletal lesion must be evaluated for the possibility that other sites are involved, including the lungs, intestinal tract, and kidneys.

In children, tuberculosis of the spine generally involves the osseous tissue of the vertebrae and not the cartilaginous growth plate. After the disease has been controlled with medication, the end plates can continue to grow. Consequently, the kyphotic deformity is reduced with time in approximately 50% of children, particularly in children who are younger than age 5 years. Similarly, if only one or two vertebrae are involved, the probability of progressive kyphosis is low. The likelihood of kyphosis increases proportionately if more than two vertebrae are involved and varies with the number of involved vertebrae.

Varicella

Varicella, commonly known as chicken-pox, is a common viral infection in children. An estimated 3.5 million cases occur annually in the United States. Serious musculoskeletal complications may include osteomyelitis, SA, necrotizing fasciitis, deep-tissue abscess, and toxic shock syndrome; these can lead to multiple limb amputations and possibly death. A high level of suspicion is necessary for potentially serious secondary infections in children who have varicella so that infection can be recognized and treated promptly. Bacterial pathogens are the cause of the complications that require surgery. Group A β-hemolytic streptococci is the most common organism found on culture.

Annotated Bibliograhy

Osteomyelitis and Septic Arthritis

Blyth MJ, Kincaid R, Craigen MA, Bennet GC: The changing epidemiology of acute and subacute haematogenous osteomyelitis in children. *J Bone Joint Surg Br* 2001;83:99-102.

This report noted that the incidence of osteomyelitis in Scotland has decreased 44% since 1990. The authors noted that *S aureus* was the most commonly isolated pathogen and that the complications rates were low (10%).

Dodman T, Robson J, Pincus D: Kingella kingae infections in children. *J Paediatr Child Health* 2000;36:87-90.

The authors note that *Kingella kingae* infection in children is more common than previously recognized. Any child with a suspected osteoarticular infection should be evaluated for the presence of the organism. Recommended empiric therapy is a third-generation cephalosporin until it can be determined whether the patient is allergic to penicillin.

Howard AW, Viskontas D, Sabbagh C: Reduction in osteomyelitis and septic arthritis related to haemophilus influenzae type B vaccination. *J Pediatr Orthop* 1999;19:705-709.

Until the early 1990s, *H influenzae B* was responsible for 5% of cases of culture-positive osteomyelitis and for 41% of cases of culture-positive SA. Since administration of the conjugated vaccine began in 1992, no case of osteomyelitis or SA has been caused by influenzae. Current empirical antibiotic therapy for hematogenous SA and osteomyelitis need cover only Gram-positive agents in vaccinated infants and children of all age groups.

Kaiser S, Jorulf H, Hirsch G: Clinical value of imaging techniques in childhood osteomyelitis. *Acta Radiol* 1998;39:523-531.

Because ultrasound can detect subperiosteal abscesses early and simply, it can be used with standard radiographs in uncomplicated cases of osteomyelitis. MRI is the modality with the highest sensitivity and specificity for detecting osteomyelitis. CT should be considered when MRI investigation is not available or when anesthesia is required but cannot be provided.

Karwowska A, Davies HD, Jadavji T: Epidemiology and outcome of osteomyelitis in the era of sequential intravenous-oral therapy. *Pediatr Infect Dis J* 1998;17:1021-1026.

The authors reviewed 146 patients with osteomyelitis. They found that decreased limb use and fever were the most common presenting symptoms and tenderness was the most common sign. *S aureus* was the most common causative organism, and *H influenzae* was not identified after 1990. Bone biopsies or aspirates were superior to blood cultures in yielding organisms. Technetium 99m Tc bone scan was the most sensitive imaging test. Complications occurred in 6.6% of patients.

Kocher MS, Zurakowski D, Kasser JR: Differentiating between septic arthritis and transient synovitis of the hip in children: An evidence-based clinical prediction algorithm. *J Bone Joint Surg Am* 1999;81:1662-1670.

The authors determined the diagnostic value of presenting variables for differentiating between SA and transient synovitis. Specifically, four independent multivariate clinical predictors were identified to differentiate the two conditions: history of fever, inability or refusal to bear weight, ESR of at least 40 mm/h, and a WBC count of more than 12,000/mm³. The predicted probability of SA was 3.0% for one predictor, 40.0% for two predictors, 93.1% for three predictors, and 99.6% for four predictors.

Lundy DW, Kehl DK: Increasing prevalence of Kingella kingae in osteoarticular infections in young children. *J Pediatr Orthop* 1998;18:262-267.

The authors note that routine immunization of infants against *H influenzae B* has caused a change in the types of bacteria historically associated with bone and joint infections in children younger than age 3 years. *H influenzae B* has lost its predominance as the most commonly identified Gram-negative pathogen and has been replaced by *K kingae*. The authors reviewed 60 children younger than age 3 years with culture-positive hematogenous septic arthritis and acute/subacute osteomyelitis, treated between 1990 and 1995, to identify the infecting organism. Gram-positive bacteria were identified in 47 patients (78.3%), and Gram-negative organisms were identified in 13 patients (21.7%). *H influenzae B* was cultured in none of the cases of septic arthritis and in only one case (1.6%) of acute osteomyelitis. *K kingae* was cultured in 10 patients (16.7%). These patients ranged in age from 10.5 to 23.5 months.

Lyon RM, Evanich JD: Culture-negative septic arthritis in children. *J Pediatr Orthop* 1999;19:655-659.

The authors reviewed 105 children treated for SA at their institution from 1990 to 1997. Seventy-six children had a clinical presentation consistent with an isolated joint infection. The joint was aspirated and fluid analyzed and cultured in all patients. Culture of the synovial aspirate identified an etiologic organism in only 30% of patients. No significant differences in most clinical and laboratory criteria existed between the culture-positive and culture-negative groups. No other diagnoses were identified. The joint was drained and comparable antibiotic therapy provided for all patients. The infection completely resolved in all patients. The authors determined that patients in the culture-negative group most likely had infections and recommended the same aggressive treatment with and without identification of a causative organism.

Pennington WT, Mott MP, Thometz JG, Sty JR, Metz D: Photopenic bone scan osteomyelitis: A clinical perspective. *J Pediatr Orthop* 1999;19:695-698.

The authors noted that patients with cold bone scans appear to have a more aggressive type of infection with higher fevers, pulse rates, ESR, lengths of stay, and rates of surgical intervention than do those with hot bone scans.

Perlman MH, Patzakis MJ, Kumar PJ, Holtom P: The incidence of joint involvement with adjacent osteomyelitis in pediatric patients. *J Pediatr Orthop* 2000;20:40-43.

In this study of 66 children with osteomyelitis, adjacent joint involvement was evident in 42% and a septic joint was evident in 33%. The most commonly involved joint was the knee. There was no difference in the incidence of adjacent joint involvement between patients younger than age 18 months and those older. The authors concluded that the incidence of adjacent joint involvement is higher than that suggested in the literature.

Rasool MN: Primary subacute haematogenous osteomyelitis in children. *J Bone Joint Surg Br* 2001;83:93-98.

This thorough review emphasizes that the lack of specific findings may make subacute osteomyelitis difficult to diagnose. The condition is believed to develop as a result of increased host resistance and decreased bacterial virulence. The radiologic features can mimic those of various benign or malignant bone tumors as well as of nonpyogenic infections; thus, biopsy and histologic confirmations are essential. Treatment with antibiotics for 6 weeks generally is successful.

Sucato DJ, Schwend RM, Gillespie R: Septic arthritis of the hip in children. *J Am Acad Orthop Surg* 1997;5: 249-260.

The authors review recent advances in the management of SA, including the effects of infection on articular cartilage, improvements in diagnostic tests, and surgical and antibiotic treatment.

Wong M, Isaacs D, Howman-Giles R, Uren R: Clinical and diagnostic features of osteomyelitis occurring in the first three months of life. *Pediatr Infect Dis J* 1995;14: 1047-1053.

In this review of 30 infants with proven osteomyelitis, the authors emphasize the fact that osteomyelitis in the neonate often is a more complex disorder than it is in the older child. Osteomyelitis was multifocal in 40% of these patients and associated with SA in 47% of patients. The long bones were affected in 80% of patients, but flat bones often were sites of clinically silent disease. Of the 30 infants, 25 (83.3%) had focal clinical signs or evidence of disseminated staphylococcal disease; five infants had no focal signs. Only 10 infants were febrile. The sensitivity of bone scanning was 84% and specificity was 89%.

Other Specific Infections and Conditions

Brown R, Hussain M, McHugh K, Novelli V, Jones D: Discitis in young children. *J Bone Joint Surg Br* 2001;83: 106-111.

In this review of 11 patients with diskitis, the presenting clinical features included refusal to walk, back pain, inability to flex the lower back, and loss of lumbar lordosis. Laboratory test results were not helpful in confirming a diagnosis, and blood and disk tissue cultures were negative. Obtaining MRI studies reduced diagnostic delay.

Chambers JB, Forsythe DA, Bertrand SL, Iwinski HJ, Steflik DE: Retrospective review of osteoarticular infections in a pediatric sickle cell age group. *J Pediatr Orthop* 2000;20:682-685.

Patients with sickle cell disease are particularly susceptible to osteoarticular infections. The physician should aspirate or biopsy the painful area in a child who appears ill and has a fever of greater than 38.2°C, pain, and swelling. Radiographs and bone scans are of limited value.

Fernandez M, Carrol CL, Baker CJ: Discitis and vertebral osteomyelitis in children: An 18-year review. *Pediatrics* 2000;105:1299-1304.

In this retrospective review of 57 children with diskitis or vertebral osteomyelitis, clinical presentation and radiographic findings were compared. The authors concluded that age and clinical presentation distinguished patients with diskitis from patients with vertebral osteomyelitis. Radiographs were sufficient for diagnosis of diskitis, but MRI was preferred for diagnosis of vertebral osteomyelitis.

Hamdy RC, Lawton L, Carey T, Wiley J, Marton D: Subacute hematogenous osteomyelitis: Are biopsy and surgery always indicated? *J Pediatr Orthop* 1996;16: 220-223.

The authors assert that benign radiologic features are demonstrated in most patients with subacute osteomyelitis and antibiotics should be the first line of treatment. Open biopsy or surgical débridement should be reserved for patients who do not respond to antibiotics or in whom aggressive radiologic features are demonstrated.

Jaakkola J, Kehl D: Hematogenous calcaneal osteomyelitis in children. *J Pediatr Orthop* 1999;19:699-704.

The authors reported on 21 skeletally immature patients (average age 2.9 years) with hematogenous osteomyelitis of the calcaneus. Local tenderness, swelling, and erythema were the most common findings. The ESR was elevated in 20 (95%) of 21 patients, whereas the C-reactive protein was abnormal in seven (47%) of 15 patients tested. Positive cultures were found in nine patients, and *S aureus* was the most prevalent causative organism. Plain radiographs showed a lytic lesion in 15 (71%) of 21 patients, whereas scintigraphy results were positive in all 16 patients who were scanned. Ten patients were treated with antibiotics alone, and 11 patients underwent surgical irrigation and débridement in association with antibiotic therapy. Three of 10 follow-up radiographs revealed residual abnormalities of the calcaneus.

Letts M, Davidson D, Birdi N, Joseph M: The SAPHO syndrome in children: A rare cause of hyperostosis and osteitis. *J Pediatr Orthop* 1999;19:297-300.

The authors reviewed their experience with a 5-year-old patient with SAPHO syndrome, a rare disorder that is characterized by synovitis, acne, pustulosis, hyperostosis, and osteitis.

Mormino MA, Esposito PW, Raynor SC: Peripelvic abscesses: A diagnostic dilemma. *J Pediatr Orthop* 1999;19:161-163.

The authors reported on their experience with acute hematogenous peripelvic infections in nine children. Eight patients had hip flexion pseudocontracture. CT scan provided the diagnosis and localization in all nine patients. Treatment included irrigation and débridement followed by intravenous and oral antibiotics in seven patients, and symptoms rapidly resolved. Two patients were treated with intravenous antibiotics only, and symptoms recurred in one.

Pollack H, Glasberg H, Lee E, et al: Impaired early growth of infants perinatally infected with human immunodeficiency virus: Correlation with viral load. *J Pediatr* 1997;130:915-922.

Stunting is an early frequent finding in perinatal HIV infection. The deleterious effect of HIV on linear growth appears to be correlated with the level of postnatal viremia.

Raj R, Verghese A: Human immunodeficiency virus infections in adolescents. *Adolesc Med* 2000;11:359-374.

In this article, the authors analyze factors that are influencing the increase of HIV infection in the adolescent population.

Ring D, Johnston CE II, Wenger DR: Pyogenic infectious spondylitis in children: The convergence of discitis and vertebral osteomyelitis. *J Pediatr Orthop* 1995;15:652-660.

In this review of 47 patients with symptoms that would be classically described as those for diskitis, the authors contend that the disorder should more accurately be termed pyogenic infectious spondylitis. They suggest that treatment with specific intravenous antibiotics is more likely to result in rapid relief of symptoms and signs without recurrence.

Sadat-Ali M, al-Umran K, al-Habdan I, al-Mulhim F: Ultrasonography: Can it differentiate between vasoocclusive crisis and acute osteomyelitis in sickle cell disease? *J Pediatr Orthop* 1998;18:552-554.

In this prospective review of 53 patients with sickle cell disease and suspected vaso-occlusive crisis or acute hematogenous osteomyelitis, 17 patients had changes on ultrasound that suggested acute osteomyelitis. Six patients had periosteal thickening and elevation with hypoechogenic regions, eight had abscesses, and three had cortical destruction. All patients with evidence of acute osteomyelitis underwent surgical drainage, and pus and positive cultures were evident in all. The authors concluded that ultrasound is an excellent tool for differentiating these two conditions.

Schreck P, Schreck P, Bradley J, Chambers H: Musculoskeletal complications of varicella. *J Bone Joint Surg Am* 1996;78:1713-1719.

The authors reported that 6% of 417 hospital admissions for varicella were for musculoskeletal complications of the disease that necessitated surgery and, in many patients, amputation. There were seven admissions for osteomyelitis, four for SA, five for necrotizing fasciitis, 10 for deep-tissue abscess, and one for toxic shock syndrome. Bacterial pathogens were identified as the cause of 25 of the 27 complications that led to surgery. Of these 25 patients, cultures revealed that the complications were caused by group A β-hemolytic streptococcus in 21 (84%).

Schultz C, Holterhus PM, Seidel A, et al: Chronic recurrent multifocal osteomyelitis in children. *Pediatr Infect Dis J* 1999;18:1008-1013.

In this article, seven new cases of chronic recurrent multifocal osteomyelitis were presented along with a review of 183 cases previously reported in the literature. The authors noted that a diagnosis of CRMO can be made if the following criteria are met: (1) a protracted course of the disease (more than 3 months); (2) evidence of chronic bone inflammation obtained by an open biopsy with exclusion of other diseases; and (3) failure of an infectious organism to provide culture results.

Sison CG, Ostrea EM Jr, Reyes MP, Salari V: The resurgence of congenital syphilis: A cocaine-related problem. *J Pediatr* 1997;130:289-292.

In this article, the authors indicate that maternal illicit drug use, specifically that of cocaine, is significantly related to the resurgence of congenital syphilis.

Song KS, Ogden JA, Ganey T, Guidera KJ: Contiguous discitis and osteomyelitis in children. *J Pediatr Orthop* 1997;17:470-477.

This article reviews the MRI findings of 16 patients with contiguous diskitis and osteomyelitis. MRI provided a specific diagnosis and defined the anatomic extent of vertebral and soft-tissue involvement. Altered signal changes were evident in the disk, adjacent vertebrae in the end plate and metaphyseal equivalent regions, and the anterior prevertebral tissues. Significant posterior spread and disk herniation were not evident. Of these patients, 14 had lumbar involvement; two had cervical involvement.

Tong CW, Griffith JF, Lam TP, Cheng JC: The conservative management of acute pyogenic iliopsoas abscess in children. *J Bone Joint Surg Br* 1998;80:83-85.

The authors described a treatment of iliopsoas abscess with intravenous antibiotics and image-guided aspiration of the abscess.

Vittecoq O, Said LA, Michot C, et al: Evolution of chronic recurrent multifocal osteitis toward spondylarthropathy over the long term. *Arthritis Rheum* 2000;43:109-119.

The authors review the long-term outcomes (mean 11.6 years) of eight children and adolescents and seven adults (mean 11.6 years) with chronic recurrent multifocal osteitis. They reported that after 10 years, chronic recurrent multifocal osteitis usually evolved to spondyloarthropathy, but with certain features not usually seen in patients with spondyloarthropathy. Specifically, these patients demonstrated unilateral sacroiliitis, a lack of family history of disease, and an absence of a link with HLA-B27.

Wang MN, Chen WM, Lee KS, Chin LS, Lo WH: Tuberculous osteomyelitis in young children. *J Pediatr Orthop* 1999;19:151-155.

In this article, 23 patients with tuberculous osteomyelitis were reviewed. At clinical presentation, the patients generally were afebrile with local swelling and painful limb disability. Delay in diagnosis was common. Laboratory data showed mild increases in WBC counts and the ESR; however, C-reactive protein levels were within normal limits in all but one patient. Radiographs demonstrated osteolytic lesions over metaphyseal areas with surrounding soft-tissue swelling. None of the patients had pulmonary tuberculosis. Bacille Calmette-Guérin vaccination was the suspected cause of tuberculosis in these young children.

Watts HG, Lifeso RM: Tuberculosis of bones and joints. *J Bone Joint Surg Am* 1996;78:288-298.

In this *Current Concepts* review, the authors discuss the evaluation of the musculoskeletal manifestations of tuberculosis.

Chapter 5

Pain Assessment and Management

Shobha Malviya, MD

Sandra I. Merkel, RN, MS

Introduction

Postoperative pain is an unpleasant sensory and emotional experience and one of the most feared symptoms for children undergoing orthopaedic surgery. Unrelieved postoperative pain is deleterious because of unchecked release of stress hormones from tissue injury, which may exacerbate the injury, delay wound healing, lead to infection and, in extreme cases, to death. Thus, the quality of analgesia may influence the incidence of complications and the length of hospital stay, thereby affecting hospital costs and use of health care resources. Effective management of postoperative pain in children requires an organized multidisciplinary approach that encompasses the entire perioperative period, beginning with preoperative education and preparation and including intraoperative analgesic techniques that continue as an integral part of the patient's postoperative care. Previous literature has alluded to undertreatment of pain in children as a result of difficulty with pain assessment, insufficient research, inadequate knowledge, and fear of opioid addiction. However, advances in pain assessment and significant strides toward effective pain management have made minimizing postoperative pain in children a realistic goal. This chapter discusses pain assessment and specific measurement tools that can be used with children and adolescents. Available techniques, strategies, and guidelines for pain management also are described, including systemic analgesia, regional analgesia, and nonpharmacologic interventions.

Pain Assessment

Accurate assessment and measurement of pain is the cornerstone of effective pain management. A preoperative history and assessment of pain is important to prepare the child and family for the expected pain and the options for pain control. This evaluation should include prior painful events, previously used methods for pain control, words that the child uses for pain and other distressors, introduction to pain assessment tools, and other information that the child or family believes may assist in managing the pain effectively.

Children vary in their cognitive and emotional development as well as in their responses to pain and therapies. Consequently, the same painful stimulus or surgical procedure does not necessarily produce the same pain behaviors or intensity ratings in all children. Therefore, careful pain assessment is essential to direct appropriate therapy. The measurement of pain in children can be accomplished with physiologic, behavioral, and self-report measures.

Physiologic Measures

Physiologic indicators, such as changes in heart rate, respiratory rate, blood pressure, and oxygen saturation, provide information about a child's response to noxious stimuli. These indicators vary among children and are altered by other stress-arousal events, such as fear and anxiety, and, therefore, should be used in conjunction with other measurements of pain, such as behavioral changes and self-report.

Self-Report of Pain

Because pain is a subjective perception, self-report of pain provides the most reliable indication of its location and intensity. Some children as young as age 3 years can identify the location of pain and use a simple tool to quantify its severity. Others, however, are unwilling to report pain because they believe they are expected to be brave or they anticipate receiving an injection or other painful therapies. A number of tools have been devised to allow young children to self-report their pain; however, results of previous studies indicate that children prefer the Wong-Baker Faces scale (Fig. 1). A number scale and a visual analog scale with word anchors can be used by children who understand the concepts of numbers and rank order. Most children older than age 7 years are able to use number

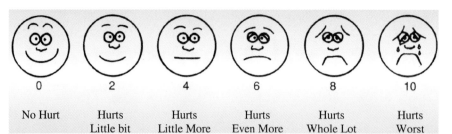

Figure 1 Wong-Baker Faces Pain Rating Scale: The examiner should point to each face using the words to describe the pain intensity, then ask the child to choose the face that best describes the pain and record the appropriate number. *(Reproduced with permission from Wong DL, Hockenberry-Eaton M, Wilson D, Winkelstein ML, Ahmann E, DiVito-Thomas PA: Whaley and Wong Nursing Care of Infants and Children, ed 6. St Louis, MO, Mosby, 1999, p 1153.)*

0	2	4	6	8	10
No Hurt	Hurts Little bit	Hurts Little More	Hurts Even More	Hurts Whole Lot	Hurts Worst

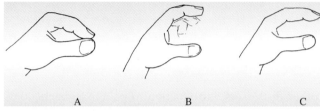

Figure 2 Finger span scale. **A,** The bottom anchor of "no pain"; **B,** The top anchor of "the most pain," and **C,** A pain estimation. *(Reproduced with permission from Merkel S, Malviya S: Pediatric pain, tools, and assessment. J Per Anesth Nurs 2000;15:408-414.)*

scales. A visual analog scale that is useful with younger children is the finger span scale. The child is asked to touch together the thumb and forefinger of one hand to represent "no pain." Stretching the thumb and index finger as far apart as possible is severe or the "worst pain." A pain estimation is communicated by holding the thumb and index finger an appropriate distance (Fig. 2). Pain intensity is based on the ratio of the observed distance to the maximum distance from the thumb to the index finger.

Behavioral Measures

Behavioral observation is the primary approach for assessing pain in children with limited verbal and cognitive skills. Behaviors such as vocalization (eg, crying and groaning), facial expression, body posture, rigidity, undue quietness, and inability to be consoled are used to determine the presence and intensity of a child's pain. Several tools that incorporate different pain behaviors are reliable and valid measures of moderate to severe pain. We devised a scale for use in children age 2 months to 7 years that includes five categories of behavior: Face, Legs, Activity, Cry, and Consolability (FLACC). The acronym FLACC facilitates recall of the five categories, and each category is scored from 0 to 2, resulting in a total score of between 0 and 10 (Table 1). The advantages of the FLACC scale include its ease of use in the busy clinical setting and its high degree of validity and reliability in children.

Because children will respond to other types of distress such as hunger and anxiety, use of behavioral observations to guide pain therapy requires consideration of the context of a child's behavior. Sleeping and withdrawn behavior can be misinterpreted as the absence of pain, when, in fact, the child may be attempting to control pain by limiting activity and interactions. A quietly sleeping child who awakens with jerky body movements and is unable to settle may be having muscle spasms. Extremity pain following injury or surgery that is unrelieved by a 50% increase in the dose of an opioid and increases significantly with movement of the extremity or digits may indicate the beginning of a compartment syndrome. Escalating opioid doses would not be effective or indicated in a child with muscle spasms or compartment syndrome.

Children who are cognitively and physically disabled and unable to report pain may be at a greater risk than other children for undertreatment of pain. Children with cerebral palsy and other neurodevelopmental disorders have behavior idiosyncrasies and patterns of facial expression that are difficult to interpret. Pain behaviors, however, are exhibited in the areas of facial expression, body position, activity, vocalization, and social interaction. Assessing pain in the newborn presents an additional challenge because many of the pain tools measure an active and robust response to pain; in fact, the premature and ill newborn may withdraw and appear to be asleep and pain-free.

Difficulties with behavioral observations arise when there is a great discrepancy between what is expected and what is observed. It is difficult to assess pain if a child exhibits pain behaviors in greater or lesser degrees in the presence of certain people or other environmental stimuli. Parents frequently are an important source of information about pain behaviors exhibited by their child and should be encouraged to contribute to the assessment of pain. Data suggest that parents can identify the presence of pain in their hospitalized child, but they may have difficulty assessing its severity.

Pain Management

Pain associated with orthopaedic surgery requires aggressive treatment with systemic and regional analgesia techniques and nonpharmacologic measures singly or in combination. Options for postoperative analgesic therapies include around-the-clock dosing, continuous opioid infusions, use of oral medications when tolerated, and combinations of different analgesic

TABLE 1 | FLACC Scale

Category	Score 0	Score 1	Score 2
	0	1	2
Face	No particular expression or smile	Occasional grimace or frown, withdrawn, disinterested	Frequent to constant frown, clenched jaw, quivering chin
Legs	Normal position or relaxed	Uneasy, restless, tense	Kicking or legs drawn up
Activity	Lying quietly, normal position, moves easily	Squirming, shifting back and forth, tense	Arched, rigid, or jerking
Cry	No cry (awake or asleep)	Moans or whimpers, occasional complaint	Crying steadily, screams or sobs, frequent complaints
Consolability	Content, relaxed	Reassured by occasional touching, hugging, or "talking to" Distractable	Difficult to console or comfort

(Reproduced with permission from Merkel SI, Lewis T, Shayevitz JR, Malviyas: The FLACC: A behavioral-scale for scoring postoperative pain in young children. *Pediatric Nurs* 1997;23:293-297.)

modalities. These options should be considered for all patients undergoing orthopaedic surgery. The treatment plan should be individualized based on the nature of the surgery and the patient's underlying medical history and previous pain experience. This section will discuss some of the treatment options available for effective analgesia following orthopaedic surgery.

Systemic Analgesia

Opioids and nonopioid adjuvants may be administered orally or parenterally to provide effective analgesia. In general, the parenteral route should be used until the patient resumes adequate oral intake.

Acetaminophen

The analgesic effects of acetaminophen result from inhibition of prostaglandin synthetase centrally. Acetaminophen is useful alone for mild pain or in conjunction with opioids for moderate to severe pain. The usual dose is 10 to 15 mg/kg orally every 4 hours or 20 mg/kg rectally. Around-the-clock dosing works well and may reduce opioid requirements in the first 24 to 48 hours after surgery or in patients on escalating doses of opioids. The daily dose for children should not exceed 75 mg/kg, and the maximum daily dose for adults is 4 g.

Nonsteroidal Anti-Inflammatory Drugs

The therapeutic effects of nonsteroidal anti-inflammatory drugs (NSAIDs) are derived from their ability to decrease levels of inflammatory mediators, such as bradykinin, substance P, thromboxane, and prostaglandins, at the site of tissue injury. The NSAIDs may be used alone to treat mild or moderate pain or in conjunction with acetaminophen and opioids to treat moderate to severe pain. Side effects include gastrointestinal upset, mucosal ulceration, and altered renal and platelet function. Because of the risk of bleeding, these drugs may be unsuitable in the early postoperative period following some operations; however, these concerns have not been addressed adequately in clinical studies.

Ketorolac tromethamine (Toradol) is effective in decreasing the dosage and side effects of opioid analgesics in children undergoing orthopaedic procedures. A randomized double-blind study comparing ketorolac with placebo in conjunction with patient-controlled analgesia (PCA) in this population, found lower pain scores during the first 36 hours after surgery, decreased use of opioids, and no increase in adverse effects in the group taking ketorolac. These children received a loading dose of ketorolac on arrival in the postanesthesia care unit and subsequent doses during the postoperative period of 0.5 mg/kg at 6-hour intervals for a maximum of eight doses. Ketorolac may be administered intramuscularly or intravenously in a dose of 0.5 mg/kg every 6 hours. Ketorolac does not have the respiratory depressant effects of opioids, but it does share the potential side effects of NSAIDs. It can cause adverse central nervous system (CNS) effects, such as somnolence, dizziness, and headache. Long-term administration can impair renal function in approximately 3% of patients and therefore should be used with caution, if at all, in patients with renal disease. Ketorolac can inhibit platelet adhesion and aggregation and prolong bleeding time by approximately 3 minutes from baseline values. Unlike with aspirin, this effect is transient with ketorolac; platelet aggregation returns to normal within 24 to 48 hours after therapy is discontinued. Guidelines from the US Food and Drug Administration suggest that the use of parenteral ketorolac be

TABLE 2 | Equipotency Table

Drug	Potency	Conversion of IV to Oral Dosing	PO Dosing Interval for Continuous Pain Relief
Morphine	1	1:3 to 5	4 to 12 hours
Fentanyl	80 to 100	Not available PO	Not available
Hydromorphone (Dilaudid)	7 to 10	1:2 to 4	4 hours
Methadone*	1	1:1 to 2	8 hours
Meperidine	0.1	1:4	3 hours
Codeine	0.1	Not recommended for IV	3 to 4 hours
Oxycodone	0.5 to 1	Not available for IV	4 to 6 hours
Hydrocodone	0.5 to 1	Not available for IV	4 to 6 hours

*Methadone has a longer half life than other opioids; therefore, dose should be reduced when switching from a short-acting opioid to methadone

limited to 5 days. Ibuprofen may offer greater flexibility in the dosage as well as increased safety and significant cost savings if a child is able to tolerate oral medications.

The cyclooxygenase-2 (COX-2) inhibitors are a new family of NSAIDs that are designed specifically to limit the side effects of bleeding and gastric ulceration encountered frequently with other NSAIDs. These drugs include celecoxib (Celebrex) and rofecoxib (Vioxx). Although they have not been approved for use in children, COX-2 inhibitors provide an excellent analgesic option in patients older than age 18 years with thrombocytopenia or gastrointestinal ulceration who could benefit from NSAID therapy. The once-a-day dosing of rofecoxib (12.5 mg to 50 mg) and the 12-hour dosing of celecoxib (100 to 200 mg/dose) may help improve patient compliance.

Benzodiazepines
Benzodiazepines are most useful for sedation, anxiolysis, and amnesia for painful procedures. Although they have no analgesic effects, their short-term use may be indicated when skeletal muscle spasms are the primary cause of pain. Because benzodiazepines potentiate the respiratory depressant effects of opioids, they should be used with extreme caution in conjunction with opioids.

Opioids
Opioid analgesics relieve pain by attaching to opiate receptor sites in the brain and spinal cord. Opioids may be administered via a number of routes and provide effective analgesia for patients with moderate to severe pain. Because intramuscular administration of opioids leads to variable absorption of the drug, it is no longer the preferred route for pain management. Intravenous administration reliably achieves a desired opioid blood level. Oral medications are best used for mild-to-moderate pain that occurs later in the postoperative course, once adequate gastrointestinal function returns. Several oral preparations of opioids have been combined with acetaminophen to increase the analgesic effect. However, the total daily dose of acetaminophen must be considered when using these combination analgesics. Dosing data and equianalgesic tables are helpful when changing opioids and routes of administration. Published tables vary in complexity and in the suggested doses. Table 2 provides a simple comparison of potency and bioavailability of opioids. Spinal axis opioids provide profound analgesia and will be discussed in the regional analgesia section of the chapter.

The common side effects of opioids include nausea, vomiting, and itching. Opioids can cause life-threatening respiratory depression in a dose-dependent manner. Other side effects include urinary retention and constipation. CNS effects include somnolence, sedation, euphoria, and dysphoria. Meperidine (Demerol) administered in high doses or for a prolonged time may cause CNS excitation as a result of the accumulation of normeperidine in the circulation. This accumulation results in tremors, twitching, and seizures. Some authors suggest that the 24-hour dose of meperidine be limited to a maximum of 500 mg in children and the duration of therapy be limited to 3 to 5 days. Hydromorphone (Dilaudid) is administered to patients who experience inadequate analgesia and side effects such as dysphoria, pruritus, or nausea and vomiting with morphine sulfate. Opioids are known to produce tolerance; when used for longer than 7 days, it may be prudent to taper the dose of the opioids to prevent withdrawal symptoms. Because clearance and protein binding are decreased, resulting in a greater free frac-

TABLE 3 | Guidelines for Patient-Controlled Analgesia Dosing

Feature	Morphine	Hydromorphone (Dilaudid)*	Fentanyl[†]
Loading dose	0.05 to 0.15 mg/kg	5 to 10 μg/kg	1 to 2 μg/kg
Infusion rate	0.01 to 0.02 mg/kg/h	2 to 3 μg/kg/h	0.1 to 0.5 μg/kg/h
Demand dose	0.02 to 0.04 mg/kg	2 to 4 μg/kg	0.2 to 0.5 μg/kg
4-hour limit	0.25 to 0.3 mg/kg	20 to 40 μg/kg	2 to 4 μg/kg
Lockout time	8 to 15 min	8 to 15 min	8 to 15 min

*Hydromorphone dose is calculated as 10 times as potent as morphine; literature indicates equivalent doses range from 7 to 10 times as potent as morphine
[†]Not recommended for routine patient-controlled analgesia use; pruritus is a problem when total dose equals 1 μg/kg/h

tion of the drug, opioids should be used with caution in infants younger than age 3 months. Furthermore, immaturity of the blood-brain barrier in infants may contribute to enhanced passage of opioids into the CNS.

Tramadol hydrochloride (Ultram) is a centrally acting synthetic analgesic with an affinity for opioid receptors. Side effects may include dizziness, somnolence, nausea, and vomiting. It is available as an oral preparation in the United States, and its efficacy is comparable to codeine for pain relief following dental extraction. Concomitant use of tramadol increases the risk of seizures in patients taking selective serotonin reuptake inhibitors, such as tricyclic antidepressants and monoamine oxidase (MAO) inhibitors.

Patient-Controlled Analgesia

PCA provides safe and effective analgesia in children as young as age 5 years. With PCA, the patient is allowed to self-administer small doses of opioids in response to changes in pain intensity. Safety features built into all PCA devices include programming features such as a lockout interval and maximum 4-hour limits. The primary advantages of PCA include avoiding delays in obtaining analgesic treatments and reducing nursing workload. Evaluation of PCA use has demonstrated a high degree of safety with appropriate use as well as patient satisfaction. In young children and those cognitively unable to make decisions about dosing, nurse-controlled analgesia (NCA) has been used with success. This technique allows nursing staff the flexibility to titrate opioids on the basis of their assessment of pain or in anticipation of painful procedures, such as physical therapy and dressing changes. The child's respiratory status, sedation, and comfort should be assessed frequently with both PCA and NCA. Most PCA devices can deliver a continuous infusion of analgesics in addition to incremental boluses. A continuous infusion maintains a therapeutic plasma opioid level,

prevents disruption of sleep, and improves pain scores; however, continuous infusion also commits the patient to a fixed amount of opioid regardless of the level of sedation. Therefore, close monitoring for oversedation may be required in patients on continuous opioid infusions. Guidelines for PCA dosing are presented in Table 3 and are based on published literature and our experience.

Adjuvant drug therapy, including the use of antidepressants such as amitriptyline and anticonvulsants such as gabapentin, is beneficial in treating neuropathic pain associated with traumatic injury or amputation. Pain relief from these agents may not be evident until these drugs have been at a therapeutic level for 1 week or longer.

Regional Analgesia

Regional anesthesia techniques provide profound analgesia with decreased opioid requirements, a rapid and pain-free recovery, early ambulation, and greater patient acceptance of continuous passive motion and physical therapy. In children, careful patient selection ensures that regional analgesia provides safe and effective pain relief.

Epidural Analgesia

A caudal block effectively provides analgesia for procedures below the level of the diaphragm. Because the landmarks are identified easily in children younger than age 8 years, this block is technically simple to perform. It is commonly indicated for lower extremity procedures such as clubfoot repair or for urologic or abdominal surgery. Bupivacaine in concentrations of 0.125% to 0.25% with 1 in 200,000 epinephrine provides effective analgesia. The duration of sensory blockade and the quality of analgesia are similar with both concentrations; however, the lower concentration produces significantly less motor blockade. Additives such as clonidine and ketamine prolong the duration and improve the quality of analgesia, although current data are insufficient to support their routine use. Morphine sulfate (50 to 75 μg/kg) administered into the epidural space provides analgesia for 12 to 24 hours, but close monitoring for respiratory depression is required for 24 hours after injection.

Lumbar epidural analgesia is indicated in older children who weigh more than 20 kg because a smaller volume per kilogram of local anesthetic is required to reach the dermatome desired than is required with caudal blocks. Local anesthetics, opioids, or a combination of the two classes of drugs can provide effective postoperative analgesia. Epidural local anesthetics provide dose-related intense analgesia, prevent muscle spasm, and allow pain-free mobilization and physical therapy while they avoid the respiratory depression associated with opioids. The disadvantages of epidural local anesthetics are related to motor and autonomic blockade and include the potential to mask perioperative complications such as compartment syndrome and pressure sores. Use of dilute solutions of local anesthetics (0.0625% to 0.1% bupivacaine) and a high index of suspicion and vigilance by the nursing staff can minimize these risks. However, the benefits of epidural analgesia should be carefully weighed prior to selection in patients at risk for compartment syndrome.

Epidural opioids have the advantage of providing analgesia without sympathetic, sensory, or motor blockade, but they do carry the risk of side effects such as respiratory depression, nausea, vomiting, and pruritus. Because of the risk of respiratory depression, systemic opioids and sedative drugs such as benzodiazepines probably should not be used in conjunction with epidural opioids. A combination of epidural opioids and local anesthetics, such as fentanyl and bupivacaine, blocks nociceptive pathways at different sites and allows lower doses of each agent to be used with fewer side effects. Results of a previous study indicate that fentanyl added to an epidural solution of bupivacaine significantly reduced the supplemental opioid requirements in children undergoing spine or lower extremity surgery. The dosages of drugs administered by the epidural route are presented in Table 4.

Epidural opioids administered for spine surgery are increasing in popularity. A single dose of morphine injected intrathecally by the surgeon prior to wound closure provides effective analgesia for 12 to 24 hours. Alternatively, the surgeon places an epidural catheter at the upper end of the incision and tunnels it lateral to the incision prior to wound closure. The catheters are left in place for 72 hours, and low-dose opioids are infused to provide effective analgesia. Close monitor-

TABLE 4 | Drugs Used for Epidural Anesthesia

Drug	Onset/Duration	Dose
Duramorph (single shot)	Onset 45 min Duration 6 to 24 (22) hours	0.03 to 0.05 mg/kg
Duramorph infusion	Onset 45 min	3 to 4 μg/kg/h
Fentanyl infusion*	Onset 5 to 15 min	0.5 to 2.0 μg/kg/h
Bupivacaine*	Onset 10 min	0.065% or 0.10% 0.1 to 0.4 mL/kg/h

*Frequently used in combination

ing, including continuous pulse oximetry and hourly documentation of respiratory rate, is required with this technique until 24 hours after the infusion has been discontinued.

Peripheral Nerve Blocks

Peripheral nerve blockade with local anesthesia allows interruption of sensory transmission along specific nerves or nerve groups. The peripheral blocks pertinent to orthopaedic surgery include brachial plexus blocks for upper extremity surgery, intercostal blocks and intrapleural catheters for thoracic surgery, and femoral, sciatic nerve, and lumbar plexus blocks (3-in-1 block) and popliteal fossa blocks for lower extremity surgery. Although these blocks are used extensively to provide analgesia in adults, limited data are available related to their use in children. Results of a study in which popliteal fossa blocks were evaluated for children undergoing foot and ankle surgery reported a 95% success rate in providing effective analgesia for 8 to 12 hours following surgery. As with any regional anesthetic technique, careful assessment of needle placement and prudent estimation of safe quantities of local anesthetic are required.

Regional analgesia is absolutely contraindicated if an infection at the site of needle puncture or sepsis or bleeding disorders are present and in patients who are taking anticoagulants. Complications of regional anesthetics include inadvertent intravascular or subarachnoid injection, local anesthetic toxicity, medication errors, and pneumothorax or hemothorax from brachial plexus and intercostal blocks.

Preemptive Analgesia

Current literature suggests that sensory signals that are generated by tissue injury during surgery can trigger a prolonged state of increased CNS excitability that may contribute to postoperative hyperalgesia. Theoretically, preemptive analgesia prevents hyperexcitability by diminishing the barrage of nociceptive inputs during surgery. The underlying principle is that therapeutic intervention is made in advance of the pain rather than in reaction to it. Results of studies in adult patients have demonstrated that when an epidural block is instituted before amputation, the incidence of phantom limb pain decreases dramatically. By using NSAIDs, local anesthetics, or opioids, singly or in combination, preemptive treatment could be directed at the periphery at inputs along sensory axons and/or at central neurons.

Nonpharmacologic Interventions

Nonpharmacologic measures provide comfort and give children a sense of control over pain and their behavior. Imagery and distraction make pain more tolerable by placing pain in the periphery of awareness. Staff and parents can use distraction by asking the child to talk about a favorite place. Questions about colors, temperature, sound, smells, weather, and people help the child focus on the favorite place instead of the distressing event. Relaxation reduces distress associated with pain. A simple relaxation technique for a young child is to breathe deeply by blowing bubbles. Physical interventions for reducing pain stimulate the skin and include application of cold, heat, or massage, exercise, and transcutaneous electrical nerve stimulation therapy. These measures are useful for ongoing pain as well as procedural pain.

Changing Practice

Frequent and routine assessment and documentation of pain is critical for its effective management and to evaluate a child's response to treatment. Pain assessment and the use of pain scales can become routine when they are coupled with other assessments as the "fifth" vital sign. Changing practice is difficult if the process of pain assessment and documentation is time consuming. Revision of flowsheets to facilitate documentation of pain scores and assessment promotes consistent measurement and monitoring.

Changes in practice occur more quickly when the innovation fits the organization's agenda or is mandated by regulation. The Agency for Health Care Policy and Research guidelines for acute pain suggest that effective pain management in infants and children requires assessment of pain intensity and evaluation of response to treatment at regular intervals using consistent and valid criteria. These guidelines also recommend that self-report measures be used whenever possible. Recognition of the wide variability in pain management practices has led the Joint Commission on Accreditation of Healthcare Organizations (JCAHO) to develop standards on pain management. The focus of these standards is to ensure that all patients with pain are identified and then treated or referred for treatment. Indeed, hospital surveyors will look for evidence of quality pain management in interviews with families, review of records, and analysis of policies and education materials for patients and staff.

Summary

Effective pain control after orthopaedic surgery in children merits high priority to promote patient comfort and satisfaction and ensure optimal surgical outcomes. The development of novel pain assessment tools, the advent of new pharmacologic agents, an increased use of regional analgesic techniques, and increasing awareness of the value of nonpharmacologic interventions have made it possible to minimize postoperative pain. New standards on pain management mandated by JCAHO focus on ensuring that patients with pain are identified, assessed, treated, and prepared for discharge. These standards should further ensure that all children receive effective pain treatment directed by frequent pain assessment and measurement. A multidisciplinary approach that involves all members of the health care team and includes input from the patient and the patient's family is essential to meet the goals of effective pain management in children.

Annotated Bibliography

Pain Assessment

Keck JF, Gerkensmeyer JE, Joyce BA, et al: Reliability and validity of the faces and word descriptor scales to measure procedural pain. *J Pediatr Nurs* 1996;11:368-374.

This study of 118 children age 3 to 18 years assessed the reliability and validity of the Faces and Word Descriptor Scales to measure pain in verbal children. Test-retest reliability and construct and discriminant validity were supported for both instruments. Most children preferred to use the Faces scale when providing self-report of pain, regardless of age.

Merkel SI, Voepel-Lewis T, Shayevitz JR, Malviya S: The FLACC: A behavioral scale for scoring postoperative pain in young children. *Pediatric Nurs* 1997;23:293-297.

The interrater reliability and reproducibility of the FLACC pain assessment tool in the postoperative period was demonstrated in this prospective study. In addition, its validity against existing tools (the nurses' global ratings of pain and the objective pain scale) was established.

Pain Management: Systemic Analgesia

Eberson GP, Pacicca DM, Ehrlich MG: The role of ketorolac in decreasing length of stay and narcotic complications in the postoperative pediatric orthopaedic patient. *J Pediatr Orthop* 1999;19:668-692.

Twenty-seven patients who underwent long-bone osteotomies or complex foot procedures received 1 mg/kg loading dose of ketorolac in the recovery room, followed by 0.5 mg/kg every 6 hours for 24 hours. The charts of 37 patients who underwent similar surgical procedures prior to the ketorolac protocol were reviewed. There were no bleeding complications in either group. The ketorolac group received fewer morphine doses, reported fewer gastrointestinal side effects, and had a shorter hospital stay.

Roelofse JA, Payne KA: Oral tramadol: Analgesic efficacy in children following multiple dental extractions. *Eur J Anaesthesiol* 1999;16:441-447.

In this prospective, double-blind study, 60 children, age 4 to 7 years, were assigned to receive either 1.5 mg/kg of tramadol drops or placebo (normal saline solution) 30 minutes before dental extraction of six or more teeth. Acetaminophen (120 mg) was given as needed postoperatively. The tramadol group reported significantly less pain than those in the placebo group at each assessment.

Sutters KA, Shaw BA, Gerardi JA, et al: Comparison of morphine patient-controlled analgesia with and without ketorolac for postoperative analgesia in pediatric orthopedic surgery. *Am J Orthop* 1999;28:351-358.

In this prospective, randomized, double-blind, placebo-controlled study, the effect of intravenous ketorolac, used to supplement morphine PCA, in 68 children undergoing orthopaedic surgery was evaluated. A loading dose of ketorolac (1 mg/kg) on arrival in the postanesthesia care unit was followed by 0.5 mg/kg at 6-hour intervals for a total of eight doses. Children in the ketorolac group had lower pain scores and received significantly less morphine than children in the placebo group. There were no significant differences between groups in opioid-induced side effects and bleeding complications.

Pain Management: Regional Analgesia

Jones MD, Aronsson DD, Harkins JM, et al: Epidural analgesia for postoperative pain control in children. *J Pediatr Orthop* 1998;18:492-496.

In this retrospective study, the use of epidural analgesia in 98 children, age 7 to 18 years, who underwent spine or lower extremity surgery was evaluated. All children received an epidural infusion of 0.0625% to 0.25% bupivacaine alone (n = 63) or with fentanyl (n = 35). Although pain scores between groups were similar, fewer children in the fentanyl group required supplemental analgesia. The side effects encountered were minor and included catheter dislodgement, pruritus, nausea, and vomiting. The authors caution that epidural analgesia may mask the early signs of compartment syndrome. Therefore, continuous epidural analgesia is not recommended in patients at risk for compartment syndrome.

Tobias JD, Mencio GA: Popliteal fossa block for postoperative analgesia after foot surgery in infants and children. *J Pediatr Orthop* 1999;19:511-514.

Results of this study demonstrated a 95% success rate of popliteal fossa blocks for postoperative analgesia in 20 children age 6 months to 12 years who underwent foot and ankle surgery. Although this technique has been used in the adult population for surgical anesthesia, limited data are available related to its use in children.

Classic Bibliography

Berde CB, Lehn BM, Yee JD, et al: Patient-controlled analgesia in children and adolescents: A randomized, prospective comparison with intramuscular administration of morphine for postoperative analgesia. *J Pediatr* 1991;18:460-466.

Goodarzi M, Shier NH, Ogden JA: Epidural versus patient-controlled analgesia with morphine for postoperative pain after orthopedic procedures in children. *J Pediatr Orthop* 1993;13:663-667.

Lee JJ, Rubin AP: Comparison of a bupivacaine-clonidine mixture with plain bupivacaine for caudal analgesia in children. *Br J Anaesth* 1994;72:258-262.

Litvak KM, McEvoy GK: Ketorolac, an injectable non-narcotic analgesic. *Clin Pharm* 1990;9:921-935.

Rice LJ: Regional anesthesia in the pediatric patient, in *International Anesthesia Research Society Review Course Lectures.* Cleveland, OH, International Anesthesia Research Society, 1994, pp 32-36.

Tyler DC: Pharmacology of pain management. *Pediatr Clin North Am* 1994;41:59-71.

US Agency for Health Care Policy and Research: *Acute Pain Management: Operative or Medical Procedures and Trauma.* Rockville, MD, US Department of Health and Human Services, 1992 (AHCPR Publication No. 92-0032).

Wedel DJ: The pediatric patient: Regional anesthesia, in Wedel DJ (ed): *Orthopedic Anesthesia.* New York, NY, Churchill Livingstone, 1993, pp 129-149.

Woolf CJ, Chong MS: Preemptive analgesia: Treating postoperative pain by preventing the establishment of central sensitization. *Anesth Analg* 1993;77:362-379.

Chapter 6

Musculoskeletal Neoplasms in Children

J. Sybil Biermann, MD

Benign Bone Tumors

Nonossifying Fibroma/Fibrous Cortical Defect

Nonossifying fibromas (NOFs), or fibrous cortical defects, usually are discovered incidentally when radiographs are obtained in children who sustain minor trauma. Most children with NOFs require no intervention; the condition will regress during adolescence. If there is concern regarding the size of the lesion and the risk of impending pathologic fracture, serial radiographs may be obtained at several month intervals. However, the risk of pathologic fracture is low if the lesion is smaller than one half the diameter of the bone.

The appearance of NOFs on plain radiographs is characteristically scalloped and eccentric, usually with a sharp sclerotic rim. However, NOFs occasionally have more aggressive features and may be mistaken for other tumors, such as aneurysmal bone cysts. This is a particular risk if a pathologic fracture has occurred; in that situation, the lesion can appear very aggressive radiographically, with periosteal new bone. Because the treatment and incidence of recurrence may differ between these types of lesions, careful pathologic analysis of the specimen is necessary. As with other musculoskeletal neoplasms, close cooperation is needed among the clinician, radiologist, and pathologist in arriving at the correct diagnosis.

Unicameral Bone Cyst

Unicameral bone cysts (UBCs) occur most frequently in the metaphyses of long bones in children (Fig. 1). The etiology of UBC remains unclear. One report suggests that a clonal abnormality was responsible for the UBC in an 11-year-old boy. Another theory suggests that the cyst develops in response to local blood flow abnormalities.

Surgical treatment of UBC may be necessary for those bones that fracture repeatedly or cysts that are of such significant size that fracture is imminent. A single percutaneous injection of a UBC with a substance such as demineralized bone matrix frequently leads to healing. A two-needle technique with a special large-bore needle can be performed under image intensification. However, the diagnosis should be established prior to percutaneous injection. The diagnosis can be confirmed if aspiration of the lesion reveals clear fluid and both the radiographs and clinical findings are consistent with the diagnosis. Injection of demineralized bone matrix or bone marrow into UBCs may replace corticosteroids injected into these lesions.

Aneurysmal Bone Cyst

The incidence of aneurysmal bone cyst (ABC) is equal in boys and girls. The median age of occurrence is 13 years with a reported annual incidence in the general population of 0.14 per 100,000. Most consistently, ABCs are medullary based and either eccentric or centric. Virtually all ABCs result in expansion of the bone and cortical thinning and lysis. Geographic bone destruction without periosteal reaction or visible matrix occurs with most ABCs (Fig. 2). Early in the course of development, the radiographic appearance of an ABC may mimic that of a UBC or other benign tumor. However, the ABC contains blood and a soft-tissue mass, in contrast to the UBC, which contains clear fluid. Fluid/fluid levels may be present on cross-sectional imaging as the red blood cells settle. MRI obtained preoperatively can be used to distinguish ABCs from UBCs. Double density fluid level, septation, a low signal on T1 images, and a high signal on T2 images usually identify a bone cyst as an ABC rather than a UBC.

Some reports suggest that ultrasound is capable of showing fluid/fluid levels in ABC; however, this technique has yet to achieve widespread use.

The etiology of ABC remains unclear. The findings of clonal abnormalities in this lesion reveal that

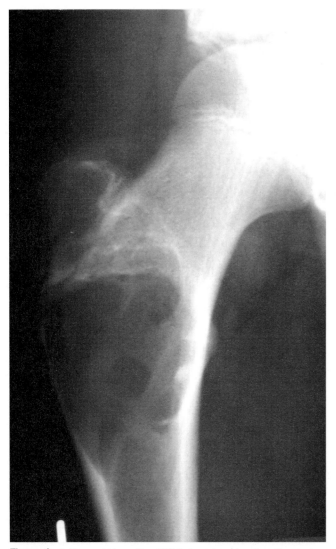

Figure 1 A 12-year-old boy with a UBC that was asymptomatic until a crack formed in the cortex of the lesion. During open curettage and bone grafting, the diagnosis was confirmed, and a plate was inserted.

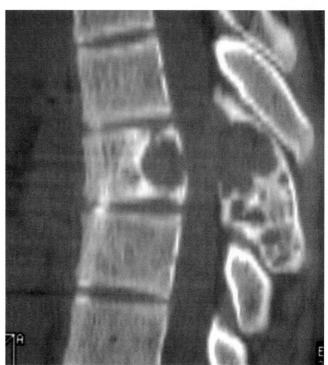

Figure 2 The painful, expansile lesion of the anterior and posterior elements of the eighth thoracic vertebra in this 14-year-old girl is characteristic of an ABC.

somatic mutations may contribute to the development of ABC; it is possible that bands 16q22 and 17p13 may harbor genes important to this process. Other findings suggest that ABC corresponds to a hemodynamic disturbance and is caused by primary or secondary venous malformation of the bone.

Local control in these lesions can be achieved with curettage and a high-speed burr in nearly 90% of patients. An 82% cure rate on initial surgery also has been reported with intralesional excision followed by cryotherapy; however, cryotherapy may be associated with a higher complication rate.

Osteochondroma

Osteochondromas (exostoses) are benign growths that usually occur at the metaphyses of long bones. Multiple hereditary exostoses (MHE) is an autosomal-dominant form of the disorder in which there are multiple exostoses. Previously, exostoses were believed to be the result of a skeletal dysplasia in which so-called "ectopic nests" of cartilage putatively formed the basis of these cartilaginous excrescences. New evidence suggests that there may be a neoplastic origin for these growths. Studies of MHE have demonstrated involvement of the EXT tumor suppressor gene family and have shown the molecular basis of this heritable process. The two genes *EXT1* and *EXT2* encode glycosyltransferases required for the biosynthesis of heparan sulfate, which is an important component of the extracellular matrix. Disturbances in the cell surface architecture as a result of defects in *EXT1* or *EXT2* likely result in the phenotypes seen in MHE. A third gene, *EXT3*, has been implicated in families with MHE but is less well studied. Progress must be made, however, in translating this knowledge into therapy for affected individuals.

Mutations in single osteochondromas have been detected in the absence of somatic mutation, further suggesting a neoplastic etiology even in solitary osteochondromas. The model of neoplastic pathogenesis of osteochondromas may replace the theory of skeletal dysplasia, which was previously used to explain the development of exostoses and their complications.

Solitary exostoses may be discovered incidentally or may be present with pain, particularly when the soft tissues are irritated. Irritation of the pes anserine bursa may result from osteochondromas arising from the proximal medial tibia. Although spontaneous regression of osteochondromas has been reported, it is extremely rare. Several local complications have been attributed to osteochondromas, including arterial compression, pseudoaneurysm of the popliteal artery, and, although rare, spinal cord compression.

Resection of solitary exostoses may be considered when complications arise, such as an osseous deformity that limits range of motion, symptomatic bursa formation, vascular injury, neurologic compromise, or malignant transformation. MRI can be ordered to diagnose or suggest the etiology for the clinical symptoms. Particular attention should be paid to the thickness of the cartilage cap, which in adults can indicate transformation of an exostosis to chondrosarcoma. The complication rate for osteochondroma removal is comparable to that of other elective orthopaedic surgical procedures. Neurapraxias are the most common complication.

Posttraumatic osteochondromatous proliferations of bone may occur. These lesions lack the characteristic features of osteochondroma, which maintains the continuity of the medullary space in the lesions. The distinct appearance of these lesions is increasingly important in light of the increasing evidence for a molecular basis of osteochondroma.

Growth deformities are associated with MHE, often affecting the forearm, knee, and ankle. However, skeletally mature patients usually are comfortable with their appearance, despite any deformity. Most deformities of the upper extremity in patients with MHE are well tolerated and lead to little loss of function. In carefully selected patients, surgery can improve appearance and provide pain relief. Some reports suggest that secondary chondrosarcomas may develop in children with MHE who have greater upper extremity involvement.

Eosinophilic Granuloma

Eosinophilic granuloma, or Langerhans' cell histiocytosis (LCH), formerly known as histiocytosis X, remains a diagnostic and therapeutic challenge. The disease is protean with multiple clinical presentations and a range of severity. The most common manifestations include osteolytic lesions and visceral involvement. Treatment options, which range from observation to surgery to aggressive chemotherapy, depend on the patient's age and the degree of the disease's involvement.

The disease etiology and pathogenesis remain unclear. Some evidence supports the disease as a neoplasm with a clonal proliferation of histiocytes. Evidence also suggests that the disease is a disorder of the immune system. Both theories may, in fact, be true; however, the details have yet to be elucidated. Epidemiologic study of LCH has revealed mild associations of the disease with infections in the neonatal period, exposure to solvents, childhood vaccinations, and thyroid disease.

The disease manifests in a range of fashions, possibly as a solitary bone lesion, multiple bone lesions, bone involvement with visceral involvement, or visceral involvement only. Bone involvement is often referred to as eosinophilic granuloma (EG). The disease may appear in bone, skin, liver, lung, lymph nodes, spleen, or bone marrow. In patients with more involved cases, the disease may be complicated by hypopituitarism and diabetes insipidus resulting from invasion of the hypothalamic-pituitary area. Despite the involvement of the pituitary gland, growth disturbances in children with LCH are uncommon; growth hormone studies should be obtained only in children who show poor or decelerating growth rates.

In general, the younger the patient's age at presentation, the more involved the disease is likely to be. Although LCH usually is not considered a malignant neoplasm, morbidity can occur in patients with extensive disease. Management of LCH varies according to the patient's age, the extent and location of disease, and the patient's response to prior therapy. Patients with isolated bone disease have the best prognosis and usually are treated with observation, corticosteroid injection, curettage, or bone grafting. Patients with systemic disease usually are treated with corticosteroids and/or cytotoxic chemotherapy. Despite treatment, progressive disease leading to death occurs in many patients with multisystem involvement. Chemotherapy for this disease has yet to be optimized.

Differentiating EG from other bone lesions has been challenging. In long bones, EG is characterized typically as a lytic, medullary-based metaphyseal or diaphyseal lesion with geographic destruction, lobular contours, periosteal reaction, no matrix, and no subarticular extension (Fig. 3). In the spine, vertebra plana in children usually indicates EG. Vertebral height generally is restored without surgical intervention. Unusual manifestations of the disease occur frequently and include epiphyseal lesions, transphyseal lesions, extracranial "button" sequestra, posterior vertebral arch lesions, dural extension of vertebral lesions, and fluid/fluid levels. This underscores the point that although some features may suggest EG, within bone, EG is protean and biopsy must confirm the diagnosis. Although some controversy remains, skeletal survey continues to be the procedure of choice for detecting and following bone lesions. Osteolytic lesions may lack osteoblastic activity and therefore not appear as abnormalities on bone scan.

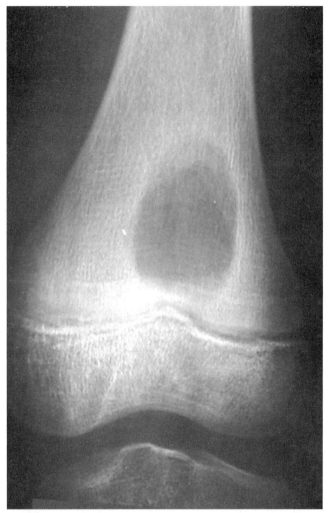

Figure 3 An EG in a 10-year-old boy is characterized by metaphyseal bone lysis with no matrix.

Fibrous Dysplasia

The etiology of fibrous dysplasia has been determined recently to be the result of postzygotic mutation in the *GNAS1* gene. All cells descended from the mutated cell can manifest features of McCune-Albright syndrome or fibrous dysplasia. Increased expression of the *c-fos* proto-oncogene, presumably a consequence of increased adenylate cyclase activity, may be important in the pathogenesis of the bone lesions in patients with fibrous dysplasia. Although this discovery has not led yet to direct therapeutic intervention, it does help explain the likelihood of recurrence and the peculiar hemimelic distribution that is often seen.

Polyostotic fibrous dysplasia can be associated with intramuscular myxomas (Mazabraud syndrome). Patients with known fibrous dysplasia who have soft-tissue masses that are of high signal intensity on T2-weighted images may be affected. Needle biopsy can confirm this diagnosis.

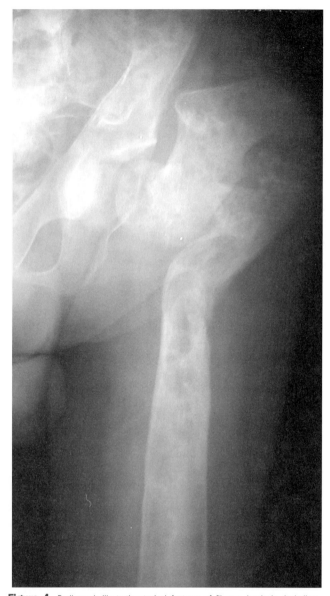

Figure 4 Radiograph illustrating typical features of fibrous dysplasia, including shepherd's crook deformity, extensive longitudinal involvement, asymmetry, and "ground-glass" appearance of the femur with loss of trabecular marking.

Surgery for the proximal femur with the classic "shepherd's crook" deformity (Fig. 4) often is performed to relieve pain and prevent further deformity. Varus deformity of the proximal femur may be treated with valgus osteotomy and internal fixation early in the course of the disease. Curettage and bone grafting of the lesion often results in resorption of the bone graft.

The administration of bisphosphonates is one of the greatest potential advances in the management of fibrous dysplasia. Intravenous pamidronate alleviates bone pain, reduces the rate of bone turnover assessed by biochemical markers, and improves the radiographic appearance. Pamidronate, given as an intravenous infusion once a month for 2 to 4 hours, is generally well tolerated generally and has few side effects. Given the increased potency and ease of administration of bisphosphonates in current use, these drugs are likely to play an increasingly important role in the management of fibrous dysplasia.

Chondroblastoma

Chondroblastoma is a benign neoplasm that occurs most commonly in the epiphysis or apophysis in a growing child or in the bones of the foot. Chondroblastoma in the proximal femoral epiphysis can present as knee pain in an adolescent.

Although chondroblastomas were believed previously to originate in cartilage, chondroblastoma cells form osteoid and fibrous matrices but not cartilaginous matrix; no type II collagen is deposited. Several chromosomal abnormalities have been detected in chondroblastoma, mostly involving chromosomes 5 and 8.

Plain radiographs usually reveal a rounded, well-marginated lytic lesion with some focal calcification in the epiphysis of a skeletally immature patient. MRI findings vary in chondroblastoma and usually reveal low signal areas on T2-weighted images, often with some high signal areas as well. Mineralization within the lesion is usually revealed on CT scan.

Treatment includes curettage, sometimes in association with an adjuvant such as phenol or liquid nitrogen. Despite the usual periarticular location of these lesions, long-term functional impairment or growth disturbances are uncommon. Chondroblastoma is considered to be a benign neoplasm; however, in rare cases malignancy, with metastases to the lungs, has been reported. Because of the possibility of metastasis, chest imaging is necessary for patients diagnosed with chondroblastoma.

Chondromyxoid Fibroma

Chondromyxoid fibroma is an extremely rare bone tumor and reports of occurrence are limited to small series of cases. Radiographically, these lesions appear as lytic, eccentric lesions in the metaphyses of long bones. The usual radiographic differential diagnosis is a nonossifying fibroma. Calcification, which is often present, is typically more evident in older patients. Chondromyxoid fibromas contain clonal rearrangements of chromosome 6. Wide local excision is recommended where possible. Intralesional treatment is associated with a 25% local recurrence rate. However, recurrence is less likely with contemporary measures of intralesional treatment, such as curettage and use of a high-speed burr.

Enchondroma

Enchondromas usually are painless lesions that occur in the metaphyses of long bones and are often found incidentally on radiographs obtained following injury. In children, enchondromas frequently are unmineralized, which gives them a radiographic appearance similar to a unicameral bone cyst. Intralesional treatment of the enchondroma results in relatively low local recurrence rates.

Enchondroma can be difficult to differentiate from its malignant counterpart, chondrosarcoma; however, chondrosarcoma is more likely to be associated with pain in the lesion, deep endosteal scalloping, cortical destruction, and soft-tissue mass. In contrast to chondrosarcomas, enchondromas are diploid. Chondrosarcoma is extremely uncommon in children; those that develop secondary lesions from enchondromas tend to do so much later in life.

Osteoid Osteoma

Osteoid osteomas are painful bone lesions, often with overlying soft-tissue swelling. Radiographs usually reveal a dense, sclerotic cortex surrounding a small lucency or nidus (Fig. 5). The nidus appears lytic, sometimes with a punctate area of mineralization in the center. High levels of prostaglandins have been reported in the center of the lesion, giving a therapeutic rationale for the use of anti-inflammatory medications for treatment of symptoms.

Surgical management of osteoid osteoma has evolved considerably over the past 2 decades. En bloc resection of the tumor is rarely, if ever, performed. Open procedures focus on removal of the nidus only; preoperative imaging accurately locates the nidus.

Several means of percutaneous removal of the osteoid osteoma have been reported recently. The osteoid osteoma can be excised percutaneously by using a power drill under CT guidance. The rate of symptom resolution is relatively high; however, complications, including fracture, can occur. Other percutaneous approaches include percutaneous radiofrequency ablation, CT-guided thermocoagulation, and, in the spine, percutaneous laser photocoagulation. Most reports of percutaneous treatment indicate that rates of symptom improvement and successful removal of the lesion are close to those for open procedures.

Some investigators recommend follow-up scintigraphy and plain radiographs to ascertain the likelihood of successful resection. Scintigraphy also may be used intraoperatively in open procedures to direct the orthopaedic surgeon.

Osteoblastoma

Osteoblastoma is a typically painful but benign bone tumor that produces osteoid, most commonly affecting the spine. Radiographically, osteoblastoma may mimic

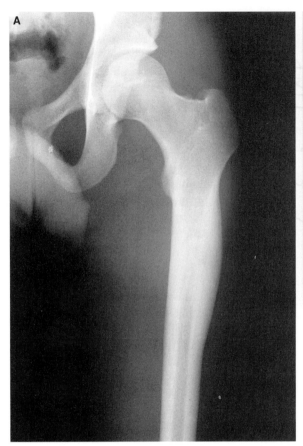

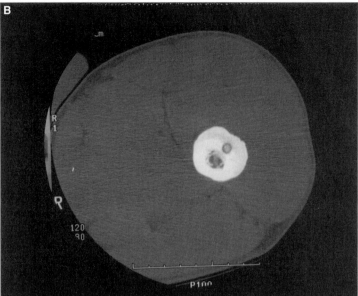

Figure 5 **A,** AP radiograph of a proximal femur reveals an osteoid osteoma. A small lucency lies within a dense, sclerotic cortex of the lateral femur. **B,** CT shows that the small intracortical lucency actually contains a small nidus of mineralization. *(Reproduced from Richards BS (ed): Orthopaedic Knowledge Update: Pediatrics. Rosemont, IL, American Academy of Orthopaedic Surgeons, 1996, pp 55-64.)*

the appearance of osteoid osteoma. Findings of spinal osteoblastoma on MRI are relatively nonspecific and varied. Because of the sensitivity of MRI to marrow edema, the lesion may be overestimated on MRI as well. Therefore, CT continues to be the imaging modality of choice for the characterization and local staging of suspected spinal osteoblastomas (Fig. 6).

Scoliosis occurs secondary to osteoblastoma and is believed to result from paravertebral muscle spasm. Histologically, the appearance of osteoblastomas may vary; however, histologic variations do not correlate with the clinical course.

Treatment of osteoblastoma usually consists of curettage and bone grafting or en bloc resection. Osteoblastomas located in the spine may require bone grafting, arthrodesis, instrumentation, or other measures of stabilization.

Malignant Bone Tumors

Ewing's Sarcoma

Ewing's sarcoma usually is evident as a painful lytic bone lesion, often with accompanying swelling. The most common sites are the diaphyses or metaphyses of long bones or the flat bones such as the pelvis or scapula. Radiographs typically reveal an aggressive, perme-

ative pattern that may be confused with infection (Fig. 7). Large soft-tissue masses may arise from the bone as well. Patients who present with systemic symptoms or an elevated serum lactate dehydrogenase when first seen have a worse prognosis.

Ewing's sarcoma typically is treated with chemotherapy, followed by surgery and/or radiation to the primary site, followed by additional chemotherapy. Successive, more intensive regimens of chemotherapy have been shown to improve survival rates. Chemotherapy dose intensification is now possible because growth factors and other agents are used to ameliorate side effects such as bone marrow and gastrointestinal toxicity.

The resected specimen must be evaluated carefully. Chemotherapy-induced necrosis is an important prognostic indicator.

The Ewing's sarcoma family of tumors has been defined genetically by specific chromosomal translocations resulting in fusion of the *EWS* gene with a member of the ETS family of transcription factors, either FLI1 in most patients, or ERG. Variation in the location of the translocation break points, which result in the inclusion of different combinations of exons from EWS and FLI1 (or ERG) in the fusion products, contributes additional molecular genetic heterogeneity. The resulting novel chimeric proteins

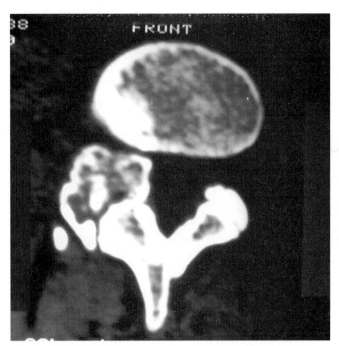

Figure 6 CT of the fifth lumbar vertebra in a 13-year-old girl with painful scoliosis. Lytic and sclerotic expansion of the superior articular process is shown. Biopsy confirmed osteoblastoma, which was treated with local resection.

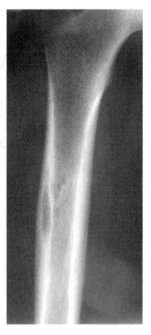

Figure 7 The permeative and reactive changes seen in this 9-year-old boy who had pain in the proximal thigh is characteristic of Ewing's sarcoma.

likely contribute to tumor development by aberrant regulation of gene expression, altering controls of cell proliferation and differentiation. Type 1, which is the most common type of EWS-FLI1 fusion transcript, is associated with a favorable prognosis and encodes a functionally weaker activator when compared with other fusion types.

These tumor-specific molecular rearrangements are useful for primary diagnosis and may be related to prognosis. Formerly, the diagnosis of Ewing's sarcoma was made on light microscopy and was somewhat subjective. The current ability to test for these novel proteins makes possible more precise diagnosis and classification within the Ewing's sarcoma group of tumors and presents the possibility of tumor-specific therapeutic targets. Expression of these proteins by tumor cells allows for decontamination of peripheral stem cells for use in bone marrow transplantation.

Survival rates for patients with nonmetastatic Ewing's sarcoma are approximately 75% to 80% at 5 years. Chemotherapy-induced necrosis is an important predictor of survival in patients with Ewing's sarcoma.

Debate continues regarding the appropriate local control modality for Ewing's sarcoma. Surgical resection with negative margins is preferred where possible, particularly if minimal morbidity will result.

Osteosarcoma

In the United States, most patients with osteosarcoma (Fig. 8) are treated with intravenous induction (neoad-

juvant) chemotherapy for several weeks, followed by surgical resection and additional chemotherapy. Surgical resection should ideally be performed with negative margins and is possible in most instances, even in the pelvis, without amputation. Limb perfusion with cytotoxic agents or hyperthermia is usually reserved for situations in which limb salvage might otherwise not be feasible or in experimental protocols.

Despite extensive attempts at identification, unifying molecular factors in osteosarcoma still need to be identified. Many cytogenetic abnormalities have been described in association with high-grade osteogenic sarcoma. P-glycoprotein overexpression in tumor cells at diagnosis is associated with a higher rate of systemic relapse and more rapid development of drug resistance. DNA ploidy continues to be studied; aneuploid osteosarcomas respond better to chemotherapy and are associated with a higher survival rate than diploid osteosarcomas tumors. Overexpression of P-53 is associated with a worse prognosis.

Survival rates for patients with nonmetastatic osteosarcoma at presentation are approximately 80%. Survival rates for patients with pelvic osteosarcoma are lower, probably because of the larger tumor size at presentation and the difficulty in achieving negative margins at the time of resection.

Approximately 15% of children with osteogenic sarcoma will have detectable metastases at presentation. Although improvements in chemotherapy have led to increased survival rates, the prognosis remains guarded in patients with recurrent disease or metastatic disease at presentation. The 5-year survival rate for patients with lung metastasis is 15% to 35%. The use of supportive agents such as granulocyte colony-stimulating

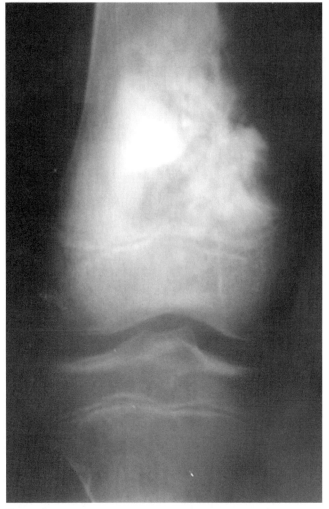

Figure 8 The osteoblastic, metaphyseal mass lesion in this 12-year-old boy is typical of osteosarcoma.

factor to limit drug toxicity allows for more aggressive approaches to osteosarcoma.

Survivors of osteosarcoma appear to be at risk for additional malignancies, most notably leukemia. Whether this increased risk is a result of chemotherapy or a reflection of a genetic propensity toward development of these neoplasms is unclear.

Limb Salvage in the Skeletally Immature Patient

Percutaneous core needle biopsy or limited open incisional biopsy should be performed initially on patients with suspected or possible bone sarcoma. To ensure that diagnostic tissue has been retrieved, frozen section diagnoses should be obtained prior to leaving the operating room. Inappropriate biopsy or curettage of suspected bone sarcomas can lead to the loss of limb-sparing options.

Appropriate surgical resection levels and the presence or absence of physeal or epiphyseal involvement are determined by the extent of marrow disease. MRI is the most sensitive test to determine the extent of marrow disease visualized on MRI; therefore, imaging should be obtained prior to biopsy of the lesion. The use of MRI allows preoperative planning, which enables the surgeon to confidently resect bone closer to the tumor. Transepiphyseal resections are possible. With the advent of improved imaging techniques and more effective chemotherapy, most patients are candidates for limb salvage.

Options for management following surgical excision of the distal femur remain essentially threefold: amputation, endoprosthesis (expandable where necessary to accommodate limb growth), and rotationplasty. Limb salvage is associated with a higher rate of local recurrence compared to amputation, but there appears to be no difference in long-term survival rates. There is slightly greater disability in patients undergoing amputation compared to limb salvage. Function following endoprosthetic reconstruction or rotationplasty is better than with amputation. Rotationplasty is not associated with any disadvantages with regard to function or quality of life compared to endoprosthetic replacement.

Patients who undergo rotationplasty have a durable reconstruction that is associated with few late complications. The main drawback to rotationplasty is appearance. Patients who undergo endoprosthetic reconstruction and survive their cancer may require additional surgical procedures, including limb lengthenings and revisions as necessary. Late complications are frequent and include aseptic loosening, infection, or prosthetic failure.

Limb salvage is possible even when resecting pelvic tumors in the skeletally immature patient by using iliofemoral or ischiofemoral fusion, hip transposition, or leaving the limb flail.

Annotated Bibliography

Nonossifying Fibroma/Fibrous Cortical Defect
Hoeffel C, Panuel M, Plenat F, Mainard L, Hoeffel JC: Pathological fracture in non-ossifying fibroma with histological features simulating aneurysmal bone cyst. *Eur Radiol* 1999;9:669-671.
Cases are presented in which a pathologic fracture through an NOF has created features in the surgical specimen that suggest an ABC, leading to a misdiagnosis.

Unicameral Bone Cyst
Killian JT, Wilkinson L, White S, Brassard M: Treatment of unicameral bone cyst with demineralized bone matrix. *J Pediatr Orthop* 1998;18:621-624.
Eleven patients with UBCs were given a single injection of demineralized bone matrix. The average time of healing was 4.5 months, and nine of 11 patients were successfully treated.

Aneurysmal Bone Cyst

Freeby JA, Reinus WR, Wilson AJ: Quantitative analysis of the plain radiographic appearance of aneurysmal bone cysts. *Invest Radiol* 1995;30:433-439.

ABCs are medullary-based most consistently, either eccentric or centric (94%), and show lysis (100%), cortical thinning (97%), enlargement of the host bone (100%), and geographic bone destruction (94%). They have well-defined edges (84%), no fallen fragment (100%), no evidence of periosteal reaction (75%), and no visible matrix (91%).

Gibbs CP Jr, Hefele MC, Peabody TD, Montag AG, Aithal V, Simon MA: Aneurysmal bone cyst of the extremities: Factors related to local recurrence after curettage with a high-speed burr. *J Bone Joint Surg Am* 1999;81:1671-1678.

Forty patients with ABCs were reviewed. Factors that appeared to be important predictors of local recurrence following curettage with a high-speed burr were young age and open growth plates. Rates of local control of almost 90% can be achieved with thorough curettage with use of a mechanical burr and without use of liquid nitrogen, phenol, or other adjuvants.

Leithner A, Windhager R, Lang S, Haas OA, Kainberger F, Kotz R: Aneurysmal bone cyst: A population based epidemiologic study and literature review. *Clin Orthop* 1999;363:176-179.

The authors performed a retrospective, population-based analysis of 94 patients with primary ABC and a literature review of 1,002 patients regarding gender and age predilection. The annual incidence of primary ABC was 0.14 per 10 (5) individuals. The male to female ratio was 1:1.04, and the median age was 13 years.

Marcove RC, Sheth DS, Takemoto S, Healey JH: The treatment of aneurysmal bone cyst. *Clin Orthop* 1995; 311:157-163.

Fifty-one patients with ABCs, some in conjunction with other lesions, were treated with intralesional excision followed by cryosurgery. A cure rate of 82% following one surgery was achieved, which was an improvement over historic controls, with a 59% local recurrence.

Sullivan RJ, Meyer JS, Dormans JP, Davidson RS: Diagnosing aneurysmal and unicameral bone cysts with magnetic resonance imaging. *Clin Orthop* 1999;366:186-190.

Investigators describe MRI features that can help distinguish ABCs from UBCs preoperatively. The presence of a double density fluid level within the lesion strongly indicated that the lesion was an ABC, as did septations within the lesion and low intensity signal characteristics on T1 images and high intensity signal characteristics on T2 images.

Vayego SA, De Conti OJ, Varella-Garcia M: Complex cytogenetic rearrangement in a case of unicameral bone cyst. *Cancer Genet Cytogenet* 1996;86:46-49.

Cytogenetic analysis of a UBC that was surgically resected in an 11-year-old boy revealed a highly complex clonal structural rearrangement involving chromosomes 4, 6, 8, 16, 21, and both 12.

Osteochondroma

Porter DE, Simpson AH: The neoplastic pathogenesis of solitary and multiple osteochondromas. *J Pathol* 1999;188:119-125.

This article describes recent findings implicating the EXT tumor suppressor gene in the etiology of MHE, as well as single exostoses.

Wirganowicz PZ, Watts HG: Surgical risk for elective excision of benign exostoses. *J Pediatr Orthop* 1997;17: 455-459.

The rate of surgical complications for exostosis is evaluted in 80 patients who underwent 285 exostectomies and other procedures. There were ten complications, mostly neurapraxias. The authors concluded that surgical risk for the management of osteochondromas is low and is comparable to the risk of other related, elective procedures.

Eosinophilic Granuloma

Arceci RJ, Brenner MK, Pritchard J: Controversies and new approaches to treatment of Langerhans' cell histiocytosis. *Hematol Oncol Clin North Am* 1998;12:339-357.

Evidence for the etiology of LCH as a neoplasm and an immune disorder are presented, as well as the use of current and potential future treatments of the disease.

Fisher AJ, Reinus WR, Friedland JA, Wilson AJ: Quantitative analysis of the plain radiographic appearance of eosinophilic granuloma. *Invest Radiol* 1995;30: 466-473.

When they compared radiographs of eosinophilic granuloma lesions with other lesions, investigators found that long bone lesions that were lytic, medullary-based metaphyseal or diaphyseal lesions with geographic destruction, lobular contours, periosteal reaction, no matrix, and no subarticular extension showed a sensitivity of 55.6% of being EG lesions.

Howarth DM, Gilchrist GS, Mullan BP, Wiseman GA, Edmonson JH, Schomberg PJ: Langerhans cell histiocytosis: Diagnosis, natural history, management, and outcome. *Cancer* 1999;85:2278-2290.

In this study, 314 patients with Langerhans' histiocytosis were reviewed. Patients with disease in the bone only fared best, with 97% of patients with solitary bone lesions rendered disease-free. In contrast, only 20% of patients with multisystem involvement progressed, despite therapy.

Howarth DM, Mullan BP, Wiseman GA, Wenger DE, Forstrom LA, Dunn WL: Bone scintigraphy evaluated in diagnosing and staging Langerhans' cell histiocytosis and related disorders. *J Nucl Med* 1996;37:1456-1460.

Of 73 patients with the histologic diagnosis of LCH, a definite lesion was reported on radiographs and subsequent biopsy-proven bone involvement in 56. For this population, the sensitivity and specificity of radiographic survey were 100% and 61%, respectively, compared to 91% and 55% for bone scintigraphy.

Kusumakumary P, James FV, Chellam VG, Ratheesan K, Nair MK: Disseminated Langerhans cell histocytosis in children: Treatment outcome. *Am J Clin Oncol* 1999;22:180-183.

In a review of 35 children with LCH, good local control was revealed in children with less involvement, but a high local recurrence rate and a high fatality rate with more extensive disease were revealed.

Fibrous Dysplasia

Chapurlat RD, Delmas PD, Liens D, Meunier PJ: Long-term effects of intravenous pamidronate in fibrous dysplasia of bone. *J Bone Miner Res* 1997;12:1746-1752.

In this open label study, 20 patients with polyostotic fibrous dysplasia were treated monthly with intravenous pamidronate. With this treatment, the severity of bone pain and the number of painful sites were significantly reduced. A radiographic response in nine patients was observed, with refilling of osteolytic lesions.

Chondroblastoma

Schuppers HA, van der Eijken JW: Chondroblastoma during the growing age. *J Pediatr Orthop* 1998;78:293-297.

A series of 116 cases of chondroblastoma were reviewed. Most patients were treated sucessfully with excochleation. Growth disturbances or functional impairments were uncommon. Metastasis developed in one patient.

Chondromyxoid Fibroma

Wu CT, Inwards CY, O'Laughlin S, Rock MG, Beabout JW, Unni KK: Chondromyxoid fibroma of bone: A clinicopathologic review of 278 cases. *Hum Pathol* 1998;29:438-446.

The authors reviewed an institutional series of 278 cases of chondromyxoid fibroma, describing usual radiographic and histologic findings. A local recurrence rate of 25% was noted, with a variety of relatively conservative surgical treatments.

Enchondroma

Bauer HC, Brosjo O, Kreicbergs A, Lindholm J: Low risk of recurrence of enchondroma and low-grade chondrosarcoma in extremities: 80 patients followed for 2-25 years. *Acta Orthop Scand* 1995;66:283-288.

Forty patients with enchondromas 40 with chondrosarcoma were treated with either biopsy alone or intralesional treatment. The 10-year local recurrence rate was 0.04 in the group with enchondroma.

Osteoid Osteoma

Donahue F, Ahmad A, Mnaymneh W, Pevsner NH: Osteoid osteoma: Computed tomography guided percutaneous excision. *Clin Orthop* 1999;366:191-196.

The authors reported on a series of 21 patients with osteoid osteoma treated with percutaneous excision under CT guidance, using a power drill. They reported a 100% resolution of symptoms with a low complication rate.

Rosenthal DI, Hornicek FJ, Wolfe MW, Jennings LC, Gebhardt MC, Mankin HJ: Percutaneous radiofrequency coagulation of osteoid osteoma compared with operative treatment. *J Bone Joint Surg Am* 1998;80:815-821.

The investigators compare treatment of patients with osteoid osteoma with conventional open surgical techniques with patients treated with percutaneous radiofrequency ablation. Eighty-seven patients who were managed with surgical excision and 38 patients who were managed with percutaneous ablation with radiofrequency were compared. The local recurrence and symptom relief in the two groups were comparable. There were no complications in the radiofrequency ablation group.

Osteoblastoma

Shaikh MI, Saifuddin A, Pringle J, Natali C, Sherazi Z: Spinal osteoblastoma: CT and MR imaging with pathological correlation. *Skeletal Radiol* 1999;28:33-40.

The MRI appearances of spinal osteoblastomas are varied and show no characteristic features. The extent of the lesion may also be overestimated on MRI as a result of extensive reactive changes and adjacent soft-tissue masses. The preferred imaging study for the characterization and local staging of suspected spinal osteoblastomas should continue to be CT.

Osteosarcoma

Grimer RJ, Carter SR, Tillman RM, Spooner D, Mangham DC, Kabukcuoglu Y: Osteosarcoma of the pelvis. *J Bone Joint Surg Br* 1999;81:796-802.

In this article, the authors described treatment of 36 patients with osteosarcoma of the pelvis. Seventeen patients were treated with chemotherapy and surgery. The survival rate in this group was 41%.

Rosito P, Mancini AF, Rondelli R, et al: Italian Cooperative Study for the treatment of children and young adults with localized Ewing's sarcoma of bone: A preliminary report of 6 years of experience. *Cancer* 1999;86:421-428.

The 3-year and event-free survival rates reported in this study (83.6% and 77.8%, respectively) are higher than previously reported and may reflect the addition of ifosfamide or the increased use of surgery for local control when compared to prior studies in the same cooperative group.

Limb Salvage in the Skeletally Immature Patient

Davis AM, Devlin M, Griffin AM, Wunder JS, Bell RS: Functional outcome in amputation versus limb sparing of patients with lower extremity sarcoma: A matched case-control study. *Arch Phys Med Rehabil* 1999;80:615-618.

Patients treated with amputations or limb salvage surgery for sarcoma resection are evaluated. A trend toward increased disability for those in the amputation group was noted, and the amputation group showed significantly higher levels of disability.

Hillmann A, Hoffmann C, Gosheger G, Krakau H, Winkelmann W: Malignant tumor of the distal part of the femur or the proximal part of the tibia: Endoprosthetic replacement or rotationplasty. Functional outcome and quality-of-life measurements *J Bone Joint Surg Am* 1999;81:462-468.

Outcomes for patients undergoing rotationplasty or endoprosthetic reconstruction following resection of distal femoral tumors are evaluated. Results indicated each group had essentially similar function or quality of life.

Schindler OS, Cannon SR, Briggs TW, Blunn GW: Stanmore custom-made extendible distal femoral replacements: Clinical experience in children with primary malignant bone tumours. *J Bone Joint Surg Br* 1997;79:927-937.

A series of cases of 18 children with expandable endoprosthetic reconstructions following tumor resection is reviewed. Patients had an average of four operations each for lengthening, and ten patients required revision at an average of 6 years.

Chapter 7

Osteogenesis Imperfecta

John S. Blanco, MD

Introduction

Osteogenesis imperfecta (OI) is a generalized disorder of connective tissue that is familiar to orthopaedic surgeons because of its primary clinical manifestation of bone fragility. Its prevalence has remained constant with an estimated incidence of one case per 25,000 individuals with little to no variability based on gender, ethnic origin, or race. Although severe cases display striking musculoskeletal abnormalities (Fig. 1), milder cases may go undiagnosed. Although this disorder has been known by several names and eponyms, it was not until 1849 that Vrolik used the term osteogenesis imperfecta to describe a newborn with multiple fractures. However, the disease predates Vrolik's description by centuries when a mummy dating back to 1000 BC was discovered with characteristic features of OI.

The phenotypic and genotypic diversity of OI is explained by the myriad of quantitative and/or qualitative type I collagen deficiencies found in patients with OI. Recent advances in the field of molecular genetics have elucidated many of the mutations responsible for the collagen abnormalities and offer new and exciting insights into future treatment options. In addition, new studies on the pharmacologic treatment of OI offer hope for patients with this connective tissue disorder.

Pathogenesis

So that OI and recent findings regarding its molecular basis are better understood, a review of the synthesis of collagen is essential. The biosynthesis of collagen is a complex, multistage process that is characterized by a number of co- and posttranslational modifications. With few exceptions, OI is caused by mutations in either the *COL1A1* gene, located on chromosome 17, or the *COL1A2* gene, located on chromosome 7. These genes are responsible for encoding the proalpha 1(I) and proalpha 2(I) chains that together form type I procollagen. Posttranslational modifications ultimately yield type I collagen, which is composed of two $\alpha 1$ chains and one $\alpha 2$ chain in a tight helical configuration. Each chain contains 338 uninterrupted triplets of glycine-X-Y, where X is often proline and Y is often hydroxyproline.

Most mutations responsible for OI are point mutations that result in the substitution of a bulky amino acid for one of the glycine residues occurring along the chain, with drastic consequences for triple helical assembly and/or stability. Other mutations include single exon splicing defects as well as large deletions, insertions, or retained introns.

Recent advances in understanding the molecular basis of OI have been used to modify the Sillence classification of the disease (Table 1). Although the Sillence classification remains the most clinically applicable classification available, the heterogeneity even among similarly classified patients can be dramatic. Interestingly, patients with the mildest and most common form of OI (type IA) have a quantitative but not a qualitative abnormality in their type I collagen resulting from the presence of a null $\alpha 1(I)$ allele. Secretion of collagen in patients with type IA OI may be reduced by as much as 80%, with intracellular degradation of collagen up to twice that found in controls. Patients with types II, III, and IV OI have varying degrees of structural abnormalities in their type I collagen molecules (Table 2).

The relationship between genotypic abnormality and its phenotypic expression is poorly understood. Factors believed to be responsible for the clinical findings in a specific patient with OI include the location and type of mutation, the extent of mutant chain incorporation into extracellular collagen fibrils, the interactions with the noncollagenous proteins present in the bone matrix, and thermal stability of the mutant collagen. However, different phenotypes ranging from type II OI to type IV OI can be produced from the same mutation. Histologic appearances of bone specimens

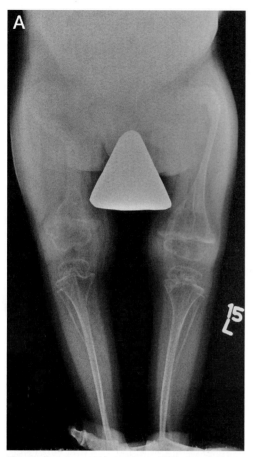
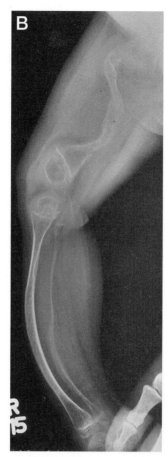
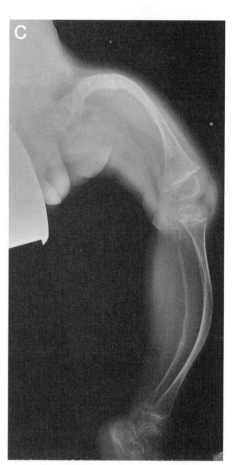

Figure 1 A 4-year-old boy with type III OI. AP and lateral views of both lower extremities demonstrate diffuse osteopenia and striking deformities of the long bones. Following intramedullary fixation of all four lower extremity segments, the patient is able to stand in full-contact hip-knee-ankle-foot orthoses. **A,** AP view. **B** and **C,** lateral views.

from patients with varying degrees of OI reveal striking differences that parallel their clinical manifestations (Fig. 2).

Clinical Manifestations

The nature and severity of the clinical features depend on the type of OI the patient has. The hallmark of the disease is bone fragility, but other clinical characteristics are present to a variable extent. These include osteopenia, progressive skeletal deformities, dentinogenesis imperfecta, joint hyperlaxity, middle ear deafness, blue sclerae, macrocephaly, triangular facies, barrel chest, short stature, and a variety of abnormalities secondary to the hypermetabolic state of the patient. Intelligence is usually normal. The features unique to the various types of OI, ranging from mild phenotypes to lethal forms, are outlined in Table 1. Patients with milder types of OI (Sillence types I and IV) often have normal lifespans. Respiratory compromise secondary to chest wall deformities and kyphoscoliosis, basilar invagination of the skull, and posttraumatic intracranial bleeding can result in premature death in patients with more severe OI. Even relatively minor head trauma warrants scrutiny in this population.

The differential diagnosis of OI from other causes of fractures and osteopenia is clinically important and is detailed in Table 3. A positive family history, abnormal dentition, blue sclerae, and diffuse osteopenia are important factors to ascertain during the physical examination. Analysis of type I collagen production from cultured dermal fibroblasts may be necessary in selected cases to confirm a questionable diagnosis.

Prenatal diagnosis of OI can be made by several techniques based on family history, recurrence risk, and the gestational age of the fetus (Fig. 3). Ultrasound can reliably identify fetuses with type II OI by 14 to 16 weeks of gestation and those with type III OI by 18 to 20 weeks of gestation using fetal limb length and limb morphology. In fetuses with milder OI that does not cause intrauterine fractures or bowing (types I and IV), ultrasound cannot be reliably used. Biochemical and molecular genetic studies of collagen synthesized from cells cultured from chorionic villus samples are advantageous in the prenatal screening of

TABLE 1 | Clinical Classification of OI

Type	Features	Inheritance
I (dominant, blue sclerae)	IA: bone fragility, blue sclerae, and normal teeth	Autosomal dominant
	IB: same as IA but with dentinogenesis imperfecta	
	IC: more severe than IB but with normal teeth	
II (lethal perinatal)	IIA: broad crumpled long bones and beaded rib; generally perinatal death	Autosomal dominant
	IIB: broad crumpled long bones but ribs show minimal or no beading; death variable from perinatal to several years	
	IIC: thin fractured cylindrical, dysplastic long bones, and thin beaded ribs; very low birth rate; stillbirth or perinatal death	
	IID: severely osteopenic with generally well-formed skeleton; normally shaped vertebrae and pelvis; perinatal death	
III (progressive deforming)	Multiple fractures at birth with progressive deformities, normal sclerae, and dentinogenesis imperfecta	Autosomal recessive
IV (dominant, white sclerae)	IVA: bone fragility, white sclerae, and normal teeth	Autosomal dominant
	IVB: similar to IVA but with dentinogenesis imperfecta	

(Reproduced with permission from Cole WG: The molecular pathology of osteogenesis imperfecta. *Clin Orthop* 1997;343:235-248.)

TABLE 2 | Biochemical Classification of Type I Collagen Mutations in OI

Protein Feature	Category of Mutation	Clinical Phenotype
Moderate reduction of normal type I collagen in tissues	Haploinsufficiency	OI-IA
Mixture of normal and mutant type I collagen molecules in tissues	Dominant negative	OI-IB:IIA-IIC:III:IVB
Severe reduction of normal type I collagen in tissues	Dominant negative	OI-IC
Very severe reduction of normal type I collagen in tissues	Dominant negative	OI-IID

(Reproduced with permission from Cole WG: The molecular pathology of osteogenesis imperfecta. *Clin Orthop* 1997;343:235-248.)

nonlethal forms of OI in those situations in which there is a positive family history. These studies can be completed within 14 days after obtaining the biopsy.

Management

Current conventional management of patients with OI centers on maximizing function, preventing fractures, and treating fractures and their sequelae. Physical therapy combined with orthotics, isotonic strengthening of muscles, and weight bearing to stimulate bone strength are all hallmarks of the rehabilitation process, depending on the severity of the disease. Treatment must be individualized and the overall goals of maximizing function, minimizing disability, fostering independence along with social integration, and maintaining overall health must always be kept in mind. Independent sitting by age 10 months predicts later walking ability.

Acute fractures are often treated nonsurgically and prevention of deformity and early weight bearing and mobilization are emphasized. Nonunions and malunions are important causes of disability and usually can be avoided by adequate immobilization. Weight bearing in lightweight splints and braces often can be resumed while fracture consolidation is completed.

Surgical treatment of nonunions often improves function, especially in the upper extremity (Fig. 4). Other indications for surgery include recurrent fractures and deformity. Children older than age 2 years

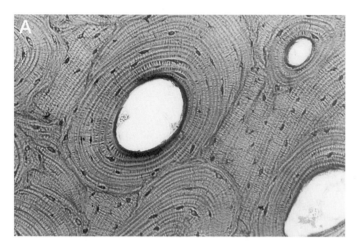

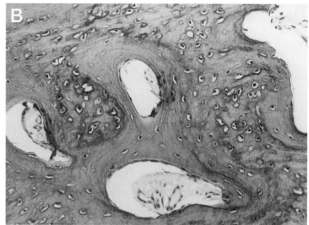

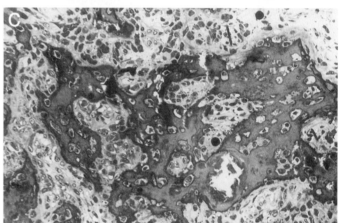

Figure 2 Histologic appearance of bone specimens from patients with OI of varying severity (hematoxylin-eosin; original magnification x65). **A,** Femoral cortex biopsy specimen from a patient with type I OI demonstrates a near-normal lamellar structure. **B,** Femoral cortex osteotomy specimen from a patient with type III OI demonstrates a mixed pattern of woven and lamellar bone. **C,** Femoral cortex specimen obtained at autopsy of a patient with type II OI demonstrates a scanty, disorganized, woven matrix with large osteocytes. *(Reproduced from Kocher MS, Shapiro F: Osteogenesis imperfecta.* J Am Acad Orthop Surg *1998;6:225-236.)*

with long bone deformities and/or frequent fractures that preclude achieving functional goals are candidates for intramedullary rodding and corrective osteotomies. Developmental delay in motor milestones alone is probably not an adequate indication for surgery. The presence of a bony canal and at least a thin cortex is a prerequisite. The most common treatment of long bone deformities remains intramedullary nail placement combined with realignment osteotomy. This can be performed open or by closed osteoclasis. The use of static or nonelongating pins results in a need for revision as the bone grows off the ends of the pins and deforms again. Telescoping nails theoretically allow for longitudinal growth; however, occasionally they do not telescope properly. Generally, complication rates are higher when the telescoping rod technique is used, although when the rods function properly, the interval for repeat surgery is longer than for static nails. The choice is based largely on the surgeon's preference. Even with recent improvements in techniques this type of surgery is technically demanding with a significant incidence of complications related to the choice of implant. However, decreased fracture incidence, ease of bracing, and improved ambulation following surgery

can be rewarding for the surgeon and beneficial for the patient and caregivers.

Spinal deformity in the patient with severe OI remains a significant problem. Its incidence is estimated at between 40% and 80% and, when combined with the frequently encountered chest wall deformities, can be a leading cause of respiratory compromise and death. Unfortunately, the incidence and severity of scoliosis seems to increase with age, even after skeletal maturity. In curves greater than 60°, vital capacity was found to decrease below 50% of predicted values. Vertebral body shape has been shown to predict spinal deformity, with the presence of six biconcave vertebrae found to correlate with development of severe scoliosis over time. Bracing is generally ineffective because of chest wall and rib deformities, and surgery is challenging and unlikely to result in correction or improved truncal height. Most authors currently recommend spinal fusion for curve magnitudes less than 45° to 50°, before curve severity makes surgery prohibitively complicated. The goal of surgery is to halt curve progression and prevent worsening of pulmonary function. Factors that make surgery difficult include poor bone quality, increased blood loss, and anesthetic risks.

TABLE 3 | Differential Diagnosis of OI by Age

Age	Diagnostic Possibilities
At birth	Hypophosphatasia
	Achondrogenesis
	Thanatophoric dwarfism
	Asphyxiating thoracic dystrophy
	Achondroplasia
	Chondroectodermal dysplasia
Infancy	"Battered baby"
	Scurvy
	Congenital syphilis
	Infantile cortical hyperostosis (Caffey's disease)
	Immobilization osteoporosis (spina bifida)
	Pyknodysostosis
	Osteopetrosis
Childhood and adolescence	Idiopathic juvenile osteoporosis
	Fibrous dysplasia
	Sarcoma (hyperplastic callus)
	Postmenopausal osteoporosis
Adult life	

(Reproduced with permission from Smith R, Francis MJO, Houghton GR (eds): *The Brittle Bone Syndrome: Osteogenesis Imperfecta.* London, England, Butterworth-Heineman, 1983.)

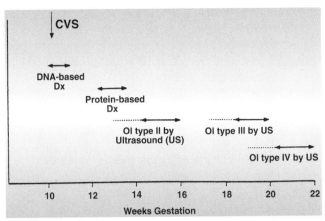

Figure 3 Timing of prenatal diagnostic studies for different forms of osteogenesis imperfecta by weeks of gestation. *(Reproduced with permission from Byers PH: Strategies and outcome of prenatal diagnosis for osteogenesis imperfecta.* Prenatal Diagnosis *1997;17:559-570.)*

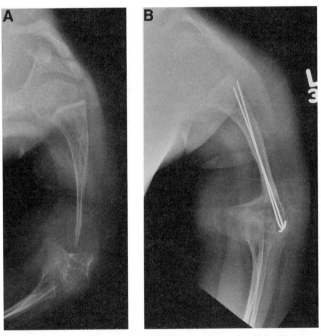

Figure 4 A 6-year-old boy with type III OI and a history of multiple distal humerus fractures. **A,** Preoperative radiograph revealing atrophic nonunion of the distal humerus. **B,** Four months after intramedullary fixation with smooth Kirschner wires. No bone grafting was performed during surgery. The humeral diaphysis enlarged following stabilization.

Basilar invagination is a common and life-threatening problem for patients with severe OI. It is now recognized as a frequent cause of death in patients with types III and IV OI. Signs and symptoms, which include headache, lower cranial nerve dysfunction, hyperreflexia, quadriparesis, ataxia, nystagmus, and scoliosis, must be recognized. A minority of patients (16%) will be asymptomatic. In a recent study, 80% of patients demonstrated radiographic progression despite successful occipitocervical fusion. Prolonged orthotic use with a Minerva brace controlled symptoms and arrested progression in these patients, but long-term results are currently unknown.

Until recently, medical management with a variety of agents has had little to no success. Treatment with calcitonin, fluoride, calcium, and vitamin supplements has been unsuccessful. Bisphosphonate compounds are synthetic analogs of pyrophosphate, a natural inhibitor of osteoclastic bone resorption, and have been successfully used in the treatment of osteoporosis and Paget's disease. Recent studies in which a variety of bisphosphonates (specifically pamidronate and olpadronate) were used, have shown promising results in the treatment of OI. In one study, 30 patients were administered pamidronate cyclically for up to 5 years. Improvements were seen in bone mineral density, cortical width, and vertebral body height with a concomitant decrease in fracture rate and no alteration in fracture healing. These studies are complicated by the commonly observed decreased incidence of fractures with age in the OI population. It is unclear what effect bisphosphonates will have on the histologic and biomechanical properties of bone. The authors stressed the importance of combining medical treatment with a comprehensive program involving physiotherapy, bracing, and corrective surgery.

In another recent study, the effects of growth hormone on patients with quantitative abnormalities in type I collagen (Sillence type I OI) were examined. After 12 months, the treatment showed improvements in growth velocity and bone density compared with a control group. Long-term, prospective, controlled trials are needed to verify these promising, albeit preliminary, results involving systemic treatment methods.

The most promising avenue of treatment of OI is in the realm of gene therapy. Bone marrow transplantation as a means of replacing mutant cells with normal cells is one method that could be used. Another approach would be to suppress mutant gene product while leaving normal product intact. This would lead to quantitative defects in collagen production and phenotypically milder cases. These approaches are not yet ready for clinical use. Specific treatment must be individualized based on the particular mutation that is present.

Much more needs to be known about the structure, formation, and turnover of type I collagen, as well as the factors that are important in determining specific phenotypic features, given a genotypic abnormality. Currently, gene therapy is in its infancy, and there are enormous technical obstacles ahead. The development of a variety of osteotropic agents to treat other conditions, such as osteoporosis, could be increasingly applicable to patients with OI. This is an extremely active and exciting time in the field of OI research.

Annotated Bibliography

Introduction

Kocher MS, Shapiro F: Osteogenesis imperfecta. *J Am Acad Orthop Surg* 1998;6:225-236.

This article provides a thorough review of the clinical manifestations and treatment options for OI.

Pathogenesis

Cole WG: The molecular pathology of osteogenesis imperfecta. *Clin Orthop* 1997;343:235-248.

A review of the molecular pathology of OI with an updated Sillence classification system and a discussion of the variability of the phenotypic expression given the genotypic abnormality.

Marini JC, Gerber NL: Osteogenesis imperfecta: Rehabilitation and prospects for gene therapy. *JAMA* 1997; 277:746-750.

This article is an excellent review of the genetics and biochemistry of OI, as well as gene therapy treatment methods.

McAllion SJ, Paterson CR: Causes of death in osteogenesis imperfecta. *J Clin Pathol* 1996;49:627-630.

An analysis of the causes of death in 79 patients with a diagnosis of OI.

Management

Antoniazzi F, Bertoldo F, Mottes M, et al: Growth hormone treatment in osteogenesis imperfecta with quantitative defect of type I collagen synthesis. *J Pediatr* 1996;129:432-439.

The authors studied 14 patients with quantitative defects in type I collagen production over a 12-month period. Half the patients received subcutaneous growth hormone (hGH) injections and the other half served as controls. The authors found increases in linear growth and increased bone turnover and mineral content in the lumbar spine in those patients receiving hGH.

Glorieux FH, Bishop NJ, Plotkin H, Chabot G, Lanoue G, Travers R: Cyclic administration of pamidronate in children with severe osteogenesis imperfecta. *N Engl J Med* 1998;339:947-952.

The authors report on 30 children with OI treated with cyclically administered intravenous pamidronate from ages 1.3 to 5 years. Increases in bone mineral density, metacarpal width, and vertebral body size as well as decreases in fracture incidence were seen.

Ishikawa S, Kumar SJ, Takahashi HE, Homma M: Vertebral body shape as a predictor of spinal deformity in osteogenesis imperfecta. *J Bone Joint Surg Am* 1996;78:212-219.

Forty-four patients with OI were studied to determine prevalence of spinal deformity and prognostic factors related to progression. The presence of biconcave vertebral body shape at six levels correlated with progression of scoliosis to greater than 50°. Based on these findings, early stabilization of scoliosis in this subset of patients may be warranted.

Luhmann SJ, Sheridan JJ, Capelli AM, Schoenecker PL: Management of lower-extremity deformities in osteogenesis imperfecta with extensible intramedullary rod technique: A 20-year experience. *J Pediatr Orthop* 1998;18:88-94.

Twelve patients with OI were treated with extensible rod techniques. The authors describe use of an overlapping Rush rod technique for the femur and offer some technical advice on placement of the Bailey-Dubow rods.

Pepin M, Atkinson M, Starman BJ, Byers PH: Strategies and outcomes of prenatal diagnosis for osteogenesis imperfecta: A review of biochemical and molecular studies completed in 129 pregnancies. *Prenat Diagn* 1997;17:559-570.

This report is based on the prenatal diagnostic studies from 129 pregnancies reviewing the indications for a variety of testing methods and their associated limitations. It provides a helpful timeline for prenatal studies based on the number of weeks of gestation.

Sawin PD, Menezes AH: Basilar invagination in osteogenesis imperfecta and related osteochondrodysplasias: Medical and surgical management. *J Neurosurg* 1997;86: 950-960.

In this study of 25 patients with a variety of osteochondrodysplasias (18 with OI) and basilar invagination, presenting complaints, treatment options, and results are discussed.

Widmann RF, Bitan FD, Laplaza FJ, Burke SW, DiMaio MF, Schneider R: Spinal deformity, pulmonary compromise, and quality of life in osteogenesis imperfecta. *Spine* 1999;24:1673-1678.

Fifteen patients with OI were studied, using spine radiographs, pulmonary function testing, and a self-assessment questionnaire, to determine the effect of scoliosis on these parameters. Curves greater than 60° adversely affected pulmonary function.

Wilkinson JM, Scott BW, Clarke AM, Bell MJ: Surgical stabilisation of the lower limb in osteogenesis imperfecta using the Sheffield Telescopic Intramedullary Rod System. *J Bone Joint Surg Br* 1998;80:999-1004.

The authors describe their expanding intramedullary rod system. Sixty lower limb segments in 24 children were reviewed at a median follow-up of 5.25 years. The implant is a variation on the Bailey-Dubow rod designed to avoid some inherent difficulties with that system.

Zionts LE, Ebramzadeh E, Stott NS: Complications in the use of the Bailey-Dubow extensible nail. *Clin Orthop* 1998;348:186-195.

The authors reviewed 40 extensible nailing procedures in 15 children with IO. Seventeen major complications resulted in 15 additional procedures. Patients at greatest risk for complications were those younger than age 5 years at nail insertion, those with tibial nails, and those in whom a technical error occurred during nail insertion.

Classic Bibliography

Binder H, Conway A, Hason S, et al: Comprehensive rehabilitation of the child with osteogenesis imperfecta. *Am J Med Genet* 1993;45:265-269.

Bullough PG, Davidson DD, Lorenzo JC: The morbid anatomy of the skeleton in osteogenesis imperfecta. *Clin Orthop* 1981;159:42-57.

Charnas LR, Marini JC: Communicating hydrocephalus, basilar invagination, and other neurologic features in osteogenesis imperfecta. *Neurology* 1993;43: 2603-2608.

Gargan MF, Wisbeach A, Fixsen JA: Humeral rodding in osteogenesis imperfecta. *J Pediatr Orthop* 1996;16: 719-722.

Sillence D: Osteogenesis imperfecta: An expanding panorama of variants. *Clin Orthop* 1981;159:11-25.

Stockley I, Bell MJ, Sharrard WJ: The role of expanding intramedullary rods in osteogenesis imperfecta. *J Bone Joint Surg Br* 1989;71:422-427.

Section 2

2

Trauma

Section Editor:
Paul D. Sponseller, MD

Section 2

Trauma

Overview

The orthopaedic surgeon caring for children who are victims of trauma must be prepared to take into account the impact of trauma on all body systems. In the chapter on patient management, guidelines are given for recognizing serious head injuries. Understanding the physiology of a head injury is critical in making decisions about fracture treatment. Because injury prevention should be a concern for the orthopaedic surgeon, this chapter also discusses airbags, safe transport, handguns, and other timely topics. The chapter on femur fractures provides a concise summary of the advantages and disadvantages of the different types of treatment for this relatively common fracture, as well as pitfalls to avoid, such as osteonecrosis of the femoral head after rigid nailing through the piriformis. The chapter on upper extremity injuries reveals that most "problem" fractures in this area involve the elbow. The assessment of vascular supply is discussed to help the surgeon determine when the fracture should be reduced emergently. The chapter on forearm and wrist fractures presents techniques for treatment as well as relative guidelines for choosing open reduction and internal fixation rather than closed treatment. Options for sedation during manipulation are discussed as well. In the chapter on injuries of the knee and tibia, current recommendations for treatment of cruciate ligament injuries are described. Age-based guidelines for surgical reconstruction are provided. Arthroscopic and open treatments are discussed as is limb salvage in severely injured extremities. Physeal injuries of the ankle are summarized in the chapter on foot and ankle injuries, and recommendations regarding open and closed treatments are provided. In the chapter on spine trauma, the different patterns of spine fractures are discussed, as well as how the greater availability of MRI and multiplanar CT has improved diagnosis of these injuries. The phenomenon of SCIWORA is receiving increased attention in the field and is discussed in this chapter.

Paul D. Sponseller, MD
Section Editor

Chapter 8

Management of the Pediatric Trauma Patient

Paul D. Sponseller, MD

Charles Paidas, MD

Overview

Trauma is one of the greatest public health problems for children and is the leading cause of mortality after the first year of life, exceeding all other causes of death combined. The incidence of trauma is higher in boys than in girls. Sociodemographic factors such as poverty and population density can also predict risk of trauma and are therefore useful in development of prevention strategies. The overall mortality of childhood trauma is less than approximately 3%; therefore, in addition to measuring fatality rates, those caring for pediatric trauma patients must measure quality of life outcomes. Injury to the head is associated with the highest percentage of both short- and long-term residual limitation. Trauma management in children has many similarities but a few important differences from trauma management in adults. The purpose of this chapter is to highlight these differences so that the orthopaedist can be an effective part of the pediatric trauma team.

An average of fewer than one pediatric trauma center per American state has been "verified" by the American College of Surgeons (ACS). Pediatric trauma patients are usually treated in centers without specialty ACS verification or state designation. Although the likelihood of survival of patients with head, multisystem, and blunt abdominal injury has been shown to be better in regions with pediatric trauma centers as opposed to nontrauma centers, this difference vanishes when pediatric trauma centers are compared with general regional trauma centers that have specialty coverage for pediatric anesthesia, intensive care, and neurosurgery. The national Pediatric Trauma Registry serves as a research and monitoring tool for outcomes of trauma in childhood. By coupling injuries with measures such as the Pediatric Trauma Score and Injury Severity Score, the registry can analyze national outcomes and population-based injury trends.

Initial Assessment and Resuscitation
Theoretical Points

There are several guiding concepts in managing pediatric trauma. Young children (especially those younger than age 4 years) have an increased metabolic rate with an oxygen demand twice that of adults. In this age group, the oropharynx is relatively small and the tongue is large; therefore, the airway is more easily obstructed. The larynx is more anterior in children than in older patients. The subglottic portion of the trachea is narrow and provides a "physiologic cuff;" therefore, uncuffed endotracheal (ET) tubes are recommended in children younger than age 8 years. In addition, the child's trachea is short; thus, an ET tube could be mistakenly inserted into the right mainstem bronchus.

Hemorrhagic shock is more easily missed in the child because of the smaller blood volume; therefore, attention must be given to small amounts of blood loss. Signs of blood volume loss in children include tachycardia, altered mental status, absent peripheral pulses, a delayed capillary refill (of more than 2 seconds), and hypothermia. The child's relatively larger body surface area increases the likelihood of hypothermia.

Practical Points

The primary survey includes checking the status of the patient's airway, breathing, circulation, disability, and exposure. Specifically, the examiner should check for hypoxia, chest wall motion, tachycardia, hypotension, and hypothermia. Time in the field should be focused primarily on securing the airway. If large-bore intravenous access is not available, intraosseous infusion may be performed using the anteromedial tibial metaphysis or the distal-lateral femur for up to 4 to 6 hours. The examiner must be alert for life-threatening injuries such as airway obstruction, tension or open pneumothorax, hemothorax, flail chest, and cardiac tamponade.

TABLE 1 | Unique Characteristics of Pediatric Trauma

Region	Pediatric Characteristics	Implications
Head/neck	Large head	Frequent head injuries
	Weak neck muscles	Airway easily obstructed; intubation difficult
	Large tongue, floppy epiglottis	
Chest	Compliant rib cage	Traumatic asphyxia possible
		Thoracic injury occult
Abdomen	Abdomen large, chest pliable	Abdominal organs vulnerable
	Abdominal muscles underdeveloped	Bladder vulnerable
	Pelvis small	
Metabolic/Physiologic	Greater surface area: mass ratio	Increased sweat loss
	Increased metabolic demand	Hypothermia
	Inability to alter stroke volume	Sudden cardiac arrest

The major emphasis should be placed on avoiding brain ischemia. Courses are available for emergency medical technicians and other care providers. Pediatric advanced life support courses can help the physician achieve improved respiration in children younger than age 18 months, especially with regard to intubation and venous access. Although chest trauma is rare in these patients (occurring in 3%), it is an indication of severe injury, with mortality of up to 40%.

The secondary survey should include a more detailed examination of systems and the ordering of diagnostic studies. Ancillary tests should be ordered according to protocol; in the obtunded patient, radiographs of the entire spine, chest, abdomen, and pelvis should be obtained. A skull film or CT scan of the head should be ordered if there is significant scalp tenderness, hematoma, or large laceration. Laboratory tests should include a complete blood count, renal function tests, amylase, type, and crossmatch. A CT scan of the abdomen is helpful in the evaluation of blunt trauma.

Unique Pediatric Aspects of Specific Injuries

Central Nervous System Injuries

Central nervous system injuries are the single most important determinants of outcome after childhood trauma. Traumatic brain injury outcome is related to both the primary injury as well as to any secondary injury that may occur, such as injuries resulting from hypotension and hypoxia. The unique characteristics of pediatric trauma and their implications are shown in Table 1.

The most widely used means of rating the status of a closed head injury is the Glasgow Coma Scale (GCS), which is composed of scores for eye opening, motor activity, and verbal response. A moderate injury is defined as one having a score of 9 to 12. For children younger than age 5 years, in whom a verbal response might not be the same as that of older patients, a modified GCS exists (Table 2). A GCS score of less than 8 is usually an indication for airway intubation.

The work-up of a closed head injury should include a CT scan if the patient experiences altered or a loss of consciousness, has a depressed skull fracture, or a GCS score of less than 8. The minimal indications for admission to the hospital include loss of consciousness for more than 5 minutes, seizure, neurologic deficit, or question of abuse. In general, children with head injury may be discharged to home if the loss of consciousness is less than 5 minutes, the GCS score is 15, the CT scan is normal, and serial examinations in the emergency department have been normal for at least 6 hours. Any questionable mental status or physical examination warrants either continued observation or admission to the hospital.

Central perfusion pressure (CPP) is defined as the mean arterial pressure minus the intracranial pressure (ICP). Normal CPP is at least 60 mm Hg. Indications for ICP measurement include a GCS score of less than 8 or a CT scan that suggests swelling, as with diffuse axonal injury. Because many orthopaedic emergencies, such as open fractures or vascular injury, require surgery on the day of injury, it is important to know the factors that influence the ICP. Inhalational anesthetic agents and ketamine increase the ICP, and barbiturates and mannitol decrease the ICP. Hyperventilation also decreases ICP by reducing carbon dioxide, producing reflex cerebral vasoconstriction. To avoid secondary brain

TABLE 2 | Pediatric Glasgow Coma Scale

Score	Older than Age 5 Years	Age 1 to 5 Years	Younger Than Age 1 Year
Best Motor Response (of 6)			(of 5)
6	Obeys commands	Obeys commands	
5	Localizes pain	Localizes pain	Localizes pain
4	Withdrawal	Withdrawal	Abnormal withdrawal
3	Flexion to pain	Abnormal flexion	Abnormal flexion
2	Extensor rigidity	Extensor rigidity	Abnormal extension
1	None	None	None
Best Verbal Response			
5	Oriented	Appropriate words	Smiles/cries appropriately
4	Confused	Inappropriate words	Cries
3	Inappropriate words	Cries/screams	Cries inappropriately
2	Incomprehensible	Grunts	Grunts
1	None	None	None
Eye Opening			
4	Spontaneous	Spontaneous	Spontaneous
3	To speech	To speech	To shout
2	To pain	To pain	To pain
1	None	None	None

ischemia resulting from hypotension and/or hypoxia, a mean arterial pressure above 80 mm Hg should be maintained. Thus, it is mandatory to restore blood volume and ensure adequate airway control prior to any treatment of traumatic brain injury.

Surgical treatment of orthopaedic injuries in children with head injuries has not been shown to improve neurologic outcome; however, surgery is usually recommended because of difficulty in managing pain and associated injuries. Important practical considerations in caring for the polytrauma patient include difficulty in managing traction and the need for frequent transportation for diagnostic tests, as well as the potential risk of agitation or spasticity. Because there is no relationship between neurologic outcome and the timing of fixation, surgery may be performed when it is best for the patient and team, either on the day of injury or at a later date if early treatment is not advisable. In general, the ICP

should be monitored if surgery is performed on a child with a traumatic brain injury.

The end of coma is defined as the patient's ability to have meaningful interaction with the environment, such as following simple commands or uttering a word. This development usually correlates with a GCS score of greater than 8 or 9. Children who have sustained traumatic brain injury should undergo neuropsychiatric evaluation to determine if special services are needed before they return to school. Brain death is defined as the absence of cerebral and brainstem function in the absence of hypothermia, shock, or pharmacologic encephalopathy. In children, brain death must be verified by two consecutive neurologic examinations 12 to 24 hours apart.

The outcome following traumatic brain injury is related to the severity of the injury. The severity is defined by the GCS score, duration of coma, and length of posttraumatic amnesia. Orthopaedic treatment for children with traumatic brain injury should

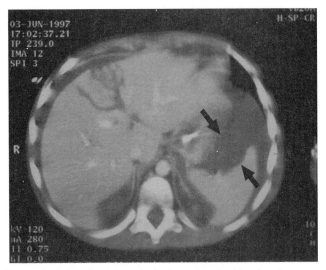

Figure 1 Fluid in the abdomen is due to a solid organ injury (*arrow*).

not be excluded during the acute phase or subsequent management. Moreover, stabilization of the skeleton will contribute to pain control and hasten early rehabilitation.

Abdominal Injuries

When children sustain blunt trauma, the abdominal organs are at increased risk because of several anatomic factors. Because the rib cage is smaller and more pliable, the abdomen begins essentially at the nipple line. The pelvis is proportionately smaller, giving less bony protection to the lower abdomen. The abdominal muscles are less well developed. The solid organs, the liver and spleen, are proportionately larger.

On physical examination, signs that should increase the suspicion of abdominal trauma include lap belt marks, ecchymosis, lacerations, and abdominal guarding. Because intraperitoneal blood is not, by itself, an indication for laparotomy in children, diagnostic

work-up for trauma in children no longer includes peritoneal lavage. Criteria for laparotomy include CT scan findings and the clinical status of the patient. Thus, CT with intravenous contrast only is currently the preferred method for diagnosis of intra-abdominal injury. The indication for CT is an obtunded patient or the presence of any of the above-mentioned physical findings. When an abdominal CT for trauma is being read, certain criteria mandate exploration, including pneumoperitoneum and fluid in the abdomen without evidence of solid organ injury (Figs. 1 and 2). Focused abdominal sonography for trauma is being used in some centers as a screening tool for blunt abdominal injury.

Treatment of isolated splenic injury is usually nonsurgical because the bleeding stops on its own. Therefore, the risk of sepsis following splenectomy can be avoided, representing a revolutionary change since 1978. Management of splenic injury involves observation in the hospital for approximately 3 to 4 days and 3 weeks of quiet home activity. Restrictions are usually lifted at 3 months. Relative indications for splenectomy include blood loss greater than one half of blood volume or unstable vital signs. Children younger than age 15 years who undergo a splenectomy should have daily antibiotic prophylaxis to prevent sepsis from encapsulated bacteria. Liver lacerations are treated according to similar principles, but they usually require a longer period of in-hospital observation. Renal injuries pose a long-term risk of hydronephrosis, decreased renal function, and hypertension. Thus, children with renal injuries require semiannual imaging and blood pressure measurements for 1 year following injury. Stable intestinal injuries may be managed by observation; otherwise, segmental resection is required. Respiratory distress and the radiographic finding of the bowel in the chest indicate diaphragmatic rupture; repair is manda-

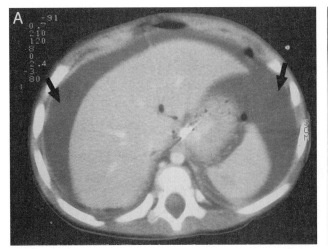
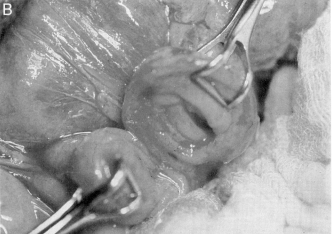

Figure 2 A, Fluid is seen in the abdomen in the absence of a solid organ injury (*arrow*). **B,** A subsequent laparotomy demonstrated intestinal injury.

tory. Any pneumoperitoneum following blunt trauma that is discovered on plain radiograph or CT scan mandates laparotomy.

Thoracic Injuries

Although rare, injuries to the thorax are due to severe trauma and should suggest a risk of associated injuries to the head and long bones. Thoracic injuries are the second leading cause of childhood mortality from trauma. Because of the increased compliance of the chest wall, a pulmonary contusion may occur without much external evidence of injury. Contusions should be treated with fluid restriction and positive pressure ventilation, if needed. Rib fractures are less common in children than in adults because of increased flexibility. In young children, rib fractures should alert the physician to the possibility of child abuse. Hemothorax may be caused by bleeding from an intercostal vessel or from the pulmonary parenchyma; tube thoracostomy is usually sufficient treatment. However, a thoracotomy should be performed if blood loss is greater than 4 mL/kg/h. Pneumothorax requires insertion of a chest tube. Although pulmonary fat embolism is rare in young children, it may be seen in teenagers, especially after a long bone fracture. Signs of fat embolism include alteration in mental status after a lucent interval, as well as the presence of petechiae, tachypnea, or tachycardia. Treatment involves respiratory support, with administration of steroids if needed.

Other Points and Complications

Deep venous thrombosis is rare in children and routine prophylaxis appears to be indicated only if the child is older than age 16 years. Multisystem organ failure is also rare in children and is not prevented by urgent fracture fixation. Therefore, the medical mandate to perform immediate fracture stabilization is not as strong in children as it is in severely traumatized adults. The risk of compartment syndrome is increased in patients with polytrauma, as well as in patients with open femur fractures. Because of generalized pain and altered responsiveness, skeletal injuries can be missed even after the secondary survey, emphasizing the need for re-examination several days after injury in the severely traumatized child. Bone scan has been recommended to screen for skeletal injury in the patient who remains obtunded for more than a few days. Nutrition should be started 24 hours or at most 72 hours after injury. Although the enteral route is preferable, peripheral nutrition should be initiated until the transition can be made. Total parenteral nutrition is reserved for the management of gastrointestinal tract problems lasting more than 10 days.

TABLE 3	Vehicle Restraint Recommendations	
Age	**Type of Restraint**
Birth to 1 year (20 lb)	Rear facing infant-only seat in back seat
1 to 4 years (20 to 40 lb)	Forward facing seat in back seat
4 to 8 years (40 to 60 lb)	Booster seat plus lap/shoulder belt in back seat
8 to 12 years (60 to 100 lb)	Lap/shoulder belt in back seat

Air bag injuries have resulted in at least 66 fatalities reported in children. Most injuries involved children who were younger than age 12 years who were sitting in the front seat of the vehicle. These injuries are believed to be due to bag velocity, which can exceed 150 mph, and the child's proximity to the bag during a crash. Injuries include friction burns, abrasions, basilar skull fractures, cervical spine injuries, and chest and facial injuries. Current recommendations include placing children in the middle of the back seat in a safety seat or three-point restraint. Infants should be seated in a rear-facing device in the back seat. Vehicle restraint recommendations for children based on age are shown in Table 3.

Early evaluation by a rehabilitation specialist should be an integral part of the injured child's evaluation. Early input from physiatrists facilitates decisions regarding treatment as an inpatient, in the home, or at a day center.

Injury Assessment

Injury severity scales are useful tools in the classification of multisystem injuries. However, the fact that more than one scale is currently in use serves as good evidence that there is no single scoring system that is appropriate for children. The Modified Injury Severity Scale (MISS) reliably predicts both morbidity and mortality rates. The MISS score is obtained by adding the severity ratings of the three organ systems that are most severely injured. Results of one study predicted that patients with a MISS score of 25 or greater had an increased risk of morbidity and mortality. Injury severity scales provide a valuable method for assessing the prognosis in children who experience multisystem trauma. Long-term disability occurs in a minority of children, generally because of head and spinal cord injuries.

Prevention

Injury has some proven risk factors; it is not a truly random event. Poverty increases injury rates; the mortality rate from injuries in children whose families have incomes below the poverty line is at least 2.6 times that of other children. For femur fractures, population density and single parenthood have also been shown to increase the risk. Among the measures proven to prevent trauma are helmets, which can reduce the severity of bicycle injury by 85%. Smoke detectors are also effective, but batteries must be checked regularly. Proper restraint in vehicles has made child transport safer; however, shoulder harnesses do not properly fit children until they are nearly adult size. The use of protocols for suspected child abuse is widespread, but continued education is required to maintain recognition of this phenomenon. Handgun legislation is evolving in many regions. Deaths resulting from injury have decreased by 26% over the past 14 years. This trend is a combination of a larger decrease in unintentional injuries that is partially offset by an increase in intentional injuries such as suicides and homicides. Prevention measures show promise for a continued drop in injury rates.

Annotated Bibliography

Overview

Baker SP, Fingerhut LA, Higgins L, et al: *Useful Statistics on Mortality Due to Trauma*. Vienna, VA, Johns Hopkins Center for Injury Research and Policy, 1996, p 18.

In this article, useful statistics on mortality resulting from trauma are presented.

Sanchez JI, Paidas CN: Childhood trauma: Now and in the new millennium. *Surg Clin North Am* 1999;79: 1503-1535.

In this article, modern practices and trends in the pediatric trauma field are described.

Initial Assessment and Resuscitation

Nichols DG, Yaster M, Lappe DG, Haller JA Jr (eds): *The Golden Hour: The Handbook of Advanced Pediatric Life Support*, ed 2. St. Louis, MO, Mosby-Year Book, 1996.

This practical handbook provides principles and protocols for acute care of the injured child.

Unique Pediatric Aspects of Specific Injuries

Christensen JR: Pediatric traumatic brain injury, in Capute AJ, Accardo PJ (eds): *Developmental Disabilities in Infancy and Childhood*, ed 2. Baltimore, MD, Paul H. Brookes Publishing, 1996, vol 1, pp 245-260.

Peak incidence of traumatic brain injuries occurs in boys in the 14 to 16 year age group. Severe traumatic brain injury is defined as having a GCS score of 3 to 8, moderate as a score of 9 to 12, and mild as a score of 13 to 15. Most children with mild traumatic brain injuries generally have no permanent sequelae. Posttraumatic amnesia (PTA) is defined as the time after injury during which the patient has no continuous memory. Duration of PTA lasting longer than 3 weeks is the most reliable predictor of cognitive impairment in mild traumatic brain injury. Memory impairment is the most common cognitive deficit following pediatric traumatic brain injury.

Gandhi RR, Keller MS, Schwab CW, Stafford PW: Pediatric splenic injury: Pathway to play? *J Pediatr Surg* 1999;34:55-59.

This prospective study of a treatment pathway with a historical control shows that isolated blunt splenic injuries in hemodynamically stable children can be safely treated with a 4-day hospital stay, 3 weeks of quiet home activity, and 3 months of light activity.

Hulka F, Mullins RJ, Leonardo V, Harrison MW, Silberberg P: Significance of peritoneal fluid as an isolated finding on abdominal computed tomographic scans in pediatric trauma patients. *J Trauma* 1998;44: 1069-1072.

In a review of 259 pediatric CT scans for trauma, it was found that extravasated oral contrast does not aid in the diagnosis of bowel injury. A child with fluid in more than one location has a 50% chance of having a bowel injury.

Prevention

Nichols DG, Yaster M, Lappe DG, Haller JA Jr (eds): *The Golden Hour: The Handbook of Advanced Pediatric Life Support*, ed 2. St. Louis, MO, Mosby-Year Book, 1996, pp 289-359.

This discussion of recent trends and promising research in injury prevention is relevant for the orthopaedist.

Rivara FP, Grossman DC: Prevention of traumatic deaths to children in the United States: How far have we come and where do we need to go? *Pediatrics* 1996;97:791-797.

The national injury death rate for children declined by 26% over the 14-year period studied. This was a result of a mixture of a large decline in unintentional injuries and an increase in intentional injuries. Further gains are possible from application of current preventive strategies.

Classic Bibliography

Beaver BL, Moore VL, Peclet M, Haller JA Jr, Smialek J, Hill JL: Characteristics of pediatric firearm fatalities. *J Pediatr Surg* 1990;25:97-100.

Buckley SL, Gottschall C, Robertson W Jr, et al: The relationships of skeletal injuries with trauma score, injury severity score, length of hospital stay, hospital charges and mortality in children admitted to a regional pediatric trauma center. *J Pediatr Orthop* 1994;14:449-453.

Davidson LL, Durkin MS, Kuhn LP, O'Connor, Barlow B, Heagarty MC: The impact of the Safe Kids/ Healthy Neighborhoods Injury Prevention Program in Harlem, 1988-1991. *Am J Public Health* 1994;84: 580-586.

Eichelberger MR, Mangubat EA, Sacco WJ, Bowman LM, Lowenstein AD: Outcome analysis of blunt injury in children. *J Trauma* 1988;28:1109-1117.

Haller JA Jr, Papa P, Drugas G, Colombani P: Nonoperative management of solid organ injuries in children: Is it safe? *Ann Surg* 1994;219:625-631.

Heinrich SD, Gallagher D, Harris M, Nadell JM: Undiagnosed fractures in severely injured children and young adults: Identification with technetium imaging. *J Bone Joint Surg Am* 1994;76:561-572.

Mayer T, Walker ML, Clark P: Further experience with the modified abbreviated Injury Severity Scale. *J Trauma* 1984;24:31-34.

Newman KD, Bowman LM, Eichelberger MR, et al: The lap belt complex: Intestinal and lumbar spine injury in children. *J Trauma* 1990;30:1133-1139.

Wesson DE, Williams JI, Spence LJ, Filler RM, Armstrong PF, Pearl RH: Functional outcome in pediatric trauma. *J Trauma* 1989;29:589-592.

Ziv I, Rang M: Treatment of femoral fracture in the child with head injury. *J Bone Joint Surg Br* 1983;65: 276-278.

Chapter 9

Trauma to the Hip and Femur in Children

David W. Gray, MD

Introduction

Treatment of femoral fractures continues to evolve toward a balanced approach between closed and open approaches in the skeletally immature patient. Using one method of management no longer applies for all femoral fractures. With the availability of many treatment options, the risks and benefits of each must be weighed for each patient. This chapter will cover fractures at all levels of the femur.

Hip Fractures

Historically, hip fractures in children have accounted for less than 1% of all pediatric fractures. Unlike in adults with osteoporosis, hip fractures in children are typically associated with high-energy trauma, unless there is an underlying pathologic process such as unicameral bone cyst or fibrous dysplasia. Although rare, hip fractures in the skeletally immature patient produce sequelae in approximately 60% of patients.

At birth, blood is supplied to the femoral head from metaphyseal vessels that are derived from the medial and lateral circumflex arteries and traverse the femoral neck. As the subcapital physis develops, these metaphyseal vessels no longer significantly penetrate the femoral head. By age 4 years, the contribution of these vessels to the blood supply is negligible. At this time the major blood supply to the femoral head is provided by the posterosuperior and posteroinferior retinacular systems derived from the medial circumflex artery. The physeal anatomy and blood supply to the proximal femur account for the high incidence of problems that follow hip fractures in children.

The classification system of Delbet reported by Colonna in 1929 is still used (Fig. 1). This system lists four types of proximal femur fractures. A type I fracture is a transepiphyseal separation of the femoral head, with or without dislocation. A type II fracture is a transcervical fracture. A type III fracture occurs at the cervi-cotrochanteric level. A type IV fracture has an intertrochanteric fracture pattern.

Type I fractures are the least common of these injuries and tend to occur in younger children, compared with other types. Dislocation of the capital femoral epiphysis occurs in almost one half of type I fractures. With dislocation of the femoral head, the rate of osteonecrosis approaches 100%.

For displaced type I fractures, closed reduction should be attempted using longitudinal traction, abduction, and internal rotation, followed by pin fixation. In patients younger than age 2 years, the reduction may be relatively stable and the injury can sometimes be treated using a spica cast alone. If there is any doubt about stability, internal fixation should be added; however, internal fixation does not supplant the need for an anatomic reduction. Open reduction will be necessary if closed reduction is unsuccessful.

For type I fractures with posterior dislocation of the capital epiphysis, the dislocation should be approached posteriorly. Conversely, if the dislocation is anterior, an anterior or anterolateral approach should be used. A CT scan can help in visualizing the location of the femoral head dislocation.

Internal fixation of a type I fracture can be accomplished by using pins or screws that, by necessity, must cross the physis. In the young child, smooth pins across the physis should be used, followed by application of a spica cast. Threaded fixation across the physis is more likely to lead to premature physeal closure and subsequent disturbance of proximal femoral growth. The capital epiphysis contributes approximately 15% of the extremity's total length. Obviously, premature physeal closure in a child nearing skeletal maturity is less significant than in a younger child. Girls typically complete skeletal growth earlier than boys, so both skeletal maturity and gender should be a consideration for smooth fixation versus threaded fixation. In a child, internal

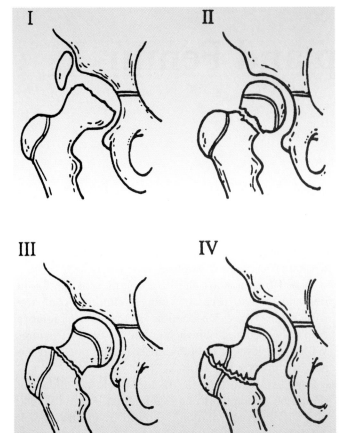

Figure 1 The hip fracture classification system of Delbet for children. Type I is a transepiphyseal separation with or without dislocation of the head from the acetabulum. Type II is a transcervical fracture. Type III is a cervicotrochanteric fracture. Type IV is an intertrochanteric fracture. *(Reproduced with permission from Hughes LO, Beaty JH: Fractures of the head and neck of the femur in children. J Bone Joint Surg Am 1994;76:283-292.)*

fixation of a type I fracture is typically supplemented with application of a spica cast.

Type II and type III fractures are the most common femoral neck fractures in the skeletally immature patient. Most of these injuries are displaced. Osteonecrosis occurs in approximately 50% of patients with type II fractures and in up to 25% of patients with type III fractures.

Nondisplaced type II and III fractures can be treated with spica cast immobilization or internal fixation and a cast. Cast immobilization alone has the best results in children younger than age 6 years. Because the loss of reduction can potentially produce coxa vara, close follow-up is mandatory if this method is chosen. In an effort to prevent displacement, an internal fixation device can be placed percutaneously using fluoroscopy and supplemented with a spica cast. Internal fixation is recommended for most nondisplaced injuries to decrease the risk of displacement and coxa vara.

Treatment of displaced type II and type III fractures is aimed at achieving anatomic reduction by closed or open means. If open reduction is needed, the capsule at the level of the intertrochanteric line should be preserved when performing a capsulotomy to protect the proximal femur's blood supply. To avoid disturbing the posterior network of the circumflex vessels, the anterolateral (Watson Jones) approach is preferred.

Internal fixation is used to stabilize the fracture following closed or open fracture reduction for a type II or type III injury. If possible, internal fixation should stop short of the physis (Fig. 2). If the metaphyseal portion of the neck cephalad to the fracture line is of sufficient size, crossing the physis can be avoided and screw fixation placed across the fracture into the upper metaphysis. Cannulated 4.0- to 4.5-mm screws often can be used in younger children, and cannulated 6.5- to 7.0-mm screws can be used in older children and teenagers. However, at times it is necessary to cross the physis with smooth pins to achieve stability and allow subsequent growth. After reduction and internal fixation, a spica cast is generally applied for patients who have undergone screw fixation in the metaphysis that does not cross the physis. In these patients, the smaller diameter of the femoral neck limits the size

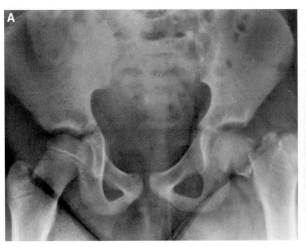

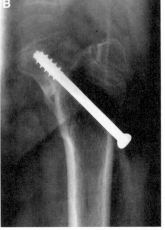

Figure 2 A, Radiograph showing a type III femoral neck fracture. **B,** The fracture was manipulated with traction and abduction on the fracture table, and a percutaneous 4-mm screw was placed. The patient was treated with a spica cast with the hip and knee in extension. There is residual medial translation of the proximal fragment that potentially could have led to varus angulation. The patient went on to uneventful healing. *(Reproduced from Richards BS (ed): Orthopaedic Knowledge Update: Pediatrics. Rosemont, IL, American Academy of Orthopaedic Surgeons, 1996, pp 229-237.)*

and number of screws that can be placed. Screw placement across the physis in the adolescent near skeletal maturity achieves improved fixation and may obviate the need for cast immobilization.

The lowest incidence of vascular insult to the proximal femur occurs with type IV fractures. The occurrence of osteonecrosis is approximately 10%. As with all femoral neck fractures in children, the initial displacement seems to most directly predict the risk of osteonecrosis. Malunion is another risk in the treatment of type IV fractures.

Type IV fractures can be treated with traction followed by application of a spica cast or with immediate spica placement with the leg abducted. If closed reduction cannot be accomplished, open reduction and internal fixation should be used to prevent varus malunion. Younger children can be treated with percutaneous cannulated screw fixation extending into the metaphysis and supplemented with a spica cast. In children older than age 8 years and in multiple-trauma patients, surgical intervention should be considered initially. Screw and side plate combinations are available in pediatric and adolescent sizes, and in these patients, screw fixation should stop short of the physis if possible. In children with screw fixation in the metaphysis that stops short of the physis, a supplemental spica cast should always be considered.

Complications of Hip Fractures

Osteonecrosis remains the most serious of the complications following hip fractures in children. An increase in the risk of osteonecrosis is associated with type I and II fractures, as well as an age of older than 10 years. Evacuation or aspiration of the hematoma has been recommended; however, the value of evacuation and a direct correlation with a reduced rate of osteonecrosis remains scientifically unclear. The factor that is most correlated with osteonecrosis is the initial fracture displacement. The next most significant factor may be the amount of time until reduction is achieved. In some patients, reduction of a displaced fracture may allow the vascular leash to reestablish blood flow, but the integrity of the vessels at the time of the injury is crucial. Displaced femoral neck fractures should be treated urgently, and every attempt at reduction and stabilization should be made within the first 24 hours following injury.

Because of a lack of alternatives, treatment of osteonecrosis following femoral neck fracture focuses on maintaining motion and containment. The femoral head can collapse relatively rapidly over a 6-month period. In some patients, an osteotomy to rotate either an uninvolved portion or a less deformed area of the femoral head into the weight-bearing region may improve congruity and symptoms. Vascularized bone grafting has been used in some patients, but the results in skeletally immature patients remain to be seen. If vascularized bone grafting shows some benefit in children, then bone scan or MRI to diagnose osteonecrosis prior to bone collapse may become warranted.

Coxa vara, premature physeal closure, and nonunion can occur following femoral neck fracture. Coxa vara can result from malunion or premature physeal closure with relative trochanteric overgrowth. The overall prevalence of coxa vara has been approximately 20%. As long as an anatomic reduction is obtained, internal fixation decreases the likelihood of varus from malunion. Even with internal fixation, the fracture can still collapse if the medial femoral neck is not aligned. It is unlikely that a hip with a neck shaft angle of less than 110° will correct with growth. Subtrochanteric valgus osteotomy is useful for those deformities that do not improve with observation.

Premature physeal closure secondary to osteonecrosis can occur even when internal fixation does not cross the physis; however, a decrease in the number of patients with premature physeal closure has been reported. This decrease may be related to the practice of avoiding crossing the physis with pins and screws when possible. Nonunion occurs in approximately 4% to 7% of patients and seems to be related to a failure to obtain or maintain an anatomic reduction. To create a compression force at the fracture site, valgus osteotomy is recommended for patients with nonunion. Chondrolysis in conjunction with osteonecrosis has also been reported.

Proximal Femoral Epiphysiolysis

Proximal femoral epiphysiolysis can occur in the newborn, typically following a breech delivery. The capital femoral epiphyseal separation has a clinical appearance of pseudoparalysis of the limb. The differential diagnosis includes infection and developmental hip dislocation. Imaging techniques, such as ultrasound and arthrogram, and hip aspiration can help confirm the diagnosis. Although MRI can be useful, it typically requires general anesthesia in the newborn. If proximal femoral epiphysiolysis is recognized initially, alignment is restored with skin traction. If it is recognized after callus formation is visible on radiographs, simple immobilization is used. Open surgical reduction is not advocated for these injuries. Because epiphyseal separations in the newborn tend to remodel if the physis does not prematurely close, observation after healing is recommended.

Hip Dislocation

Traumatic hip dislocation may occur after relatively minor trauma in younger children. Approximately one half of dislocations in children younger than age 10 years are related to low to moderate levels of trauma, such as tripping or falling. However, in adolescents, a higher energy injury is needed to produce a dislocation. Most hip dislocations are posterior, and it is necessary to look for associated fractures of the proximal femur and acetabulum.

Closed reduction is usually successful. Excellent analgesia or anesthesia is needed so that hip stability following reduction can be assessed. Concentric reduction is mandatory. Because intra-articular fragments might be present, any suspected widening of the joint space should be assessed with CT. Open reduction is used in patients in whom concentric reduction is not achieved or who have unstable closed reduction or displaced acetabular rim or wall fractures. In patients younger than age 6 years, immobilization with a spica cast is often used following reduction. Older children can be managed with a cast, brace, or protected ambulation with crutches.

Osteonecrosis occurs in up to 10% of patients with hip dislocation. Factors for the risk of osteonecrosis include the time to reduction of the dislocation and the amount of energy involved in the trauma. Treatment of osteonecrosis is similar to that discussed with hip fractures. Coxa magna can be a late radiographic finding following hip dislocation.

Subtrochanteric Femur Fractures

Subtrochanteric femur fractures in children are those fractures that occur 2 cm or more distal to the lesser trochanter. The proximal fragment is markedly flexed, abducted, and externally rotated. If traction or spica cast immobilization is used, the distal fragment must be matched to this position. Because these fractures can be very difficult to manage by closed methods, surgery is commonly performed. The guidelines and principles of treatment are the same as those for diaphyseal femur fractures.

Diaphyseal Femur Fractures

Fractures of the femoral diaphysis are common injuries in children that can occur in distinctly different settings; the mechanism of injury can vary from a playground accident to a high-energy injury such as a motor vehicle accident. In children younger than age 1 year, approximately 40% of femoral fractures are related to nonaccidental trauma.

Treatment

A variety of treatment options have obtained good results in children. Treatment methods include early application of a spica cast, traction followed by application of a spica cast, external fixation, flexible intramedullary rods, interlocking nails, and compression plate fixation. Except for reamed antegrade nails, all of these modalities have a role in fracture treatment in the skeletally immature patient. The choice of treatment depends on several factors, including age, weight, mechanism of injury, open versus closed fracture, ipsilateral tibial fracture, neurovascular injury, head injury, multiple trauma, pathologic fractures, and social environment.

Traction

Traction followed by casting has been a very traditional and reliable method of care. The patient is placed in traction for 2 to 4 weeks until early consolidation occurs, and then a cast is applied. Because of expected later femoral overgrowth, the fracture fragments are allowed to overlap 1 to 1.5 cm.

Skin traction is used in a child who weighs less than 30 lb. Because Bryant's traction can potentially cause neurovascular compromise, variations on split-Russell traction have become quite popular. In the older child, 90-90 skeletal traction works effectively. The hip and knee are flexed to 90° and a short leg cast is applied to support the foot and ankle in a neutral position. The distal femur is the preferred pin site because it allows direct pull without transmitting the traction forces across the knee. Pin placement in the proximal tibia creates a risk of injury to the tibial physis near the tubercle and growth disturbance. Knee subluxation and dislocation have been reported following proximal tibial pin traction in the skeletally immature patient.

Early Application of a Spica Cast

Good results from traction followed by casting can be expected in children younger than age 10 years; however, the overall trend among pediatric orthopaedists across the country continues to move away from traction. The combination of initial traction discomfort, parent anxiety generated with the child's pain, prolonged hospital stay, social issues, and economic costs both to society and the family have propelled this trend. Early application of a spica cast either on the day of injury or within the first couple of days has now replaced traction as the primary mode of treatment at pediatric institutions across the country.

Because early spica cast treatment obviates the need for prolonged traction, the hospital stay is minimized. Early cast application provides significant economic savings when compared with inpatient hospital traction. Surgery followed by traction in a spica cast is

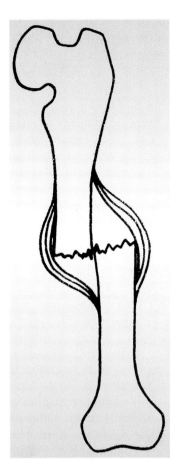

Figure 3 The extent of periosteal and muscular stripping is the main determinant of shortening potential when a femoral fracture is treated in a spica cast.

three times as expensive as immediate application of a spica cast alone.

The concerns with early application of a spica cast have centered on its ability to maintain adequate alignment. The acceptable amount of angulation in a cast is less than 10° of varus or valgus, 20° of posterior or anterior bowing (the femur has approximately 10° of anterior bowing normally). The cast has little ability to maintain the length of the fractured femur. The main barrier to shortening is provided by the integrity of the periosteal and muscular cuff (Fig. 3). Therefore, it is important to protect the periosteal and muscular cuff from excessive soft-tissue disruption caused by treatment with a spica cast. The main proven predictor of this shortening is an overlap of more than 3.0 cm either at rest or with gentle axial compression. Some shortening in the cast is acceptable because of femoral overgrowth. In children age 2 to 10 years, the overgrowth averages 1.0 cm. There can also be slight overgrowth of 0.2 to 0.5 cm of the tibia on the ipsilateral leg. Considering the overgrowth as well as the fact that shortening of 1.0 cm at maturity is well tolerated, the amount of shortening in a cast should not exceed 2.5 cm on follow-up radiographic examination.

For cast application to be effective, attention to detail is required. Either a below-knee or above-knee cast is applied first. The knee should be bent at least 60° but no more than 90°. The knee flexion helps maintain the traction on the leg to minimize fracture shortening. The cast should extend over the trochanter onto the buttock on the injured side. With inadequate knee flexion and a lack of trochanteric cast coverage, progressive shortening is more likely to occur. The injured thigh should be molded both on the anterior and lateral portions of the cast. After cast application, the lateral border of the thigh should be flat. Placement of a lateral mold controls the fracture's tendency to shift into varus; an anterior mold controls the sagittal plane and prevents excessive anterior bowing of the femur. Placing the foot in the cast is not necessary to control rotation. As long as the thigh is molded and the knee flexed, the foot can be safely left out of the cast. Leaving the foot free also helps prevent a possible cast sore on the heel.

Excessive shortening in the cast does develop in some patients. These patients require cast removal and subsequent treatment with traction, an external fixator, or other means of surgical stabilization. In patients with fractures secondary to high-energy trauma, more soft-tissue and periosteal stripping occurs, allowing for potentially greater shortening of the fracture fragments. Greater disruption of the soft-tissue envelope compromises stability. Radiographs obtained weekly during the first 3 weeks following injury are necessary to monitor the patient for excessive angulation and shortening.

Not all patients are suitable candidates for early spica cast treatment. Patients with multiple trauma have other injuries that may be difficult to care for in a cast. Maintaining control of the fracture fragments by spasticity following a head injury is complicated. Some children age 6 to 10 years are large enough that it is either too difficult to apply a molded cast or too hard for the family to lift and care for them. Most experts are reluctant to apply a spica cast for children who weigh more than 75 to 100 lb. The "floating knee" is another example of a clinical situation in which rigid fixation of at least one fracture simplifies the treatment and improves the result.

Surgery

Although early application of a spica cast and traction followed by casting can provide good results for many fractures, there is a role for surgery. Generally, patients between age 10 and 12 years are best managed with surgical fixation. Essentially all adolescent patients should be treated surgically because traction and cast application are not as reliable for them. Children younger than age 10 years may require surgery in instances of multiple trauma, head injury, open fractures, neurovascular injury, ipsilateral tibia fracture,

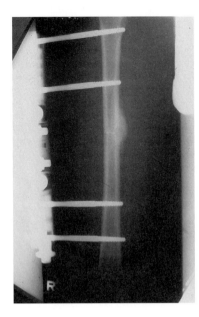

Figure 4 External fixation is a more satisfactory method of treatment of femoral fractures in children than in adults. Usually, two pins above and two pins below the fracture provide successful results.

The duration of external fixation averages about 12 to 16 weeks. Prior to frame removal, radiographs should show excellent callus formation and at least three cortices of bridging callus. As fracture healing progresses, the stiffness of the frame should be decreased or the frame should be "dynamized."

Secondary fractures can occur in patients treated with external fixation. The risk of refracture varies from 2% to 12%. Most refractures occur at the original fracture site within a week of frame removal. Fractures through a pin site have also been reported, both with the frame in place and after frame removal. The surgeon should consider the relationship between the diameter of the patient's femur and that of the pins used. If there is any concern about the amount of callus visible, cast, brace, or cast bracing should be considered. The short transverse fractures have been noted in some series to have higher refracture rates compared to longer oblique patterns.

Nailing Techniques

Intramedullary rod fixation has been quite successful in adults and its use has been extended to adolescents and older children. Locked intramedullary fixation is most useful in skeletally mature adolescents. Although reamed intramedullary antegrade nails have been used in younger patients, there are complications, specifically osteonecrosis (Fig. 5). There are no reliable salvage procedures for these patients. Another potential problem of antegrade reamed nails is trochanteric growth arrest with subsequent coxa valga. The current consensus is that use of the reamed antegrade nail through the piriformis fossa should be limited to those patients who have completed their skeletal growth with complete closure of the proximal femur physis.

and excessive shortening of the fracture fragments. The proximity of the fracture to either the knee or subtrochanteric region can influence whether surgery is necessary because of the difficulty of a cast alone holding a satisfactory reduction.

External Fixation

External fixation of femoral fractures is quite useful in children and can be applied relatively easily with minimal blood loss. Often, only two pins above and two pins below the fracture are needed (Fig. 4) unless there is concern that severe comminution or loss of the soft-tissue envelope from an open injury may prolong fracture healing. In these patients, it may be advisable to use three pins on each side of the fracture. The fractures can be placed out to length or overlapped 1.0 to 1.5 cm depending on the patient's age and the surgeon's preference. Progressive weight bearing is encouraged once callus is visible. Depending on the school and family environment, some children can return to school with the fixator. Patients are also allowed to shower or swim.

As with any treatment, there are disadvantages to external fixation. Proper pin care is necessary, and pin-tract inflammation and infection can occur in up to 10% of patients. The combination of the fracture and the pins in the lateral soft tissues of the thigh tend to limit knee range of motion. Some patients have full range of motion with the external fixator in place, while others have significantly limited motion. Patients tend to regain motion within 6 weeks following frame removal. Occasionally, gentle manipulation may be needed just prior to removal of the frame if the patient has very limited active range of motion.

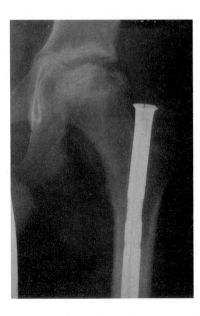

Figure 5 Osteonecrosis is seen in a large 12-year-old boy whose femoral fracture was treated with a rigid intramedullary nail through a piriformis entry site. Osteonecrosis has been reported in patients younger than age 15 years with this treatment.

Elastic or flexible intramedullary nailing has gained acceptance for the treatment of some pediatric femoral fractures, given the concerns about osteonecrosis with reamed nailing in the older child. Several variations are used with this technique. The nails can be placed retrograde or antegrade, and no reaming is done. The distal retrograde insertion is proximal to the physis. Proximally, a nail can be inserted through the trochanter; however, there is a risk of trochanteric growth arrest. Alternatively, a nail can be inserted through the lateral proximal femur just distal to the trochanteric apophysis. A single nail, such as a Rush rod, in the canal can help achieve some alignment, but a cast is required to augment the fixation because a single rod provides no rotational stability. Ender-type rods or flexible titanium rods can be placed in the canal using either a C or S configuration to achieve three-point fixation within the bone. The surgeon can bend these rods and insert them so they spring out at the fracture site to give three-point control while holding the fracture reduction. Alternatively, multiple (more than two) rods can be stacked into the canal to create more rigidity. The use of these nailing techniques requires patience and planning.

Truly elastic nailing techniques using two titanium rods allow some motion at the fracture site (Fig. 6). Some surgeons prefer a knee immobilizer or cast initially. Full weight bearing is generally delayed at least 4 to 6 weeks until early callus is visible on radiographs.

The advantage of using these nailing techniques is the reliable callus formation when the appropriate patient is selected. The best fracture patterns for these techniques are middiaphyseal transverse or short oblique fractures with little to no comminution. This same transverse fracture pattern that often has an extended healing time with external fixation typically heals readily with elastic or flexible nails.

The drawbacks to these nailing techniques are obvious and include rotational instability, risk of shortening of a comminuted fracture, and angulation of the fracture on the nails. If adequate stability cannot be achieved in some fractures, cast immobilization may be necessary. Long oblique fractures, severely comminuted fractures, and fractures near the metaphyseal-diaphyseal junction are not very suitable to this type of fixation. Fractures of the cortex at the insertion site of the nails have been reported. The development of a bursa at the insertion site over the tip of the rod just above the knee is common. When this local tissue irritation occurs, the rods typically require removal.

Variations of Ender nails with an additional loop on the end of the rod are available. The loop allows a screw to be placed across the femur through the rod at the insertion site. This ability to "lock" the rod on one end may allow these rods to handle some of the more difficult fracture patterns.

Plate Compression

Another option for the treatment of femoral fractures in children is compression plate fixation. However, diaphyseal fractures are now more frequently being treated with the other modalities, so the indications for plate fixation seem to be narrowing. Fractures of the subtrochanteric area or the area near the distal diaphyseal-metaphyseal junction can sometimes be more readily handled by plate fixation. Plate fixation has also been advocated for patients with associated head injuries because plate fixation in the setting of spasticity is better tolerated than external fixation.

With compression plating, broad 4.5-mm plates should be used, if possible. If there is any evidence of medial comminution at the fracture site, the patient should be cautioned that unprotected weight bearing may lead to plate breakage. There is also a risk of fracture through a screw hole after plate removal. Other disadvantages of open reduction with plate fixation include a long lateral scar on the thigh and increased blood loss compared to external fixation and closed elastic nailing.

Complications

Limb-length discrepancies have not been a problem in published series for most patients treated surgically for femoral fractures. Most patients have length equality

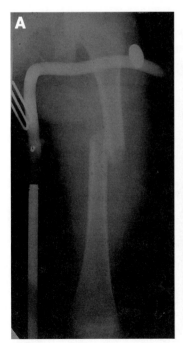
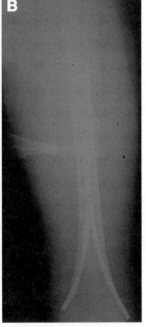

Figure 6 Flexible intramedullary nails offer a successful treatment option for transverse or short oblique diaphyseal fractures in children. **A,** Transverse diaphyseal fracture. **B,** Short oblique diaphyseal fracture.

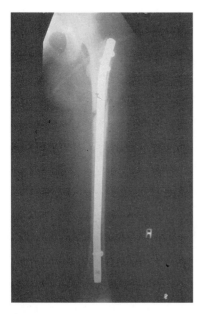

Figure 7 If necessary, an intramedullary nail may be placed through the greater trochanter in a larger adolescent who has reached skeletal maturity.

within 0.5 to 1 cm after 1 year. However, in some series, a small number of patients may have a significant difference of 2.5 cm or more. Unfortunately, predicting those individual patients who will have significant overgrowth is not possible.

Lower limb lengths should be followed after femoral fractures have healed, regardless of the treatment used. Approximately 78% of the overgrowth occurs in the first 18 months, and 85% of all patients have reached their maximum discrepancy by 42 months after fracture healing. These patients may need periodic follow-up to determine whether lower limb-length discrepancy will be a clinical problem.

Summary
In summary, in infants and children up to age 6 years, early spica cast application is reliable and should be

the treatment of choice. If the injury is a result of a high-energy accident that requires several days of observation, split-Russell skin traction can be used until application of a cast is appropriate. Excessive femoral shortening in the cast (greater than 2.5 cm) can be corrected by conversion to traction or external fixation. In this group, other clinical issues such as multiple trauma, an open fracture, head injury with spasticity, or a "floating knee" may be more easily managed with external fixation. Elastic nailing may be applicable to some patients; however, fracture pattern and femoral canal size are the limiting factors.

Children age 6 to 10 years have more treatment options. Early spica cast application can be used successfully in this group. Excessive shortening can be managed by conversion to a different treatment. In this group, patient size and the family's ability to care for the child in a cast must be considered. These factors, along with multiple trauma, head injury, open fractures, and "floating knee" may be reasons to consider other treatment modalities. External fixation, flexible intramedullary rodding, and compression plating are excellent options. Reamed intramedullary nailing is not advocated in this age group because of the risk of osteonecrosis.

Children age 10 years through adolescence are best managed with surgery. Stabilization can be provided with external fixation, flexible intramedullary rods, or compression plating. Antegrade reamed locked nailing systems inserted through the piriformis fossa are best reserved for those patients who have reached skeletal maturity with closed femoral physes. Nails inserted through the tip of the greater trochanter may be an option; however, great care must be taken to remain out of the fossa and away from the medial circumflex

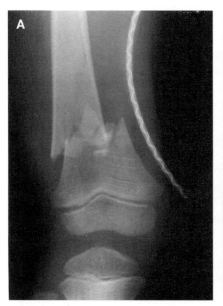
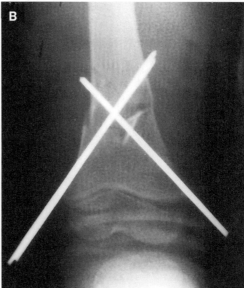

Figure 8 A, An AP radiograph of a supracondylar femur fracture. **B,** This fracture was unstable and difficult to hold by closed methods. Crossed pin fixation was performed and a cast applied. Although plate fixation could be used for this patient, a cast would probably be required because of the small distal fragment available for screws above the physis. Restriction of knee range of motion caused by half pins through the iliotibial band distally and the risk of intra-articular sepsis from pin penetration of the joint capsule make external fixation an unsatisfactory treatment option in this patient. *(Reproduced from Richards BS (ed): Orthopaedic Knowledge Update: Pediatrics. Rosemont, IL, American Academy of Orthopaedic Surgeons, 1996, pp 229-237.)*

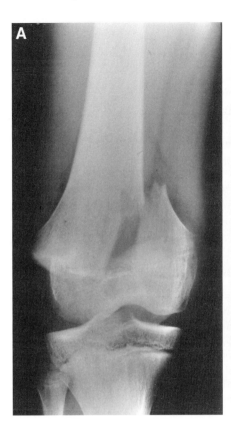
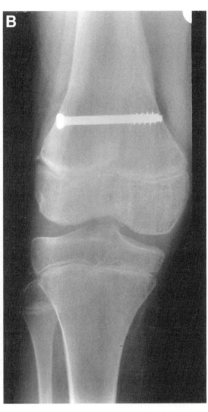

Figure 9 A, Salter-Harris type II distal femur fracture. **B,** This fracture could not be reduced by closed manipulation. The lateral side remained displaced with a gap between the epiphysis and metaphysis. A lateral approach to the distal femur allowed removal of the intervening soft tissue, and the fracture was anatomically reduced. Lateral exposure screw fixation to the large metaphyseal fragment was performed and a cast applied. More than one screw could have been used. Screws can also be placed from the medial side. *(Reproduced from Richards BS (ed): Orthopaedic Knowledge Update: Pediatrics. Rosemont, IL, American Academy of Orthopaedic Surgeons, 1996, pp 229-237.)*

vessels (Fig. 7). The guidelines for femoral fracture treatment are the same as in adults once the child reaches skeletal maturity. Antegrade reamed nails are the primary means of treatment.

Supracondylar Femur Fractures

Supracondylar femur fractures that occur just above the level of the gastrocnemius insertion typically produce apex-posterior angulation between the two fragments. Adequate alignment with cast application or traction can be achieved only if the knee is flexed to reduce the pull of the gastrocnemius. Achieving and maintaining alignment by closed methods can be difficult. The proximal fragment can be "buttonholed" through the quadriceps mechanism. The acceptable amount of angulation in a cast is less than 10° of varus or valgus, 10° of posterior bowing, and 20° of anterior bowing; however, as the child approaches the final 2 years of skeletal growth, even less angulation is acceptable.

If a satisfactory reduction cannot be maintained, treatment options include crossed pin or screw fixation with cast application (Fig. 8). Open reduction with a plate system such as a blade plate, screw plate combination, or compression plate also can be performed. If the distal femoral physis remains open, plate systems should remain proximal to the physis. Monolateral external fixation can be used; however, it is not as ideal. A circular frame may be used at this location.

Loss of knee motion with pins in the distal iliotibial band can exacerbate the development of adhesions in the quadriceps mechanism. Another drawback to external fixation at a distal level is joint sepsis secondary to inadvertent penetration of the capsule by the distal pins.

Distal Femoral Physeal Fractures

Distal femoral physeal fractures are most commonly caused by a hyperextension or valgus force. Angular and growth disturbances are common sequelae of these injuries and occur in up to 30% of patients. In children younger than age 10 years, the physis and periosteum are thicker and a greater force, such as a fall from a window or motor vehicle accident, is required to produce a fracture at this location. As the patient nears skeletal maturity, adolescent sports injuries become the common mechanisms of injury to the distal femoral physis.

Distal femoral physeal fractures in newborns also have been reported in relation to a breech delivery. These injuries can be managed with skin traction or cast immobilization. If a limb-length discrepancy or angular deformity occurs, it resolves in most infants; however, severe deformity does develop in some children.

The most widely used classification of fractures in children and adolescents is the Salter-Harris classification. Nondisplaced injuries can be managed in a well-molded long leg cast or hip spica cast with the knee slightly flexed. Because of the risk of neurovascular compression, the knee should not be positioned in extreme flexion to hold the reduction.

Displaced Salter-Harris type I and II fractures require reduction. To obtain reduction, manual longitudinal traction is followed by gentle correction of residual angulation and translation. Because forceful manipulation may further damage the physis, adequate sedation or anesthesia is required. Fractures that result from a valgus force are more stable than those from hyperextension. Percutaneous smooth pin fixation across the physis is often used to help maintain the reduction. To avoid the physis if the metaphyseal spike is larger than 2.5 cm, pin or screw fixation across the metaphyseal fragment can be used (Fig. 9). These forms of internal fixation are not rigid, so a cast is necessary. Depending on the patient's age and the fracture pattern, sufficient healing 4 to 6 weeks following injury may allow early range of motion.

When smooth pins are placed from the epiphysis through the metaphysis, proper positioning of the intra-articular pin is important. The starting point of the pin should be proximal on the epiphysis in a plane slightly posterior to the midpoint of the femoral condyle. The pins should cross above the physis in the metaphysis and engage the opposite cortex. The pins are then buried because of the risk of septic arthritis from an intra-articular pin tract if the pin is left percutaneously. These buried pins require later removal, often with anesthesia. Alternatively, smooth pins can be placed from proximal to distal, avoiding inadvertent intra-articular placement of a percutaneous pin.

Displaced Salter-Harris type III and IV fractures require anatomic reduction and fixation with pins or screws. Open reduction may be necessary. Screw fixation can be placed between the two epiphyseal regions or between the metaphyseal spike and the femoral metaphysis. The physis should be avoided with threaded fixation. Application of a cast is needed. Range of motion is started within 4 to 6 weeks.

Complications of Distal Femoral Physeal Fractures

Following a distal femoral physeal fracture, angular deformity and limb-length discrepancy are major concerns. Because angular correction during growth is not a dependable phenomenon in children and adolescents with these fractures, they should be aligned without residual angulation. Physeal bar formation can cause significant lower limb-length discrepancies. Growth arrest is not as closely linked to the Salter-Harris classification as it is to the initial severity of the injury and the amount of displacement. Patients with all types of distal femoral physeal injuries require close observa-

tion to ensure that a physeal bar and growth arrest do not develop. Radiographs obtained at 6 months and 1 year after healing can alert the physician to early physeal problems. Radiographs should be coned and centered on the growth plates. Park-Harris growth lines parallel to the physis indicate the rate and evenness of growth. If there is no evidence of growth arrest or angular deformity after the first year, the patient can be followed annually with a clinical examination until skeletal maturity. Some patients will need reconstructive procedures such as bar resection, contralateral epiphyseodesis, lengthening, or angular correction by osteotomy.

Annotated Bibliography

Hip Fractures

Cheng JC, Tang N: Decompression and stable internal fixation of femoral neck fractures in children can affect the outcome. *J Pediatr Orthop* 1999;19:338-343.

In this retrospective look at 14 fractures of the femoral neck, no cases of osteonecrosis were reported. Seven transcervical fractures with displacement were included, of which six were treated with closed reduction, aspiration of the hematoma, and screw fixation, and one was treated with open reduction and screw fixation. All were treated within 24 hours of injury. The article describes the role of aspiration of the hematoma and whether it may have a positive influence on development of osteonecrosis.

Femoral Shaft Fractures

Aronson J, Tursky EA: External fixation of pediatric femur fractures. *J Pediatr Orthop* 1996;16:342-346.

In this update of an earlier article, 132 femoral fractures were treated by external fixation for both multiple trauma and single extremity injuries. Patients were encouraged to bear weight progressively. To avoid refracture, the authors determined that complete consolidation and bridging of the fracture should be visible prior to fixator removal. Time in the external fixator averaged 11.4 weeks. There were two refractures and one fracture through a pin tract (2.1%).

Buehler KC, Thompson JD, Sponseller PD, Black BE, Buckley SL, Griffin PP: A prospective study of early spica casting outcomes in the treatment of femoral shaft fractures in children. *J Pediatr Orthop* 1995;15:30-35.

In this article, the authors indicate that telescoping of the fracture of less than 3 cm at the time of reduction predicts a 95% chance of acceptable length maintenance at healing.

Ferguson J, Nicol RO: Early spica treatment of pediatric femoral shaft fractures. *J Pediatr Orthop* 2000;20:189-192.

In this prospective study, excellent results were obtained with immediate spica cast treatment in children younger than age 10 years. The authors' major concern was the shortening that occurred in eight of 101 fractures. Four patients in whom more than 2 cm of shortening developed were converted to traction; all had less than 1.5 cm of discrepancy 6 months after injury. Another four patients had fractures that shortened but were not converted to any other treatment; these patients had 2.1 to 2.3 cm of shortening 6 months after injury. The authors reported no major problems with angular or rotational malalignment.

Hutchins CM, Sponseller PD, Sturm P, Mosquero R: Open femur fractures in children: Treatment, complications, and results. *J Pediatr Orthop* 2000;20:183-188.

Forty-three patients with open femoral fractures were studied. Union took longer in these fractures than in closed fractures. Infections were a problem only in type III fractures and occurred in half of this group. Compartment syndrome of the ipsilateral leg was also common.

Skaggs DL, Leet AI, Money MD, Shaw BA, Hale JM, Tolo VT: Secondary fractures associated with external fixation in pediatric femur fractures. *J Pediatr Orthop* 1999;19:582-586.

In this article, refractures after external fixation of the femur were reported in eight of 66 patients. Five fractures were through the original fracture site and occurred within 1 week of frame removal. Three fractures occurred through pin sites. To avoid a secondary fracture at the original site, bridging callus formation on at least three cortices was desired. The authors made no correlation between femoral diameter and pin diameter in those patients with pin-site fractures.

Stans AA, Morrissy RT, Renwick SE: Femoral shaft fracture treatment in patients age 6 to 16 years. *J Pediatr Orthop* 1999;19:222-228.

In this journal article, 85 femoral fractures were reviewed in which multiple treatment modalities were used. The fewest complications and the lowest cost were seen in children younger than age 10 years who had immediate spica cast treatment. Every other treatment option cost approximately three times the amount of the immediate spica cast treatment. The best callus formation was seen in the group that had flexible intramedullary rodding; the least amount of callus was seen in the groups that had plating and external fixation. The shortest average time to full weight bearing was seen in the group with flexible nailing (8 weeks), followed closely by the groups with immediate spica cast treatment, traction and cast, and plating (all at 10 to 12 weeks). The group with external fixation averaged 22 weeks until full weight bearing.

Distal Femur Fractures

Thomson JD, Stricker SJ, Williams MM: Fractures of the distal femoral epiphyseal plate. *J Pediatr Orthop* 1995;15:474-478.

The authors reported that in 30 fractures of the distal femoral epiphyseal plate, best results were achieved with anatomic reduction and fixation. Pin fixation prevented displacement of the fracture after reduction. In fractures treated with closed manipulation and cast alone, more than 40% subsequently became displaced. Complications including growth arrest were most frequent in displaced fractures.

Classic Bibliography

Beaty JH, Austin SM, Warner WC, Canale ST, Nichols L: Interlocking intramedullary nailing of femoral shaft fractures in adolescents: Preliminary results and complications. *J Pediatr Orthop* 1994;14:178-183.

Forlin E, Guille JT, Kumar SJ, Rhee KJ: Transepiphyseal fractures of the neck of the femur in very young children. *J Pediatr Orthop* 1992;12:164-168.

Forlin E, Guille JT, Kumar SJ, Rhee KJ: Complications associated with fracture of the neck of the femur in children. *J Pediatr Orthop* 1992;12:503-509.

Heinrich SD, Drvaric D, Darr K, MacEwen GD: Stabilization of pediatric diaphyseal femur fractures with flexible intramedullary nails: A technique paper. *J Orthop Trauma* 1992;6:452-459.

Heinrich SD, Drvaric DM, Darr K, MacEwen GD: The operative stabilization of pediatric diaphyseal femur fractures with flexible intramedullary nails: A prospective analysis. *J Pediatr Orthop* 1994;14:501-507.

Hughes LO, Beaty JH: Fractures of the head and neck of the femur in children. *J Bone Joint Surg Am* 1994;76:283-292.

Mileski RA, Garvin KL, Crosby LA: Avascular necrosis of the femoral head in an adolescent following intramedullary nailing of the femur: A case report. *J Bone Joint Surg Am* 1994;76:1706-1708.

Shapiro F: Fractures of the femoral shaft in children: The overgrowth phenomenon. *Acta Orthop Scand* 1981;52:649-655.

Ward WT, Levy J, Kaye A: Compression plating for child and adolescent femur fractures. *J Pediatr Orthop* 1992;12:626-632.

Beaty JH, Kumar A: Fractures about the knee in children. *J Bone Joint Surg Am* 1994;76:1870-1880.

Lombardo SJ, Harvey JP Jr: Fractures of the distal femoral epiphyses: Factors influencing prognosis. A review of thirty-four cases. *J Bone Joint Surg Am* 1977; 59:742-751.

Riseborough EJ, Barrett IR, Shapiro F: Growth disturbances following distal femoral physeal fracture-separations. *J Bone Joint Surg Am* 1983;65:885-893.

Chapter 10

Injuries of the Arm and Elbow

Paul D. Sponseller, MD

The orthopaedic surgeon's care for injuries to different regions of the child's upper extremity is influenced by several factors, one of which is the amount of growth remaining in these areas. Because of the great amount of growth and remodeling potential, injuries to the upper end of the humerus usually heal and remodel with careful observation. Injuries about the elbow are more likely to require precise, often surgical, reduction. A second factor that influences care is the vulnerability of the neurovascular structures, which are relatively tethered around the elbow. A third factor is the prediction of deformity. A fracture that heals in 10° to 15° of varus in the proximal humerus would produce no noticeable deformity, even if it were not to remodel, while a similar fracture in the distal humerus would be quite evident. We continue to try to understand the natural history of various fractures in an attempt to isolate those that require action and carry out that action in the safest fashion. This chapter provides an overview of current thinking and recent developments concerning injuries of the humerus and elbow.

Fractures of the Humerus

Fractures of the proximal humerus are usually classified as Salter-Harris type I injuries in neonates and infants, metaphyseal fractures in preadolescents, and Salter-Harris type II or III injuries in adolescents. These fractures likely result from the lower resistance of the physis to failure in newborns and adolescents. At birth, a neonate may sustain a type I fracture of the humerus from abduction-external rotation forces during delivery. The infant may have pseudoparalysis of the extremity, giving the impression of an Erb's palsy; however, the location of the tenderness reveals the site of the injury. Although the shoulder may appear to be dislocated on radiographs, ultrasound reveals an intact, well-located epiphysis separated from the metaphysis. Treatment includes immobilizing the arm to the infant's side with an elastic bandage for 2 weeks.

Although rare, shortening or a varus deformity of the humerus may develop in the long term.

Adolescents most commonly sustain type II proximal humeral physeal fractures. These fractures result from a hyperextension force to the shoulder in abduction. Physeal growth arrest and neurovascular injury are rare with this type of injury. Because of the active growth and remodeling potential, anatomic reduction of these fractures is not necessary. Usually, fracture alignment improves once the patient is upright and muscle spasm has subsided. Reduction is not usually indicated unless the patient is within 2 years of skeletal maturity and the fracture angulation exceeds approximately 25°. All other type II fractures may be treated with a sling and swathe. When active treatment is needed, such as in an older adolescent or a patient with multiple injuries, closed or open reduction with percutaneous pin fixation is recommended.

The same mechanism of injury causes fractures of the proximal humeral metaphysis; however, these injuries tend to affect preadolescents. Nonsurgical treatment is the rule, typically with a sling and swathe or hanging cast. The remodeling potential is great. Radiographs should be scrutinized for underlying abnormalities such as unicameral bone cysts or fibrous dysplasia. Midshaft fractures of the humerus are uncommon in children. In children younger than age 3 years, intentional injury accounts for approximately 20% of these injuries. Treatment with a functional humeral brace and sling yield excellent long-term results.

The Elbow

Elbow injuries usually require exacting treatment, which begins with proper diagnosis. Elevation of the posterior fat pad, even in the absence of a demonstrable fracture, signals an occult intracapsular fracture in more than 75% of children. Supracondylar, proximal ulnar, lateral condylar, or proximal radial fractures are most likely to be the cause of the elevated fat pad.

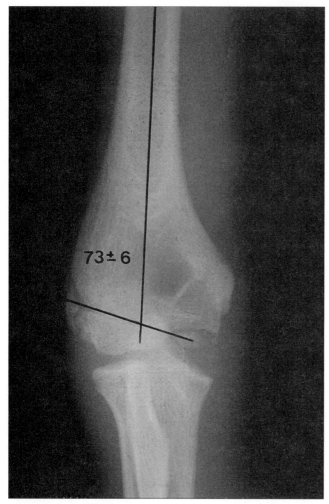

Figure 1 The normal Baumann's angle, formed by the capitellar physis and the long axis of the humerus, is 73° ± 6°.

TABLE 1 | Classification of Supracondylar Humerus Fractures and Most Common Sequelae

Type	Description	Complications
I	Nondisplaced	Missed diagnosis
II	Displaced with an intact hinge	Angulation into varus
III	Completely displaced	Vascular or neurologic damage Cubitus varus Compartment syndrome

sile failure in immature metaphyseal bone. More than 95% of these are extension injuries. Treatment is guided by classification of the fracture. A type I fracture is nondisplaced, type II is angulated but with an intact posterior cortex, and type 3 is completely displaced with no bony contact (Table 1). The less common flexion-type injury results from a fall directly on the flexed elbow. Approximately 5% of supracondylar fractures are associated with a fracture of the forearm.

Clinical Findings
In some type I fractures, especially the buckle or greenstick types typically seen in younger children, the patient may be irritable, but there may be no other evidence of a fracture, and a pulled elbow may be mistakenly diagnosed. Diffuse medial and lateral swelling should alert the examiner of the possibility of a fracture. The same mechanism of injury and clinical appearance may occur with a distal humeral physeal fracture, an injury that is most common in toddlers. By contrast, in some severe type III fractures, the fracture edge may cause the skin to pucker, suggesting that the brachialis muscle and possibly subcutaneous tissue have been displaced or torn and the neurovascular structures subjected to similar trauma. Results of a careful evaluation of the anterior interosseous, median, radial, and ulnar nerves should be recorded. Because of the severity of these injuries, the function the patient had before treatment must be documented. The anterior interosseous nerve appears to be the most commonly injured; and function can be tested by asking the patient to make a circle with the thumb and index finger, looking for flexion at the distal interphalangeal joints of each digit. Circulation should be assessed by pulse, capillary refill, color, temperature, muscle strength, and pain on passive stretch of the digits.

Radiographic Findings
When evaluating a supracondylar fracture reduction radiographically, angular malalignment must be identified using the limited view of the fracture region that

Children with an elevated posterior fat pad should be treated in a sling or a splint to promote comfort and relieve parental anxiety, as well as remove the slight risk of displacement. A recent paper defined the normal range of Baumann's angle, which is formed by the capitellar physis and long axis of the humerus, as 73° ± 6°, with little variation from side to side or with age or gender (Fig. 1). Because the normal range is broad, a radiograph of the contralateral elbow should be obtained when a fracture of the distal humerus is diagnosed, especially if the Baumann's angle of the fractured side falls at the extremes of the normal range.

Supracondylar Fractures of the Humerus
Epidemiology and Classification
Supracondylar fractures of the humerus are among the most common elbow injuries in children. They occur most often during the first decade of life and have a peak incidence in children age 5 to 7 years. The presence of the olecranon fossa decreases resistance to ten-

the radiograph provides because it may not be possible to see the elbow extended. Baumann's angle (between the lateral condylar physis and the long axis of the distal humerus) should be 73° ± 6°. Note that there is very little difference in Baumann's angle between sides in children (mean, 2°). The lateral condylar physis should be approximately 15° to 20° from perpendicular to the humeral shaft without excessive overlap or impaction of one column of the distal humerus or distraction of the other. On the lateral view, the anterior cortical line of the distal humerus should intersect the middle of the capitellum.

Treatment

Closed treatment is appropriate for type I fractures and those type II fractures in which the angulation in the coronal plane is less than approximately 5° and the hyperextension can be corrected easily. These type II fractures must be followed closely to rule out displacement. Although more severely displaced fractures also may be treated with closed reduction and a cast, the incidence of vascular problems and late malposition increases significantly. For these fractures, reduction and pin fixation has gained widest acceptance. Results of recent studies show no difference between urgent treatment (occurring within 8 hours) and elective treatment. Reduction should be performed aided by fluoroscopy and should consist of longitudinal traction/countertraction to bring the fracture into apposition, followed by angular and translational adjustment (Fig. 2). In hyperextension fractures, once this "docking" is achieved, the elbow is flexed and the distal fragment pushed with the physician's thumb to complete the realignment. If the fracture cannot be reduced, especially if there is a persistent gap between the fracture fragments, periosteum, muscle, nerve, and/or artery may be interposed. Interposition is especially likely when the fracture is initially widely displaced or the skin is tented. A maneuver to "milk" the impaled brachialis muscle from the spike of the fracture is performed by grasping the brachialis muscle while the patient's arm is held in countertraction and lifting the muscle from the spike of the proximal fragment (Fig. 3). If this maneuver is not successful, open reduction may be indicated. Although in the past, open reduction was believed to lead to increased stiffness, recent studies show that 94% of patients lose less than 15° of motion compared with the contralateral side; therefore, the surgeon should not hesitate to open the fracture and remove the interposed structures when necessary.

Following reduction, pins are then inserted percutaneously to stabilize the fracture. Placement of one pin each from the medial and lateral sides is mechanically strongest, but two pins placed laterally also are satisfactory if the surgeon prefers (Fig. 4). Pins inserted with the elbow hyperflexed may be easier in the absence of a skilled assistant; however, this position causes the ulnar nerve to be in close proximity to the medial epicondyle. Pins inserted with the elbow held in traction in minimal flexion requires two hands and a skilled assistant but may lessen the risk of ulnar nerve injury. The most common errors that occur with pin fixation include (1) failure to achieve an anatomic reduction before pin fixation, (2) placing the pins too close to the fracture site, (3) allowing the pins to exit through the fracture, and (4) failure to engage two cortices with each pin. Traction is a satisfactory treatment option for displaced fractures; the fractures may be aligned with the elbow in extension or overhead in 90° of flexion and held with an olecranon pin. However, traction is rarely practiced in North America because prolonged hospitalization is needed.

When a child with a supracondylar humeral fracture has no radial pulse, other indicators of perfusion, such as capillary refill, temperature and color of the extremity, and motor function distal to the elbow should be evaluated. Many times, the pulse will return when the fracture is reduced. However, if the pulse does not return, proper treatment depends on the clinical evidence of perfusion. An arteriogram is not needed because the location of the problem is known. If the forearm and hand do not appear well perfused, exploration by a skilled vascular surgeon is needed, addressing the entrapment, intimal tear, or transection of the brachial artery. Usually, an anterior approach is best. If ischemia has lasted more than 6 hours, a fasciotomy of the forearm should be performed. However, if the hand appears to be viable despite absence of a pulse, careful observation is one treatment option. This non-surgical approach is supported by the fact that there often is adequate collateral circulation despite damage to the brachial artery and late evidence of occlusion or stenosis in 40% of repaired arteries, with no reports of clinical sequelae. If observation is elected, the surgeon must ensure that there are no signs of ischemia. However, most surgeons prefer open exploration if the radial pulse is absent, because clinical adequacy of perfusion is often unclear in the absence of a pulse and vascular compromise may develop insidiously. Sometimes, a step as simple as extracting or untethering an entrapped brachial artery restores the pulse. A complete or an intimal tear usually is treated with a vascular graft.

Of patients with a supracondylar fracture, 8% have an associated neurologic injury. Treatment is the same as described above, and most patients recover spontaneously. Exploration and neurolysis are indicated if recovery is not seen on clinical examination or electromyography at 5 to 6 months following injury. By con-

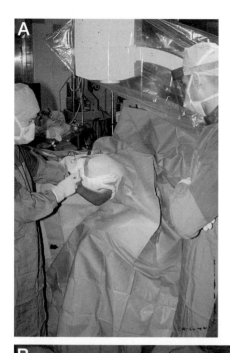

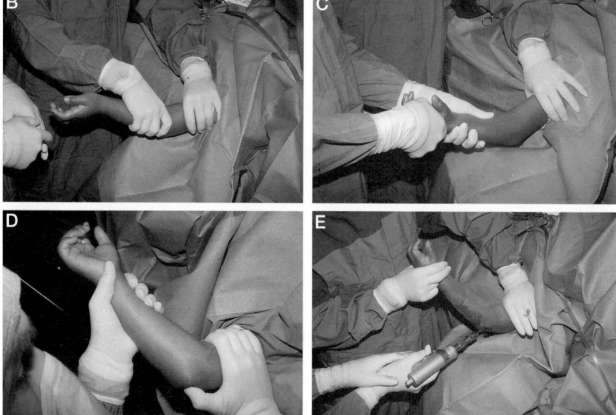

Figure 2 Sequence illustrating a technique for closed reduction and percutaneous pin fixation of a displaced supracondylar humerus fracture. **A,** The patient is moved to the side of the operating table, the C-arm is brought next to the table, and the patient's arm is rested on the large flat receiving end. **B,** Translation and angulation are reduced with the elbow in extension. **C,** Longitudinal traction in slight flexion is applied. **D,** Firm pressure by the thumb on the olecranon completes the reduction. **E,** The pins are inserted while traction is maintained in slight flexion to allow both visualization and stabilization of the fracture.

trast, if a neurologic deficit results from reduction and pinning, the nerve should be surgically explored to ensure that it is not trapped within the fracture site or by the pin.

Associated forearm fractures occur with 5% of supracondylar fractures. As long as the supracondylar fracture has been stabilized, forearm fractures can be treated by closed reduction. If forearm fractures are difficult to manage, internal fixation may be necessary.

Angular deformity, most commonly cubitus varus, following supracondylar fracture usually results from an incomplete reduction rather than a later growth deformity (Fig. 5). A varus-valgus malalignment of more than

American Academy of Orthopaedic Surgeons

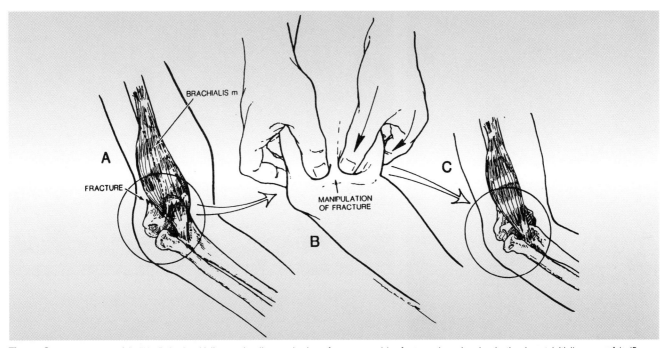

Figure 3 The technique of "milking" the brachialis muscle allows reduction of a supracondylar fracture when closed reduction is not initially successful. *(Reproduced with permission from Archibeck MJ, Scott SM, Peters CL: Brachialis muscle entrapment in displaced supracondylar humerus fractures: A technique of closed reduction and report of initial results. J Pediatr Orthop 1997;17:298-302.)*

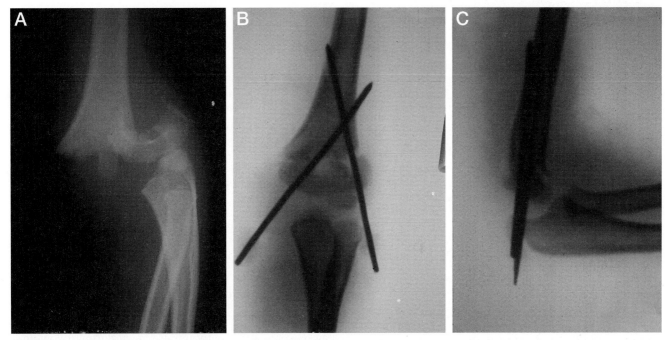

Figure 4 A, Type III supracondylar fracture of the humerus. **B** and **C,** The fracture was reduced by closed manipulation and held with two pins placed percutaneously. The medial pin enters the prominence of the medial epicondyle at an angle of approximately 45°; the lateral pin enters more distally at an angle of 30°.

10° is usually noticeable and is made more apparent with an extension at the fracture site of more than approximately 15°. Although there is no proven functional deficit from moderate malalignment, the deformity is noticeable and most families prefer correction if the deformity exceeds these parameters. Manipulation of the fracture site may be successful up to 10 to 14 days following injury; after this, results should be inspected after fracture healing and an osteotomy performed, if necessary. Osteotomy is performed in the supracondylar region of the humerus, excising a wedge or creating a dome osteotomy. Stable internal fixation is the key to maintaining correction and may be achieved by using crossed pins or small plates.

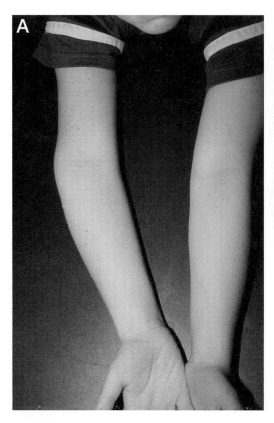
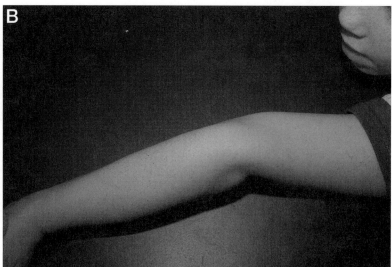

Figure 5 Malunion of a supracondylar fracture usually produces a characteristic varus deformity **(A)** and hyperextension **(B)**.

Physeal Fractures of the Distal Humerus

Physeal fractures of the distal humerus occur most often in very young children but also may occur in children up to age 6 years. Although difficult childbirth may result in physeal fractures, child abuse must be considered in the infant or toddler with this injury. Clinically and radiographically, a physeal fracture resembles an elbow dislocation (Fig. 6). In the child whose capitellum has not yet ossified, there may be no indication that the distal humerus is displaced. The key to the correct diagnosis is to remember that elbow dislocations are extremely rare in children younger than age 6 years. The distal humeral physeal fracture may be classified as a Salter-Harris type I or II injury. In a type II injury, the metaphyseal fragment is most often lateral and may resemble a lateral condyle fracture on radiographs. The distinction between a distal humeral physeal fracture and a lateral condylar fracture may be made, however, by the more circumferential swelling seen in the type II physeal fracture and the presence of medial and lateral tenderness. In addition, in a type II injury, the radius and ulna are translated as a unit with the entire distal humeral fragment; in a lateral condylar fracture, the ulna does not shift. If the diagnosis is not clear, MRI, ultrasound, or an arthrogram may confirm the correct diagnosis. If MRI is necessary, the elbow should be splinted in extension to allow the most interpretable image.

Treatment of the newborn or older child with a minimally displaced physeal fracture should consist of closed reduction and immobilization of the elbow in flexion to allow the thick periosteal hinge to hold the reduction. Minimally displaced physeal fractures occur through the broad metaphyseal surface, not the thin supracondylar bone; therefore, they are more stable than supracondylar fractures. Usually, immobilization for 3 to 4 weeks is all that is necessary. In a child with significant displacement, the fracture should be treated like a supracondylar fracture with closed reduction and percutaneous pin fixation. Because the medial epicondyle is not ossified in young children, fixation with two lateral pins is recommended. Osteonecrosis of the trochlea, presumably as a result of interruption of the lateral trochlear transphyseal vessels has been reported. In a study of children younger than age 3 years, varus deformity was seen during follow-up in most patients and was believed to be caused by a combination of incomplete reduction and osteonecrosis of the trochlea. Results were best in children who were treated with closed reduction and percutaneous pin fixation.

Intercondylar Fractures of the Distal Humerus

Intercondylar fractures, also called T- or Y-condylar fractures, of the distal humerus are more common than supracondylar fractures in adolescents, when the

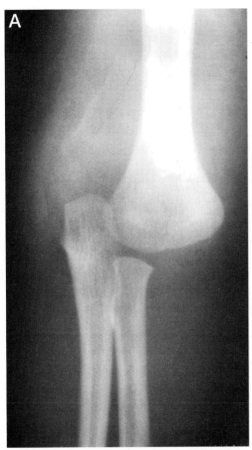
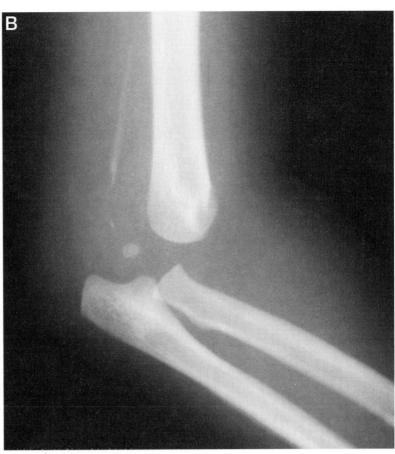

Figure 6 A, The AP radiograph of an 18-month-old infant with a 2-week-old physeal separation of the distal humerus that resembles an elbow dislocation. The radius and ulna are translated together. **B,** The lateral view demonstrates the true nature of the injury, showing the displacement of the capitellum and the periosteal reaction that follows the epiphyseal displacement. The patient's injuries were believed to be intentional.

metaphyseal bone is less plastic, but they also occur in children as young as age 8 years. The nondominant extremity is significantly more likely to be injured. Although nerve dysfunction is common with these fractures, function usually is recovered spontaneously. Patients age 10 years or younger may sometimes be treated with closed reduction and percutaneous pin fixation. No matter what the patient's age, articular displacement should be less than 2 mm or open reduction should be performed. Open reduction is usually necessary for children older than age 10 years. A posteromedial (Bryan-Morrey) approach preserves greater range of motion than a triceps-splitting approach, and the exposure is adequate for those injuries in which the intra-articular component is a single fracture line. For patients with significant intra-articular comminution, an olecranon osteotomy offers excellent visualization (Fig. 7). In patients with ulnar nerve dysfunction, decompression or transposition is recommended. Rigid fixation and early continuous passive motion minimize stiffness in teenagers. In one study, the plates and screws irritated more than one third of patients, but irritation was relieved with implant removal.

Lateral Condylar Fractures

Lateral condylar fractures commonly result in suboptimal outcomes. To some extent, this may be because the lateral condyle is mostly cartilaginous, and the rather innocuous initial appearance of the injury may result in undertreatment. Two important principles regarding lateral condylar fractures help in selecting the proper treatment method. First, nonunion may develop with displacement of more than 2 mm because the fracture is almost completely intra-articular. Second, reduction of a displaced fracture is rarely obtained or maintained in a cast because there are no external means of applying a reduction force.

In lateral condylar fractures, the cleavage plane is usually oblique, which may not be fully appreciated on AP or lateral radiographs. Oblique views are helpful if an occult lateral condylar fracture is suspected. Neurovascular injuries are not commonly associated with these fractures.

If the fracture is displaced less than 2 mm in all radiographic views, immobilization in a cast and close observation is appropriate. To detect and promptly

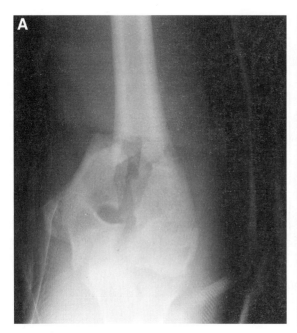

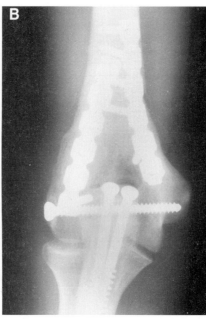

Figure 7 A, Intercondylar or T-condylar fracture in a boy age 15 years who fell on his elbow. **B,** Anatomic reduction and rigid fixation to allow early range of motion are the objectives of treatment. Because of the intra-articular nature of the fracture, it is treated in the same manner in children and adults.

treat any displacement of the fragment, radiographs should be obtained at 5 and 10 days following injury. A fiberglass splint or cast allows a better radiographic visualization of the fracture than plaster. If there is any question of the amount of displacement or compliance with follow-up instructions, pin fixation would provide a better outcome.

If the initial radiograph reveals displacement of 2 mm or more between the fracture fragments, reduction and pin fixation is necessary. An arthrogram may help to document the congruity of the joint surface. If the fracture has an intact cartilaginous hinge at the articular surface and occurred less than 48 hours earlier, a closed reduction and percutaneous pinning can be attempted. If a closed anatomic reduction cannot be achieved, an open reduction should be performed.

Pin Fixation of Lateral Condylar Fractures

A minimally displaced fracture is reduced by placing percutaneous pressure on the fragment perpendicular to the plane of the fracture, which is usually oriented posterolaterally. To prevent redisplacement, two widely spaced or divergent pins should be used. One or both pins may need to traverse the capitellum cartilage. If a closed anatomic reduction cannot be achieved, open reduction through a lateral Kocher incision is necessary. Dissection should be neither distal nor posterior to the fracture but limited to the region around the fracture because the blood supply to the lateral crista of the trochlea enters from the posterior side. The metaphysis should not be extensively exposed. If visualization of the joint is necessary, it should be anterior. The entry sites for the pins should be posterolateral. Growth will not be affected by the

temporary presence of a pin across the epiphysis. The normal tilt to the distal humerus also should be restored. The pins should engage both cortices and may back out if the far cortex is not engaged. The patient may begin elbow range of motion exercises at 4 to 6 weeks, and the pins may be removed at 6 weeks.

Complications

Delayed Union or Nonunion

If a fracture is treated only with a cast, and union is not achieved within 8 weeks, bone and grafting in situ across the metaphyseal fragment is indicated. Internal fixation may be used, and excessive dissection should be avoided. The bone graft should be packed gently into the fracture cleft after the edges are freshened, and a bone peg may be inserted into the humeral metaphysis. Late nonunion (after 12 weeks) may create a dilemma. If the nonunion remains in good position and the patient is pain-free, the nonunion may be left untreated to avoid loss of elbow motion that grafting might cause. Progressive cubitus valgus with tardy ulnar nerve palsy may develop in some lateral condylar fractures, a condition that usually evolves over many years. If this progressive shift into valgus occurs, the ulnar nerve should be transposed and the fracture grafted in situ. The fracture should not be anatomically reduced, because this may cause stiffness or osteonecrosis. If the patient has a tardy ulnar palsy, anterior transposition of the ulnar nerve should be performed. In patients with cubitus valgus, varus osteotomy is indicated if there is instability with loading or cosmetic concerns. Osteotomy will not resolve a nerve palsy or improve elbow range of motion.

Cubitus varus may develop in some patients. Cubitus varus may result from malreduction of the fracture, overgrowth of the condyle secondary to hyperemia, or osteonecrosis of the lateral portion of the trochlea. Problems resulting from cubitus varus are less severe than those from cubitus valgus. A "fishtail" or inverted-V appearance of the distal humerus may occur because of undergrowth of this avascular segment; however, its clinical importance is not believed to be great.

Medial Epicondylar Fractures

Avulsion of the medial epicondyle occurs most often in children between age 9 and 14 years and results from valgus stresses to the elbow. A medial epicondylar fracture sometimes occurs with an elbow dislocation, and the epicondylar fragment may become entrapped within the joint during reduction. The ossification center of the medial epicondyle should be differentiated from that of the trochlea. Applying tension through the flexor-pronator mass with the patient's forearm supinated and the wrist and fingers extended may free the entrapped epicondyle from the joint. Because of significant soft-tissue disruption, fractures associated with a dislocation are more difficult to treat.

Isolated displacement of the medial epicondyle is well tolerated by the patient unless significant repetitive or forceful loading is anticipated in the future. Results of long-term follow-up studies have shown that the presence of a displaced fragment does not cause significant discomfort, and fibrous union of the epicondyle functions satisfactorily. Therefore, open reduction only is indicated for an entrapped medial epicondylar fragment within the joint that fails to be extracted with manipulation or a displaced medial epicondylar fragment in the dominant arm when significant valgus loading is expected (as with tennis or baseball). Acute ulnar neuritis or palsy may occur with these avulsions but usually resolves spontaneously.

If surgical fixation is indicated, the patient is placed prone with the arm on a hand table or supine with the arm abducted and externally rotated to allow access to the posteromedial side, and a tourniquet is applied. A posteromedial Kocher-J incision is made, the fracture fragments and nerve are identified, and the fracture edges are cleared. If the fragment is incarcerated in the joint, the flexor-pronator mass is followed until it leads to the bone fragment. After reduction, a threaded pin provisionally fixes the fragment in place before it is definitively stabilized with an appropriately sized compression screw. Excessive compression with the screw must be carefully avoided or the medial epicondyle may be crushed. Countersinking the screw head or using a washer with the screw may prevent damage. An anterior transposition of the ulnar nerve is not nec-

essary. Range of motion exercises are begun 4 to 6 weeks after surgery, and the screw is removed only if it is significantly prominent. Permanent complications, other than the occasional prominence or mild restriction of extension, are rare. The same problems but with less restriction of extension can result with nonsurgical treatment.

Elbow Dislocations

Elbow dislocations occur most commonly in children older than age 6 years; however, they are not as common as supracondylar humeral fractures. Both injuries are caused by hyperextension of the elbow with abduction. Associated fractures including radial head, medial epicondylar, lateral condylar, and coronoid avulsion fractures commonly occur with elbow dislocations. Radial neck fractures must be identified before reduction to prevent displacement. Although an elbow dislocation is usually reduced under sedation in the emergency department, at times it may be necessary for the dislocation to be reduced in the operating room if the patient also has a radial neck fracture or a medial epicondyle fracture that remains in the joint, preventing a congruous reduction.

Neurologic injury occurs in approximately 10% of elbow dislocations and usually involves the ulnar nerve. Most nerve injuries resolve spontaneously. Radial nerve abnormalities are rare, but median nerve injury may result if the nerve becomes entrapped in the joint or behind the medial epicondyle. Arterial injuries with elbow dislocation are rare. Decreased range of motion follows most elbow dislocations but usually is not severe.

After reduction of an uncomplicated elbow dislocation, circulation and muscle function should be monitored, usually by close observation at home. The decision whether to hospitalize the patient depends on the amount of soft-tissue injury and the parents' ability to monitor the child. Elbow range of motion exercises should begin within 2 weeks of treatment.

Although most patients have a stable elbow after rehabilitation, a small percentage have recurrent elbow dislocations and posterolateral instability. In virtually all patients with recurrent elbow dislocations, the initial episode occurred in childhood. The responsible pathology is an attenuated posterolateral capsule. In patients who are symptomatic, repair is necessary and may be performed by reattaching the capsule securely to the lateral epicondyle.

Patients who have sustained multiple traumatic injuries or head injuries also may have late untreated elbow dislocations. If treatment is delayed for longer than 1 week, open reduction should be performed. Open reduction may be performed successfully as late as 2 years after the dislocation. Following open reduction, the patient should begin early controlled joint range of motion exercises. In addition, nonsteroidal anti-inflammatory drugs should be prescribed to prevent heterotopic ossification. Patients with very late recognized dislocations who have a reasonable range of motion in the dislocated position (an arc greater than 60°) should be treated nonsurgically.

Trauma may result in an isolated radial head dislocation. The radial head may dislocate and spontaneously reduce, manifesting only a posterior fat pad sign seen on radiographs. If this is suspected, the elbow should be immobilized and reduction documented at follow-up 2 weeks later. On both AP and lateral radiographs, the axis of the proximal radius should intersect the middle of the capitellum. A radial head dislocation may also occur with a plastic deformation of the ulna, which, at times, is quite subtle. A traumatic dislocation must be differentiated from a congenital dislocation. A congenital dislocation has a more rounded appearance to the radial head, incongruity with the capitellum, relative overgrowth of the radius, and hypoplasia of the capitellum. There also may be synostosis of the proximal radius to the ulna. Because a successful outcome is not likely, a congenital dislocation should not be reduced. However, if a traumatic dislocation is detected early, closed reduction is usually successful. Any subtle ulnar plastic or greenstick deformity must be corrected at the same time. In patients in whom dislocation is not recognized until several weeks or more later, open reduction and stabilization of the radial head using an annular ligament reconstruction should be considered. In this method, a strip of triceps fascia is harvested with its attachment to the ulna maintained, then it is woven around the radial neck and through one or two tunnels in the ulna. The ligamentous reconstruction should centralize the radial head in its articulation with the proximal ulna, not pull it eccentrically (Fig. 8). Any residual angulation of the ulna should be corrected concurrently by osteotomy.

Traumatic dislocations of the radial head have been successfully reduced as late as 7 years after injury, as long as a normal concavity of the radial head articular surface remains.

Fractures of the Proximal Radius and Ulna

The normal articular surface of the radial head forms an angle of approximately 80° with the long axis of the radius. This mild valgus angulation is best viewed on an AP radiograph. Knowledge of the normal angle helps with interpretation of fracture displacement.

Radial neck fractures are classified into three patterns, as follows: valgus force to the extended forearm resulting in an isolated fracture, a shearing force during elbow dislocation or reduction, and fracture-dislocations that result from complex mechanisms such as variations of Monteggia fractures. In fractures that result from a valgus force, an associated olecranon fracture or avulsion of the medial epicondyle often occurs. Radial neck fractures associated with dislocation usually are not impacted and have a greater amount of translation. In some of these injuries, the radial head has "flipped" 180°, resulting in an articulation between the fractured surface of the radial neck and the capitellum. Compartment syndrome also has occurred with this fracture.

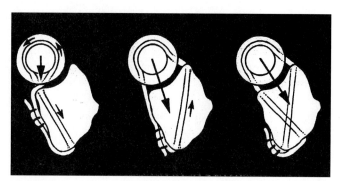

Figure 8 Three techniques of reconstructing the annular ligament using a strip of triceps fascia. Because they produce more of a symmetric restraining vector, the techniques shown in the center and at the right are preferred. *(Reproduced with permission from Seel MJ, Peterson HA: Management of chronic posttraumatic radial head dislocation in children. J Pediatr Orthop 1999;19:306-312.)*

The remodeling potential of radial neck fractures is surprisingly good (Fig. 9); however, the proximal radius is very sensitive to surgery, and growth disturbance or significant stiffness may result. Simple immobilization followed by early motion is the recommended treatment of radial neck fractures in which there is less than 30° angulation (Table 2). Closed reduction alone is indicated for fractures with an angulation between 30° and 50°. Closed reduction with percutaneous pin fixation is indicated for fractures with more than 50° of angulation that cannot be reduced by manipulation alone. Open reduction should be reserved for intra-articular fractures or severely displaced fractures that cannot be reduced with closed methods.

Closed reduction of radial neck fractures can be attempted using several methods. In one method, the fracture is manipulated with the elbow in extension. The elbow is rotated until the maximum deviation of the fracture can be palpated or visualized with fluoroscopy, then a varus stress is applied to open the lateral side, and digital pressure is applied over the angulated fragment. A second method involves manipulation with the elbow in flexion. The physician places a thumb anteriorly over the displaced radial head and forces the fragment into place with pronation. Both of these techniques are difficult if the radial head fragment is severely impacted.

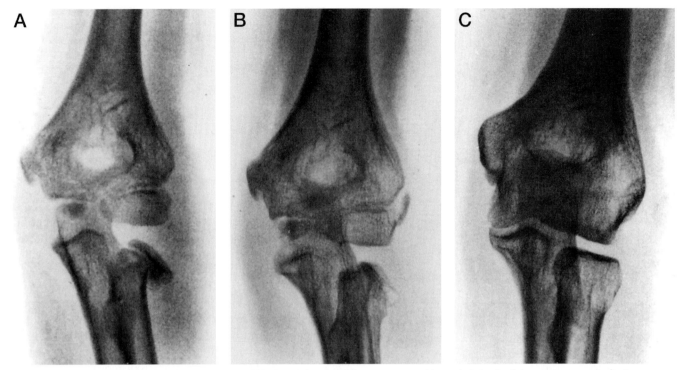

Figure 9 **A,** Radial neck fracture in a 9-year-old girl with 40° of angulation. **B,** The fracture was treated by manipulation, but little reduction was maintained. **C,** Follow-up 14 years later revealed that the fracture had remodeled completely. *(Reproduced with permission from Vocke AK, von Laer L: Displaced fractures of the radial neck in children: Long-term results and prognosis of conservative treatment.* J Pediatr Orthop *1998;7:217-222.)*

TABLE 2	Treatment Options for Displaced Radial Neck Fracture

Observation if angulation is less than 30°

Manipulation in flexion

Manipulation in extension

Manipulation with a smooth K-wire

Manipulation with an intraosseous K-wire (Metaizeau technique)

Open reduction

Severely angulated radial neck fractures are most commonly reduced using a percutaneous Steinmann pin to lever the fragment back into place. This procedure is performed in the operating room and aided by fluoroscopy. The patient's forearm is rotated until the maximum fracture profile is seen, then a Kirschner wire (K-wire) is introduced percutaneously into the radial head (Fig. 10). Irritation of the posterior interosseous nerve is avoided by introducing the K-wire posteriorly near the ulna. The K-wire, used in combination with some axial traction on the arm, pushes the radial head back into place. The Metaizeau technique disimpacts and rotates the proximal fragment using an intramedullary 1.4- to 1.8-mm K-wire with a short

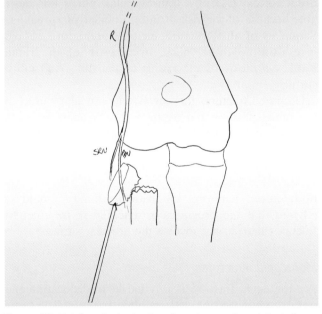

Figure 10 Technique showing insertion of percutaneous pin posterior to the superficial radial nerve to reduce a displaced radial neck fracture. Alternatively, the pin could be inserted obliquely across the fracture and used for fixation if needed.

curve in it that is introduced through the distal radial metaphysis and passed proximally (Fig. 11).

Open reduction through a lateral approach may be necessary for a severely angulated fracture that cannot be reduced with closed or percutaneous methods. If the reduction is stable through a reasonable range of

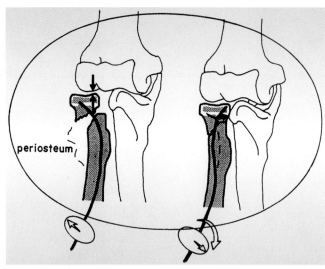

Figure 11 *The Metaizeau technique of reducing a displaced radial neck fracture. (Reproduced with permission from Gonzalez-Herranz P, Alvarez-Romera A, Burgos J, Rapariz JM, Hevia E: Displaced radial neck fractures in children treated by closed intramedullary pinning (Metaizeau technique). J Pediatr Orthop 1997;17:325-331.)*

TABLE 3	Monteggia Classification and Preferred Position	
Type	**Description**	**Immobilization**
I	Anterior dislocation	Hyperflexion; supination
II	Posterior	Flexion and midposition of rotation
III	Lateral	Flexion and midposition of rotation
IV	Divergent	Flexion

rotation, no fixation is needed; however, an unstable reduction requires fixation, preferably using an intraosseous technique. A percutaneous K-wire is passed from the proximal-lateral corner of the proximal radius and across the fracture site to engage the distal cortex. Use of a transcapitellar pin is less desirable because of the risk of intra-articular pin breakage. Sequelae of this fracture include premature growth arrest of the radial neck, overgrowth of the radial head, synostosis of the radius to the ulna, and elbow stiffness.

Displaced fractures that involve the articular surface of the radial head should be treated with open reduction and internal fixation. Because much of the proximal radial epiphysis is not ossified, the size of the articular fragments is underestimated on radiographs. The risk of stiffness and growth disturbance is greater with this type of fracture; therefore, the patient's family should be advised that the prognosis is generally worse than for fractures that do not involve the articular surface.

Monteggia Fractures

A Monteggia fracture is a radial head dislocation that occurs in conjunction with an ulnar fracture. The radial head dislocates in the direction of the apical ulnar angulation. Approximately 70% of Monteggia fractures are classified as type I fractures, defined as an ulnar fracture with anterior dislocation of the radial head. A type II fracture involves posterior dislocation and comprises only 5% of Monteggia fractures. A type III fracture involves lateral dislocation and comprises 25% of Monteggia fractures. A type IV fracture is rare and is a fracture of both the ulna and radius with a disloca-

tion of the radius. Isolated radial head dislocations without an obvious ulnar fracture or ulnar shaft fractures with an associated radial neck fracture are called Monteggia-equivalent lesions.

Most Monteggia fractures in children may be treated with closed reduction (Table 3). The strong ulnar periosteum usually allows a satisfactory ulnar reduction that in turn allows the radial head to be reduced. However, a relatively oblique, comminuted, or otherwise hard-to-control ulnar fracture may require primary stabilization. In type I injuries, the radial head dislocation should be reduced with the elbow flexed and fully supinated. In type II injuries, the elbow should be extended and the forearm placed in 45° of pronation. In type III injuries, the elbow should be flexed to 90° with supination. Type IV injuries are usually treated with the elbow in flexion. Closed reduction of the radial head usually can be obtained as late as 2 weeks after the fracture. Imperfect reduction of the ulna, an infolded annular ligament, or buttonholing of the radial head through the joint capsule may prevent reduction of the radial head. Initial treatment of unsatisfactory closed reductions consists of internal fixation of the ulna followed by open reduction of the radial head, if necessary. Radial head dislocations may be reduced up to 7 years after the injury and still achieve satisfactory range of motion. Ulnar angulation must be corrected and can be stabilized with an intramedullary rod.

Complications of Monteggia fractures include restriction of motion, recurrent dislocations, and nerve palsy. Most commonly, the radial or posterior interosseous nerve is injured, usually in type III injuries. Spontaneous neural recovery can be expected.

Olecranon Fractures

Olecranon fractures are rare in children. The fractures occur at a slightly older age in children (9 years) than supracondylar fractures, and 20% of patients have associated fractures about the elbow. Most olecranon fractures are obvious on radiographs (Fig. 12), but the

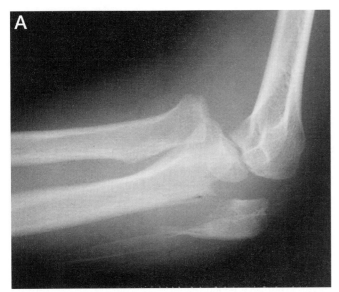

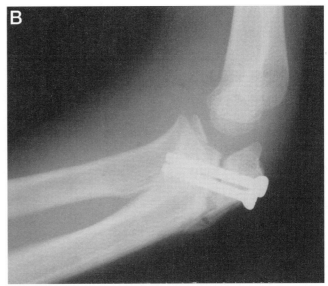

Figure 12 **A,** Closed reduction of an olecranon fracture with dislocation of the elbow. **B,** Reduction was followed by percutaneous pin fixation.

extent of displacement may be underestimated. Some fractures are occult, presenting only with an elevated posterior fat pad. A "sleeve" fracture, which is an apophyseal avulsion that occurs with the elbow flexed, is a subtle form of this injury. Lateral radiographs may only reveal a small metaphyseal fleck of bone. Olecranon fractures displaced 3 mm or more on plain radiographs need reduction and fixation. Tension band wires provide predictably good results.

Elbow Capsular Contracture

Children rarely lose significant range of motion following elbow fractures; however, there are exceptions. If elbow range of motion is less than 30° to 130°, which is considered the useful arc of elbow flexion-extension needed for activities of daily living, significant impairment may result. Initial treatment should include static and dynamic splinting. If range of motion does not improve, surgical release of the capsular contracture may be indicated. This procedure is performed through a lateral incision, including the entire anterior or posterior capsule as needed and removing any fragments that prevent motion. In one study of nine children, a mean improvement of 50° was noted after open surgical release of the capsular contracture.

The successful treatment of pediatric elbow fractures depends on the physician's understanding of ossification and fracture patterns, and knowing which fractures are at risk for nonunion, stiffness, or growth disturbance. Good judgment is needed to select the proper treatment.

Annotated Bibliography

Fractures of the Humerus

Rockwood CA Jr, Wilkins KE, Beaty JH, Green DP (eds): *Fractures in Children*, ed 4. Philadelphia, PA, JB Lippincott, 1996, vol 3.

This definitive reference provides excellent information on the history, anatomy, treatment, and complications of fractures in children.

Shaw BA, Murphy KM, Shaw A, Oppenheim WL, Myracle MR: Humerus shaft fractures in young children: Accident or abuse? *J Pediatr Orthop* 1997;17: 293-297.

This retrospective review was undertaken because of the common belief that humeral shaft fractures in children younger than age 3 years are often caused by abuse. Only 18% of 34 fractures in this study were classified as probable abuse. No aspect of the fracture pattern was pathognomonic of abuse. Thus, a complete history, physical and appropriate radiographic examination are necessary before any conclusions can be made.

Fractures of the Distal Humerus

Archibeck MJ, Scott SM, Peters CL: Brachialis muscle entrapment in displaced supracondylar humerus fractures: A technique of closed reduction and report of initial results. *J Pediatr Orthop* 1997;17:298-302.

A technique of disengaging or "milking" the brachialis muscle from the proximal humerus in displaced supracondylar fractures is described. This technique may be useful in patients in whom the fracture is difficult to reduce.

Copley LA, Dormans JP, Davidson RS: Vascular injuries and their sequelae in pediatric supracondylar humerus fractures: Toward a goal of prevention. *J Pediatr Orthop* 1996;16:99-103.

The authors describe a case of supracondylar fracture in which the patient had a delayed loss of pulse and subsequent Volkmann contracture. In 17 other patients, steps were taken to restore the pulse, and no ischemic sequelae resulted.

Fleuriau-Chateau P, McIntyre W, Letts M: An analysis of open reduction of irreducible supracondylar fractures of the humerus in children. *Can J Surg* 1998;41:112-118.

Open reduction of displaced supracondylar fractures was performed on 41 patients whose fractures could not be reduced under anesthesia. Findings during surgery included entrapment of the brachialis muscle alone in 35% of patients, with the radial median nerve in an additional 5%, and with the brachial artery in 10%. Wide displacement of the fracture fragments with loss of cortical contact and bruising or puckering of the skin were frequent preoperative findings. Range of motion returned to within 15° of normal or better in 94% of patients. The pulse should be carefully monitored in patients with these physical findings, and open reduction should be performed if the pulse is lost or closed reduction is unsuccessful.

Iyengar SR, Hoffinger SA, Townsend DR: Early versus delayed reduction and pinning of type III displaced supracondylar fractures of the humerus in children: A comparative study. *J Orthop Trauma* 1999;13:51-55.

Fifty-eight patients were retrospectively classified into two groups treated with reduction and pin fixation. One group was treated within 8 hours of the injury; the other was treated more than 8 hours after injury. Both groups did equally well, suggesting that elective treatment can be performed to save hospital resources.

Keenan WN, Clegg J: Variation of Baumann's angle with age, sex and side: Implications for its use in radiological monitoring of supracondylar fracture of the humerus in children. *J Pediatr Orthop* 1996;16:97-98.

This review of 577 radiographs of the elbow in children without fracture showed that the normal Baumann's angle is 73° ± 6°. There is a minimal (2°) variation between sides or with age or gender.

Oh CW, Park BC, Ihn JC, Kyung HS: Fracture-separation of the distal humeral epiphysis in children younger than three years old. *J Pediatr Orthop* 2000;20:173-176.

Twelve patients with fracture of the distal humerus epiphysis that was treated with different methods were followed up for a mean of 2 years. Cubitus varus that was believed to result from osteonecrosis of the trochlea was seen in seven patients. However, follow-up was not long enough to determine the long-term importance of any osteonecrosis. Best results were achieved with closed reduction and percutaneous pin fixation.

Re PR, Waters PM, Hresko T: T-Condylar fractures of the distal humerus in children and adolescents. *J Pediatr Orthop* 1999;19:313-318.

In 17 T-condylar fractures of the distal humerus, the Bryan-Morrey approach was preferred to the triceps splitting because it allowed the patient greater range of motion. Results of olecranon osteotomy were good in patients with significant comminution. Early motion is recommended.

Sabharwal S, Tredwell SJ, Beauchamp RD, et al: Management of pulseless pink hand in pediatric supracondylar fractures of the humerus. *J Pediatr Orthop* 1997;17:303-310.

Thirteen patients with a pulseless but clinically well-perfused hand associated with a supracondylar fracture of the humerus underwent procedures to restore a pulse. The patients were followed at a mean of 31 months, and a history, magnetic resonance angiogram, and doppler ultrasound were obtained. At follow-up, two patients had an occluded artery and four had stenosis, but each patient had a pulse. None of the patients had symptoms of cold or exercise intolerance or growth disturbance.

Skaggs DL, Mirzayan R: The posterior fat pad sign in association with occult fracture of the elbow in children. *J Bone Joint Surg Am* 1999;81:1429-1433.

An occult fracture was revealed on repeat radiographs 3 weeks after injury in 76% of children with posterior fat pad elevation but no initial finding of fracture. The most common fractures were supracondylar or lateral condylar humeral or proximal ulnar fractures.

Elbow Dislocations

Weisman DS, Rang M, Cole WG: Tardy displacement of traumatic radial head dislocation in childhood. *J Pediatr Orthop* 1999;19:523-526.

A late diagnosis of radial head dislocation was made in 10 of 110 patients who either had an isolated injury or a Monteggia fracture-dislocation. In eight of the 10 patients, the dislocation could be seen on early radiographs, but in two of the 10 patients, the dislocation was clearly reduced at the initial visit following a traumatic injury and dislocated on a later visit. The authors theorize that in these two patients, the dislocation reduced spontaneously and later dislocated again.

Fractures of the Proximal Radius and Ulna

Vocke AK, Von Laer L: Displaced fractures of the radial neck in children: Long-term results and prognosis of conservative treatment. *J Pediatr Orthop* 1998;7: 217-222.

In this review of 38 children with displaced radial neck fractures, follow-up occurred at 2 to 20 years (mean, 11 years) following injury. Of these patients, 23 were treated with simple cast immobilization, seven with closed reduction, and eight with open reduction. All fractures with angulation of up to 50° that were treated nonsurgically reduced spontaneously. Functional disturbance was found in four patients and this problem was attributed to spontaneous radioulnar synostosis in one patient, growth disturbance in one patient, and stiffness in two patients. Three of the four patients with limitation had undergone open reduction. The authors recommend simple immobilization for fractures with angulation up to 50°, closed reduction with a pin in those with greater angulation, and open reduction only for patients with a completely displaced fragment in the joint.

Gonzalez-Herranz P, Alvarez-Romera A, Burgos J, Rapariz JM, Hevia E: Displaced radial neck fractures in children treated by closed intramedullary pinning (Metaizeau technique). *J Pediatr Orthop* 1997;17:325-331.

Excellent results were obtained in 94% of patients with displaced radial neck fractures who were treated with a rotated retrograde intramedullary K-wire.

Peters CL, Scott SM: Compartment syndrome in the forearm following fractures of the radial head or neck in children. *J Bone Joint Surg Am* 1995;77:1070-1074.

Compartment syndrome was reported in three patients following fracture of the radial head or neck resulting from a fall. This seemingly unlikely complication occurred even though one of the three patients had a minimally displaced fracture.

Monteggia Fractures

Seel MJ, Peterson HA: Management of chronic post-traumatic radial head dislocation in children. *J Pediatr Orthop* 1999;19:306-312.

Open reduction provided good to excellent results in children with chronic posttraumatic radial head dislocation as long as the normal concavity of the radial head was preserved. Surgery was performed up to 7 years after injury.

Olecranon Fractures

Gaddy BC, Strecker WB, Schoenecker PL: Surgical treatment of displaced olecranon fractures in children. *J Pediatr Orthop* 1997;17:321-324.

Satisfactory results were obtained in 35 children following treatment of displaced olecranon fractures. Patients with displacement of less than 3 mm were treated with immobilization for 3 weeks; open reduction and internal fixation was performed on patients with greater displacement.

Classic Bibliography

Bernstein SM, McKeever P, Bernstein L: Percutaneous reduction of displaced radial neck fractures in children. *J Pediatr Orthop* 1993;13:85-88.

Culp RW, Osterman AL, Davidson RS, Skirven T, Bora FW Jr: Neural injuries associated with supracondylar fractures of the humerus in children. *J Bone Joint Surg Am* 1990;72:1211-1215.

Flynn JC: Nonunion of slightly displaced fractures of the lateral humeral condyle in children: An update. *J Pediatr Orthop* 1989;9:691-696.

Fowles JV, Slimane N, Kassab, MT: Elbow dislocation with avulsion of the medial humeral epicondyle. *J Bone Joint Surg Br* 1990;72:102-104.

Josefsson PO, Danielsson LG: Epicondylar elbow fracture in children: 35-year follow-up of 56 unreduced cases. *Acta Orthop Scand* 1986;57:313-315.

Mih AD, Wolf FG: Surgical release of elbow-capsular contracture in pediatric patients. *J Pediatr Orthop* 1994;14:458-461.

Pirone AM, Graham HK, Krajbich JI: Management of displaced extension-type supracondylar fractures of the humerus in children. *J Bone Joint Surg Am* 1988;70: 641-650.

Voss FR, Kasser JR, Trepman E, Simmons E Jr, Hall JE: Uniplanar supracondylar humeral osteotomy with preset Kirschner wires for posttraumatic cubitus varus. *J Pediatr Orthop* 1994;14:471-478.

Chapter 11

Forearm and Wrist Fractures

Peter M. Waters, MD

Introduction

A child's growing years are a period of high risk for forearm fractures. Forearm fractures are the most common long bone fractures in children, accounting for 45% of all childhood fractures and 62% of upper extremity fractures. Approximately 75% to 84% of forearm fractures occur in the distal third; 15% to 18%, in the middle third; and less than 5%, in the proximal third. Less commonly, children sustain injuries to the distal radioulnar joint, carpal bones, or intercarpal ligaments. The most common carpal bone fracture is of the scaphoid; yet this fracture accounts for only 0.45% of all upper extremity fractures in children.

A current understanding of the best methods of treatment for forearm fractures is important for almost all orthopaedic surgeons. Recent developments include a better understanding of the effect of malunion in both-bone fractures and the indications for intramedullary fixation in some of these fractures.

Diaphyseal Fractures of the Radius and Ulna

Types of Fractures

Diaphyseal fractures are classified as plastic deformation, buckle or torus, greenstick or incomplete, or complete fractures. Approximately 50% of diaphyseal fractures are greenstick fractures and most often occur in children younger than age 8 years. Greenstick fractures most commonly have apex volar malangulation and supination rotational deformity. Incomplete fractures have apex dorsal malangulation and pronation rotational deformity and occur less commonly. The principle of treatment of closed reduction in both greenstick and incomplete fractures is the same: correct the malrotation first, then the malangulation. Complete fractures are more common in the preadolescent and adolescent age groups and tend to be unstable.

The forearm rotates an average of 150° to 180°, with the mechanical axis of rotation extending from the proximal radius to the distal ulna. Rotational malalignment of a forearm fracture directly results in a loss of this rotation in a ratio of at least 1:1. In middle third diaphyseal fractures with malrotation, this loss of rotation may have a ratio as high as 2:1. Bayonet apposition of one or both bones of the forearm is acceptable as long as the fragments are parallel.

Frontal or sagittal angulation also limits forearm rotation. Angular deformity greater than 20° significantly decreases pronation and supination. Fortunately, an angular deformity will remodel in children, but remodeling depends on the patient's age, proximity of the fracture to the physis, amount of deformity, and direction of the angular deformity. Remodeling of an angular deformity of the radius may be as much as 10° per year. Remodeling potential and outcome may be better assessed by the index of axis deviation than by measurement of the amount of angulation alone. Axis deviation is the deviation of the fracture apex from a straight line between the proximal and distal articular surfaces and is calculated from reference tables. However, the clinical outcome of forearm rotation does not always correlate with the degree of malunion. Criteria for acceptable reduction of diaphyseal fractures have not been definitively established and clearly depend on the patient's age and location of the fracture. Fractures of the proximal third of the radius tend to be the least forgiving of malangulation deformities. Fracture remanipulation following an axis deviation measurement of greater than 5 in younger patients and 3 in near-skeletally mature patients has been recommended.

By definition, torus or buckle fractures are stable; cortical failure occurs only in compression and not in tension. Immobilization in a short arm cast for 3 to 4 weeks provides pain relief and prevents further injury. If both cortices are fractured, there is a risk that

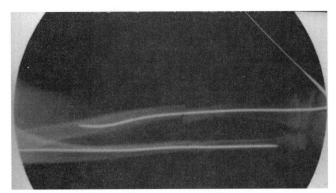

Figure 1 Radiograph of intramedullary fixation of diaphyseal radial and ulnar fractures.

TABLE 1	Indications for Considering Internal Fixation of Forearm Fractures

Diaphyseal fractures

    Irreducible fracture (after closed or open reduction)
    Unstable fracture in adolescent
    Displaced segmental fracture
    Fracture associated with unstable Monteggia, Galeazzi, or
       supracondylar fracture
    Refracture

Metaphyseal fractures

    Neurovascular compromise
    Significant soft-tissue swelling or injury
    Concomitant fracture of the elbow
    Loss of reduction

Physeal fractures

    Median nerve injury
    Intra-articular fracture (displaced)
    Loss of reduction

malangulation will occur gradually, and a well-molded long arm cast should be used. Greenstick fractures generally are stable after a closed reduction and can be treated in a long arm cast with appropriate three-point molding, use of an interosseous mold, and a straight ulnar border. Because most greenstick fractures have apex volar malangulation and supination malrotation, the malrotation should first be corrected by pronating the forearm, followed by correction of the apex volar angulation using three-point molding. Often, these fractures can be manipulated with conscious sedation in the ambulatory setting. Nitrous oxide and parenterally administered narcotic-benzodiazepine combinations are the most commonly used agents and may be supplemented by a hematoma block. Use of ketamine as an anesthetic during reduction of these fractures is reliable, safe, and effective. It is particularly helpful if there is a portable flouroscopy unit available to immediately assess the reduction.

Treatment

Displaced complete diaphyseal fractures are difficult to reduce with closed treatment and frequently are unstable. Closed reduction requires aligning the distal fragment with the proximal fragment by correcting the malrotation, angulation, and translation sequentially. If both bones are displaced, it often is best to reduce the ulna first. However, there is a high incidence of loss of reduction with this method. More recently, unstable diaphyseal forearm fractures have been treated with intramedullary fixation. The intramedullary device can be placed percutaneously after successful closed reduction. The ulnar pin is passed from proximal to distal, while the radial pin is placed from distal to proximal, with the entry site proximal to the distal radial physis (Fig. 1). The type of intramedullary device may be a smooth Steinmann pin (usually 5/64" or 0.064"), Rush rod (3/32", 1/8", or 3/16"), or elastic intramedullary nail (2 mm or 2.5 mm). The diameter of the rod should be approximately one third that of the intramedullary canal. The ends of the rods may be buried

or left protruding through the skin. Despite the seeming simplicity of this method, minor complications, such as migration of the rod, loss of reduction, or infection, are not uncommon. Rotational alignment is not as well controlled with rods as it is with plates. There seems to be no clear superiority of rods over plates in children. Plates provide better control of the fracture; however, they require a larger incision, longer operative time for surgery, and are more difficult to remove.

The considerations for open reduction are listed in Table 1.

Fractures of the Distal Radius and Ulna
Metaphyseal Fractures

The distal radius is involved in 75% to 84% of pediatric forearm fractures. Most of these radial fractures are metaphyseal and associated with metaphyseal ulnar fractures. Although closed reduction and immobilization in a long arm cast is indicated for fractures with greater than 10° of malalignment, several recent studies indicate a high incidence of loss of reduction with closed treatment of these fractures. Poor casting techniques, isolated radial fractures, associated displaced ulnar fractures or plastic deformation, and initial malangulation of greater than 30° have been implicated as causes. The need for repeat closed reduction has been cited to be as high as 34%. Percutaneous pin fixation eliminates the need for repeat reduction of difficult distal radial frac-

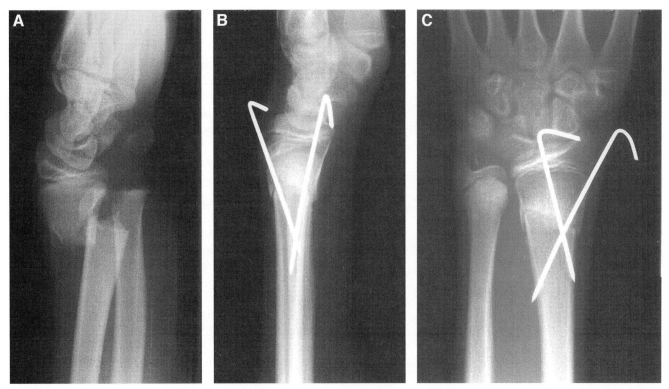

Figure 2 **A,** A displaced metaphyseal fracture of the distal radius. **B** and **C,** The fracture was treated with percutaneous fixation. Care must be taken to avoid the radial sensory nerve and, if possible, the distal radial physis.

tures, but it does carry with it the issues of anesthesia, problems with pin placement or infection, and scarring. Malunited fractures will remodel in the flexion/extension plane and, to a lesser extent, in the radial deviation/ulnar deviation plane. However, rotational malunion will not remodel. Currently, what represents an acceptable alignment after reduction is controversial but clearly depends on the patient's age, fracture location, and other injuries.

Percutaneous pinning may be indicated for fractures associated with neurovascular compromise, significant soft-tissue swelling, initial angulation of greater than 30°, displacement of more than 50% of the diameter of the radius, or concomitant fractures of the elbow. A smooth Kirschner wire (K-wire) is inserted obliquely from distal to proximal, starting in the radial metaphysis just proximal to the physis (Fig. 2). During insertion, the radial sensory nerve must be avoided. This may be done by using a 5- to 10-mm incision and clearing the pin track. A second, crossing K-wire can be inserted from between the third and fourth dorsal extensor compartments while avoiding the extensor pollicus longus tendon at the level of Lister's tubercle.

Distal Radial Physeal Fractures

Most distal radial physeal fractures are Salter-Harris type II injuries that occur in the adolescent. Displace-

ment typically is dorsal with apex volar angulation. Atraumatic closed reduction and immobilization in a long arm cast is indicated for fractures with greater than 10° of malangulation. The most significant concerns associated with these fractures are future growth arrest and acute neurovascular compromise. The incidence of associated nerve injuries was 8% in one prospective study. Another retrospective series reported that patients with signs or symptoms of median nerve injury at the time of presentation would be best managed with percutaneous pin fixation rather than cast immobilization, in order to reduce the risk of forearm compartment syndrome, acute carpal tunnel syndrome, or median neuropathy. A single oblique smooth K-wire inserted from the radial styloid distally and directed to the ulnar aspect of the radial metaphysis proximally provides sufficient fixation. As with metaphyseal fractures, the radial sensory nerve must be avoided during pin insertion. If left percutaneous, the K-wire can be readily removed in the office after 4 weeks. A concern regarding the risk of pin placement across the physis is growth arrest. Smooth, small-diameter pins should be used and removed at 3 to 4 weeks to lessen this concern.

Growth arrest is related to two factors: the amount of initial trauma affecting the physis and iatrogenic injury. To avoid iatrogenic physeal arrest, patients with redisplacement or late presentation should not undergo

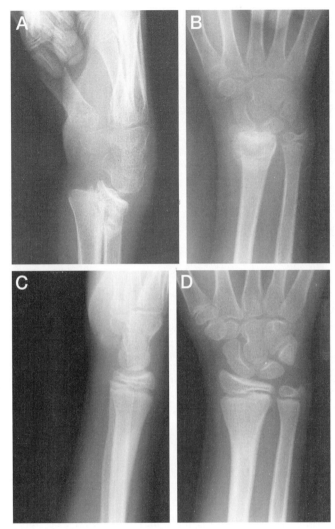

Figure 3 **A** and **B,** Radiographs of an 11-year-old boy who presented late with a significantly displaced Salter-Harris type II distal radial physeal fracture. **C** and **D,** Remodeling was monitored with growth, and subsequent radiographs 1 year after the fracture showed anatomic alignment of the radius with open physes. *(Reproduced from Richards BS (ed): Orthopaedic Knowledge Update: Pediatrics. Rosemont, IL, American Academy of Orthopaedic Surgeons, 1996, pp 251-257.)*

repeat reduction after 7 days. Late open reduction should be avoided for the same reason.

Because these fractures displace in the plane of motion of the wrist joint and are near the physis, there is tremendous potential for remodeling of a malunion in the younger adolescent (Fig. 3). If the malunion does not remodel with growth, a dorsal opening wedge osteotomy with bone graft and internal fixation may be needed for the skeletally mature patient with greater than 10° of apex dorsal malangulation. Finally, patients with displaced physeal fractures should be examined 1 to 2 years after the fracture to rule out growth disturbance. If a radial growth arrest does occur, the continued ulnar growth can result in distal radioulnar joint incongruity, ulnocarpal impaction, and a triangular fibrocartilage complex (TFCC) tear. If the radial growth arrest is recognized early, it can be resolved by

physeal bar resection or ulnar epiphysiodesis, depending on the clinical situation and patient's age.

Salter-Harris type III and IV fractures are rare but require anatomic reduction to restore articular and physeal congruity. Open reduction is indicated for those fractures in which closed reduction has failed. Wrist arthroscopy used in adolescents can aid and assess closed reductions and percutaneous fixation.

Galeazzi Fractures

A Galeazzi fracture is defined as a distal radial fracture and distal radioulnar joint disruption. True Galeazzi injuries are rare in children. More common is a Galeazzi equivalent, with an ulnar physeal fracture associated with a distal radial metaphyseal or physeal fracture. Anatomic reductions of both radial and ulnar fractures are required to restore normal function. In children, reduction often can be achieved using a closed method. Inability to achieve a closed reduction of the ulnar physeal fracture may result from extensor tendon or periosteal interposition. If so, an open reduction is required. Late instability is rare following this fracture, but premature ulnar physeal arrest and shortening has been reported in up to 55% of patients with distal ulnar physeal fractures.

Carpal Injuries

Triangular Fibrocartilage Complex Tears

Persistent ulnar-sided wrist pain in an adolescent with an ulnar styloid nonunion or hypertrophic union often represents ulnocarpal impaction. It may be associated with a peripheral TFCC tear. In patients in whom nonsurgical management is not successful, excision of the nonunion or hypertrophic union and repair of the TFCC tear reduces pain and improves motion and function.

Unresolved ulnar-sided wrist pain may indicate an unrecognized TFCC tear, which can be confirmed by diagnostic arthroscopy of the wrist. Wrist arthrography and MRI have less sensitivity and specificity when compared with wrist arthroscopy in prospective studies comparing multiple imaging techniques. The development of the 2.5- to 3.0-mm diameter arthroscopes and small instruments has offered easy access to the radiocarpal, midcarpal, and radioulnar joints. Isolated tears of the TFCC are now being diagnosed with increasing frequency in adolescents. Arthroscopic repair of peripheral TFCC tears has been successful in adolescents.

Scaphoid Fractures

Most scaphoid fractures in the skeletally immature patient are fractures of the waist or avulsions of the

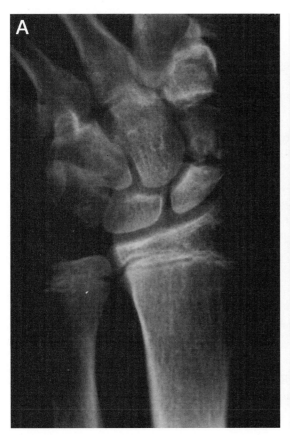
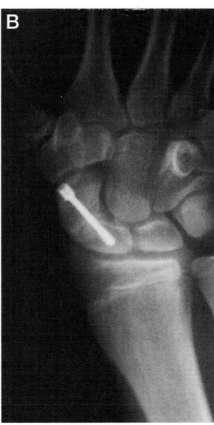

Figure 4 **A,** Scaphoid nonunion in a skeletally immature patient. **B,** Treatment with an iliac crest bone graft and Herbert screw fixation was successful. *(Reproduced from Richards BS (ed):* Orthopaedic Knowledge Update: Pediatrics. *Rosemont, IL, American Academy of Orthopaedic Surgeons, 1996, pp 251-257.)*

distal pole. These fractures rarely are displaced, probably because of the relatively thick rim of nonossified cartilage. These fractures readily heal with immobilization in a thumb spica cast for 4 to 8 weeks with minimal risk of nonunion or osteonecrosis (ON). However, scaphoid waist fractures carry the same risks of nonunion and ON in the child and adolescent as they do in the adult. Scaphoid waist fractures should be assessed with tomograms for fracture displacement. Nondisplaced fractures require immobilization in a thumb spica cast for 3 to 6 months until they have healed. The issue of whether to immobilize the fracture in a long arm or short arm thumb spica cast is unresolved. Recently, these fractures have been treated with percutaneous cannulated screw fixation; however, the efficacy of this technique is still unknown. An established nonunion in a child or adolescent should be treated with open reduction, bone grafting, and, possibly, internal fixation (Fig. 4). The issue of whether a bipartite scaphoid, even if bilateral, is congenital or posttraumatic is unresolved; however, if a bipartite scaphoid is symptomatic, it should be treated as a nonunion with open reduction and bone grafting. Proximal pole scaphoid fracture nonunions complicated by ON rarely occur in adolescents. Distal radial vascularized bone grafting can be successful in this rare, complicated injury.

Adolescent Wrist Pain

Most adolescents with chronic wrist pain do not have a traumatic intercarpal ligamentous or TFCC tear. Many of these adolescents have generalized ligamentous laxity and pain from midcarpal wrist instability. These patients often respond positively to a prolonged strengthening program. On rare occasions, the source of the chronic pain is an underlying scapholunate ligamentous tear. Most of these injuries are partial ligament tears with chondral impingement in the scaphoid or lunate fossa of the radius. Arthroscopic débridement of the partial tear and associated chondral injury has been successful in management of most of these rare injuries.

Annotated Bibliography

Diaphyseal Fractures of the Radius and Ulna
Cullen MC, Roy DR, Giza E, Crawford AH: Complications of intramedullary fixation of pediatric forearm fractures. *J Pediatr Orthop* 1998;18:14-21.

Eighteen complications occurred in 20 patients, including hardware migration, infection, loss of reduction, nerve injury, synostosis, and delayed nonunion.

McCarty EC, Mencio GA, Green NE: Anesthesia and analgesia for the ambulatory management of fractures in children. *J Am Acad Orthop Surg* 1999;7:81-91.

In this journal article, the authors discussed the goal of anesthesia as an analgesic and as a means to provide anxiety relief in the ambulatory fracture management of children. Different techniques were presented along with the important factors to consider in the choice of a particular technique. The authors cautioned that with any technique, proper monitoring and safety are important.

McCarty EC, Mencio GA, Walker LA, Green NE: Ketamine sedation for the reduction of children's fractures in the emergency department. *J Bone Joint Surg Am* 2000;82:912-918.

In this article, this dissociative anesthetic was shown to produce a reliable, safe anesthetic state in 85 upper extremity fractures requiring reduction in the emergency department. Its use is most appropriate in children younger than age 11 years. Contraindications included respiratory disease, hypertension, and psychiatric disorder.

Shoemaker SD, Comstock CP, Mubarak SJ, Wenger DR, Chambers HG: Intramedullary Kirschner wire fixation of open or unstable forearm fractures in children. *J Pediatr Orthop* 1999;19:329-337.

In this retrospective series, 32 diaphyseal fractures were treated with intramedullary K-wire fixation. The authors reported nine complications in eight patients that included refracture, loss of reduction with premature K-wire removal, and infection. Excellent results were reported in 31 patients.

Van der Reis WL, Otsuka NY, Moroz P, Mah J: Intramedullary nailing versus plate fixation for unstable forearm fractures in children. *J Pediatr Orthop* 1998;18: 9-13.

In this retrospecive review of 28 fractures that were treated with plates and 18 treated with rods, no significant difference in the functional result, rate of union, or complications was found. Intramedullary fixation required shorter operative time, smaller incisions, and allowed easier hardware removal.

Vrsansky P, Bourdelat D, Al Faour A: Flexible stable intramedullary pinning technique in the treatment of pediatric fractures. *J Pediatr Orthop* 2000;20:23-27.

The authors' report 12 years worth of experience in 308 pediatric fractures of all types treated with intramedullary flexible rod fixation. Approximately one third of the fractures were forearm fractures.

Younger AS, Tredwell SJ, Mackenzie WG: Factors affecting fracture position at cast removal after pediatric forearm fracture. *J Pediatr Orthop* 1997;17:332-336.

The authors measured axis deviation to assess quality of reduction and loss of reduction factors. Loss of reduction was more often the cause of malalignment than position of the fracture after initial reduction. The authors recommended remanipulation for an axis deviation of greater than 5 in younger patients and greater than 3 in near-skeletally mature patients.

Triangular Fibrocartilage Complex Tears

Terry CL, Waters PM: Triangular fibroacartilage injuries in pediatric and adolescent patients. *J Hand Surg Am* 1998;23:626-634.

In this retrospective series, 29 pediatric patients with posttraumatic TFCC tears are described. More than one half of the TFCC injuries were associated with previous distal radius fractures. Coexisting pathology was very common with ulnar styloid nonunion, ulnocarpal impaction, distal radial deformity, and intercarpal ligament tears. Treatment options and recommendations are described for all these conditions.

Scaphoid Fractures

Mintzer CM, Waters PM: Surgical treatment of pediatric scaphoid fracture nonunions. *J Pediatr Orthop* 1999;19:236-239.

The authors present a case series of thirteen skeletally immature patients with scaphoid nonunions treated with open reduction, bone grafting, and Herbert screw fixation. Average time between fracture and surgery was 16.7 months, with average surgical follow-up at 6.9 years. All of the nonunions healed radiographically without a carpal instability pattern. All but one patient had an excellent clinical result.

Wulff RN, Schmidt TL: Carpal fractures in children. *J Pediatr Orthop* 1998;18:462-465.

The authors describe 33 children with scaphoid fractures and one child each with triquetrum, trapezoid, hamate, and capitate fractures. All of the scaphoid fractures were nondisplaced, and all but one united with conservative treatment.

Classic Bibliography

Doman AN, Marcus NW: Congenital bipartite scaphoid. *J Hand Surg Am* 1990;15:869-873.

Gibbons CL, Woods DA, Pailthorpe C, Carr AJ, Worlock P: The management of isolated distal radius fractures in children. *J Pediatr Orthop* 1994;14:207-210.

Golz RJ, Grogan DP, Greene TL, Belsole RJ, Ogden JA: Distal ulnar physeal injury. *J Pediatr Orthop* 1991; 11:318-326.

Holmes JR, Louis DS: Entrapment of pronator quadratus in pediatric distal-radius fractures: Recognition and treatment. *J Pediatr Orthop* 1994;14:498-500.

Letts M, Rowhani N: Galeazzi-equivalent injuries of the wrist in children. *J Pediatr Orthop* 1993;13:561-566.

Mani GV, Hui PW, Cheng JC: Translation of the radius as a predictor of outcome in distal radial fractures of children. *J Bone Joint Surg Br* 1993;75:808-811.

Proctor MT, Moore DJ, Paterson JM: Redisplacement after manipulation of distal radial fractures in children. *J Bone Joint Surg Br* 1993;75:453-454.

Waters PM, Kolettis GJ, Schwend R: Acute median neuropathy following physeal fractures of the distal radius. *J Pediatr Orthop* 1994;14:173-177.

Chapter 12

Knee Injuries and Tibial Fractures

Steven L. Buckley, MD

Knee Injuries

Most knee injuries in children are simple contusions and abrasions. These minor injuries must be differentiated from more serious ligament injuries, meniscal lesions, or occult fractures. It has been increasingly recognized that knee hemarthrosis in children often represents a serious injury such as a torn cruciate ligament or meniscus, or an osteochondral fracture. The physical examination, imaging studies, and treatment options carry different implications for children than for adults. The orthopaedic surgeon must understand these differences and apply them in his or her clinical practice.

Ligament Injuries

Ligament injuries of the knee occur less frequently in children than in adults; however, distal femoral and proximal tibial physeal fractures and anterior tibial eminence fractures occur more frequently. Physeal fractures are caused by stress concentration within the physes when bending or twisting forces are applied across the knee. The unique arrangement of the knee ligament-physeal complex produces this stress concentration. The ligaments arise from the epiphyses of the distal femur, proximal tibia, and proximal fibula except for the superficial portion of the medial collateral ligament (MCL), which inserts distally into the tibial metaphysis.

Medial Collateral Ligament Injuries

The physical examination helps differentiate physeal injury from ligament injury. A physeal fracture produces circumferential swelling and tenderness that is located at the level of the physis. An MCL injury produces swelling and tenderness that is localized to the region of the ligament. Clinical instability to valgus stress may be secondary to either a physeal or MCL injury. Radiographic stress views may help differentiate these injuries, although stable nondisplaced physeal fractures may not open when stressed. MRI also may help differentiate these injuries. In equivocal cases, a 3-week period of immobilization may be necessary to differentiate these injuries. Following immobilization, an injury to the distal femoral or proximal tibial physes demonstrates radiographic evidence of periosteal new bone and/or physeal widening. An unprotected physeal injury may displace; therefore, a suspected physeal fracture must be immobilized. Although rare, a collateral ligament injury and a physeal fracture may occur together.

MCL injuries are treated according to injury severity. Grade I injuries are stable and may be treated symptomatically. Grade II injuries show mild instability, and grade III injuries show severe instability to valgus stress. All types of injury respond well to nonsurgical treatment. A brief period of immobilization of a few days to 3 weeks, based on pain and patient discontent, followed by 3 to 6 weeks of unlimited motion in a hinged knee brace and rehabilitation allow a rapid return to preinjury activities. If an MCL injury and an anterior cruciate ligament (ACL) injury occur together, the ACL injury dictates treatment.

Anterior Cruciate Ligament Injuries

Intrasubstance ACL tears are uncommon in children younger than age 14 years and often result from deceleration, external rotation, and valgus stress to the knee. The patient may feel or hear a pop at the time of injury accompanied by a sensation that the knee has subluxated. At the time of injury, continued participation in activities usually is not possible. A hemarthrosis develops quickly, and clinical swelling is present within hours. The Lachman test is the most sensitive examination to detect acute ACL insufficiency. The anterior drawer and pivot shift tests are difficult to perform in acute injuries because of muscle guarding and pain. The joint line should be carefully palpated for tenderness, which may indicate an associated meniscal injury. Associated meniscal injury affects more than 40% of

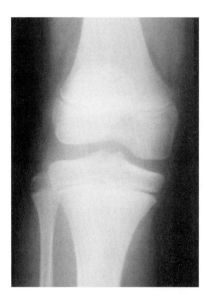

Figure 1 AP view of the knee with wide open physes. Because of skeletal immaturity, this patient is at risk for premature physeal closure if the ACL is reconstructed using transphyseal tunnels and a bone-tendon-bone-patellar tendon graft.

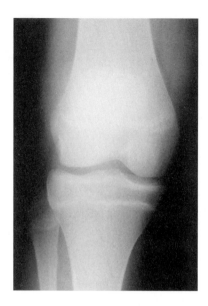

Figure 2 AP view of the knee with closing physes. Because this patient is nearing skeletal maturity, the ACL could be reconstructed using transphyseal tunnels and a bone-tendon-bone-patellar tendon graft.

children and adolescents with ACL tears. Collateral ligament and physeal injuries also must be ruled out. An avulsion fracture of the tibial eminence should be evaluated radiographically. MRI or diagnostic arthroscopy may help document ligament disruption, meniscal injury, and osteochondral lesions. However, MRI is unable to predict intra-articular pathology in children and young adolescents as well as it can in adults. Results of nonsurgical treatment of ACL injuries generally are poor in children and adolescents. Unfortunately, the open physes in children limit surgical options (Fig. 1). Primary ligament repair and extra-articular reconstruction that avoids injury to the physes have both resulted in persistent instability and poor long-term outcomes. Intra-articular ligament reconstruction using tibial and femoral tunnels drilled through open physes may be successfully performed in adolescents nearing skeletal maturity who have limited risk for abnormal growth (Fig. 2). In younger patients, however, the risk of physeal injury from transphyseal tunnels is greater; therefore, primary treatment should consist of physical therapy, bracing, and activity limitation. Surgical reconstruction should be delayed until the patient is near skeletal maturity. The proper timing for surgery can be determined when the patient has reached Tanner stage IV or V and/or a bone age of 14 years in girls and 15 years in boys. If nonsurgical treatment fails and the patient experiences instability with activities of daily living, the ligament can be reconstructed using the semitendinosus and gracilis tendons with or without physis-sparing bone tunnels. During reconstruction, the tendons are detached proximally at their musculotendinous junctions and left attached distally. The grafts are passed over a groove or through a tunnel on the anterior aspect of the tibial epiphysis, avoiding the physis, and then pulled to the over-the-

top position of the distal femur to avoid injury to the physes. In a similar procedure, the medial one third of the patella tendon is left attached distally and the proximal end is passed over the top of the lateral femoral condyle (Fig. 3). Although experience with these techniques is limited, initial reports are encouraging. More recently, a procedure has been described in which the distal portion of the hamstring or patellar tendon graft is passed through a tibial transphyseal tunnel. This technique did not result in premature or asymmetric closure of the physis in the small number of patients studied. However, this technique should be used with caution until surgeons gain more experience with its use and its safety is established. Bone-tendon-bone–patellar tendon grafts should be reserved for patients whose physes are closing or already closed (Fig. 4).

Posterior Cruciate Ligament Injuries

Because posterior cruciate ligament (PCL) injuries are rare in children and adolescents, the natural history of this injury is unknown. PCL injuries occur secondary to forced posterior displacement of the tibia on the femur with the knee flexed 90° or to knee hyperextension. Following an acute injury, knee motion is painful and weight bearing difficult. The PCL is extrasynovial; therefore, there may be no knee effusion. Tenderness may be isolated to the posterior aspect of the knee and proximal calf; joint line tenderness may indicate meniscal pathology. Posterior sag of the proximal tibia and results of the posterior drawer test may not be obvious in acute injuries; however, the quadriceps active drawer test helps detect acute PCL injuries. For this test, the patient is supine on the examination table with the knee flexed 70° and the foot flat on the table. The patient then contracts the quadriceps muscle. In

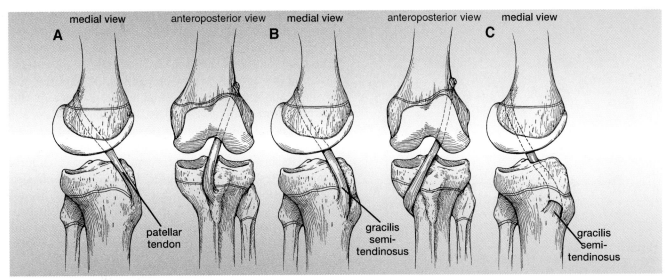

Figure 3 Options for ACL reconstruction in children include nontransphyseal or partial transphyseal techniques. **A** and **B**, Views of a nontransphyseal technique. **C**, Medial view of a partial transphyseal technique. *(Reproduced from Stanitski CL: Anterior cruciate ligament injury in the skeletally immature patient: Diagnosis and treatment. J Am Acad Orthop Surg 1995;3:146-158.)*

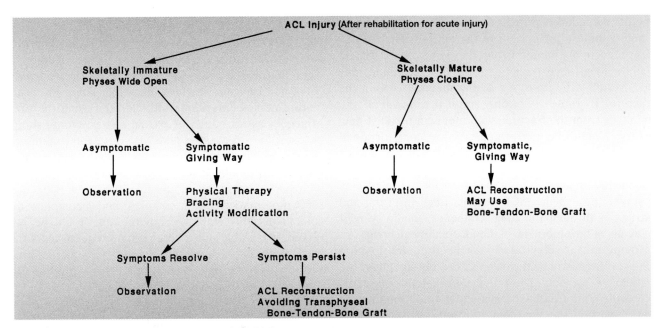

Figure 4 Algorithm showing symptoms and treatment of ACL injuries.

the presence of PCL insufficiency, the tibial plateau moves anteriorly. Accompanying collateral ligament injuries also must be ruled out. Stress radiographs or MRI may be necessary to distinguish between a physeal fracture and ligament disruption. Radiographs also must be carefully evaluated for avulsion fractures from either the femur or tibia. Displaced avulsion fractures are best treated with open reduction and internal fixation using intraepiphyseal sutures or screws. Diagnostic arthroscopy may help document intra-articular injuries. Isolated intrasubstance tears in the skeletally immature patient should be treated without surgery. Ligament reconstruction in children with chronic symp-

tomatic PCL insufficiency should be avoided until skeletal maturity to prevent injury to the physes.

Tibial Eminence Fractures

Most ACL equivalent injuries in children are avulsion fractures of the anterior tibial eminence. Before the tibial physis closes, the ACL is more resistant to traction forces than the intercondylar eminence. Avulsion from the femoral insertion is rare. Associated injuries to the collateral ligaments and menisci commonly occur. An acute hemarthrosis accompanies associated anterior joint laxity. Nondisplaced fractures should be

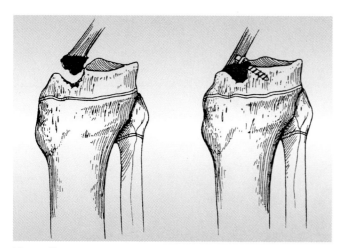

Figure 5 Screw fixation technique for tibial eminence fractures. The screw should engage and buttress the fragment; however, it should not cross the physis. *(Reproduced from Stanitski CL: Anterior cruciate ligament injury in the skeletally immature patient: Diagnosis and treatment. J Am Acad Orthop Surg 1995;3: 146-158.)*

immobilized, and elevated or displaced fractures should be reduced. Fractures that are somewhat elevated without displacement of the entire fragment may be reduced by immobilizing the knee in extension. Failure to achieve reduction with this technique may be a result of interposition of the meniscus within the fracture. In these situations, surgical removal of the meniscus from the fracture, with meniscal repair if necessary, should be performed. Arthroscopy or open reduction and internal fixation provide the best means of anatomically reducing completely displaced fracture fragments. Internal fixation may be achieved by placing a suture through the ACL near its tibial insertion and passing it through the tibial eminence, finally tying it over an anterior bridge of tibial epiphyseal bone. An intraepiphyseal screw also may be used for fixation (Fig. 5). Screws should not cross the physis unless the patient is an adolescent nearing skeletal maturity. Regardless of treatment, many patients demonstrate mild laxity on the Lachman and anterior drawer tests but do not report instability.

Meniscal Injuries

Meniscal injuries are uncommon in children and young adolescents. However, because knee pain, giving way, and locking are common in older children and adolescents, meniscal injury is frequently considered in the differential diagnosis. Other possible diagnoses include patellar instability, osteochondritis dissecans, a loose body, inflammatory arthritis, and hip disease. A history of a twisting injury with a joint effusion, joint line tenderness, positive results on a McMurray test, and extension block frequently are associated with meniscal injury, but also may occur with many other conditions.

Loose bodies, fractures, and osteochondritis dissecans are demonstrated on plain radiographs. Although MRI helps diagnose soft-tissue injuries such as discoid menisci and displaced meniscal tears, these studies should be interpreted with caution in children and young adolescents. In T1-weighted MRI scans in children, normal menisci tend to have increased signals and may resemble a partial or intrameniscal tear. In a recent study, clinical examination was judged superior to MRI in predicting arthroscopic findings in children and adolescents with injured knees. Serial physical examinations that take place during a 2- to 6-week period following injury help exclude minor soft-tissue injuries that usually resolve quickly. In patients with persistent symptoms, arthroscopic examination may be necessary.

Injured menisci have greater healing potential in children than in adults; therefore, meniscal tears in children should be repaired when possible, including tears in the less vascular white-white zone in physically immature patients who are age 12 years or younger. In a recent study, all 26 patients age 17 years or younger who underwent arthroscopic meniscal repair reported complete healing. Of the repaired meniscal tears, 22 were in the red-red zone, six were in the red-white zone, and one was in the white-white zone. Physically mature adolescents should be managed using the same principles as for adults. A partial meniscectomy should be used for irreparable tears. Because total meniscectomy in children and adolescents leads to degenerative arthritis of the knee, it should be avoided. Arthroscopy with partial resection of the meniscus should be used for symptomatic tears in complete and incomplete discoid menisci. A stable peripheral rim should be preserved, if possible, for load bearing. Meniscal tears that occur with ACL disruption should be repaired when possible. Open physes may preclude simultaneous intra-articular ligament reconstruction.

Patellar Fractures and Dislocations

Fractures of the patella are unusual because of the large cartilage-to-bone ratio in children and the patella's increased mobility. Children may sustain patellar sleeve fractures, which occur through unossified cartilage and include only a small piece of calcified bone in the fracture fragment. The fracture fragment may appear very small on radiographs. Patellar sleeve fractures may involve the proximal, distal, or medial aspects of the patella. Patellar tenderness following injury should raise suspicion of a fracture. If the fracture is displaced and the retinaculum is torn, a palpable defect may be apparent or the patient may be unable to actively extend the knee. Management of pediatric patellar fractures does not differ significantly from that of fractures in adults. Nondisplaced fractures should be immobilized, and displaced fractures should be treated with open reduction and internal fixation, using a technique such as the tension band wire technique. With a bipartite patella, fracture may occur at the bone-cartilage junction.

Acute patellar dislocations may result from a direct blow to the knee or a twisting injury. Most dislocated patellae spontaneously reduce, and the patient may provide a history of the knee "going-out" but be unaware that the patella actually dislocated. If the patient heard or felt two pops at the time of injury, a patellar subluxation or dislocation very likely occurred. Patients with indirect injuries and generalized ligamentous laxity might not have an effusion. Furthermore, joint fluid might escape from a torn joint capsule into surrounding tissues and prevent accumulation of fluid within the knee. The patient may have tenderness along the medial border of the patella or the adductor tubercle. Plain radiographs should be obtained to evaluate for osteochondral fractures or loose bodies. If present, these lesions should be examined arthroscopically. Small fragments should be removed, whereas larger fragments may be managed with internal fixation using suture material, pins, or Herbert screws. Concomitant ACL and MCL injuries may occur with patellar dislocation and must be ruled out. Some authors recommend routine arthroscopic examination for patients with major effusions, loss of full extension, flexion less than 90°, and pain. In many of these patients, occult articular and osteochondral injuries that cannot be seen on radiographs may be identified.

Management of an initial dislocation should include a 1- to 3-week period of immobilization, based on pain and patient discontent, followed by a quadriceps rehabilitation program. Approximately 15% to 20% of pediatric patients experience recurrent patellar dislocations. The highest recurrence rates occur in patients with predisposing factors such as femoral condyle hypoplasia, shallow femoral sulcus, an increased quadriceps angle, atrophy of the vastus medialis, or generalized joint laxity. Generally, as the patient's age advances into the third decade, the frequency of subsequent dislocations decreases. The incidence of osteoarthritis does not appear to be higher in children and adolescents who have experienced multiple patellar dislocations. Interestingly, in a recent study, osteoarthritis was found to be more likely to develop in a patient who experienced a single traumatic patellar dislocation than in a patient who experienced multiple atraumatic patellar dislocations. In patients with recurring patellar dislocations, the primary indications for patellar realignment surgery should be symptom relief and lifestyle considerations. Surgery should be considered only if a nonsurgical treatment program consisting of physical therapy, activity modification, and patellar bracing has been unsuccessful.

Before surgical intervention is considered, the physician must determine whether the patient has tight lateral restraints, medial patellofemoral laxity, and an increased quadriceps angle. The passive patella tilt test assesses tightness of the lateral restraints. The lateral edge of the patella is elevated from the lateral condyle with the knee extended. A 0° or negative patella tilt angle indicates excessive lateral tightness. The passive patella glide test determines the amount of medial patellofemoral laxity. The patella is pushed laterally with the knee in extension. Lateral subluxation of the patella of greater than 50% indicates insufficient medial restraints. A quadriceps angle of greater than 10° in boys and 15° in girls indicates an increased lateral vector of force for the patella. To determine the active quadriceps angle, the patient contracts the quadriceps muscles with the knee extended. The patella normally moves straight superior or lateral to superior in a 1:1 ratio. Abnormal lateral pull results in a movement that is more lateral than superior. The pull of the lateral retinaculum is decreased by a lateral release alone, which may be considered in the patient with recurrent patellar dislocation and tight lateral restraints. Medial reefing and vastus medialis advancement are used to treat insufficient medial restraints, and distal realignment procedures are performed to correct an abnormal quadriceps angle. Tibial tubercle transfer is to be avoided in skeletally immature patients because of the risk of physeal damage and growth arrest. The Galeazzi procedure (semitendinosus tenodesis) or the Roux-Goldthwait procedure may be used in the skeletally immature patient who needs distal realignment. Frequently, management of recurrent patellar dislocations requires that the lateral release, medial reefing, and distal realignment all must be performed. Surgical outcome is less predictable in patients with connective tissue laxity such as may occur with Ehlers-Danlos syndrome or Down syndrome.

Tibial Tuberosity Fractures

Fractures of the tibial tuberosity are uncommon avulsion injuries that occur in older adolescents. Type I fractures are characterized by an avulsion of a small fragment of the tuberosity. Type II fractures involve the entire anterior tuberosity with extension proximally to the level of the horizontal portion of the proximal tibial physis. Type III fractures, or Salter-Harris type III fractures, involve the entire tuberosity with extension proximally into the articular surface. Patients have pain, swelling, and tenderness over the tuberosity, and patella alta may be present. The presence of patella

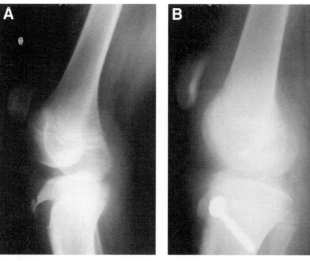

Figure 6 **A,** Lateral view of a displaced type III tibial tuberosity fracture. **B,** Postoperative radiograph after the fracture was reduced and stabilized with a cancellous screw.

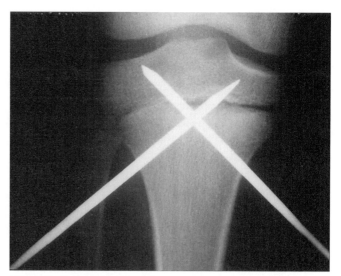

Figure 7 AP radiograph of the tibia obtained intraoperatively demonstrating percutaneous fixation technique of a proximal tibial physeal fracture. Smooth Steinmann pins placed from distal to proximal to prevent intracapsular penetration were used to reduce and stabilize the fracture. The pins were cut and buried beneath the skin to reduce the risk of infection.

alta, compared with the normal uninjured side, and a significant bony prominence indicate the need for surgical treatment of type I fractures. Displaced type II and III fractures require open reduction and internal fixation. In these fractures, a cancellous interfragmentary screw may be placed through the tuberosity into the metaphysis (Fig. 6). Because this injury occurs in patients who are near skeletal maturity, growth arrest with secondary genu recurvatum is rare. Compartment syndrome is an uncommon complication of tibial tuberosity fractures that should be ruled out in patients with excessive postinjury pain or neurologic deficits.

Tibial Fractures

Proximal Tibial Epiphyseal Fractures

Fractures of the proximal tibial epiphysis are usually secondary to hyperextension of the knee and occur in older children and adolescents. Most are Salter-Harris type I and II injuries.

Patients have pain, swelling, and tenderness at the level of the physis distal to the joint line. In angulated extension fractures, recurvatum is distal to the tuberosity. Because the vascular trifurcation is tethered to bone in this area, popliteal artery injuries may occur with this fracture. Therefore, a careful neurovascular evaluation is essential. Angulated and displaced fractures are obvious on radiographs; however, nondisplaced fractures must be diagnosed clinically. If a nondisplaced fracture is suspected because of swelling and tenderness at the level of the proximal tibial physis, 3 to 4 weeks of immobilization is warranted. Radiographs obtained 2 to 3 weeks following injury demonstrate periosteal new bone and physeal widening if a fracture has occurred.

Most Salter-Harris type I and II fractures may be treated with closed reduction and immobilization. Hyperextension injuries are reduced by flexing the knee and applying a cast with the knee in flexion. After 3 weeks, the knee is gently extended and another cast applied. Total immobilization should not exceed 6 weeks. Displaced fractures may be treated with closed reduction and percutaneous pinning with the knee immobilized in extension (Fig. 7). Salter-Harris type III and IV fractures may be treated with closed reduction and Kirschner wire or cannulated screw fixation; however, if closed reduction is not possible, open reduction and internal fixation should be performed. Threaded internal fixation devices should not cross the physis. The most common complications of these fractures are physeal arrest with secondary angular deformity and limb-length discrepancy. Angular deformity occurs in 30% of patients and limblength discrepancy in 20% of patients. Children who sustain proximal tibial physeal injuries should be followed for at least 1 year to track possible development of these complications.

Proximal Tibial Metaphyseal Fractures

Fractures of the proximal tibial metaphysis are usually nondisplaced fractures that occur in younger children, most often the result of a valgus stress to the tibia. Although the fractures may appear to be innocuous, they can result in a late progressive valgus deformity, which is more common in greenstick and complete fractures and unusual in buckle fractures. If an acute valgus deformity is noted, the fracture should be

TABLE 1 | Classification and Antibiotic Treatment of Open Tibial Fractures

Classification	Empiric Antibiotics
Type I—An open fracture with a clean wound less than 1 cm long	Cephalosporin
Type II—An open fracture with a wound more than 1 cm long without extensive soft-tissue damage, flaps, or avulsions	Cephalosporin
Type III—An open segmental fracture, an open fracture with extensive soft-tissue damage, a traumatic amputation, or an open fracture caused by a farm injury	Cephalosporin and aminoglycosides
A—Extensive soft-tissue laceration with adequate bone coverage	
B—Extensive soft-tissue injury with periosteal stripping and exposed bone	
C—Vascular injury requiring repair	

reduced and immobilized. If soft-tissue interposition prevents a successful closed reduction, open reduction should be performed. Parents should be advised that a late valgus deformity might develop within a year of the injury. Development of a late tibial valgus deformity is not influenced by the presence or absence of a fibula fracture. The valgus deformity most likely is secondary to asymmetric growth of the proximal tibial physis. Patients with a posttraumatic tibial valgus deformity should be followed through skeletal maturity. Spontaneous angular correction occurs in most patients. Surgery to correct a late valgus deformity should be postponed for at least 2 to 3 years following the injury and should be reserved for symptomatic patients. If an osteotomy is performed in a skeletally immature patient, slight overcorrection with rigid fixation should be obtained because the valgus deformity tends to recur. Bracing is not an effective means of correcting a late valgus deformity.

Fractures of the Tibial and Fibular Diaphyses

Closed fractures of the tibia and fibula in children have fewer complications, heal faster, and have less morbidity than those in adults. As long as significant shortening, angulation, and rotation are prevented, long-term sequelae are unusual. Infants may sustain a nondisplaced oblique fracture of the distal tibia, or "toddler's fracture," as a result of an innocuous injury such as tripping over a toy or falling from a short height. These fractures heal quickly and can be treated with a short leg weight-bearing cast. More significant trauma is necessary to fracture the tibia in older children. Displaced or angulated tibial and fibular fractures should be reduced and immobilized in an above-the-knee cast until healed. Remodeling is not predictable; therefore, angulation of greater than 5° should not be accepted initially in adolescents. As much as 10° of angulation

may be accepted in younger children. Valgus angulation and apex posterior angulation are the least likely types to remodel. Because rotational malalignment does not remodel, it is not acceptable. The fractured tibia overgrows an average of 5 mm in children age 2 to 10 years. Because tibial overgrowth is minimal, shortening of more than 1 to 1.5 cm is not acceptable in acute fractures. Unstable tibial fractures may be treated with external fixation or percutaneous pin fixation and cast immobilization until radiographs reveal evidence of healing. Although the presence of open physes precludes the use of rigid intramedullary rod fixation, flexible intramedullary rods may be used in transverse fractures, provided that the physes are not violated during rod insertion. With ipsilateral femur and tibial fractures, at least one and perhaps both of these long bones should undergo rigid fixation. With these injuries, overgrowth of both the femur and tibia may result in a limb-length discrepancy.

Although open tibial fractures in children are associated with osteomyelitis and delayed union, the occurrence of nonunion and the need for late amputation are uncommon. With current treatment methods in children, serious soft-tissue injuries heal, and patients can recover from osteomyelitis and achieve a solid union. Compared with younger children, adolescents experience more complications following open tibial fractures. A higher rate of osteomyelitis and a longer time to fracture union was recently reported in children age 12 years and older with open tibial fractures than in younger children. The classification of injury severity described by Gustilo and Anderson (Table 1) helps in predicting complications and selecting appropriate antibiotics for children with open tibial fractures.

Complications can be minimized with prompt initiation of treatment. Antibiotics and tetanus prophylaxis should be initiated in the emergency department, and the wound should be covered with a sterile dressing. A broad-spectrum cephalosporin is used for types I and II open fractures, and aminoglycoside should be added for type III open fractures. Penicillin is added for children who sustain lawn mower injuries or other injuries that occur in a farm environment. Resuscitation in the emergency department, if necessary, is followed by irrigation and débridement of the fracture in the operating room. Most types I and II fractures can be stabilized with cast immobilization. External fixation or transcutaneous crossed pins combined with cast immobilization can be used for type III open fractures and fractures with unstable fracture patterns. Management of soft-tissue and arterial injuries is the same in children as in adults. Free muscle flaps may be successfully used in children. The small caliber of children's blood vessels does not preclude successful repair or grafting of vascular injuries. Although the indications for primary amputation are not clearly defined in children, the mangled extremity severity score (MESS) used for adults appears to be applicable to children and adolescents. An open tibial fracture with an avascular lower extremity, disruption of the posterior tibial nerve, and an insensate foot is probably best treated with primary amputation.

Annotated Bibliography

Ligament Injuries

Bisson LJ, Wickiewicz T, Levinson M, Warren R: ACL reconstruction in children with open physes. *Orthopedics* 1998;21:659-663.

Nine patients with wide open physes underwent intra-articular ACL reconstruction using semitendinosus and gracilis tendon grafts passed through the tibial physis and over the top of the femoral condyle. Results were excellent in seven patients. The grafts ruptured in two patients, one at 10 months and one at 3 years. There was no clinically significant limb-length discrepancy, angular deformity, or radiographic evidence of physeal injury.

Cohen DM, Jasser JW, Kean JR, Smith GA: Clinical criteria for using radiography for children with acute knee injuries. *Pediatr Emerg Care* 1998;14:185-187.

In this article, 254 patients who went to the emergency department with acute knee injuries were retrospectively reviewed to evaluate clinical criteria for selective radiography of the knee. Point tenderness was not statistically associated with fracture. The authors determined that inability to bear weight in the emergency department (37% fracture rate) and inability to flex the knee to 90° (52% fracture rate) were associated with a fracture. The authors concluded that the number of radiographs would have decreased by 73% and no fractures would have been missed if the criteria of inability to bear weight or flex the knee to 90° had been applied.

Lo IK, Bell DM, Fowler PJ: Anterior cruciate ligament injuries in the skeletally immature patient. *Instr Course Lect* 1998;47:351-359.

This is an excellent review of the evaluation and treatment of ACL injuries in skeletally immature patients. Surgical methods that are discussed include primary repair, extra-articular reconstruction, nontransphyseal intra-articular reconstruction, and intra-articular transphyseal graft tunnels.

Lo IK, Kirkley A, Fowler PJ, Miniaci A: The outcome of operatively treated anterior cruciate ligament disruptions in the skeletally immature child. *Arthroscopy* 1997;13:627-634.

Five skeletally immature children with midsubstance tears of the ACL and "wide" open growth plates were treated with intra-articular reconstruction with passage of the distal portion of the tendon graft through 6-mm or smaller holes in the open tibial physis. None of the patients demonstrated evidence of asymmetric physeal closure or limb-length discrepancy at a minimum follow-up of 4.5 years.

Matelic TM, Aronsson DD, Boyd DW Jr, LaMont RL: Acute hemarthrosis of the knee in children. *Am J Sports Med* 1995;23:668-671.

Arthroscopy for acute traumatic hemarthrosis of the knee was performed on 21 patients between age 10 and 17 years. An osteochondral fracture of the femoral condyle or patella was found in 67% of the patients. These fractures were not demonstrated on preoperative radiographs in five of the 14 patients with osteochondral fractures. Only two patients (10%) had ACL injuries.

McDermott MJ, Bathgate B, Gillingham BL, Hennrikus WL: Correlation of MRI and arthroscopic diagnosis of knee pathology in children and adolescents. *J Pediatr Orthop* 1998;18:675-678.

MRI of the knee and subsequent arthroscopy were performed on 53 patients between age 4 and 17 years with knee pathology. MRI had a lower sensitivity, specificity, positive predictive value, and accuracy for the pediatric group (age 4 to 14 years) than for the adolescent group (age 15 to 17 years). However, greater negative predictive value was demonstrated on MRI for the pediatric group than for the adolescent group. The authors concluded that MRI is much less accurate in predicting intra-articular pathology in pediatric patients than in adolescents or adults.

Mizuta H, Kubota K, Shiraishi M, Otsuka Y, Nagamoto N, Takagi K: The conservative treatment of complete tears of the anterior cruciate ligament in skeletally immature patients. *J Bone Joint Surg Br* 1995;77:890-894.

Eighteen skeletally immature patients were treated nonsurgically for ACL tears. At a minimum follow-up of 36 months, all patients were symptomatic. Results were excellent in one patient, good in one, fair in eight, and poor in eight. Only one patient returned to her preinjury level of athletics. The authors concluded that results of nonsurgical treatment for ACL injuries in children is poor.

Pressman AE, Letts RM, Jarvis JG: Anterior cruciate ligament tears in children: An analysis of operative versus nonoperative treatment. *J Pediatr Orthop* 1997; 17:505-511.

Forty-two patients between age 5 and 17 years sustained ACL disruption. Of these patients, 13 were treated without surgery, six were treated with primary repair, and 23 were treated with intra-articular reconstruction. The best outcomes, based on clinical examination, knee score, and results from the KT-1000 arthrometer, were seen in the patients treated with intra-articular reconstruction. No limb-length discrepancies or angular deformities resulted from iatrogenic physeal injury.

Stanitski CL: Correlation of arthroscopic and clinical examinations with magnetic resonance imaging findings of injured knees in children and adolescents. *Am J Sports Med* 1998;26:2-6.

Physical examination, MRI, and arthroscopy were performed on 28 patients between age 8 and 17 years with knee injuries. A positive correlation (78.5%) was found between clinical and arthroscopic findings. A negative correlation was found between arthroscopic and MRI findings (78.5%) and between clinical and MRI findings (75%). The authors concluded that accuracy, positive predictive value, negative predictive value, sensitivity, and specificity were more favorable with the clinical examination than with the MRI.

Tibial Eminence Fractures

Mah JY, Adili A, Otsuka NY, Ogilvie R: Follow-up study of arthroscopic reduction and fixation of type III tibial-eminence fractures. *J Pediatr Orthop* 1998;18: 475-477.

Arthroscopic-assisted reduction of tibial eminence fractures was performed in nine children. At an average follow-up of 3.5 years, all of the patients demonstrated excellent subjective knee function without objective evidence of knee laxity or instability.

Meniscal Injuries

Mintzer CM, Richmond JC, Taylor J: Meniscal repair in the young athlete. *Am J Sports Med* 1998;26:630-633.

Twenty-nine arthroscopic meniscal repairs in 26 patients between age 11 and 17 years were performed and followed for a minimum of 2 years. The clinical healing rate was 100%. All patients had a full range of motion with no effusion, joint line tenderness, or McMurray sign. The authors concluded that the prognosis of meniscal repair in young patients is excellent.

Takeda Y, Ikata T, Yoshida S, Takai H, Kashiwaguchi S: MRI high-signal intensity in the menisci of asymptomatic children. *J Bone Joint Surg Br* 1998;80:463-467.

MRI examinations were performed on 108 asymptomatic knees in children. A high signal within the menisci was demonstrated in 66% of the knees, compared with 29% in adults. A high signal within the meniscus of a child or adolescent may not indicate pathology.

Patellar Fractures and Dislocations

Letts RM, Davidson D, Beaule P: Semitendinosus tenodesis for repair of recurrent dislocation of the patella in children. *J Pediatr Orthop* 1999;19:742-747.

Reconstruction with semitendinosus tenodesis was performed in 26 knees with recurrent patellar dislocations. At a minimum follow-up of 2 years, 23 of the knees were asymptomatic, three were painful, one had become dislocated again, and medial subluxation of the patella had developed in one.

Maenpaa H, Lehto MU: Patellofemoral osteoarthritis after patellar dislocation. *Clin Orthop* 1997;339:156-162.

Eighty-five patients were evaluated for osteoarthritic changes within the patellofemoral joint at a minimum of 6 years following patellar dislocation. Predisposing factors for patellar instability, such as abnormal quadriceps angle, positive apprehension test, quadriceps muscle atrophy, or generalized joint laxity, were not associated with arthritic changes. Patellofemoral joint degeneration was found in 22% of the affected knees and 11% of the unaffected knees. Arthritic changes developed in 29% of knees without subsequent patellar dislocation and in only 13% of knees with occasional redislocations. Arthritic changes developed in 35% of patients who underwent late surgery for pain or instability.

Stanitski CL: Patellar instability in the school age athlete. *Instr Course Lect* 1998;47:345-350.

This is an excellent review of the evaluation, diagnosis, and treatment of patellar instability in the young patient.

Stanitski CL, Paletta GA Jr: Articular cartilage injury with acute patellar dislocation in adolescents: Arthroscopic and radiographic correlation. *Am J Sports Med* 1998;26:52-55.

Forty-eight adolescents with acute, noncontact patellar dislocations were evaluated radiographically and arthroscopically. Radiographic evidence of articular injury was seen in 11 patients (23%) and results of arthroscopy revealed articular injury in 34 patients (71%). Poor results following patellar dislocation may represent unrecognized articular injury.

Tibial Tuberosity Fractures

Buckley SL, Smith GR, Sponseller PD, Thompson JD, Robertson WW Jr, Griffin PP: Severe (type III) open fractures of the tibia in children. *J Pediatr Orthop* 1996;16:627-634.

In this review of 20 patients between age 2 and 16 years with type III open tibia fractures, all fractures healed and there were no late amputations. Children with severe open fractures of the tibia have a good prognosis for limb salvage with modern techniques for open fracture management.

Grimard G, Naudie D, Laberge LC, Hamdy RC: Open fractures of the tibia in children. *Clin Orthop* 1996;332: 62-70.

In this review, 90 open fractures of the tibia were irrigated and débrided in the operating room. Seventeen wounds (19.8%) were primarily closed, and 69 wounds (80.2%) were left open. There were no deep infections. The average time to union was 4.5 months. There were 10 delayed unions and seven nonunions. Patient age and the fracture grade were the only variables associated with time to fracture union. Children older than age 12 years with open tibial fractures have a higher risk of delayed union or nonunion than children younger than age 6 years with the same injuries.

Kreder HJ, Armstrong P: A review of open tibia fractures in children. *J Pediatr Orthop* 1995;15:482-488.

In this review of 56 open tibial fractures in 55 children, 14% of the fractures became infected. Neurovascular injury and a delay to surgery of more than 6 hours were the most important variables for the development of infection. The patient's age was the most important variable for time to fracture union.

McCarthy JJ, Kim DH, Eilert RE: Posttraumatic genu valgum: Operative versus nonoperative treatment. *J Pediatr Orthop* 1998;18:518-521.

In this review of 15 patients with posttraumatic genu valgum, 10 patients were treated without surgery and five patients were treated with surgery. In both groups, the valgus deformity had improved at follow-up without significant difference between the two groups.

Skaggs DL, Kautz SM, Kay RM, Tolo VT: Effect of delay of surgical treatment on rate of infection in open fractures in children. *J Pediatr Orthop* 2000;20:19-22.

Surgical irrigation and débridement can be delayed for 6 hours or longer without an increased incidence of infection in children with type I or II open fractures who are given early parenteral antibiotics.

Tuten HR, Keeler KA, Gabos PG, Zionts LE, MacKenzie WG: Posttraumatic tibia valga in children: A long-term follow-up note. *J Bone Joint Surg Am* 1999;81:799-810.

In this article, seven children were managed without surgery for progressive valgus deformity that had occurred within 12 months after satisfactory healing of a proximal tibial metaphyseal fracture. The patients were followed for a minimum of 10 years; the average time of follow-up was 15 years, 3 months. All patients demonstrated spontaneous improvement of the metaphyseal-diaphyseal and mechanical tibiofemoral angles. A corrective osteotomy was performed on one patient after skeletal maturity because of pain believed to be caused by malalignment. The authors concluded that patients with posttraumatic tibia valga should be followed through skeletal maturity and surgical intervention should be reserved for those patients with symptoms secondary to malalignment.

Yang JP, Letts RM: Isolated fractures of the tibia with intact fibula in children: A review of 95 patients. *J Pediatr Orthop* 1997;17:347-351.

Of 76 fractures with initial angular deformity, deformity recurred in 32 after closed reduction, occurring within 21 days of the initial injury. Cast wedging or a second reduction was performed in 15 of these children. The authors recommend that children with an isolated tibial fracture and intact fibula undergo weekly radiographic examination for the first 3 weeks following injury.

Classic Bibliography

Bohn WW, Durbin RA: Ipsilateral fractures of the femur and tibia in children and adolescents. *J Bone Joint Surg Am* 1991;73:429-439.

Buckley SL, Smith G, Sponseller PD, Thompson JD, Griffin PP: Open fractures of the tibia in children. *J Bone Joint Surg Am* 1990;72:1462-1469.

Engebretsen L, Svenningsen S, Benum P: Poor results of anterior cruciate ligament repair in adolescence. *Acta Orthop Scand* 1988;59:684-686.

Grogan DP, Carey TP, Leffers D, Ogden JA: Avulsion fractures of the patella. *J Pediatr Orthop* 1990; 10:721-730.

Kreder HJ, Armstrong P: The significance of perioperative cultures in open pediatric lower-extremity fractures. *Clin Orthop* 1994;302:206-212.

Maguire JK, Canale ST: Fractures of the patella in children and adolescents. *J Pediatr Orthop* 1993;13: 567-571.

McCarroll JR, Shelbourne KD, Porter DA, Rettig AC, Murray S: Patellar tendon graft reconstruction for midsubstance anterior cruciate ligament rupture in junior high school athletes: An algorithm for management. *Am J Sports Med* 1994;22:478-484.

McManus F, Rang M, Heslin DJ: Acute dislocation of the patella in children: The natural history. *Clin Orthop* 1979;139:88-91.

Ogden JA, Tross RB, Murphy MJ: Fractures of the tibial tuberosity in adolescents. *J Bone Joint Surg Am* 1980;62:205-215.

Parker AW, Drez D Jr, Cooper JL: Anterior cruciate ligament injuries in patients with open physes. *Am J Sports Med* 1994;22:44-47.

Salter RB, Best TN: Pathogenesis of progressive valgus deformity following fractures of the proximal metaphyseal region of the tibia in young children. *Instr Course Lect* 1992;41:409-411.

Shelton WR, Canale ST: Fractures of the tibia through the proximal tibial epiphyseal cartilage. *J Bone Joint Surg Am* 1979;61:167-173.

Stanitski CL, Harvell JC, Fu F: Observations on acute knee hemarthrosis in children and adolescents. *J Pediatr Orthop* 1993;13:506-510.

Willis RB, Blokker C, Stoll TM, Paterson DC, Galpin RD: Long-term follow-up of anterior tibial eminence fractures. *J Pediatr Orthop* 1993;13:361-364.

Wroble RR, Henderson RC, Campion ER, El-Khoury GY, Albright JP: Meniscectomy in children and adolescents: A long-term follow-up study. *Clin Orthop* 1992;279:180-188.

Zionts LE, MacEwen GD: Spontaneous improvement of post-traumatic tibia valga. *J Bone Joint Surg Am* 1986;68:680-687.

Chapter 13

Foot and Ankle Injuries

R. Dale Blasier, MD, FRCSC

Introduction

Foot and ankle injuries in children are very common and may result from minor play activity, falls, sports competition, recreational vehicle accidents, motor vehicle accidents, and even penetrating trauma. Most injuries require little treatment and have a benign prognosis. A few injuries, especially those involving higher energy or direct penetration, may result in long-term growth or functional problems. An awareness of the pitfalls of treatment will help to ensure the best possible result.

Ankle Injuries

Fractures of the Distal Tibia and Fibula

The bone quality of the distal tibia and fibula in children is different from that of adults. The cortical bone is somewhat more flexible than in adults and the metaphyseal bone is softer, more spongy, and able to absorb considerable energy prior to failure. Fractures of the distal tibia and fibula can result from a direct blow or twisting injury to the lower leg. Most fractures result from a sudden injury, but repetitive microtrauma can result in stress fracture. Fractures in adults tend to be complete; however, younger children often sustain buckle fractures in which the spongy metaphyseal bone fails during compression. In complete injuries, severe pain and deformity make the diagnosis obvious. In compression-type injuries, the child will have less pain and will often limp and be unable to bear weight. There will be tenderness at the site of the fracture. Radiographs will generally confirm the diagnosis, although occasionally radiographs will appear negative initially. Radiographs "coned down" on the region of tenderness, as well as oblique views, may show the injury. If there is a high index of suspicion, a bone scan will reveal the fracture; however, plain radiographs will usually show the lesion within 10 to 14 days as new bone formation is seen.

Treatment consists of immobilization and limited weight bearing until healing is complete, usually 3 to 4 weeks. Fractures angulated greater than 15° should be reduced under anesthesia. Fractures displaced into recurvatum should be immobilized in equinus to prevent aggravation of the recurvatum. Heel cord tightness will not develop in children. The long-term natural history is excellent for healing and remodeling.

Physeal Injuries of the Distal Tibia and Fibula

As a result of the relative weakness of the physes and the strength of the ligaments in children, growth plate injuries are more common than ligament rupture. The physes are susceptible to crush, shear, and distraction injuries. Injuries result from twisting, falls, and direct blows to the ankle. Pain and difficulty bearing weight are the usual symptoms, although deformity may be seen occasionally. Plain radiographs almost always confirm the diagnosis. Nondisplaced Salter-Harris type I fractures may appear normal on radiographs, so a clinical diagnosis based on localized tenderness over the physis is required. Oblique views may be necessary to show fractures of the epiphysis. CT or MRI may be used if necessary to delineate the three-dimensional pattern of the fracture.

Salter-Harris type I and II fractures have a good prognosis for healing and rarely result in any late-growth derangement. Treatment consists of closed reduction with the assistance of analgesics or relaxing agents. Flexion of the knee helps relieve muscle tension in the calf prior to reduction. External rotation deformity is common with these injuries and must be corrected. The thigh-foot angle can be used to assess this deformity. Cast immobilization for 3 to 6 weeks is usually sufficient.

Salter-Harris types III and IV injuries, which involve both the physis and the articular surface, require more aggressive treatment (Fig. 1). Many of these injuries involve the medial malleolus. Because

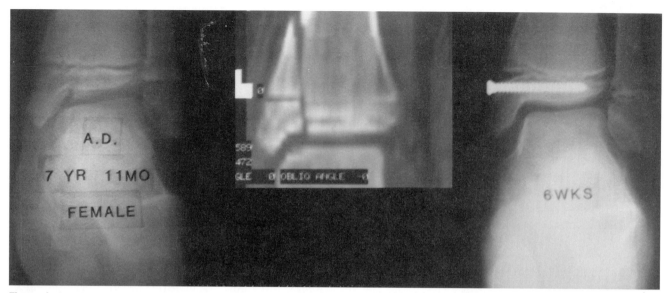

Figure 1 Salter-Harris type IV fracture. Although it is difficult to see in plain radiographs, CT reconstructions show step-off across the physis. Open reduction and internal fixation was required to align the growth plate and joint surface. *(Reproduced from Richards BS (ed): Orthopaedic Knowledge Update: Pediatrics. Rosemont, IL, American Academy of Orthopaedic Surgeons, 1996, pp 267-272.)*

the tough, fibrous periosteum around the distal tibia and fibula limits displacement, few of these fractures are completely displaced. Treatment is aimed at maintaining a smooth articular surface and eliminating displacement across the physis, which may result in late growth arrest or deformity. If plain radiographs clearly demonstrate less than 2 mm of gap in the articular surface and no displacement along the physis, these fractures may be immobilized in a cast and followed closely. Surgery should be performed for larger displacement. If the fracture displacement is greater than 2 mm or cannot be determined on plain radiographs, CT helps delineate the internal nature and extent of fracture. Specific indications for open reduction internal and fixation of epiphyseal injuries include a gap in the joint surface greater than 2 mm; a step off of the joint surface greater than 1 mm; malalignment of the physis with significant growth (more than 1 year) remaining; and open fracture. These fractures should be reduced anatomically to decrease the risk of growth arrest and intraarticular incongruity. Fixation with pins or screws is appropriate.

With proper treatment, epiphyseal injuries have a good prognosis for healing, return to function, and further growth. Occasionally, physeal injuries will result in late growth derangement, such as shortening or angulation of the leg, even with proper treatment. In these patients, late surgical reconstruction will likely be required. At the time of injury, parents should be warned about the possibility of future growth problems.

Ankle Ligament and Chondral Injuries

In children, the relatively weak physes are likely to fail before ligaments rupture; however, ligament injuries are still quite common, especially laterally. Less frequently, the deltoid ligament may be injured. These injuries result from twisting, especially in external rotation, inversion (most commonly), or eversion (less commonly) forces. Associated forceful pronation may injure the tibialis posterior tendon and the ligaments of the medial arch. Tenderness is localized over the injured ligaments, not the distal fibular or tibial physes. Swelling, ecchymosis, and inability to bear weight are common. Radiographs may be completely normal or reveal minor avulsion fractures where ligament attaches to bone. Although it is generally unnecessary, MRI evaluation may reveal bone bruising adjacent to the ankle, but the significance of this finding is unclear. Plain radiographs should be inspected for osteochondral fractures and osteochondritis dissecans, which commonly accompany ligament injuries. Nondisplaced chondral lesions can be treated with simple immobilization. If they are displaced or free in the joint, surgical removal may be required. Juxta-articular avulsion fractures generally can be treated with immobilization. No surgery is required unless there is a large displaced fracture, which is rare. Bone bruises seen on MRI require no specific treatment, but associated injuries such as ligament injuries or fractures should be treated in the usual manner. Pure ligament sprains can be treated with rest, ice, elevation, and immobilization. With improvement of pain and swelling, mobilization and strengthening should be instituted with an expectation of return to full function. In the long term, ligament injuries and avulsion fractures have a benign course. Symptomatic ankle instability that requires surgery is very rare in children. Nondisplaced osteochondral lesions have a good prognosis for healing. Displaced lesions may cause mechanical symptoms that require excision or fixation. Bone bruises are not associated with late problems.

Foot Injuries
Calcaneal Fractures

For several reasons, children with calcaneal fractures fare better than adults. The calcaneus is largely cartilaginous in young children, so it is more resilient than in adults. Additionally, remodeling is possible with growth. Calcaneal fractures in children generally result from high-energy injuries, such as falls and motor vehicle accidents; however, in toddlers, nondisplaced calcaneal fractures may result from minor trauma. The diagnosis is made on the basis of plain radiographs, which readily reveal displaced fractures. A toddler's fracture may not be readily identified early, but a fracture line can be seen on radiographs, usually within 7 to 10 days. A bone scan can be obtained if radiographs are negative and there is a high index of suspicion, but, generally, scintigraphy is not necessary for this benign condition in small children. If a fracture that extends into the subtalar joint is identified, CT should be ordered to delineate the location and extent of displacement.

Treatment of nondisplaced fractures is generally focused on symptom relief, including immobilization and non–weight-bearing until healing is seen. Open reduction and internal fixation should be considered if there is avulsion of a significant fragment or joint incongruity, usually in teenagers or adolescents (Fig. 2). Nondisplaced and nonarticular fractures have a good prognosis for full recovery. Arthrosis or limitation of subtalar motion can be seen after displaced articular fractures.

Talar Fractures

The child's talus is relatively resistant to fracture because it is largely cartilaginous. Talar fractures can occur in the neck area, in the body, or as avulsions from the medial or lateral ligament complexes. Talar injuries usually result from forced dorsiflexion, which fractures the talar neck, or crushing injuries, which may fracture the talar body. Injuries often result from falls or motor vehicle accidents. The diagnosis is suggested by the history, pain and swelling in the ankle, and radiographs. Plain radiographs do not always reveal the fracture acutely if it is nondisplaced.

Most nondisplaced fractures or minor avulsion injuries heal with simple immobilization. Open reduction and internal fixation should be considered for displaced fractures of the neck or body (Fig. 3). In the

long term, nondisplaced fractures and avulsion injuries have a good prognosis. As with adults, there is a risk of osteonecrosis of the talar body after talar neck fracture in children. If this happens, talar flattening and ankle stiffness are likely. Younger children appear to have a better prognosis than older children following this complication.

Subtalar Dislocation

Subtalar dislocations are unusual in children and, unless suspected, may be overlooked. These dislocations generally occur as a result of a fall or high-energy twisting injury. The diagnosis is suggested by the appearance of a deformed foot with localized pain and swelling. Radiographs usually will reveal the dislocation; however, a tendency to focus on the associated fractures may divert attention from the dislocation itself.

Treatment consists of attempted closed reduction and immobilization. If the dislocation is irreducible or the diagnosis delayed, open reduction may be performed to extract interposed tissue. If the reduction is unstable, the talonavicular joint should be pinned. Long-term results are generally good if treatment is instituted early.

Midfoot Injuries
Midtarsal Dislocation

Midtarsal injuries are rare in children because of their low body mass, a relatively short lever arm to apply force to the midtarsal joint, and a tendency to dissipate torsional forces in the distal tibia. Midtarsal dislocation occurs as a result of a forceful forefoot supination, which disrupts the calcaneocuboid joint and may fracture or dislocate the navicular or cuneiform bones. History, pain, localized swelling at the midtarsal joint, and fracture of associated midtarsal bones raise the suspicion of midtarsal dislocation. The key to diagnosis is disruption of the calcaneocuboid joint, which is best seen on lateral or oblique radiographs. The AP view may be entirely normal, despite the dislocation.

Treatment consists of closed or open reduction with pinning of the calcaneocuboid joint, followed by immobilization. Results are good with early treatment.

Tarsometatarsal Joint Injuries

In both children and adults, the base of the second metatarsal is contained in a mortise. The first cuneiform-second metatarsal ligament holds the second metatarsal in place. When a strong force is applied to the forefoot, there are no physes in the proximal lesser metatarsals through which to dissipate force, so Lisfranc's joint gives way. Generally, this occurs as a result of a forceful forefoot plantar flexion with or without rotation. Clinical sus-

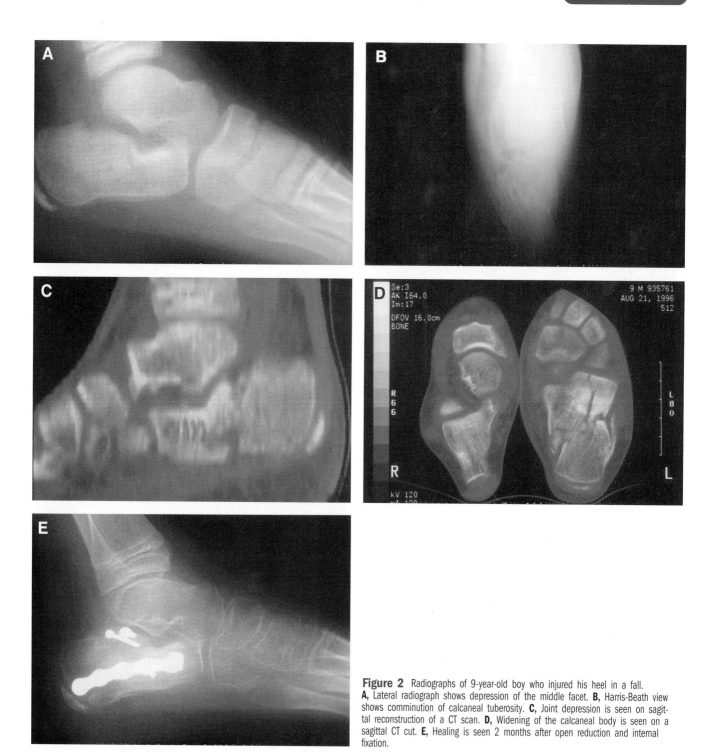

Figure 2 Radiographs of 9-year-old boy who injured his heel in a fall. **A,** Lateral radiograph shows depression of the middle facet. **B,** Harris-Beath view shows comminution of calcaneal tuberosity. **C,** Joint depression is seen on sagittal reconstruction of a CT scan. **D,** Widening of the calcaneal body is seen on a sagittal CT cut. **E,** Healing is seen 2 months after open reduction and internal fixation.

picion based on a history of forefoot plantar flexion suggests the diagnosis. The radiographic findings, which are a key to the diagnosis, include separation of the first and second metatarsals; displacement of the second metatarsal from the mortise; lateral translation of the lesser metatarsals; or a "nutcracker fracture" of the cuboid. The base of the first metatarsal may not completely dislocate. The proximal growth plate may fail, allowing displacement at the metaphysis rather than through the joint. An intra-articular fracture may be seen at the lesser metatar-

sals, and there may be a complete dislocation or divarication injury, in which the first metatarsal displaces medially and the lateral metatarsals displace laterally.

With no displacement, treatment consists of immobilization with monitoring for late displacement. With displacement, treatment with reduction and pinning is indicated. If closed reduction is not attainable, open reduction should be performed. The results are good if this disruption is recognized early and anatomically reduced.

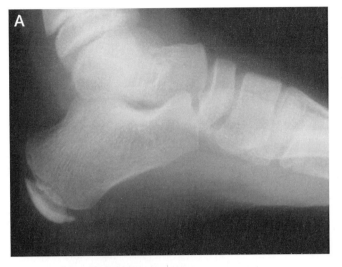

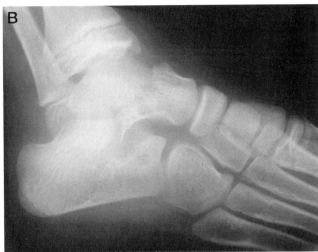

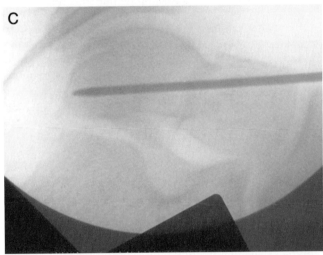

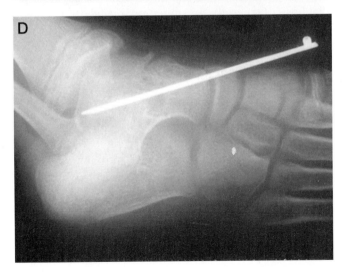

Figure 3 Radiographs of a 7-year-old girl who was injured in a tornado. **A,** Lateral radiograph of ankle shows talar neck fracture. **B,** Oblique view shows displacement. **C,** Lateral spot image reveals percutaneous pin placement. **D,** At 3 weeks, callus formation is seen. **E,** Oblique view at 6 months shows healing without osteonecrosis.

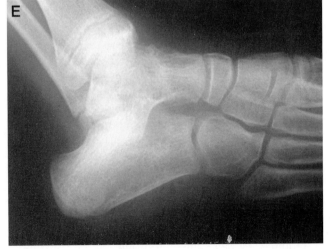

Forefoot Injuries

Because the physis or metaphyseal bone is likely to fail prior to dislocation, dislocations in the toes are relatively rare in children. In children, the physis of the distal phalanx lies just proximal to the nail fold, and if this physis fails, it may disrupt the skin and nail fold at the dorsum of the toe, resulting in an open fracture, the so-called "Seymour lesion." Forefoot injuries in children result from crushing or stubbing injuries. Routine examination and radiographs suggest the diagnosis. Fractures may occur through the metatarsals or phalanges. Dislocations of the phalanges or metatarsophalangeal joints are unusual.

Simple immobilization of nondisplaced fractures is adequate treatment, with few exceptions. Dislocations require reduction. Epiphyseal injuries of the phalanges are treated with simple immobilization, except for displaced Salter-Harris type III and IV fractures of the proximal phalanx of the great toe. Treatment of a Seymour lesion consists of irrigation and débridement, repair of the nail fold, and reduction of the fracture. Long-term results for all these fractures are generally good.

Mutilating Injuries

Mutilating injuries can be a difficult management problem in children. Although the prognosis for healing is favorable in children, injury of the growing foot may lead to severe or progressive deformity long after wound management problems have resolved. Mutilating injuries often result from powered machinery, especially lawn mowers, motor vehicle accidents, and severe crushing injuries. Diagnosis of these injuries is generally obvious. Partial or complete amputations are frequent. Compression and shear of soft tissues are common, and tissue viability may be in question. The use of Doppler flow detectors and pulse oximetry may help to determine the viability of distal structures. Failure to bleed after lancing the skin with a needle or blade suggests inadequate arterial inflow. Arteriography is rarely useful in the foot. Intact denervated or devascularized parts often result in problems if retained. The family's desire to retain the dysfunctional foot or toes may prolong healing and rehabilitation.

Life-threatening conditions should be treated first. Mutilating wounds are often contaminated and require removal of particulate debris in the operating room. Obviously nonviable tissue should be excised sharply. Initial débridement should be conservative because tissue with marginal viability may survive given the healing powers of children. Skeletal injuries should be stabilized to enable management of soft-tissue injuries. Because of the very small vessel size at the foot and ankle, revascularization of injured parts often is impractical. Bone, joint, tendons, and neurovascular structures must be covered as soon as possible to prevent necrosis by dessication. Vascularized flap coverage for these structures often is required. Because discomfort and stiffness are not as prominent in children as in adults, cross-leg flaps are well tolerated in children. Permanent disability is likely after these injuries, although most children adapt well. Multiple surgeries are often necessary for skin coverage, revision, and reconstruction. Amputations should be considered only as a last resort, but may be preferable to a poorly functioning foot that requires multiple surgical revisions.

Soft-Tissue Injuries

Peroneal Tendon Subluxation

The peroneal tendons are restrained in a bony groove posterior to the lateral malleolus by the superior peroneal retinaculum. The distal fibular growth plate is adjacent. Hyperdorsiflexion of the ankle may result in acute subluxation of the peroneal tendons around the lateral aspect of the lateral malleolus. This is more likely in children with generalized ligamentous laxity. A history of lateral pain after a hyperdorsiflexion injury of the ankle suggests the diagnosis. Often, the tendons can be repetitively subluxated anterolaterally with active ankle dorsiflexion. Although minor bony avulsions within the retinaculum have been described on radiographs, radiographs generally are not helpful. Subluxation can result from acute rupture of the retinaculum or chronic retinacular laxity.

For acute injuries, treatment consists of immobilization to allow retinacular healing and for recurrent subluxation, repair or reconstruction of the retinaculum.

Compartment Syndrome

Youth does not eliminate susceptibility to compartment syndrome. As in the adult foot, the child's foot has nine fascial compartments that are prone to contained swelling. Compartment syndrome can result from a crush injury or significant fracture, or as a result of reperfusion after temporary loss of arterial inflow. A history of injury or reperfusion suggests the diagnosis. Generally, examination reveals tense swelling and pain that are out of proportion to what would be expected for the musculoskeletal injuries. Pallor, pulselessness, and paresthesia are late signs and not particularly helpful for making an acute diagnosis. A clinical suspicion followed by compartmental pressure measurement is the key to making the diagnosis.

Regardless of etiology, treatment is immediate surgical release of the involved compartments. Elevation of the limb is not particularly helpful and may restrict tissue perfusion. After fasciotomy, time should be allowed for the swelling to subside, and then delayed closure or skin grafting is appropriate. Good results are generally seen after early diagnosis and treatment. Delayed treatment likely results in contracture of toes, deformity, and foot dysfunction.

Foreign Bodies

Because children are likely to go barefoot indoors and out, they are more susceptible to foreign bodies in the foot. A history and identification of a puncture wound suggests the diagnosis. Radiographs will not help find radiolucent foreign bodies. Radiopaque foreign bodies such as nails, needles, and some types of glass may be seen on radiographs. Radiolucent bodies, such as most glass, splinters, and toothpicks are more challenging to locate. Ultrasound may be useful in localizing foreign bodies. Treatment begins with ensuring that a foreign body actually is present. Wound exploration should be done in the operating room where anesthesia and hemostasis can be obtained. Specific intraoperative measures for localizing a foreign body include the use of fluoroscopy for radiopaque lesions or real-time ultrasound for radiolucent lesions. The wound should be expanded, irrigated, and débrided. If there is any contamination, the use of antibiotics after foreign body removal should be considered. If there has not been a recent immunization, tetanus prophylaxis should be provided. Generally, long-term results are excellent with adequate and early treatment.

Annotated Bibliography

Fractures of the Distal Tibia and Fibula

Rapariz JM, Ocete G, González-Herranz P, et al: Distal tibial triplane fractures: Long-term follow-up. *J Pediatr Orthop* 1996;16:113-118.

Triplane fractures can be detected on plain radiographs, but CT scanning is required to determine the configuration of the fracture. Closed reduction should be attempted for displaced fractures. Open reduction is reserved for fractures that cannot be closed reduced to within 2 mm displacement. The prognosis is suprisingly good.

Walker RN, Green NE, Spindler KP: Stress fractures in skeletally immature patients. *J Pediatr Orthop* 1996;16:578-584.

Stress fractures are not uncommon in active children. In this series of 34 fractures, 50% resulted from sports activities. Stress fractures were seen in the distal tibia, fibula, and metatarsals. These stress reactions could be detected on MRI before they could be seen on plain radiographs, but even plain radiograph results were positive early due to a rapid healing response. Bone scans were not often necessary. Delay in diagnosis was common, but treatment was effective. No complications or nonunions were seen.

Physeal Injuries of the Distal Tibia and Fibula

Carey J, Spence L, Blickman H, Eustace S: MRI of pediatric growth plate injury: Correlation with plain film radiographs and clinical outcome. *Skeletal Radiol* 1998;27:250-255.

MRI evaluation of the growth plate may be useful when radiographs are negative but skeletal injury is strongly suspected. MRI is particularly useful prior to the appearance of ossification centers or to create a detailed "road map" for surgery. T2-weighted fast-field echo sequences with off-resonance saturation may improve visualization of nonossified epiphyses.

Ankle Ligament and Chondral Injuries

Alanen V, Taimela S, Kinnunen J, Koskinen SK, Karaharju E: Incidence and clinical significance of bone bruises after supination injury of the ankle. *J Bone Joint Surg Br* 1998;80:513-515.

In a prospective study of 95 patients with inversion injury of the ankle without fracture, 27% were found to have bone bruises on MRI. Most bruises were in the talus, typically in the medial part. The clinical course of patients with bone bruises was no different from those without bruises. The authors concluded that bone bruises are common in uncomplicated injuries, do not require treatment, and have minor, if any, clinical significance.

Higuera J, Laguna R, Peral M, Aranda E, Soleto J: Osteochondritis dissecans of the talus during childhood and adolescence. *J Pediatr Orthop* 1998;18:328-332.

Eighteen patients with osteochondritis dissecans were followed long term. Nonsurgical treatment consisting of not bearing weight for 1.5 months in a cast, followed by 3.5 months out of a cast frequently provided good results. Indications for surgery included failure to respond to conservative treatment, lesions with thick sclerotic edges, and loose articular fragments.

Calcaneal Fractures

Inokuchi S, Usami N, Hiraishi E, Hashimoto T: Calcaneal fractures in children. *J Pediatr Orthop* 1998;18:469-474.

Calcaneal fractures occur much less frequently in children than in adults. The fractures are often missed. In this study, most fractures (60%) were extra-articular. Surgery may be required for avulsion of the tendo Achilles insertion or displaced intra-articular fractures.

John SD, Moorthy CS, Swischuk LE: Expanding the concept of the toddler's fracture. *Radiographics* 1997;17:367-376.

Nondisplaced impacted fractures and greenstick fractures may be difficult to diagnose acutely on plain radiographs. Toddler's fractures can occur in young children involving the fibula, metatarsals, and tarsal bones. Physical examination, oblique radiographs, bone scintigraphy, and delayed radiographs are helpful for making the diagnosis.

Midtarsal Dislocation

Hosking KV, Hoffman EB: Midtarsal dislocations in children. *J Pediatr Orthop* 1999;19:592-595.

Midtarsal dislocations are unusual in children but may occur as a result of forceful forefoot supination. The diagnosis should be suspected if a fracture of the midtarsal bones is detected. The calcaneocuboid joint is routinely disrupted, and this is best visualized on lateral and oblique radiographs. Accurate reduction and pin fixation are recommended.

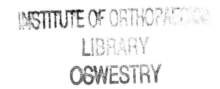

Mutilating Injuries

Mooney JF III, DeFranzo A, Marks MW: Use of cross-extremity flaps stabilized with external fixation in severe pediatric foot and ankle trauma: An alternative to free tissue transfer. *J Pediatr Orthop* 1998;18:26-30.

After severe foot and ankle trauma, soft-tissue defects may require tissue transfer. The morbidity and difficulty of free flap coverage can be avoided by the use of cross-leg or cross-foot flaps. External fixation between limbs provides stability until healing and flap detachment. Donor sites are split-thickness skin grafted. Joint stiffness is not a problem. Secondary debulking and recontouring are not necessary.

Foreign Bodies

Leung A, Patton A, Navoy J, Cummings RJ: Intraoperative sonography-guided removal of radiolucent foreign bodies. *J Pediatr Orthop* 1998;18:259-261.

Ultrasonography is useful for locating radiolucent foreign bodies, not only preoperatively, but also intraoperatively, using a sterile transducer probe sheath. Glass particles are readily identified by a "comet tail" artifact, other materials by acoustic shadowing. This technique is considerably more efficient than routine wound exploration.

Chapter 14

Spine Trauma

Brian E. Black, MD

Transport of Injured Small Children

A child with a loss of consciousness, lacerations to the head, face, or chest, extensive blunt trauma and pain in the axial spine, or paralysis must be treated in the field with a high suspicion of cervical injury. Emergency medical services personnel should perform and document a complete neurologic examination before moving the child. The child should be moved as a unit to ensure that his or her position is not changed.

Because the most common level of injury in the small child involves the occiput C1-C2 complex, flexion of the neck in the infant and small child is contraindicated during immobilization and transport. With these injuries, if the odontoid process is intact and the atlantoaxial ligaments are disrupted, spinal cord compression may occur if the child's neck is flexed. Children have a disproportionately large head in relation to the torso; therefore, the neck can be inadvertently flexed if a small child is transported positioned flat on a spine board. Inadvertent flexion can be prevented by transporting the child in a special position that maintains extension of the neck. Either the child's torso should be elevated or the head should be recessed.

Causes of Spine Trauma in Children

Physical Differences Between Children and Adults

Radiologic Differences

Distinctive radiographic differences are seen when the infant's and child's spine is compared with the adult's spine. Many of these differences are due to primary and secondary ossification centers and synchondroses (Table 1).

In addition, the child's vertebral bodies are rounded and slightly wedged anteriorly. Notching of the anterior and posterior vertebral body in the child is normal and results from the locations of the entry of the nutrient vessels and the ring apophyses.

Increased Elasticity

The child's and infant's spine has increased elasticity when compared with the adult's spine. The bones and ligaments in the child's spine are able to tolerate four times more elongation than the spinal cord. Therefore, spinal cord injury without radiographic abnormality (SCIWORA) may occur.

Multiple contiguous or noncontiguous fractures also are more common in the child because of the increased elasticity, which allows the energy of the injury to dissipate over multiple segments.

Periosteal Tube Fracture

An apparent spinal dislocation in the child younger than age 8 years heals with closed reduction as a result of an intact periosteal tube that is connected to a nondisplaced cartilage apophysis or nonossified vertebral fracture (Fig. 1). Small children with this fracture pattern may be treated with closed reduction as long as other injuries do not require open treatment. Older children and adults have less potential for spontaneous healing.

Immobilization

Children tolerate immobilization better than adults do. A prolonged period of rest and external immobilization has a low risk of complications in children.

Posttraumatic paralytic thoracolumbar spinal deformity always occurs in children younger than age 10 years with traumatic quadriplegia and paraplegia. Although bracing delays curve development and progression, these deformities typically require eventual surgical correction and stabilization.

Child Abuse

Child neglect and abuse must be considered when pediatric spine injuries are evaluated. Whiplash/shaken-child syndrome should be suspected in children with intracranial and intraocular hemorrhages and spinal cord injury. Other signs of child abuse such as multiple

TABLE 1	Normal Parameters of Pediatric Cervical Spine

Ossification Centers and Synchroses	Normal Parameters
Dens-basion distance	≤ 12 mm
C1 facet-occipital condyle distance	≤ 5 mm
Atlantodens interval	≤ 4 mm
Pseudosubluxation of C2 on C3	≤ 4 mm
Pseudosubluxation of C3 on C4	≤ 3 mm
Retropharyngeal space	≤ 8 mm
Torg ratio (canal to vertebral body)	≥ 0.8

Odontoid synchondrosis-lucent growth junction at waist of dens fuses by age 6 years
Neurocentral synchondroses-lucent growth junctions in atlas fuse by age 7 years
"Wedging" of cervical vertebral bodies—normal until age 12 years

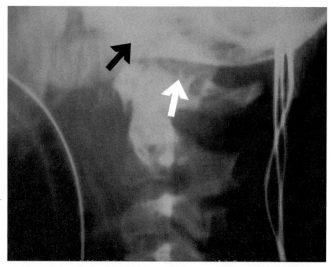

Figure 1 Atlanto-occipital dislocation in a patient with partial hemiparesis. Although the landmarks of the foramen magnum are indistinct, the occipital condyles (*black arrow*) are translated anterior to the C1 facets (*white arrow*).

bruises, retinal hemorrhage, or other fractures should be sought during the physical examination and radiographic assessment.

Air Bag Injuries

Since their introduction, air bags in motor vehicles have been responsible for saving thousands of lives. However, children age 12 years and younger are at risk for significant spinal cord injury and death from air bag deployment. Future air bag technology is expected to deploy the air bag less aggressively; however, until the new technology is available, children age 12 years and younger should not ride in the motor vehicle's front passenger seat when an air bag is functional.

Spine Injuries

Upper Cervical Spine Injuries

Atlanto-Occipital Dislocation

The atlanto-occipital articulation in children has little bony stability and relies on ligamentous integrity. Atlanto-occipital dislocation is rare and often results in death. Some children who survive are ventilator dependent and remain quadriplegic. These injuries are very unstable and require halo immobilization. Some patients may become stable following a halo immobilization. Fusion is required for patients who fail to stabilize with halo immobilization. An occiput-C1 fusion can be performed in the neurologically intact patient; an occiput-C2 fusion can be performed in the neurologically impaired patient.

Atlas Fractures

Fractures of the atlas do not commonly occur in the pediatric population. Although significant force can damage the spinal cord, neurologic compromise is uncommon because this level of the spinal canal is already capacious and further enlarged by the spreading bony fragments in this fracture pattern. CT offers the most precise imaging of these injuries, and proper gantry alignment is recommended to evaluate whether any lesions were missed on plain radiographs. Nonsurgical treatment is recommended.

Atlantoaxial (C1-C2) Disruptions

The lesions that involve the atlantoaxial articulation include traumatic ligamentous disruption, rotatory subluxation and/or dislocation, and odontoid epiphyseal separation or dens fractures. Steel's rule of thirds is an important anatomic principle regarding this level of the spine and states that the odontoid, spinal cord, and free space each occupy one third of the available space enclosed by the ring of C1. With an intact odontoid and atlantoaxial instability, the free space diminishes with flexion (Fig. 2). Initial management of an acute ligamentous disruption of the atlantoaxial articulation includes placement in a Minerva or halo cast or vest in extension for 8 to 12 weeks. With persistent or recurrent instability, posterior C1-C2 fusion is indicated. The etiology of atlantoaxial rotatory subluxation or dislocation may be traumatic or inflammatory. Subluxation also may develop spontaneously with an unknown etiology. Most of these conditions are mild and resolve spontaneously. Some patients have a fixed C1-C2 subluxation that is described as a "cock-robin" appearance. Fortunately, neurologic deficit and vertebral artery

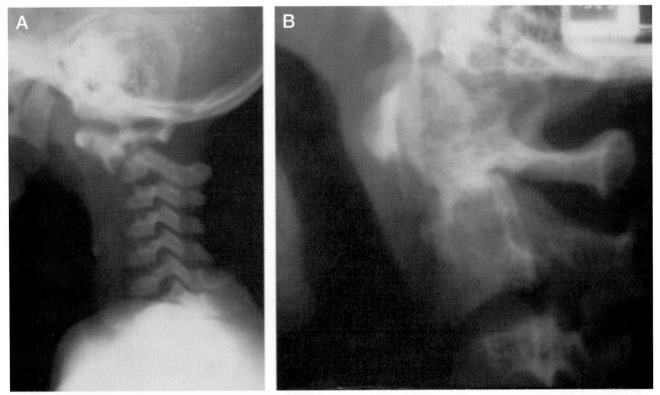

Figure 2 **A,** An odontoid fracture in a 5-year-old with no neurologic injury. **B,** The fracture was reduced by extension in a Minerva cast and healed in a good position.

compromise are rare. An open-mouth odontoid radiograph demonstrates asymmetry between the lateral masses of C1 and the dens. On a lateral radiograph, the anterior atlas may appear to have an abnormal wedge shape. Axial CT imaging is recommended to evaluate the extent of subluxation. Dynamic axial CT imaging is useful for evaluating the rigidity of the deformity. If the subluxation is

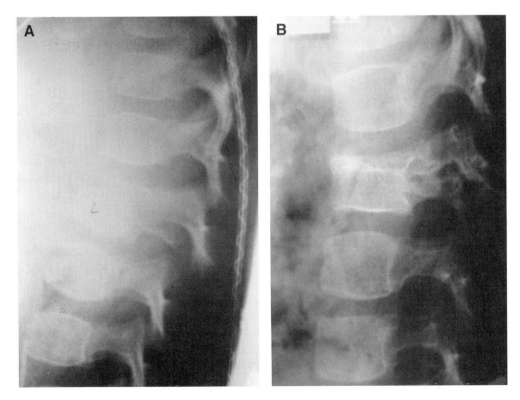

Figure 3 **A,** A lap belt injury in a 2-year-old child resulted in an apparent L2-L3 Chance dislocation. **B,** At healing, double laminae are evidence of a previous periosteal tube fracture mechanism.

diagnosed early, it may be reduced by rest and exercise, then immobilized for a brief period. For a subluxation that is more than 1 week old, traction with a cervical halter or possibly a halo is necessary, followed by immobilization in a hard collar or halo vest. Surgical fusion of C1-C2 is required for patients with neurologic involvement in whom reduction cannot be achieved and maintained.

Dens Injuries
Fracture of the dens in children usually results from significant trauma. Most dens injuries can be diagnosed on plain radiographs. Patients report instability and may hold their head with two hands to prevent motion. Most pediatric odontoid fractures heal with closed reduction and application of a halo vest or Minerva cast after 4 months of immobilization. If persistent motion is present at the fracture site, posterior C1-C2 arthrodesis is indicated.

Os odontoideum may result from nonunion of an odontoid fracture. Posterior stabilization and fusion is indicated in patients with a persistently hypermobile os odontoideum.

Hangman's Fracture
Pedicle fractures of C2, or hangman's fracture, can result from an acute flexion or acute extension injury. These injuries are usually isolated and heal well after closed reduction and placement in a halo vest or cast for 8 weeks. If significant C2-C3 disk disruption or nonunion occurs, posterior C1-C3 arthrodesis is indicated.

C2-C3 Subluxation and Dislocation
In children, C2-C3 subluxation and dislocation must be differentiated from pseudosubluxation. Patients with true injury typically have had significant trauma to the head, face, neck, and chest and report pain. MRI may be helpful to assess for spinal cord and soft-tissue injury. The spinal laminar line typically is undisturbed in patients with pseudosubluxation but is disrupted in patients with true subluxation. In children younger than age 8 years, true C2-C3 subluxation has a high potential for healing with closed reduction and immobilization in a halo vest. In older children, the healing potential with closed management is poor and fusion generally is required.

Middle to Lower Cervical Injuries
Lower cervical injuries are more prevalent in older children and adolescents than upper cervical injuries. Closed reduction and immobilization in a halo vest may be attempted in younger children. If cord compression and neurologic deficit are present, surgical decompression and stabilization are recommended. Such surgical intervention

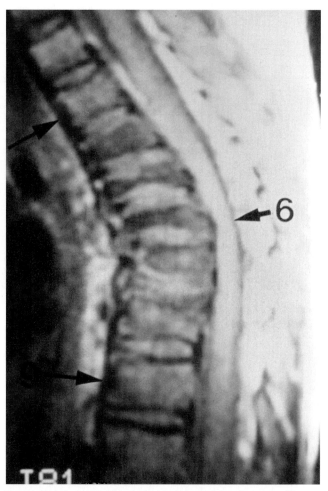

Figure 4 A 5-year-old child sustained multiple contiguous fractures at T4 through T8 from a lap belt injury. The injury resulted in paraplegia.

may allow for some spinal cord recovery in incomplete injuries, or for nerve root recovery.

Thoracic and Lumbar Injuries

Apparent Dislocations in Small Children
Thoracic and lumbar dislocations in the small child have greater healing potential than in the older child and adult, possibly because they represent periosteal tube or physeal vertebral injury rather than a true dislocation. Periosteal tube or physeal injuries have a favorable healing potential with nonsurgical treatment (Fig. 3).

Multiple Fractures and Spinal Cord Injury Without Radiographic Abnormality
The increased flexibility of the child's spine allows the energy of the injury to dissipate over multiple levels, resulting in multiple contiguous or noncontiguous fractures (Fig. 4).

SCIWORA lesions may occur in the child with spine trauma secondary to the increased flexibility.

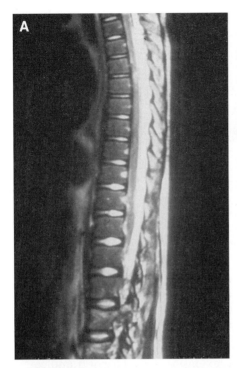
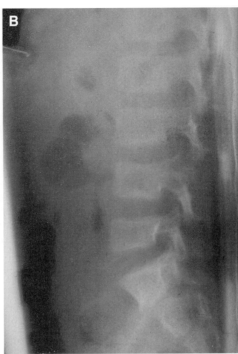

Figure 5 A complete spinal cord injury at T4 in a 6-year-old child. **A,** Plain radiographs and MRI show no bony or ligamentous injury; however, the MRI shows cord edema at this level. **B,** The phenomenon of multiple non-contiguous spine injuries is also shown by the flexion-distraction injury at L3-4.

Delayed onset of neurologic deficit has been reported. MRI to evaluate patients with SCIWORA is recommended (Fig. 5). MRI also should be used for patients in whom head injury or prolonged intubation prevents the spine from being fully assessed or "cleared." If a physical examination to rule out tenderness and neurologic injury cannot be performed, the patient should be treated as if an injury were present. If the patient's condition does not improve in a few days, MRI can be used to definitively assess the spine.

Burst Fractures
Burst fractures are rare in children but more common in adolescents. The mechanism of injury may be a fall or motor vehicle accident. Treatment is the same in children as in adults. Because significant canal compromise and kyphosis may be tolerated without sequelae, the indications for surgery are controversial. Surgical fixation and decompression is indicated only in the presence of severe kyphosis or neurologic injury resulting from cord impingement from fragments displaced from the middle column into the canal.

Lap Belt Injury
Lap belt injuries are a common cause of thoracic and lumbar fractures and dislocations in children. In these injuries, the fulcrum of flexion is at the level of the lap belt placement. Patients may have a lap belt sign, which is a strip of ecchymosis at the level of the lap belt placement (Fig. 6). Patients with a lap

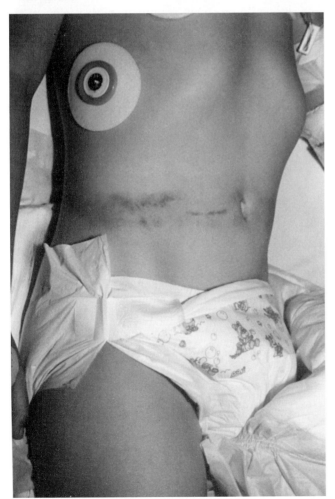

Figure 6 Lap belt sign reveals ecchymosis at the level that the lap belt had been placed.

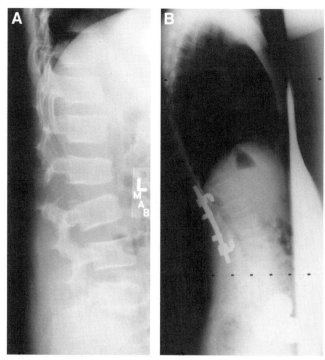

Figure 7 **A,** Lap belt fracture-dislocation at L2-L3 with associated visceral injuries in an 11-year-old boy. **B,** The fracture was treated with open reduction with posterior compression instrumentation.

TABLE 2 | Vehicle Restraint Recommendations

Age	Type of Restraint
Birth to 1 year (20 lb)	Rear facing infant-only seat in back seat
1 to 4 years (20 to 40 lb)	Forward facing seat in back seat
4 to 8 years (40 to 60 lb)	Booster seat plus lap/shoulder belt in back seat
8 to 12 years (60 to 100 lb)	Lap/shoulder belt in back seat

belt sign must be evaluated for associated neurologic, spinal, and visceral injuries. In patients younger than age 9 years, lap belt Chance fractures or apparent dislocations in neurologically intact patients can be treated with closed reduction and hyperextension casting. If the patient has a spinal cord or nerve root injury, open reduction (with decompression, if necessary) and surgical stabilization should be considered (Fig. 7). In young children with severe associated injuries, prolonged cast immobilization in hyperextension may be contraindicated. In these children, open treatment with wiring of the spinous processes or posterior compression instrumentation is recommended. During reduction, the spinal cord should be monitored. Proper positioning and use of restraints in the motor vehicle can reduce the risk of lap belt injury (Fig. 8, Table 2).

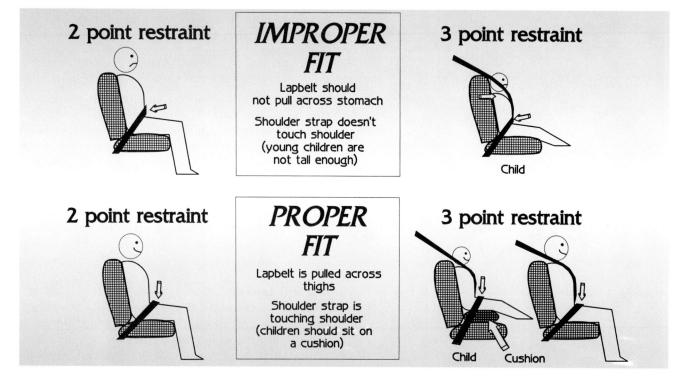

Figure 8 Illustration demonstrating fitting of two- and three-point restraints. *(Reproduced with permission from Black BE, O'Brien E, Sponseller PD: Thoracic and lumbar spine injuries in children: Different than adults.* Contemp Orthop *1994;29:253-260.)*

Annotated Bibliography

Air Bag Injuries

McCaffrey M, German A, Lalonde F, Letts M: Air bags and children: A potentially lethal combination. *J Pediatr Orthop* 1999;19:60-64.

In this review of 13 children in Canada who were injured by air bags, 12 children sustained relatively minor injuries. One child died following an occiput-C1 dislocation.

Spine Injuries

Odent T, Langlais J, Glorion C, Kassis B, Bataille J, Pouliquen JC: Fractures of the odontoid process: A report of 15 cases in children younger than 6 years. *J Pediatr Orthop* 1999;19:51-54.

In this review of 15 children with fractures of the odontoid process, eight patients had neurologic involvement and six had MRI changes in the spinal cord at the cervicothoracic junction. The injury was believed to be caused by anterior displacement of the upper spine resulting in spinal cord stretch at the spinal apex of the cervical and thoracic spine. Fractures managed nonsurgically fused with no problem; however, surgical treatment resulted in complications in three patients. Average follow-up was 4 years, 3 months.

Sponseller PD, Cass JR: Atlanto-occipital fusion for dislocation in children with neurologic preservation: A case report. *Spine* 1997;22:344-347.

In this retrospective review of patients with atlanto-occipital dislocations, a technique is described for fusing only the occiput to C1, which is indicated in neurologically intact patients following dislocation at this level.

Copley LA, Dormans JP: Cervical spine disorders in infants and children. *J Am Acad Orthop Surg* 1998;6:204-214.

In this article, normal values as well as treatment of developmental and traumatic problems of the cervical spine are discussed.

Dormans JP, Criscitiello AA, Drummond DS, Davidson RS: Complications in children managed with immobilization in a halo vest. *J Bone Joint Surg Am* 1995;77:1370-1373.

In this article, the differences in management of the child in a halo vest are discussed. Of the 37 patients 3 to 16 years who were immobilized in a halo vest, the vest was applied following arthrodesis of the cervical spine in 24 patients and following trauma in 13 patients. Complications included pin-site infections and loosening of the pins and occurred in 25 patients.

Classic Bibliography

Aufdermaur M: Spinal injuries in juveniles: Necropsy findings in twelve cases. *J Bone Joint Surg Br* 1974;56:513-519.

Birney TJ, Hanley EN Jr: Traumatic cervical spine injuries in childhood and adolescence. *Spine* 1989;14:1277-1282.

Black BE, O'Brien E, Sponseller PD: Thoracic and lumbar spine injuries in children: Different than in adults. *Contemp Orthop* 1994:29:253-260.

Hadley MN, Zabramski JM, Browner CM, Rekate H, Sonntag VK: Pediatric spinal trauma: Review of 122 cases of spinal cord and vertebral column injuries. *J Neurosurg* 1988;68:18-24.

Herzenberg JE, Hensinger RN, Dedrick DK, Phillips WA: Emergency transport and positioning of young children who have an injury of the cervical spine: The standard backboard may be hazardous. *J Bone Joint Surg Am* 1989;71:15-22.

Mayfield JK, Erkkila JC, Winter RB: Spine deformity subsequent to acquired childhood spinal cord injury. *J Bone Joint Surg Am* 1981;63:1401-1411.

Pang D, Wilberger JE Jr: Spinal cord injury without radiographic abnormalities in children. *J Neurosurg* 1982;57:114-129.

Rathbone D, Johnson G, Letts M: Spinal cord concussion in pediatric athletes. *J Pediatr Orthop* 1992;12:616-620.

Rumball K, Jarvis J: Seat-belt injuries of the spine in young children. *J Bone Joint Surg Br* 1992;74:571-574.

Torg JS, Pavlov H, Genuario SE, et al: Neurapraxia of the cervical spinal cord with transient quadriplegia. *J Bone Joint Surg Am* 1986;68:1354-1370.

Section 3

Lower Extremity

Section Editor:
Steven L. Buckley, MD

Section 3

Lower Extremity

Overview

Recent literature has provided much new information about problems with the lower extremity in children. Slipped capital femoral epiphysis remains the most common significant hip problem in adolescents, and early diagnosis and internal fixation remain the mainstay of management. The chapter on Legg-Calvé-Perthes disease raises the possibility that a coagulation abnormality may be a cause of the disease in some children. In the chapter on developmental dysplasia of the hip, emphasis is placed on the importance of early diagnosis in providing effective treatment and minimizing complications. The chapter on congenital and acquired tibial deformities describes available treatments for these conditions as well as some of the complications that can occur. The controversies surrounding limb lengthening for short stature are described in the limb-length inequality chapter. In the knee disorders chapter, the problems with MRI as a diagnostic tool in pediatric patients are described. The chapter on clubfoot presents different methods of correction, along with a meta-analysis that reviews the results of these procedures. The chapter on flexible flatfoot and tarsal coalition presents the limited treatment options for patients who remain symptomatic following resection and the benefits of a medial closing wedge calcaneal osteotomy or calcaneal lengthening osteotomy in patients with severe hindfoot valgus. The benefits of multiple procedures versus a standard surgical procedure for juvenile and adolescent bunion deformities are described in the chapter on miscellaneous foot disorders.

Steven L. Buckley, MD
Section Editor

Chapter 15

Slipped Capital Femoral Epiphysis

John C. Eldridge, MD

Introduction

Slipped capital femoral epiphysis (SCFE) is a disorder of the growing femur in which the proximal femoral epiphysis slips posteriorly on the femoral neck. The disorder causes hip pain and a distinctive gait in the early stages and may damage the hip, leading to early degenerative hip disease in adulthood. Complications of a SCFE, such as chondrolysis and osteonecrosis (ON), may cause early hip pain and dysfunction. The early recognition and prompt treatment of SCFE may prevent many of the problems associated with the disorder and help to preserve the longevity of the hip joint.

Demographics

Children with SCFE do not always have classic symptoms. Knowing which patient is most likely to be affected is the first step to an early diagnosis. SCFE is the most common hip problem in adolescents, with a worldwide incidence of 2 per 100,000 individuals. Polynesian children are the most likely to have SCFE, with a prevalence 4.5 times that of white children. Indonesian and Indo-Mediterranean children are least likely to have a slip, with a prevalence ratio of 0.5 and 0.1, respectively, compared with white children. Low-risk populations may increase their risk by adopting the lifestyle of those in the high-risk category, especially by extreme obesity.

Geographic variation is present within the United States as well. The prevalence rate is 10 per 100,000 individuals in Connecticut but only 2.1 per 100,000 individuals in the Southwest. This may be related to race distribution because black children are 2.25 times more likely to have SCFE than white children in the same region. Boys are more often affected than girls with a ratio of 1.43:1. This, too, differs with geography and race; the Indo-Mediterranean children show a ratio of 4.25:1 of boys over girls.

Body weight may be the most important factor in SCFE. Morethan 60% of children with SCFE are above the 90th percentile for weight. In addition, SCFE develops in obese children at a younger age than in lighter weight children.

Etiology

There is no single etiology known for SCFE as yet. Most cases occur in relation to the pubertal growth spurt, suggesting a hormonal influence on the physis. The association with obesity also suggests a mechanical overload on the structures of the hip. Other possibilities have included structural abnormalities in the configuration of the hip, immunologic abnormalities, and environmental causes.

SCFE can be compared to a physeal fracture of the proximal femur. Abrupt forces can cause a fracture to occur through the metaphyseal surface of the physis, allowing the epiphysis to slip. SCFE is not usually associated with significant injury; the forces of displacement occur gradually. The orientation of the proximal femoral physis changes during early adolescence, increasing in obliquity and assuming a more vertical position to the proximal femur. Thus, weight-bearing forces on the physis change from compression to increasing shear. The physis has less strength in shear and is more vulnerable to failure, especially with increasing weight.

The physis thickens with the onset of puberty. Initially, the increase in testosterone stimulates the growth of the physis and only later stimulates closure. Growth hormone (GH) also stimulates physeal growth, while estrogen stimulates closure without the marked growth phase. Rapid physeal growth increases the thickness of the calcified cartilage columns, outpacing metaphyseal ossification and causing an increase in relative physeal height. A delay in ossification would markedly increase the thickness of the physis and decrease the strength. Ossification requires thyroid hormone, vitamin D, and adequate calcium. Hypothyroidism and renal osteodystrophy, therefore, decrease the stability of the proximal femoral physis and make a slip more likely. Approximately 7% of patients with SCFE have an endocrinopathy, most commonly hypothyroidism. Many of these patients also have short stature and delayed growth plate closure, traits that help to identify them. However, most children with SCFE do not have associated hormonal abnormalities, although subclinical vitamin D deficiency has been suggested. Osteodystrophy and endocrine disorders should be kept in mind in children with bilateral SCFE and an unusual clinical presentation.

The occurrence of SCFE in several children taking GH led to a search for the role of GH in proximal femoral physeal dysfunction. Results of repeated testing of serum GH levels were normal in patients with SCFE; however, levels can be quite variable in healthy children. The mediator of GH function, insulin-like growth factor I and its binding proteins, have more stable levels but also show no abnormalities in association with SCFE. Thus, a relationship between GH and SCFE has not been established.

Decreased femoral anteversion is associated with chronic SCFE and is more frequent in black children. No relationship, however, has been shown for acetabular or tibial version. A deeper acetabulum, as determined by the center-edge Wiberg's angle, is more frequent in children with SCFE, both white and black. Overall, black children have greater center-edge angles than white children. The shear stress on the proximal femoral physis is calculated to be greater with a deeper acetabulum, making the child more vulnerable to failure of the physis.

Radiation of physes for nearby malignancies is known to cause physeal dysfunction, including SCFE. Injury to endocrine glands caused by radiation may produce hormone deficiencies that make the child more vulnerable to SCFE. Chemotherapeutic agents may enhance the effects of radiation on the physes, adding to the possibility of later hip problems. Children with postradiation SCFE tend to be of normal weight and are less likely to have bilateral disease. In these children, the slipped epiphyses are usually chronic and mild compared with idiopathic cases and often occur at a younger age. With them, the physis takes longer to close after treatment, which may lead to a recurrent slip if the femur grows past the fixation device.

Pathophysiology

The final pathway for SCFE is a separation of the physis from the metaphysis, leading to the abrupt or gradual posterior displacement of the epiphysis. The stability of the physis is due to the orientation, shape, and intrinsic strength of the physis. The orientation of the proximal femur and hip determine the amount of compression or shear forces on the physis. The increasing obliquity of the physis that occurs with the adolescent growth spurt places a strain on the physis, as does retroversion of the femur and deepening of the acetabulum. The structure of the physis provides stability through the undulating shape of its junction with the metaphysis, as well as the perichondral ring of fibrocartilaginous tissue. The zone of hypertrophy in the physis consists of elongating columns of chondrocytes which blend into the zone of provisional ossification. This junction, and the long chondrocyte columns, are the weak areas of the physis and are the location of failure in SCFE. The endocrine environment affects the quality and height of the cartilage columns, and failure of ossification can increase the thickness of the weak provisional zone. Thus, the intrinsic strength of the physis may change, making the hip more susceptible to shear forces.

Electron microscopic evaluation of shearing physeal fractures demonstrate that the interconnections of chondrocyte columns provide resistance to failure. Although failure occurs at the junction of the hypertrophic and provisional calcification zones, the fracture line may meander through the zones. The chondrocyte columns appear to be individual mechanical units that remain intact after shear fractures. Thus, conditions that affect the integrity of the chondrocyte structure alter the susceptibility to failure of the physis.

Biopsies from the metaphyseal and physeal areas of the hip in patients with SCFE reveal thickening of the hypertrophic zone, scattered clusters of chondrocytes in the metaphysis, and loss of the orderly arrangement of chondrocyte columns in the hypertrophic zone. An abnormal arrangement and concentration of proteoglycan and glycoprotein in the cartilage matrix of the hypertrophic zone is seen as well. Defects in the supporting collagen structure and unexpected chondrocyte death are noted on electron microscope evaluation. Many of these findings are similar to histologic changes in the tibial physis of patients with Blount's disease. It is not known whether the microscopic changes occur in response to mechanical overload of the physis or are the primary cause of physeal failure.

Clinical Presentation

Children with SCFE typically are obese and report pain and limping, more often on the left side, of several months' duration. These children are usually in the preteen to early teen years, averaging age 12 years for girls and 13.5 years for boys. They can bear weight but usually show outturning of the affected leg. Many children have a history of mild trauma that they believe is the cause of the hip pain.

Approximately 85% of SCFE cases can be described as chronic, in which symptoms have been present for at least 3 weeks. Most patients have an even longer history of symptoms, averaging nearly 5 months. SCFE with symptoms of less than 3 weeks' duration is described as acute. The pain and limited motion are generally more severe in patients with acute SCFE. Other terms that are often used to describe SCFE include preslip, characterized by mild hip pain and no radiographic slip, and acute-on-chronic, in which an abrupt change in pain has occurred in a chronic slip. The latter type has not correlated well with treatment decisions.

Classification of SCFE by stability is more useful in the office situation. An unstable slip is characterized by an abrupt onset of severe pain with inability to bear full weight. These patients often report hip and groin pain and are quite uncomfortable. Fluoroscopy studies show true instability of the epiphysis with gross motion on movement of the femur. This type of SCFE can be compared to acute physeal fracture, and the risk of ON may be as high as 50%. Patients with stable slips have only mild groin or medial knee pain and can bear weight, but sometimes they limp or use crutches. Most often, the symptoms in these patients are chronic. Fluoroscopy studies reveal no gross motion of the epiphysis, and there is usually evidence of callus or remodeling. The risk of ON is much lower in stable slips. Age and weight are individual factors in each type but are not differentiated between the types.

Reports of knee pain should be taken seriously in children in the early teenage years. Approximately 15% of patients with SCFE report pain only in the distal thigh and medial knee. Many more complain of both groin and knee pain. Most patients with only knee pain report a longer duration of symptoms, suggesting a more chronic onset. The time to diagnosis also may be longer if evaluation is limited to knee studies. Thus, the evaluation of a child with knee pain should always include a thorough examination of the lower extremity, including the hip.

The hip examination of a child with SCFE reveals pain with internal rotation. The posterior movement of the epiphysis results in relative external rotation and extension of the femur. This change in hip alignment results in decreased hip flexion, increased external rotation with flexion, and an external rotation with gait on the affected side. Pain revealed on examination is related both to hip instability and synovitis. A child with a mild slip may have considerable pain but little change in hip range of motion, whereas a child with a severe, stable slip may have more deformity than pain and very noticeable external rotation.

The left hip is affected in 60% of patients. At least 22% of slips are bilateral, but not all are simultaneous. Approximately 60% of bilateral SCFE is seen at presentation; in the remainder of patients, a second slip occurs over the next 18 to 24 months. However, long-term studies of patients treated for SCFE have shown asymptomatic contralateral slips. Bilaterality may be as high as 80%, and nearly 30% of patients with asymptomatic slips have arthrosis in the affected hip.

Imaging

When SCFE is suspected, AP and true lateral hip radiographs are required. Although the frog-lateral view is most often used, the position can be painful and cause displacement in an acute slip. In early SCFE, the AP view may show widening of the physis and periphyseal irregularity. In a more severe slip, the physis may appear thinned as the epiphysis moves posterior to the femoral neck, but this should not be mistaken for a closing physis. The overlap of the epiphysis and the metaphysis may result in the appearance of increased density in the most proximal metaphysis. Subtle displacement may be detected by using Klein's line, a line drawn along the superior neck of the femur on the AP view. This line should intersect the lateral edge of the epiphysis but will pass laterally to it in a patient with SCFE. The lateral view is very sensitive for epiphyseal displacement and shows the posterior position more clearly than the AP view. The initial radiographs often show considerable remodeling in patients with chronic SCFE. New bone formation is seen at the medial edge of the metaphysis with erosion, or rounding-off, along the exposed superior edge.

AP and lateral radiographs are not as accurate in the diagnosis of early SCFE, prior to displacement. In the preslip stage, diagnostic sensitivity for both views is 80% and for AP views, only 66%. Ultrasound can show early changes in the hip and surrounding tissues with a 95% sensitivity. CT can detect subtle displacement, and MRI can show early alterations in the physis, prior to displacement. The bone scan can detect small changes in bone vascularity and has been recommended for pretreatment evaluation of patients with SCFE. Unstable slips have shown decreased uptake on pretreatment scans, but not all unstable slips progress to ON. Synovitis of the hip associated with SCFE increases periarticular vascularity, which is also seen on the bone scan. The role of the bone scan before or after treatment of SCFE is not yet clear.

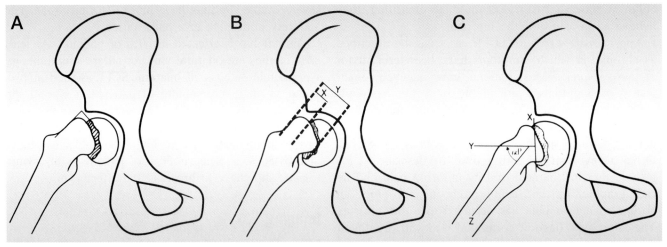

Figure 1 Schematic representations of slip severity measured on the frog-lateral radiograph. **A,** Absolute epiphyseal displacement. **B,** Percent epiphyseal displacement. **C,** Lateral head-shaft angle. *(Reproduced with permission from Cohen MS, Gelberman RH, Griffin PP, et al: Slipped capital femoral epiphysis: Assessment of epiphyseal displacement and angulation. J Pediatr Orthop 1986;6:259-264.)*

Classification

Classification of SCFE can be based on clinical or radiographic parameters. The clinical classifications of stable and unstable SCFE, as well as acute, chronic, and acute-on-chronic, were discussed earlier. Radiographic classifications include slip severity and slip angle. Severity is based on the amount of epiphyseal displacement seen on AP or lateral radiographs. A mild slip is displaced less than one third the neck width; moderate, one third to one half the neck width; and severe, more than one half the neck width (Fig. 1).

The slip angle measures the magnitude of the slip by measuring the angular displacement of the epiphysis on the femoral neck femur. A line drawn along the center of the neck is compared to the perpendicular bisector of the epiphysis. A slip angle of less than 30° is considered mild; a slip of 30° to 50° moderate; and a slip angle of more than 50° severe. The slip angle also can be measured on the CT scan.

Treatment

The early diagnosis of SCFE provides an opportunity to stabilize the epiphysis and prevent malalignment of the hip and early onset of arthrosis. Treatment is urgent. Even in stable slips, a simple twist or fall can cause severe displacement of the hip and lifelong problems. The child should not bear weight on the affected leg until it is treated. The primary goal of treatment is to stabilize the slip until physeal closure. The most frequently used technique for stabilization is placement of a single screw across the physis; other techniques include spica cast immobilization, multiple pins or screws, and bone-peg epiphysiodesis. A wide array of reconstructive osteotomies are available to treat mal-

alignment of the proximal femur after physeal closure, if necessary.

Screw Fixation

Single-screw fixation is a widely accepted primary treatment of SCFE. Previous multiple-pin fixation resulted in frequent pin penetration into the hip joint and articular damage. Usually, a single cannulated screw, 6.5 mm or greater diameter, is placed from the metaphysis into the epiphysis. This requires insertion along the anterior femoral neck perpendicular to the posteriorly displaced epiphysis. Often, this can be done through a very limited incision into the anterolateral thigh. The incision and path for the guide wire can be determined with fluoroscopy (Fig. 2). A guide wire is positioned on the skin so that, under fluoroscopy, it is perpendicular to the physis and in the center of the epiphysis on the AP view. A line is drawn on the skin along the wire. This is repeated on the lateral view. The incision is made at the intersection of the lines, and the guide wire bisects the angle as it approaches the femoral neck. The wire and screw placement is guided by fluoroscopy to avoid placing unnecessary holes in the femoral neck.

The best position for screw placement is in the center of the epiphysis in both AP and lateral views. The tip should not be closer than 5 mm to the subchondral bone of the femur. The anterolateral quadrants of the femoral head should be avoided to prevent damage to the intraepiphyseal vessels by the screw. The guide wire may advance during drilling and can be monitored with fluoroscopy as the drill is used. Transient pin penetration appears to cause little damage; however, care must be used to prevent penetration of the screw into the hip joint. The hip can be moved through

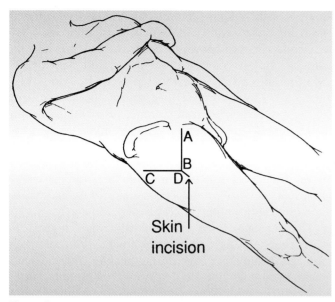

Figure 2 Technique and landmarks used to mark the position of the skin incision for pin placement. A-B represents line overlying femoral head and neck (bisecting femoral head and lying perpendicular to physis) as visualized on AP fluoroscopic image. C-D represents line overlying femoral head and neck (also bisecting femoral head and lying perpendicular to physis) as visualized on lateral image. *(Reproduced from Aronsson DD, Karol LA: Stable slipped capital femoral epiphysis: Evaluation and management. J Am Acad Orthop Surg 1996;4:173-181.)*

a range of motion under fluoroscopy to ensure that the screw is positioned well within the epiphysis. Although placement of a second screw has been recommended for unstable hips, in other situations, the benefit of secure fixation may be outweighed by the increase in complications.

Bone-Peg Epiphysiodesis

Open bone-peg epiphysiodesis accelerates physeal closure by applying a peg of bone across the physis. Although the incidence of complications is low with this procedure, the exposure and surgical procedure are more extensive. The excellent results of single-screw fixation have markedly reduced the indications for the use of open procedures.

Cast Immobilization

Spica cast immobilization of SCFE is not recommended in routine cases. The cast does not provide rigid immobilization, and the slip may progress in the cast. Complications, especially chondrolysis, are not necessarily reduced with cast treatment. The physis is not closed by immobilization, and the slip may recur after cast removal. Cast treatment has better results in patients with metabolic bone disease who are awaiting correction of the primary metabolic disease. Screw fixation of dystrophic bone may not be secure and can be combined with spica cast application.

Manipulative Reduction

Manipulation of the hip prior to screw fixation is not recommended because of the possible increase in the risk of ON. The risk of ON is higher in unstable SCFE, but often the hip will reduce spontaneously during positioning for surgery. This incidental reduction does not show a deleterious effect on bone scan studies, but in situ fixation generally is better accepted. Forceful reduction is contraindicated because of the risk of vascular damage and ON. Stable slips undergo remodeling and adaptation of the soft tissue; by contrast, abrupt realignment may damage vascular tissue. The resulting ON may cause devastating damage to the hip, while malalignment often can be salvaged with reconstructive surgery.

Fixation of the Contralateral Hip

SCFE occurs bilaterally in at least 22% of patients and perhaps in as many as 80%. Children with radiographic evidence of SCFE in the contralateral hip, even if asymptomatic, should undergo in situ fixation. When the contralateral hip is normal clinically and radiographically, fixation is not currently recommended. However, the association of late arthrosis with asymptomatic SCFE in the contralateral hip may justify a more aggressive approach. SCFE caused by an endocrinopathy or osteodystrophy is more likely to be bilateral. When screw fixation is indicated in the affected hip in these cases, the contralateral hip also should be treated.

Osteotomy

Screw fixation of SCFE can prevent further displacement and encourage physeal closure, but it cannot correct deformity of the proximal femur. Reconstructive osteotomies of the proximal femur are performed in an attempt to prevent early degenerative joint disease of the hip. The true deformity is in the subcapital femoral neck, but osteotomies in this area are associated with high rates of ON and chondrolysis. Osteotomies performed in the intertrochanteric or subtrochanteric areas result in fewer complications; however, they must be designed to correct angular deformity and translation. Long-term results of osteotomies are difficult to assess because of the poor long-term natural history of severe SCFE.

Cuneiform Osteotomy

Cuneiform osteotomy is performed in the subcapital femoral neck. The deformity correction is best when performed near the apex of the deformity. The cuneiform osteotomy takes advantage of the extrametaphyseal circulation to the epiphysis prior to physeal closure. The lateral epiphyseal vessels course through to the posterior periosteum of the femoral neck. A wedge of bone is resected, which corrects the deformity, but does not interrupt the posterior periosteum or cause tension on the lateral epiphyseal vessel. However, rates of ON range from 20% to 35% and should be of concern even to surgeons experienced in femoral osteotomies. A cuneiform osteotomy should be considered only for a very limited range of indications.

Base-of-Neck Osteotomy

As the osteotomy site moves distally on the femoral neck, the correction is less complete, but the incidence of ON decreases. The base-of-neck osteotomy is a wedge resection at the junction of the femoral neck and intertrochanteric region. This osteotomy works best for moderate deformities because it cannot correct complete epiphyseal displacement. Other deformities are produced by this procedure, including shortening of the femoral neck and relative trochanteric overgrowth, both of which may increase the patient's limp. ON and chondrolysis are possible significant complications of surgery.

Osteotomy at the Trochanteric Level

Intertrochanteric and subtrochanteric osteotomies are made outside the hip capsule and have a low complication rate. Both are multiplanar osteotomies, designed to correct external rotation and varus, if present. The most immediate effect of osteotomy is restoration of more normal hip range of motion and gait. The long-term benefits of reduction in degenerative joint disease are more difficult to document due to the nature of long-term studies and the natural history of SCFE.

Intertrochanteric and subtrochanteric osteotomies can be stabilized with rigid internal fixation, making cast immobilization unnecessary and allowing for early weight bearing. ON and chondrolysis rates are generally less than 10% and may be related more to the initial treatment of the slip than the osteotomy. The compensatory femoral shaft malalignment may make later joint replacement challenging.

Complications
Chondrolysis

Chondrolysis is an acute arthritis of the hip of unknown etiology. The articular surface of the hip undergoes necrosis with a vigorous synovial reaction. The child reports severe hip pain, usually after fixation of the SCFE. Examination reveals little hip motion, and adduction contracture often gives the false appearance of a limb-length discrepancy. Radiographic exam-

ination usually shows more than a 50% reduction in joint hip space, with juxta-articular osteoporosis.

Chondrolysis is known to occur without previous hip disease, but it is most often associated with SCFE. Multiple-pin fixation of the hip is related to a high incidence of chondrolysis because of the severe damage an implant penetration can cause within the hip joint. Single-screw fixation with attention to the position of the screw has greatly reduced, but not eliminated, the incidence of chondrolysis. Chondrolysis also is reported after fracture, infection, and rheumatologic illnesses. It also occurs occasionally with spica cast immobilization, both for SCFE and trauma.

The damage caused by chondrolysis is a nonspecific cartilage necrosis and joint synovitis. Fibrocartilage replaces hyaline cartilage during healing, and the synovium undergoes fibrosis. Hip range of motion can be severely limited. Treatment is based on maintaining active and passive range of motion while the condition progresses. Anti-inflammatory medication may improve pain and synovitis. Resolution may take several years, with gradual improvement in motion and radiographic appearance. Often, however, the result is poor with persistent pain and stiffness.

Osteonecrosis

ON is a devastating complication of SCFE, with a partial or total loss of blood supply to the epiphysis and destruction of the weight-bearing surface. Unstable SCFE is much more likely to be followed by ON, affecting as many as 47% of patients. However, chronic SCFE has an incidence of less than 3%. Ischemia has been demonstrated by bone scan prior to treatment of unstable SCFE, whereas it is not routinely seen in chronic SCFE. Incidental reduction of unstable slips does not seem to increase the rate of ON, but forceful reduction of stable SCFE is related to a high incidence of subsequent ON. Segmental ON may occur after pin placement into the anterolateral and posterolateral epiphyses. The blood supply to this area may be damaged, especially with multiple pin placement into the upper hemisphere of the femoral head.

Patients with ON present with a recurrence of hip pain, usually several months after treatment of SCFE. The extent of femoral head involvement may not be apparent initially and may only include a small segment. Collapse of the femoral head may result in exposure of the screw tip and more damage to the hip joint. Removal of the exposed screw prior to closure of the physis could lead to further slipping of the epiphysis. In this case, replacement of the screw into a more healthy area is appropriate. After ON is discovered, the child should rest the hip and avoid weight bearing on the affected leg by using crutches. Anti-inflammatory medication may improve pain and irritation and facilitate physical therapy. Although improvement may occur, complete head involvement often leaves a very poor result. Osteotomy or arthrodesis may be needed.

Pathologic Fracture

Fracture may occur through the hole left by placement or removal of fixation devices. The risk is increased if the screw head is at or below the lesser trochanter. The use of cannulated screws has decreased the incidence of fracture through lateral cortical entry sites because a small guide wire is used for initial alignment prior to drilling. Multiple pin fixation often leaves several larger holes as pin position is adjusted. Removal of internal fixation after fixation or osteotomy may leave stress risers that result in later fracture.

Long-term Considerations

In situ fixation of SCFE quickly reduces pain and improves weight bearing, so many children try to resume activities within weeks after successful stabilization. Most, however, still have reduced hip flexion and an externally rotated leg on the side of the slip, despite pain relief. Hip range of motion spontaneously improves in most children within 6 months with a reduction in the gait abnormality. The incidence of ON and chondrolysis is low. Gradual deterioration in hip function may occur over the lifetime of the patient, in proportion to the degree of proximal femur malalignment. The onset of degenerative joint disease is earlier in the hip affected by SCFE and often requires joint replacement. Objective analyses of hip function show very good long-term results, especially with mild slips.

The results of aggressive treatment of SCFE usually are worse than in situ fixation. Forceful manipulation of SCFE to realign the proximal femur results in ON in approximately 35% of patients. Osteotomy of the femoral neck for realignment results in ON in approximately one third of children. Chondrolysis and ON occur more frequently after reduction or osteotomy and are associated with rapid deterioration of the hip and very poor long-term results.

Changes are noted in the relationship of the proximal femur and acetabulum in the years following SCFE. After in situ fixation, the change in range of motion over time would suggest remodeling of the epiphysis and shaft, restoring the anatomic relationship. Indeed, radiographs show rounding off of the anterior and superior metaphyses, as well as changes in the acetabulum (Fig. 3). These changes may well be the result of impingement of the femoral neck on the rim and internal surface of the acetabulum, eroding the bone, but improving the radiographic appearance (Fig.

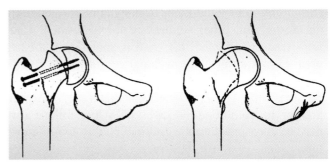

Figure 3 Schematic representation of remodeling of the proximal femoral metaphysis. Bone is resorbed from the anterosuperior aspect of the femoral neck, and new bone is formed appositionally on the posteroinferior surface. *(Reproduced with permission from Siegel DB, Kasser JR, Sponseller P, Gelberman RH: Slipped capital femoral epiphysis: A quantitative analysis of motion, gait, and femoral remodeling after in situ fixation. J Bone Joint Surg Am 1991;73:659-666.)*

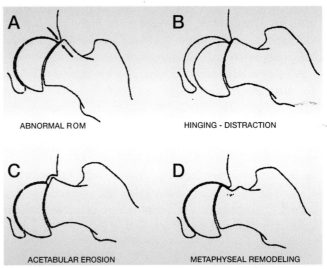

Figure 4 Potential consequences of impingement in SCFE. Abnormal motion and hinging (**A** and **B**) are a direct result of impaction. Remodeling may be acetabular or femoral (**C** and **D**), but note that femoral metaphyseal remodeling causes a portion of the femoral head to be nonarticular metaphysis (inclusion). *(Reproduced with permission from Rab GT: The geometry of slipped capital femoral epiphysis: Implications for movement, impingement, and corrective osteotomy. J Pediatr Orthop 1999;19:419-424.)*

4). The change in hip range of motion with SCFE, external rotation with flexion, may result from impingement of the newly exposed femoral metaphysis. Erosion of that ridge may allow the metaphysis to enter the acetabulum, improving the range of motion, but possibly shortening the longevity of the hip.

Conclusion

Slipped capital femoral epiphysis is a common cause of hip pain in obese children during early adolescence. Degenerative hip disease occurs earlier in hips affected by SCFE and is proportional to the severity of the slip. Early diagnosis and in situ fixation have excellent long-term results. SCFE should be suspected in obese preadolescents or adolescents who present with acute or chronic hip and knee pain. Radiographs are generally diagnostic, and other studies are rarely needed. Caution is necessary when the child is young, thin, or has open physes at an older age, and consideration should be given to endocrine, renal, or postradiation causes for the slip. The incidence of bilaterality is often greater in nonidiopathic cases of SCFE. Bilaterality may require prophylactic fixation of the contralateral hip.

Screw fixation can be minimally invasive, but extreme caution should be used to avoid persistent screw penetration of the femoral head. Fluoroscopy can aid in identifying penetration prior to leaving the operating room. Reduction of the proximal femoral deformity and early femoral neck osteotomy should be avoided because of the high rate of ON and chondrolysis. Unstable hips have a very high incidence of ON, and patients' families should be warned of possible poor outcome.

Although degenerative joint disease may occur earlier after in situ fixation, the long-term results of in situ fixation are very good. The results of reconstructive procedures to realign the proximal femur are difficult to compare because of the high rate of complications in severe SCFE, increased rates of ON and chondrolysis after osteotomy, and the good results of screw fixation. The incidence of bilaterality may be greater than currently suspected, but prophylactic contralateral hip fixation is still not recommended.

Annotated Bibliography

Demographics

Loder RT: The demographics of slipped capital femoral epiphysis: An international multicenter study. *Clin Orthop* 1996;322:8-27.

In this retrospective, multicenter analysis of 1,630 children with SCFE, the high prevalence of SCFE in Polynesian children and low prevalence in Indo-Mediterranean children were identified. Age, gender, and physical characteristics were similar throughout the world. More than 60% of children with SCFE were above the 90th percentile for weight.

Stasikelis PJ, Sullivan CM, Phillips WA, Polard JA: Slipped capital femoral epiphysis: Prediction of contralateral involvement. *J Bone Joint Surg Am* 1996;78: 1149-1155.

In a retrospective review of 50 children with unilateral SCFE, the characteristics of those in whom a contralateral slip developed were evaluated. The authors found that, for boys, younger age at presentation of the first slip was predictive of bilateral involvement.

Etiology

Gunal I, Ates E: The HLA phenotype in slipped capital femoral epiphysis. *J Pediatr Orthop* 1997;17:655-656.

This is a retrospective review of six children with short-term SCFE. The authors found a relationship in this group with HLA-DR4, but not with HLA-B12, as had been previously reported. The small number of patients in the study made the relation to inflammatory disease difficult.

Kitadai HK, Milani C, Nery CA, Filho JL: Wiberg's center-edge angle in patients with slipped capital femoral epiphysis. *J Pediatr Orthop* 1999;19:97-105.

The authors measured the center-edge angle of 104 patients with SCFE, comparing a subgroup of 58 patients with controls. They found that patients with SCFE had deeper acetabulae than did the controls, but the center-edge angle was not predictive of severity.

Loder RT, Hensinger RN, Alburger PD, et al: Slipped capital femoral epiphysis associated with radiation therapy. *J Pediatr Orthop* 1998;18:630-636.

In this retrospective analysis of 32 children with radiation-associated SCFE, the authors found that the age at presentation of SCFE was related to a younger age at treatment with radiation and that a greater dosage was associated with a greater likelihood of a slip.

Nicolai RD, Grasemann H, Oberste-Berghaus C, Hovel M, Hauffa BP: Serum insulin-like growth factors IGF-I and IGFBP-3 in children with slipped capital femoral epiphysis. *J Pediatr Orthop B* 1999;8:103-106.

Measurements of growth factors were made in 19 healthy children with SCFE; 10 of 19 children were above the 97th percentile for weight. The serum concentrations of growth mediators were normal, showing no relationship between growth factors and SCFE.

Stanitski CL, Woo R, Stanitski DF: Acetabular version in slipped capital femoral epiphysis: A prospective study. *J Pediatr Orthop B* 1996;5:77-79.

This study compared CT scan measurements of the pelvis of 60 children with SCFE to normal values. The acetabular version was the same for SCFE and control values.

Stanitski CL, Woo R, Stanitski DF: Femoral version in acute slipped capital femoral epiphysis. *J Pediatr Orthop B* 1996;5:74-76.

This study compared CT scan measurements of the femurs of seven children with SCFE to standard values. Children with chronic SCFE had less anteversion than normal, but those with acute SCFE did not differ from control values.

Pathophysiology

Weiner D: Pathogenesis of slipped capital femoral epiphysis: Current concepts. *J Pediatr Orthop B* 1996;5:67-73.

This article is a review of the literature on the pathogenesis of SCFE. Biomechanical and biochemical factors are considered.

Williams JL, Vani JN, Eick JD, Petersen EC, Schmidt TL: Shear strength of the physis varies with anatomic location and is a function of modulus, inclination, and thickness. *J Orthop Res* 1999;17:214-222.

In this bench research article, shearing fractures of bovine proximal tibia were studied. Ultimate physeal strength was inversely related to physeal thickness, and intrinsic physeal strength was a significant factor. Visible displacement of the physis implied complete instability.

Clinical Presentation

Matava MJ, Patton CM, Luhmann S, Gordon JE, Schoenecker PL: Knee pain as the initial symptom of slipped capital femoral epiphysis: An analysis of initial presentation and treatment. *J Pediatr Orthop* 1999;19: 455-460.

This retrospective review analyzed the presenting complaint of 106 patients with SCFE. A primary report of knee pain, a longer delay to diagnosis, and a more severe femoral deformity were seen in 15% of children. The presence of knee pain alone may delay the diagnosis because the knee might be investigated before the hip.

Imaging

Jerre R, Billing L, Hansson G, Karlsson J, Wallin J: Bilaterality in slipped capital femoral epiphysis: Importance of a reliable radiographic method. *J Pediatr Orthop B* 1996;5:80-84.

This retrospective radiographic study of 100 patients with SCFE assessed the incidence of bilaterality. Evidence of bilateral SCFE was found in 59% of patients; 71% of these patients were asymptomatic. There was no evidence of a second slip during adolescence in 18% of patients. A standard radiographic view improved measurement.

Rhoad RC, Davidson RS, Heyman S, Dormans JP, Drummond DS: Pretreatment bone scan in SCFE: A predictor of ischemia and avascular necrosis. *J Pediatr Orthop* 1999;19:164-168.

In this prospective study of 73 hips with bone scan prior to treatment of SCFE, stable slips all had normal scans; however, 60% of unstable slips showed ischemia prior to treatment.

Strange-Vognsen, H, Wagner, A, Dirksen, K, et al: The value of scintigraphy in hips with slipped capital femoral epiphysis and the value of radiography and MRI after 10 years. *Acta Orthop Belg* 1999;65:33-38.

In this prospective study of 33 hips with bone scan prior to treatment of SCFE, no patient was found to have decreased uptake, regardless of hip stability or displacement. Postoperative scans showed one patient with decreased uptake after osteotomy.

Treatment

Schai PA, Exner GU, Hansch O: Prevention of secondary coxarthrosis in slipped capital femoral epiphysis: A long-term follow-up study after corrective intertrochanteric osteotomy. *J Pediatr Orthop B* 1996;5:135-143.

This is a retrospective study of 51 hips treated with early intertrochanteric osteotomy for severe SCFE. Good results at an average follow-up of 24 years were seen in 55% of patients; 45% of patients had decreased motion and degenerative arthritis. The complication rate was low. The average age at review was 37 years for women and 39 years for men.

Smith JT, Price C, Stevens PM, Masters KS, Young M: Does pediatric orthopedic subspecialization affect hospital utilization and charges? *J Pediatr Orthop* 1999;19:553-555.

This article reviews the charges and length-of-stay data for 334 children with femur fractures and 63 children with SCFE. The authors found that care by subspecialists resulted in shorter hospitalizations and decreased charges than care by general orthopaedists.

Complications

Lubicky JP: Chondrolysis and avascular necrosis: Complications of slipped capital femoral epiphysis. *J Pediatr Orthop B* 1996;5:162-167.

This is a review of current information and studies on the complications of chondrolysis and osteonecrosis. No new data are presented.

Long-term Considerations

Bellemans J, Fabry G, Molenaers G, Lammens J, Moens P: Slipped capital femoral epiphysis: A long-term follow-up, with special emphasis on the capacities for remodeling. *J Pediatr Orthop B* 1996;5:151-157.

This study is a retrospective review of 59 hips treated with in situ fixation, followed at an average of 11 years. No clinical symptoms were seen in 90% of patients, and 83% of patients showed no degeneration of the hip on radiographs. The authors describe metaphyseal remodeling on radiographic measurement.

Goodman DA, Feighan JE, Smith AD, Latimer B, Buly RL, Cooperman DR: Subclinical slipped capital femoral epiphysis: Relationship to osteoarthrosis of the hip. *J Bone Joint Surg Am* 1997;79:1489-1497.

The femurs of 2,665 adult skeletons were examined for postslip morphology. In 8% of hips, changes of SCFE were seen and affected by osteoarthritis more frequently than in controls. The authors suspect postslip morphology as a major risk factor in osteoarthritis and that the onset of degenerative change may be later than previously suspected.

Hagglund G: The contralateral hip in slipped capital femoral epiphysis. *J Pediatr Orthop B* 1996;5:158-161.

The author analyzes previously reported data, suggesting that SCFE is bilateral in 40% to 80% of patients. He recommends prophylactic fixation because of the low risk of surgery and high rate of arthrosis in untreated SCFE. No new data are presented.

Jerre R, Billing L, Karlsson J: Loss of hip motion in slipped capital femoral epiphysis: A calculation from the slipping angle and the slope. *J Pediatr Orthop B* 1996;5: 144-150.

This study is a retrospective measurement of the range of motion of 128 hips at an average of 32 years after SCFE. The authors found that after observation or in situ fixation, there was no significant loss of range of motion, but with osteotomy, external rotation was decreased. They concluded that osteotomies should be reserved for extreme bony malalignment.

Rab GT: The geometry of slipped capital femoral epiphysis: Implications for movement, impingement, and corrective osteotomy. *J Pediatr Orthop* 1999;19: 419-424.

This article reports a computer analysis of the relationship of the proximal femur and acetabulum in SCFE. The author describes the model of damage by metaphyseal impingement and the correlation with slip severity. Consideration is given to corrective osteotomies.

Classic Bibliography

Carney BT, Weinstein SL, Noble J: Long-term follow-up of slipped capital femoral epiphysis. *J Bone Joint Surg Am* 1991;73:667-674.

Siegel DB, Kasser JR, Sponseller P, Gelberman RH: Slipped capital femoral epiphysis: A quantitative analysis of motion, gait, and femoral remodeling after in situ fixation. *J Bone Joint Surg Am* 1991;73:659-666.

Chapter 16

Legg-Calvé-Perthes Disease

Peter A. DeLuca, MD

Legg-Calvé-Perthes disease (LCPD) was first described independently in 1910 by the three named investigators, and despite the passage of nearly a century, its etiology and appropriate management remain controversial. The sequence of femoral head fragmentation and repair is most widely considered to be the result of an idiopathic osteonecrosis, although some theories of etiology exist that have not been proven. There is no strong evidence of a genetic predisposition. Social and environmental associations include older parental age, difficult birth presentations, stature within the low range of normal, lower socioeconomic status, and residence in an urban setting.

Clinical Picture

LCPD generally occurs in children between age 4 and 8 years, but it can occur in children through the extremes of age 2 to 12 years. It is four or five times more common in boys than in girls, and it may be bilateral in approximately 10% of cases. There is no difference in age of presentation, bilaterality, or degree of involvement between the sexes.

Pain usually is not severe in patients with LCPD. Parents typically seek medical attention because the child has a prolonged limp, usually with an intermittent ache in the groin, thigh, or knee. Atrophy of the gluteal and thigh muscles may be noted if the condition has been present for an extended period of time. Although it is common for a child with LCPD to have synovitis at some time during the course of the disease, fewer than 3% of children with acute synovitis and a normal radiograph later have the fragmentation characteristic of LCPD. However, children with a prolonged or recurrent irritable hip and a greater than 2-year delay in skeletal age may represent a small at-risk group. A delay in bone age averaging 21 months and short stature occur in 90% of children with LCPD. Laboratory studies are normal in children with LCPD.

Differential Diagnosis

The differential diagnosis of LCPD in a child with unilateral osteonecrosis should be suggested by a history of prior trauma, surgery, or infection. In bilateral LCPD, both hips usually do not become symptomatic at the same time. Rather, if the contralateral hip appears abnormal on the initial radiograph, it usually is at a different stage of involvement. Bilateral symmetric involvement in a child of short stature should raise suspicion for hypothyroidism, which is also more common in patients with Down syndrome, renal compromise, or one of the generalized epiphyseal dysplasias, such as multiple epiphyseal dysplasia or spondyloepiphyseal dysplasia. Radiographs of the epiphyses of the knees, wrists, and spine should be obtained to rule out a skeletal dysplasia. Other causes of unilateral or bilateral osteonecrosis include steroid use and hemoglobinopathy.

Imaging

Because the prognosis in LCPD relates to age at presentation and the degree of involvement, the initial radiographic assessment should include AP and frog-lateral views of the pelvis and a posteroanterior view of the wrist to determine bone age. A radiograph of the pelvis with the hips abducted helps determine what portion of the femoral epiphysis is involved (ie, beneath the subchondral fracture) and to what degree the epiphysis centers or "contains" itself within the acetabulum. This information is important for determining treatment.

Although a finding of osteonecrosis on MRI warrants concern, there is not enough knowledge about the long-term clinical correlation of MRI findings. Because of the increased sensitivity of this technology, an abnormal MRI scan in some patients might even represent a transient ischemic episode. However, because the anatomic resolution of this modality is improving, the future use of MRI is almost certain to find a niche in the management of LCPD.

TABLE 1 | Classifications Used in LCPD

Name	Purpose	Description	Comments
Catterall	Predict outcome at healing	Involved area: I: anterocentral II: centro-superior III: centro-superolateral IV: whole head	High interrater variability
Herring (lateral pillar)	Predict outcome at healing	Flattening of lateral one third: A: minimal B: one third to one half C: greater than one half	
Stulberg	Predict risk of osteoarthritis after healing	I, II: spherical, congruous III, IV: aspherical, congruous V: aspherical, incongruous	
Mose (sphericity)	Predict risk of osteoarthritis after healing	More than 2 mm deviation from perfect circle on AP and lateral views	

A pin-hole collimated technetium Tc 99m bone scan obtained early in the course of the disease can help demonstrate the extent of avascularity. The appearance of vascularization of the lateral column may indicate a good prognosis. Some authors have found that serial studies are valuable in determining the need for treatment.

Etiology

Vascular disturbance or disordered epiphyseal cartilage is theorized to cause LCPD. Ischemia may represent the primary pathologic event; however, no distinct cause of such ischemia has been identified. Vascular compromise may be caused by secondary smoke or increased intracapsular pressure from sustained synovitis. Some studies have found coagulation abnormalities such as protein C deficiency in groups of children with LCPD. However, other studies show no evidence of inherited thrombophilia in most patients with LCPD. The theory of deficient epiphyseal cartilage is supported by the finding that most patients with LCPD have a delayed bone age and short stature. The prolonged healing time, more than 2 years in many patients, also may be a sign of cartilage abnormality.

Classification

The most commonly used classification systems are those described by Catterall and Herring (Table 1). These systems are based on the extent of epiphyseal involvement, which has prognostic significance. The Catterall radiographic classification is based on the degree of fragmentation of the epiphysis. In groups I and II, the anterior and superior portions of the epiphysis are involved, but the lateral portion (pillar) is preserved; and in groups III and IV, the lateral pillar is involved. Unfortunately, the Catterall classification has poor interobserver consistency, and, because fragmentation may take 6 to 8 months to occur, its prognostic value is limited.

Salter and Thompson attempted to simplify a prognostic classification based on the early appearance subchondral fracture (crescent sign), which they believed to forecast the extent of involvement. Their group A hips (in which the crescent sign involved less than one half of the epiphysis, are characterized by no involvement of the lateral pillar. This group corresponds to hips in Catterall groups I and II. Salter and Thompson group B hips, which correspond with Catterall III and IV hips are more extensively involved and demonstrate pillar fragmentation.

Herring and associates have proposed the more consistently applied "lateral pillar" classification in an effort to improve interobserver agreement and provide more useful prognostic information. They hypothesized that loss of epiphyseal height was the key factor in allowing subluxation and deformity. Their group A hips have no lateral pillar involvement, whereas their groups B and C hips do have lateral pillar involvement (Fig. 1). In group B, more than 50% of the epiphyseal height is maintained, compared with less than 50% in group C.

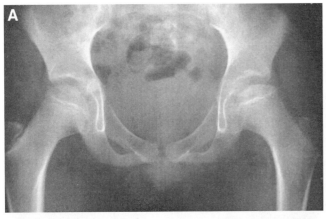

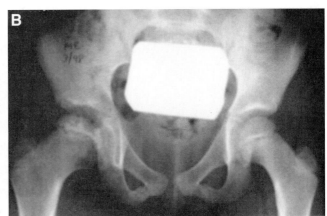

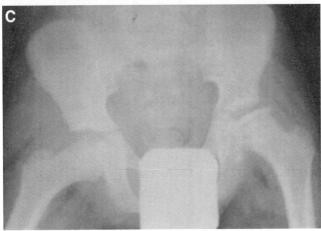

Figure 1 Herring lateral pillar classification. **A,** Group A—lateral pillar is not involved. **B,** Group B—lateral pillar is involved; more than 50% of pillar height is maintained. **C,** Group C—lateral pillar is involved; less than 50% of pillar height is maintained.

Prognostic Factors

Lateral extrusion of more than 20% of the epiphysis correlates with poor long-term prognosis. Onset of LCPD after age 8 years also correlates with a poor outcome. Although girls were once believed to have a worse prognosis, this theory has been disproven.

The age at presentation may not be as much of a prognostic factor as the degree of involvement and early deformity. A spherical head has a more favorable prognosis than one with early deformity. Hips in Herring group A generally have an excellent outcome, while hips in group C generally have a poor prognosis. Stulberg rated hips at maturity as having congruency between the femoral head and acetabulum (class I, II), aspherical congruency (class III, IV), and aspherical incongruency (class V). Stulberg's radiographic parameters of sphericity, shortened femoral neck, and steepness of the acetabulum are poorly defined and lack intrarater reliability. A number of studies have demonstrated deformity at skeletal maturity (Stulberg III, IV) in almost all hips in group C, regardless of age at presentation. Hips in group B in children younger than age 9 years at onset have favorable deformity ratings at skeletal maturity. Initial deformity as graded by

arthrography has helped some investigators predict outcome in group B hips.

Evolution of Deformity

When there is significant loss of height of the lateral pillar, as seen with some Herring group B hips and most Herring group C hips, femoral head deformity results. The reparative (revascularization) process is associated with collapse of the anterolateral epiphysis. The portion of the epiphyseal cartilage receiving nutrition through the synovium might enlarge, especially in the presence of synovitis. Adductor spasm or contracture results in a stiff, adducted position of the hip. Abduction beyond this position may force the flattened lateral portion of the epiphysis under the lateral edge of the acetabulum, resulting in "hinge abduction" and pain, a limp, and further deformity of the femoral head. An AP radiograph with the hip abducted or dynamic arthrography can define this position. The flattened, ovoid, or saddle deformities of LCPD are seen mainly in the older population. The less frequently involved medial epiphysis remains contained within the acetabulum and generally maintains a round, congruous shape that may be used during late

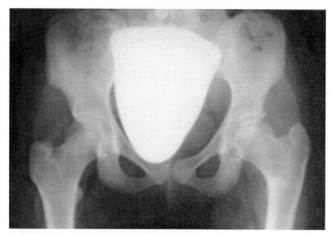

Figure 2 Resultant coxa vara with elevation of the greater trochanter following a varus osteotomy.

TABLE 2 | Treatment Options for Patients With LCPD
Nonsurgical Treatment
Activity restriction
Abduction casts
Abduction brace
Traction
Surgical Treatment
Before healing
Redirectional surgery
Adductor tenotomy
Medial capsulotomy
Femoral varus osteotomy
Innominate rotational osteotomy
Nonredirectional surgery
Shelf procedure
Chiari osteotomy
After healing
Femoral valgus osteotomy
Trochanteric transfer
Contralateral epiphysiodesis

reconstruction of the saddle deformity by valgus osteotomy.

The epiphyseal deformity is not the only factor that may result in alteration in the shape of the proximal femur. Secondary effects of LCPD on the growth plate also result in deformity. Partial disruption of the physis occurs in up to 70% of patients and may be one problem that can be demonstrated on early MRI. If the disruption occurs throughout the physis, a shortened femoral neck and relative trochanteric overgrowth are the result. If the physeal disturbance is eccentric, a slight change in angulation of the femoral neck may occur over time.

In some patients, as the fragmented epiphyseal ossification begins to coalesce and heal, an osteochondral fragment may fail to unite, forming a lesion resembling osteochondritis dissecans. However, this occurs in fewer than 3% of patients, and often is only a radiographic finding. If symptomatic, this lesion can be drilled if the articular surface is intact, or removed if it becomes a loose body.

Natural History

After the epiphysis heals, most patients have relatively little, if any, pain during the remainder of childhood. A persistent limp most likely remains if the trochanter is elevated with respect to the epiphysis, resulting from physeal growth disturbance or femoral varus osteotomy (Fig. 2). Shortening of the involved femur rarely exceeds 2 cm unless an osteotomy, which causes some loss of length, has been performed.

Although there is significant interobserver variability in both the Catterall and Stulberg classification systems, almost all long-term follow-up studies have shown that several factors appear to be pertinent to the patient's ultimate prognosis. These factors include the degree of involvement of the epiphysis; the

patient's age at onset; the amount of deformity at presentation, especially collapse and extrusion of the lateral one third of the epiphysis; and congruity of the hip at skeletal maturity.

Children younger than age 6 years at onset have a favorable prognosis, as do children of any age with Herring group A hips. When prognosis is based on epiphyseal involvement, poor results (60% to 80%) are found with hips in Catterall groups III and IV, which correspond with hips in Herring groups B and C. Hips graded as greater than 2 mm out of round or as incongruent at skeletal maturity are at higher risk for poor results. Although most adolescents function well clinically despite poor radiographic findings, long-term studies reveal that by follow-up at age 45 years, more than one half of these individuals have disabling osteoarthritis. Most patients become symptomatic after age 40 years.

Treatment

The objectives of treatment are to minimize the development of epiphyseal flattening and lateral extrusion

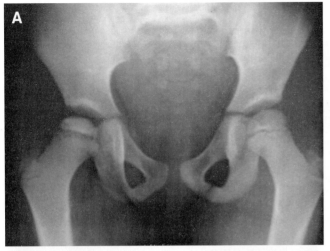

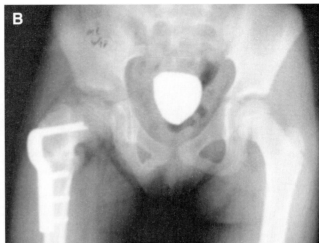

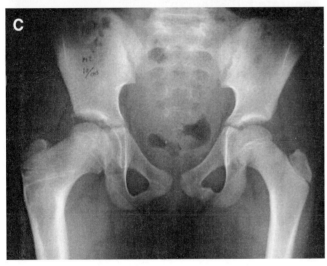

Figure 3 **A,** Herring group 2 LCPD in a 7-year-old girl in which most of the lateral pillar is intact. **B,** Following a femoral varus osteotomy. **C,** Three years postoperatively, the neck-shaft angle and epiphysis have been adequately restored.

and thereby decrease the incidence of late osteoarthritis (Table 2). Secondary objectives are to educate the parents about the healing process and prognosis and help patients through periods of synovitis and decreased range of motion. Treatment of synovitis consists of short-term bed rest, skin traction, abduction cylinder casts, protected weight bearing, anti-inflammatory medication, and physical therapy. Occasionally, adductor tenotomy followed by a cast in abduction helps restore abduction and achieve containment, especially in the older patient with subluxation. This procedure may be performed as a preliminary stage to osteotomy to obtain a well-covered hip.

All children should be followed carefully during the fragmentation stage, and failure to maintain abduction past neutral and a functional range of motion indicates the need for rest, treatment with abduction, and physical therapy. Hips in Herring group A have a good outcome in all age groups; therefore, further treatment is not required. Recent studies reveal that bone age is more useful than chronologic age in deciding which hips in Herring group B might benefit from surgery.

LCPD in children with a bone age of 6 years or younger usually has a good outcome without treatment, whereas in children with older bone ages and hips in Herring group B, results are better following surgery to improve containment. Although group C hips have the worst prognosis, they also have a better outcome following surgery to improve containment.

Methods of surgical containment include femoral varus and/or Salter innominate osteotomy. The varus osteotomy is somewhat more commonly used, but it causes additional shortening and increases the risk of a permanent limp resulting from persistent varus. Results are similar with both methods regarding sphericity. When performing a femoral osteotomy, the surgeon should try to avoid creating a neck-shaft angle of less than 115° (Fig. 3). Restoration of the neck-shaft angle by approximately 20° usually occurs if the physis has not been damaged. If significant varus is surgically created, a concomitant trochanteric epiphyiodesis may be performed. Although some authors propose containment by "derotation," or decreasing the angle of anteversion, in actuality, the proximal femoral segment

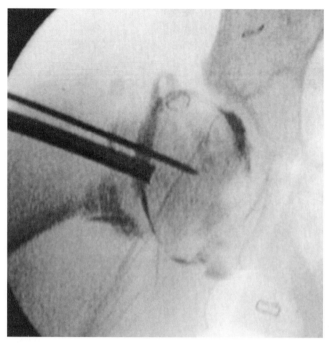

Figure 4 Intraoperative arthrogram confirms containment of the epiphysis under the acetabular labrum. Flattening of the femoral head is already visible.

does not turn in to the acetabulum with this procedure, but the distal segment turns out more. Before the hip is realigned with either a femoral or innominate osteotomy, the surgeon should be certain that the hip can be contained. The use of abduction traction, abduction casts, adductor tenotomy, or medial release and capsulotomy represent increasingly invasive methods to achieve containment. Hip arthrography under anesthesia may help determine the true shape of the epiphysis and the degree of containment and congruency to be expected by either femoral or iliac realignment osteotomy (Fig. 4). If the arthrogram reveals a significantly enlarged or incongruous epiphysis, especially in an older patient, shelf augmentation or Chiari osteotomy seems to be useful. These procedures focus on minimizing further epiphyseal extrusion in older patients in whom the temporary incongruity produced by a femoral or innominate osteotomy cannot be remodeled or an already deformed femoral head does not fit into the existing acetabulum.

Management in children older than age 9 years is controversial. Most of these children have extensive femoral head involvement but little hope for acetabular remodeling. Although surgery may offer the best attempt at containment, the long-term results frequently are poor.

Late Sequelae

Patients should be followed past the healing stage. Those patients in whom hinge abduction persists dur-

ing or after the healing phase may be candidates for valgus osteotomy to increase abduction and improve gait (Fig. 4). Cheilectomy is a less satisfactory option because it may increase hip stiffness.

If early growth cessation causes limb-length inequality, serial radiographs to plot limb length are indicated and epiphysiodesis is an option. A limp resulting from abductor weakness following epiphyseal healing may be managed with a valgus osteotomy or a trochanteric transfer. A trochanteric transfer may be performed if the primary problem is a short femoral neck. Symptomatic osteochondritis dissecans occasionally may require treatment with excision of the loose fragment.

Annotated Bibliography

Clinical Picture

Guille JT, Lipton GE, Szoke G, Bowen JR, Harcke HT, Glutting JJ: Legg-Calvé-Perthes disease in girls: A comparison of the results with those seen in boys. *J Bone Joint Surg Am* 1998;80:1256-1263.

In this comparison study of 105 girls and 470 boys, no difference was revealed regarding age of onset, bilateral involvement, Catterall or the lateral pillar classification, or Stulberg rating in those children who had reached skeletal maturity. Girls had a shorter potential period for remodeling of the femoral head (average, 3.4 years) compared with boys (average, 5.9 years).

Herring JA (ed): *Legg-Calvé-Perthes Disease.* Rosemont, IL, American Academy of Orthopaedic Surgeons, 1996.

This monograph provides an overview of the clinical knowledge base and treatment options of LCPD.

Differential Diagnosis

Keenan WN, Clegg J: Perthes' disease after "irritable hip": Delayed bone age shows the hip is a "marked man." *J Pediatr Orthop* 1996;16:20-23.

The authors report that in 13 children age 4 to 8 years with a prolonged or recurrent irritable hip syndrome and normal radiographs, only those with more than 2 years delay in bone age were eventually indentified to have been in the early phase of LCPD. Screening with wrist bone age and repeat radiographs or MRI was recommended for this group to allow early treatment.

Imaging

de Sanctis N, Rega AN, Rondinella F: Prognostic evaluation of Legg-Calvé-Perthes disease by MRI: Part I. The role of physeal involvement. *J Pediatr Orthop* 2000;20:455-462.

MRI findings in 24 patients with LCPD revealed a good correlation with the Stulberg rating at follow-up 5.4 years later. Factors rated for reliability included the extent of epiphyseal necrosis, lateral extrusion, physeal involvement, and metaphyseal changes. The physeal involvement had the highest predictive value.

Reinker KA: Early diagnosis and treatment of hinge abduction in Legg-Perthes disease. *J Pediatr Orthop* 1996;16:3-9.

In this article, hinge abduction occurred early in the course of LCPD in 19 of 106 hips. Hinging frequently occurred about a nonossified portion of the femoral head, making detection difficult. Failure of the lateral corner of the epiphysis to move under the edge of the acetabulum on an internally rotated and abducted radiograph is prima facie evidence. Confirmation is easily obtained by arthrography.

Song HR, Lee SH, Na JB, et al: Comparison of MRI with subchondral fracture in the evaluation of extent of epiphyseal necrosis in the early stage of Legg-Calvé-Perthes disease. *J Pediatr Orthop* 1999;19:70-75.

In this study, MRI was compared with radiographs in 20 patients who had a subchondral fracture line. The extent of the subchondral fracture line on the radiograph is more accurate in predicting the amount of eventual necrosis than is the extent of necrosis visible on MRI, which does not have a consistent correlation.

Tsao AK, Dias LS, Conway JJ, Straka P: The prognostic value and significance of serial bone scintigraphy in Legg-Calvé-Perthes disease. *J Pediatr Orthop* 1997;17: 230-239.

In this article, 44 consecutive patients with LCPD underwent serial pinhole magnification technetium Tc 99m phosphate bone scintigraphy. Average follow-up occurred at 4.4 years. The bone scintigraphy classification characterized two groups: the A pathway and the B pathway. Early lateral column formation was only in patients in the A pathway. Pathway A included 20 hips, required no surgery, and had an average Mose classification of 1.2 and a Catterall score of 2.4. Pathway B included 20 hips, an average Mose classification of 5.2, and a Catterall score of 3.5. In pathway B, 18 patients had head-at-risk signs, and 11 patients required surgery. Bone scintigraphy classification preceded the radiographic head-at-risk signs by an average of 3 months, allowing earlier treatment, and correlated with subsequent femoral head involvement.

Etiology

Gallistl S, Reitinger T, Linhart W, Muntean W: The role of inherited thrombotic disorders in the etiology of Legg-Calvé-Perthes disease. *J Pediatr Orthop* 1999;19: 82-83.

The authors report that of 44 patients with LCPD, only three (6.8%) had positive results for activated protein C resistance, and one patient (2.2%) showed a deficiency of protein C activity. These results do not support inherited thrombophilia as a cause of osteonecrosis.

Glueck CJ, Crawford A, Roy D, Freiberg R, Glueck H, Stroop D: Association of antithrombotic factor deficiencies and hypofibrinolysis with Legg-Perthes disease. *J Bone Joint Surg Am* 1996;78:3-13.

Coagulation abnormalities were demonstrated in 33 of 44 unselected patients (75%) with LCPD. Of these patients, 23 had thrombophilia, and 19 had protein C deficiency. Other coagulation abnormalities included protein S deficiency in four patients, a high level of lipoprotein (a) in seven patients, and hypofibrinolysis in three patients.

Hayek S, Kenet G, Lubetsky A, Rosenberg N, Gitel S, Weintroub S: Does thrombophilia play an aetiological role in Legg-Calvé-Perthes disease? *J Bone Joint Surg Br* 1999;81:686-690.

In this study of 62 patients, the authors found no correlation between thrombophilia and LCPD.

Mata SG, Aicua EA, Ovejero AH, Grande MM: Legg-Calvé-Perthes disease and passive smoking. *J Pediatr Orthop* 2000;20:326-330.

The authors reported that the odds ratio for development of LCPD was 5.3 in the presence of a passive smoking environment as determined by a case-control study of 90 patients and 83 controls. These findings were statistically very significant.

Classification

Farsetti P, Tudisco C, Caterini R, Potenza V, Ippolito E: The Herring lateral pillar classification for prognosis in Perthes' disease: Late results in 49 patients treated conservatively. *J Bone Joint Surg Br* 1995;77:739-742.

The authors followed 49 patients with LCPD from the fragmentation stage to the Stulberg rating at maturity in an attempt to identify the prognostic value of the Herring classification when used with age, especially for patients with group B hips. Reconstruction of the femoral head was successful in 10 of the 11 hips in group A. Deformity developed in all group C hips regardless of age of onset. In group B, all patients younger than age 9 years did well, and most patients older than age 9 years were classified as Stulberg III and IV.

Ismail AM, Macnicol MF: Prognosis in Perthes' disease: A comparison of radiological predictors. *J Bone Joint Surg Br* 1998;80:310-314.

The authors reported that classification during the fragmentation stage of LCPD in 73 patients with 81 affected hips showed that the Herring grade and arthrographic sphericity were the best predictors of final outcome and that combining these two values further increased the predictive value. One half of the patients were treated surgically. Using the Stulberg classification to assess outcome, all but one patient in Herring group A achieved an excellent outcome. None of the hips in Herring group C had a normal appearance at maturity and the outcome was not significantly influenced by the age at onset or the arthrographic appearance.

Neyt JG, Weinstein SL, Spratt KF, et al: Stulberg classification system for evaluation of Legg-Calvé-Perthes disease: Intra-rater and inter-rater reliability. *J Bone Joint Surg Am* 1999;81:1209-1216.

This study questions the reliability of the Stulberg system of classification and the validity of any treatment decisions, outcome evaluations, or epidemiologic studies based on this classification. Nine evaluators independently used the Stulberg system to evaluate the radiographs of skeletally mature patients with LCPD. Intraobserver reliability was fair but interobserver reliability was poor, even after instruction.

Natural History

Weinstein SL: Long-term follow-up of pediatric orthopaedic conditions: Natural history and outcomes of treatment. *J Bone Joint Surg Am* 2000;82:980-990.

The author summarized long-term follow-up to maturity of patients with LCPD who have had either no treatment or brace treatment. Generally favorable results are found at 20 to 40 years follow-up, unless the femoral head is flattened and irregular, the neck is deformed, or the trochanter is overgrown.

Treatment

Kim HT, Wenger DR: Surgical correction of "functional retroversion" and "functional coxa vara" in late Legg-Calvé-Perthes disease and epiphyseal dysplasia: Correction of deformity defined by new imaging modalities. *J Pediatr Orthop* 1997;17:247-254.

Combined femoral valgus-flexion-internal-rotation femoral osteotomy plus simultaneous triple innominate osteotomy was performed in five patients with LCPD. This procedure was designed to correct the "functional coxa vara" and hinge abduction, establish a more normal articulation between the posteromedial portion of the femoral head and the acetabulum, correct external rotation deformity of the distal limb, and improve joint congruity and anterolateral femoral head coverage in hips with associated acetabular dysplasia.

Kim HT, Wenger DR: "Functional retroversion" of the femoral head in Legg-Calvé-Perthes disease and epiphyseal dysplasia: Analysis of head-neck deformity and its effect on limb position using three-dimensional computed tomography. *J Pediatr Orthop* 1997;17:240-246.

The authors studied femoral head and neck deformity in 17 patients (22 hips) with LCPD and epiphyseal dysplasia, using three-dimensional CT. They determined that the deformed femoral head can be divided into two portions, the false head, which protrudes anterolaterally and inferiorly, and the true head, the posteromedial superior portion, which represents the original articulating femoral head. The remodeled segment results in "functional retroversion," which causes an externally rotated gait. Results of this study contradict previous reports of increased anteversion in patients with LCPD.

Kitakoji T, Hattori T, Iwata H: Femoral varus osteotomy in Legg-Calvé-Perthes disease: Points at operation to prevent residual problems. *J Pediatr Orthop* 1999;19:76-81.

In this article, the authors analyzed proximal femoral growth following femoral varus osteotomy in 46 patients, once they reached skeletal maturity. Trochanteric prominence remained despite mean remodeling of the neck-shaft angle by 20.4°. Trochanteric prominence and genu valgum were common. The authors determined that postoperative containment is more important than postoperative femoral neck-shaft angle and the amount of surgical varus should be individualized.

Matan AJ, Stevens PM, Smith JT, Santora SD: Combination trochanteric arrest and intertrochanteric osteotomy for Perthes' disease. *J Pediatr Orthop* 1996;16:10-14.

In this study of 28 patients who underwent unilateral femoral varus osteotomy, those who received prophylactic trochanteric arrest at the time of the osteotomy (average 7.5 years) had greater articulotrochanteric distance, better range of motion, less abductor weakness, less pain, and superior activity levels at a follow-up of 4.8 years. The authors include a detailed discussion of surgical technique.

Moberg A, Hansson G, Kaniklides C: Results after femoral and innominate osteotomy in Legg-Calvé-Perthes disease. *Clin Orthop* 1997;334:257-264.

In a retrospective study of the surgical management of patients with LCPD classified as Catterall group 3 or 4, 16 femoral osteotomies (group A) and 18 innominate osteotomies (group B) were compared with regard to clinical and radiographic results. The average follow-up was 6 years in group A and 8 years in group B. All patients were asymptomatic, and the clinical results were equal. Radiographs revealed equal measurements of femoral head sphericity, Mose's index, and epiphyseal quotient; however, the coverage of the femoral head by the acetabulum (center edge angle) was better in group B.

Classic Bibliography

Catterall A: The natural history of Perthes' disease. *J Bone Joint Surg Br* 1971;53:37-53.

Herring JA, Neustadt JB, Williams JJ, Early JS, Browne RH: The lateral pillar classification of Legg-Calvé-Perthes disease. *J Pediatr Orthop* 1992;12:143-150.

Herring JA: The treatment of Legg-Calvé-Perthes disease: A critical review of the literature. *J Bone Joint Surg Am* 1994;76:448-458.

Salter RB, Thompson GH: Legg-Calvé-Perthes disease: The prognostic significance of the subchondral fracture and a two-group classification of the femoral head involvement. *J Bone Joint Surg Am* 1984;66:479-489.

Stulberg SD, Cooperman DR, Wallensten R: The natural history of Legg-Calvé-Perthes disease. *J Bone Joint Surg Am* 1981;63:1095-1108.

Yrjonen T: Prognosis in Perthes' disease after noncontainment treatment: 106 hips followed for 28-47 years. *Acta Orthop Scand* 1992;63:523-526.

Chapter 17

Developmental Dysplasia of the Hip

Gregory A. Mencio, MD

Nomenclature

The term developmental dysplasia of the hip (DDH) has replaced the more traditional term congenital dislocation of the hip because it more accurately reflects the variable characteristics of this complex disorder. The spectrum of conditions includes those clearly identifiable at birth (prenatal, teratologic dislocation); others that become apparent during the first year of life (postnatal instability); and those that are clinically silent during childhood but become symptomatic during adolescence or early adulthood (subluxation, acetabular dysplasia) (Table 1).

Incidence

The incidence of DDH varies with factors such as sex, age, race, and definition of the condition. The rate of neonatal hip instability (positive Barlow or Ortolani test results) is approximately 1 per 100 to 250 live births. Established dislocations occur in approximately 1 in 1,000 infants and late dislocation, subluxation, and acetabular dysplasia in approximately 4 per 10,000 individuals.

Etiology

Physiologic, genetic, and mechanical factors have been implicated in the etiology of DDH. Ligamentous laxity, which is hormonally mediated in women (estrogen and/or relaxin) or familial (in either sex), generally is believed to play a role. The incidence of DDH has been observed to be as high as 34% in family history and sibling and twin studies, supporting the role of genetic influence. The increased incidence of DDH that occurs with conditions typically associated with abnormal intrauterine position and fetal crowding, ie, breech position, oligohydramnios, congenital recurvatum/dislocation of the knee, congenital muscular torticollis, and metatarsus adductus, suggests a mechanical basis.

Diagnosis

Screening

Neonatal clinical screening programs reduce the number of missed diagnoses of dislocations in children of walking age and are economically beneficial. However, not all cases of developmental dysplasia are detectable at birth. Therefore, screening programs must be ongoing, and children should be periodically examined until they are of walking age.

The adjunctive use of ultrasound is neither cost effective nor practical in the routine screening of all newborns. In addition, its use is controversial even in children with risk factors for DDH. Ultrasound generally is acknowledged as being too sensitive and nonspecific as a screening modality, leading to increased diagnostic and unnecessary therapeutic efforts while only marginally reducing the incidence of late cases compared to clinical screening alone. The presence and severity of abnormal ultrasound findings in newborns with clinically normal examinations do not correlate with the ultimate status of the hip.

Alternatively, ultrasound screening delayed to after age 6 weeks or plain radiographs obtained at age 4 months for selected infants with risk factors for DDH by virtue of a positive family history and clinical parameters, such as breech presentation, foot deformity, or a persistent click, is advocated as a more cost-effective alternative to global ultrasound screening.

Physical Examination

The clinical findings of DDH vary with age and reflect the underlying pathoanatomy of the condition. In the neonate up to approximately age 2 to 3 months, the dysplastic hip is usually unstable, and the diagnosis of DDH is based on results of the classic provocative Barlow and Ortolani maneuvers. A positive Barlow result is a hip that is reduced but able to be dislocated with adduction and downward pressure on the flexed

TABLE 1 | Variants of DDH

Variant	Characteristics
Teratologic hip	Fixed dislocation that occurred prenatally and often is associated with neuromuscular disorders
Unstable hip	Femoral head is reduced in the true acetabulum but can be fully (dislocated) or partially (subluxated) removed
Dislocated hip	Femoral head does not articulate with any portion of the true acetabulum and may or may not be reducible
Subluxated hip	Femoral head contacts only a portion of the true acetabulum
Acetabular dysplasia	Acetabulum is shallow and femoral head is subluxated or normal

femur. A positive Ortolani result is a hip that is dislocated but reducible with abduction and forward pressure on the flexed femur.

By age 3 months, the hip with the positive Barlow result stabilizes while the dislocated hip can no longer be reduced with the Ortolani maneuver. The muscles about the dislocated hip have adaptively shortened in response to the higher resting position of the femoral head, and limited hip abduction becomes the predominant finding. The femur is clinically foreshortened (a positive Galeazzi sign), and there may be asymmetry of thigh skinfolds. The greater trochanter is cephalad to Nélaton's line, the line between the anterosuperior iliac spine and the ischial tuberosity. The unstable articulation between the hip and the pelvis may cause the hip to "piston." In the child of walking age, the most obvious findings are abnormal stance (excessive lordosis, pelvic obliquity) and Trendelenburg gait as a result of limb-length inequality, hip flexion contracture, and abductor muscle insufficiency.

Imaging
Radiography
The cartilaginous nature of the femoral head and acetabulum in neonates and young infants may result in unreliable radiographic diagnoses of hip subluxation or dislocation. The surgeon must extrapolate from immature osseous landmarks to interpret findings on plain radiographs. Moreover, radiographs of the pelvis do not allow evaluation of important soft-tissue structures such as the labrum and capsule. Shenton's, Perkins' and Hilgenreiner's reference lines and acetabular index and center-edge angles help in evaluating AP radiographs of the infant's pelvis (Fig. 1). An AP radiograph is warranted to evaluate for teratologic dislocation of the hip or other possible congenital anomalies of the upper femur, pelvis, or spine in any neonate or infant with a fixed irreducible dislocation, limited hip abduction, or obvious limb-length discrepancy.

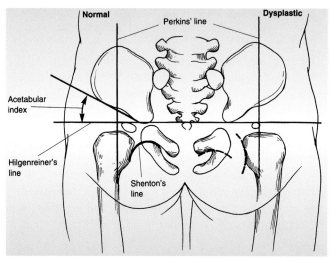

Figure 1 Standard reference lines and angles used to interpret pelvic radiographs in DDH. The femoral ossific nucleus normally is located in the lower, inner quadrant formed by the intersection of Hilgenreiner's (horizontal) and Perkins' (vertical) lines. Shenton's line is a continuous arc along the inferior border of the femoral neck and superior margin of the obturator foramen, which is disrupted when the femoral head is dislocated. The acetabular index measures the inclination of the acetabulum. Normal values for a newborn are less than 30° (average 27.5°). *(Reproduced from Guille J, Pizzutillo P, MacEwen G: Developmental dysplasia of the hip from birth to six months. J Am Acad Orthop Surg 1999;8: 232-242.)*

Ultrasound
Ultrasound plays an important role in the early diagnosis of DDH. Although its role as a routine screening examination is controversial, it is useful as an adjunct in patients with equivocal physical findings and to document and monitor hip reduction during treatment. It is most useful in children younger than age 6 to 8 months, before the femoral head begins to ossify, although it can effectively be used until approximately age 1 year. Ultrasound is not invasive and does not expose the child to ionizing radiation. It allows visualization of the cartilaginous femoral head, the nonossified portion of the acetabulum, and the soft-tissue structures, the labrum and capsule. As the femoral head begins to ossify, visualization of the acetabulum by ultrasound becomes progressively difficult, and plain radiographs become better suited to evaluate the hip.

Both morphology and stability of the hip joint can be assessed with ultrasound. Graf's method emphasizes assessment of the morphology of the hip based on static measurements of the acetabulum in the coronal plane. In this technique, the angle subtended by reference lines through the iliac bone and tangential to the osseous roof of the acetabulum, referred to as the alpha angle, represents the hard bony roof and reflects the depth of the acetabulum. A second angle, the beta angle, subtended by a line drawn through the labrum and intersecting the iliac reference line, represents the cartilaginous roof of the acetabulum and indirectly reflects the position of the femoral head. These measurements do not predict later acetabular dysplasia in hips that are otherwise clinically reduced and stable. In the dynamic method proposed by Harcke, the joint is evaluated in the transverse plane while being stressed with modified Barlow and Ortolani maneuvers. Instability of the hip is measured by the amount of displacement of the femoral head from the acetabulum.

Arthrography

Arthrography is still the gold standard for demonstrating soft-tissue impediments in DDH. However, it is an invasive procedure that requires deep sedation or general anesthesia. For this reason, ultrasound has supplanted arthrography for diagnostic purposes, although arthrography remains a useful adjunct for assessing hip stability and concentricity following closed or open reduction. It is also a useful guide for surgical decision making in patients with more complicated DDH when secondary reconstructive procedures are contemplated.

Computed Tomography and Magnetic Resonance Imaging

Neither CT nor MRI plays a major role in the primary diagnosis of DDH, although both have other uses. CT of the acetabulum is quite useful in assessing hip position in the spica cast following closed or open reduction. Imaging of only the acetabulum minimizes radiation exposure. Because the hip is immobilized, sedation is unnecessary. CT and MRI data can be reformatted with software to produce three-dimensional reconstructions of the hip joint. By manipulating these images, the effects of proposed reconstructive procedures can be simulated preoperatively.

Treatment

The goal of treatment is to obtain and maintain concentric reduction of the hip without disrupting the blood supply to the capital femoral epiphysis. In most infants, treatment goals can be accomplished using closed methods (Fig. 2). In the older child, particularly after achieving walking age, surgical reduction and/or concomitant osteotomies may be necessary (Fig. 3).

Closed Reduction
Pavlik Harness

In infants up to age 6 months, gentle closed reduction usually can be achieved by positioning the hip in flexion and abduction. The Pavlik harness is a dynamic splint that provides the desired flexed-abducted position necessary to maintain reduction of the femoral head, yet it allows a safe range of hip motion. The harness is easy to apply, adjustable, and relatively inexpensive. The Pavlik harness also can be used to treat a dislocated hip that is not initially reducible (a negative Ortolani test result) provided that the femoral head can be directed toward the acetabulum. In this situation, treatment with the harness should be abandoned if the hip does not reduce by 2 to 3 weeks. This technique is most effective in infants younger than age 6 months.

The Pavlik harness is applied with the chest strap at or slightly below the nipple line. The anterior straps are located at the anterior axillary line and control hip flexion, which ideally should be between 100° and 110°. The posterior straps attach at about the tip of the scapula. Their purpose is to restrict adduction of the hip by maintaining abduction of approximately 50° to 70°. With the hip reduced, it is necessary to determine the range of flexion and abduction through which the hip is stable and verify that this position does not result in excessive soft-tissue tension. Insufficient flexion or abduction can result in loss of reduction, excessive flexion can cause injury to the femoral nerve or inferior dislocation, and excessive abduction may result in osteonecrosis (ON); therefore, attention to the principles of positioning is important.

Reduction of the hip should be confirmed with a radiograph or by ultrasound. Continued use of the harness in the event of a nonconcentric reduction can exacerbate dysplasia of the posterolateral portion of the acetabulum and complicate subsequent closed or open reduction. The harness should be worn continuously until the hip is stable. Part-time wear should continue until acetabular remodeling is complete. Treatment with the Pavlik harness is effective in achieving reduction more than 90% of the time. The incidence of ON is low (less than 5%), particularly when treatment is initiated before age 3 months and excessive abduction is avoided. The most common pitfall associated with the device is failure to obtain reduction, which often is not initially recognized. Risk factors for an adverse outcome with the harness include an inability to reduce the hip (a negative Ortolani test result) prior to application of the device, bilaterality, and age older than 7 weeks when treatment is started.

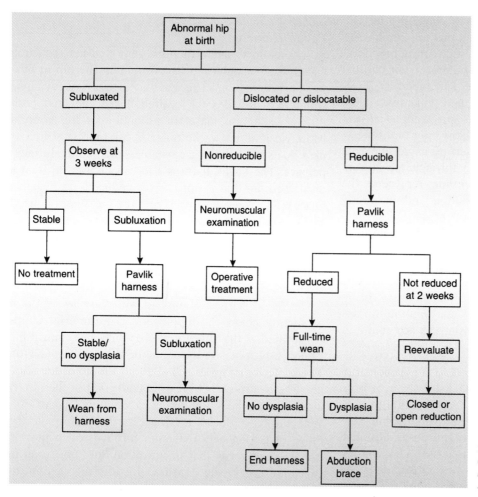

Figure 2 Algorithm for management of DDH in the infant up to age 6 months. *(Reproduced from Guille J, Pizzutillo P, MacEwen G: Developmental dysplasia of the hip from birth to six months. J Am Acad Orthop Surg 1999;8: 232-242.)*

Traction

Closed or open reduction is necessary in infants in whom Pavlik harness treatment fails and in infants older than age 6 months who are too large for the harness. Closed reduction has been the preferred method of treatment in children up to age 24 months provided it can be achieved without excessive force. However, treatment can be protracted in children older than age 12 months, and secondary femoral or acetabular procedures are usually necessary to address residual deformity. The role of traction prior to closed reduction of the hip is controversial. It has been widely held that traction stretches the contracted soft tissues around the hip, facilitates a gentler reduction of the femoral head, and reduces the incidence of ON. Opponents of prereduction traction argue that infants who are immobilized in the "human" position, in which the hips are flexed between 90° and 100°, abducted 45°, and neutrally rotated, and undergo an adductor tenotomy at the time of hip reduction do not have a higher rate of ON than those treated with prereduction traction. Regardless of whether or not prereduction traction is used, the position of immobilization is one of the most important factors regarding the prevention of ON.

Avoiding forced abduction of the femur protects the blood supply of the femoral head, while flexing the hip and knee relaxes the muscles across the hip joint, decreasing pressure on the femoral head. Even proponents disagree as to the most beneficial type of traction (skin versus skeletal), direction of pull (overhead versus longitudinal, divarication versus in-line), amount of weight, and duration of treatment. Results of two of three recent studies have shown no difference in the rates of successful closed reduction or ON in comparable groups of infants treated with and without traction.

Closed Reduction With Arthrography

Whether or not preliminary traction is used, closed reduction of the hip should be performed under general anesthesia with arthrographic guidance. This approach permits an objective visual and tactile assessment of the hip following reduction. The quality of the reduction can be determined by arthrography and objectively defined by the width of the dye column between the femoral head and acetabulum and the status of the limbus (Fig. 4). Impediments to reduction include the following: constriction of the inferior cap-

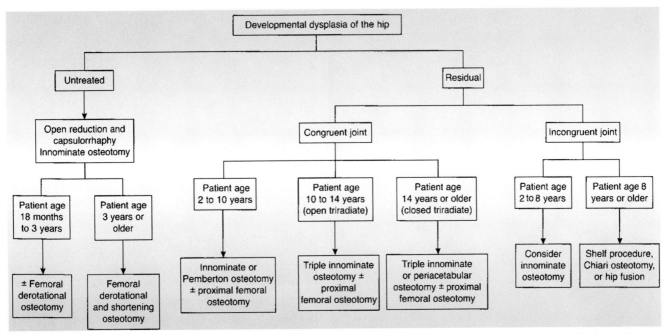

Figure 3 Algorithm for treatment of untreated DDH and residual acetabular dysplasia in the child older than age 18 months. *(Reproduced from Gillingham B, Sanchez A, Wenger D: Pelvic osteotomies for the treatment of hip dysplasia in children and young adults. J Am Acad Orthop Surg 1999;7:325-337.)*

sule and contracture of the iliopsoas, causing an hourglass-shaped narrowing of the isthmus to the acetabulum; infolding and hypertrophy of the labrum (neolimbus), obstructing the superior boundary of the acetabulum; thickening and superior migration of the transverse acetabular ligament, limiting the inferior margin; and elongation of the ligamentum teres and proliferation of fibrofatty tissue (pulvinar), filling the depths of the acetabulum. Any or all of these findings may be present and usually become more pronounced as the child matures. Hips with less than 5 mm of contrast material between the femoral head and acetabulum and those in which the limbus is not interposed are expected to have an acceptable outcome. The stability of the reduction in abduction and adduction, flexion and extension, internal and external rotation (stable zone), and the "safe zone," which is defined as the difference between maximum abduction of the hip and the minimal amount of abduction necessary to maintain the reduction, can be determined. If the adductors are tight, percutaneous tenotomy of the adductor longus effectively widen the safe zone and minimize the risk of immobilizing the hip in a position that may result in ON.

After the hip has been reduced, the infant is immobilized in a spica cast with the hips in the human position. Plain radiographs, ultrasound, or CT documents the reduction. Of the three modalities, CT provides the best visualization of the posterior aspect of the acetabulum. Unlike with ultrasound, CT does not require modification of the cast, and it can be performed with radiation exposure as low as for plain radiography.

Cast immobilization is continued for approximately 3 to 4 months with interim changes, followed by nighttime abduction bracing until the acetabular dysplasia resolves.

Open Reduction

Regardless of the child's age, indications for open reduction include nonconcentric reduction or hip instability requiring excessive positioning (safe zone is narrower than stable zone) to maintain reduction. Open reduction may be performed in older children to avoid the prolonged casting time associated with the nonsurgical approach. During open reduction, the obstacles that prevent seating of the femoral head in the acetabulum are removed, and the hip is stabilized with capsulorrhaphy. Open reduction may be performed with either the anterior or medial approach.

Anterior Approach

The anterior approach is the most versatile and commonly used method for surgical reduction of the dislocated hip. It is appropriate at any age and may be used in virtually all situations. This approach is preferred in children older than age 18 months and generally is required in any dislocation in which the hip cannot manually be brought to the level of the acetabulum. With this approach, the anatomic interval is between the sartorius and tensor fascia lata muscles, and the dissection is more extensive than with either of the medial approaches. The anterior approach provides excellent exposure of the acetabulum and access to all of the impediments to reduction. Capsulorrhaphy can

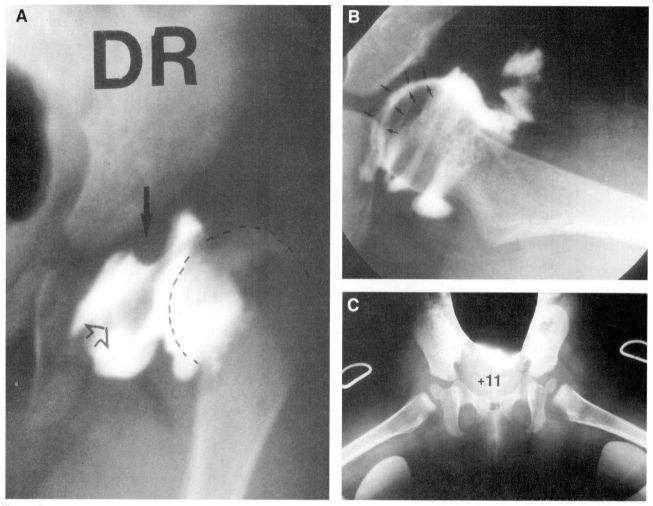

Figure 4 **A,** Arthrogram of a 6-month-old girl with DDH prior to attempted closed reduction of the hip demonstrates the hypertrophied labrum (*solid arrow*), ligamentum teres (*open arrow*) and capsular narrowing. **B,** Concentric reduction is demonstrated by thin (5 mm) column of contrast (*multiple arrows*). **C,** Plain radiograph of the pelvis in abduction splint 5 months following closed reduction of the hip showing growth of the femoral ossific nucleus and remodeling of the acetabulum.

be performed, providing immediate stabilization of the hip. If necessary, a pelvic osteotomy may be performed through the same incision.

Medial Approach

The medial adductor approach of Ludloff allows direct access to all of the primary obstacles to hip reduction except the labrum. There are two routes to the hip via the medial approach, and each is defined by the interval of dissection relative to the adductor brevis muscle. In the anteromedial approach, the interval is anterior to the adductor brevis and then either anterior or posterior to the pectineus. In the posteromedial approach, the plane of dissection is deep to the adductor brevis. With this approach, tight hip adductors, a contracted iliopsoas tendon, the constricted inferior portion of the capsule, and the transverse acetabular ligament can be released. Capsulorrhaphy is not possible; therefore, cast immobilization is used to stabilize the hip until the capsule tightens. The posteromedial approach generally

is not suited to reduce hip dislocations in older children in whom the femoral head has migrated proximally, the labrum is a significant obstacle to reduction, and secondary skeletal deformity may dictate the need for concurrent pelvic or femoral osteotomy. In these situations, the anterior approach is more effective.

Femoral Shortening

Femoral shortening effectively reduces soft-tissue tension across the hip joint. It has supplanted traction as an adjunct to open reduction of the hip joint. Femoral shortening is routinely used in children older than age 2 years, but it is appropriate any time there is excessive soft-tissue tension about the hip. The proximal femur is exposed through a lateral approach, and a subtrochanteric osteotomy is performed. With hip reduction, the amount of overlap of the proximal and distal ends of the osteotomy can be used to gauge the amount of bone to be resected. Derotation and/or varus correction may be performed if excessive femoral anteversion or coxa valga is part of the patho-anatomy. The osteotomy is internally fixed, usually with a plate and screws.

Secondary Procedures

Dislocation of the hip often is accompanied by increased femoral anteversion and acetabular dysplasia (anterolateral deficiency). These secondary skeletal deformities typically are more severe in children older than age 2 years and may prevent stable reduction of the hip or preclude biologic remodeling of the joint after a successful reduction. Secondary surgical procedures, such as femoral osteotomy, pelvic osteotomy, or both, may facilitate reduction of the hip, address persistent subluxation or deformity of the proximal femur, or correct residual acetabular dysplasia (Fig. 3).

In children older than age 3 years, open reduction, femoral shortening, and redirectional osteotomy of the innominate bone usually are performed simultaneously to achieve concentric reduction, prevent ON, and address the secondary acetabular pathology. In younger children, controversy exists regarding both the choice and timing of secondary procedures. Some surgeons are concerned that the risk of ON may be greater when open reduction and pelvic osteotomy are performed simultaneously. However, several reports suggest that simultaneous open reduction and innominate osteotomy can be safely performed with superior results compared with open reduction alone or open reduction followed by delayed innominate osteotomy.

Acetabular remodeling allows correction of acetabular dysplasia following reduction of the hip or osteotomy of the proximal femur. Remodeling of the acetabulum is most dramatic within 6 to 12 months following hip reduction. The potential for improvement also depends on the amount of acetabular growth remaining. Remodeling is most predictable in children younger than age 4 years; is somewhat unpredictable between age 4 and 8 years; and is virtually nonexistent thereafter.

Femoral Osteotomy

A femoral osteotomy may be performed at the time of open reduction to correct excessive femoral anteversion or coxa valga. Correction of excessive femoral anteversion allows the hip to be reduced without extreme internal rotation and is consistent with the principle of a tension-free reduction. Overcorrection of anteversion can result in posterior instability of the hip, particularly if a redirectional acetabular osteotomy is performed at the same time. In children with residual acetabular dysplasia following reduction, a proximal femoral osteotomy may be performed as a staged procedure until age 4 years, with the expectation that

redirecting the femoral head into varus will indirectly stimulate acetabular remodeling. A varus derotational osteotomy of the proximal femur also may be performed at any age to correct subluxation of the hip, provided that plain radiographs show that the femoral head is reduced in an abducted, internally rotated position.

Pelvic Osteotomy

A pelvic osteotomy allows a more direct approach to resolving acetabular dysplasia. It augments the stable zone of the hip at the time of open reduction and corrects acetabular dysplasia that fails to remodel following reduction of the hip. A pelvic osteotomy should be considered in children older than age 3 years because of the unpredictable remodeling capacity after this age. In adolescents and adults with residual subluxation and painful acetabular dysplasia, the rationale for treatment is to improve the hip's biomechanical function in hopes of preventing or reversing deterioration of the hip joint. Pelvic osteotomy achieves this by increasing the contact area between the femoral head and acetabulum, thereby reducing the point loading that occurs at the edge of the dysplastic acetabulum, relaxing the capsule and soft tissues about the hip, and improving the abductor moment arm. The treatment of asymptomatic acetabular dysplasia in older children and adolescents is controversial. Most surgeons avoid major pelvic procedures in asymptomatic adolescents with radiographic acetabular dysplasia.

There are two types of pelvic osteotomies: reconstructive procedures and salvage procedures. Reconstructive procedures use hyaline cartilage to restore the articular surface, and salvage procedures use the joint capsule supported by bone or bone graft as the weight-bearing surface. Reconstructive procedures redirect the position of the acetabulum to effect coverage of the femoral head, or they reshape the acetabulum to address abnormal morphology. The surgical prerequisites for both types of procedures include a hip that is concentrically and congruently reduced or capable of being reduced by open reduction or femoral osteotomy and normal or near-normal range of motion. In adolescents and adults, a perfectly concentric reduction may not be possible because of the presence of more established, adaptive skeletal changes; however, the joint space should be preserved.

Reconstructive Procedures
The two types of reconstructive pelvic osteotomies are redirectional osteotomies or reshaping (configuration changing) osteotomies. Redirectional osteotomies (Fig. 5) involve complete cuts through the innominate bone and require fixation until the osteotomy is healed. The single innominate osteotomy of Salter is ideal if there is deficiency of the

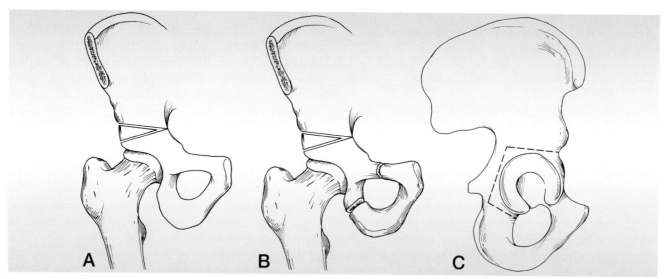

Figure 5 Redirectional osteotomies. **A,** Single innominate (Salter). **B,** Triple innominate (Steel). **C,** Pericapsular (Ganz). *(Reproduced from Gillingham B, Sanchez A, Wenger D: Pelvic osteotomies for the treatment of hip dysplasia in children and young adults. J Am Acad Orthop Surg 1999;7:325-337.)*

anterolateral acetabulum and lack of coverage of the anterolateral portion of the femoral head. The single innominate osteotomy can be expected to provide approximately 20° to 25° of lateral coverage and approximately 10° to 15° of anterior coverage. In older patients who may have limited mobility of the symphysis pubis or need additional coverage, the triple innominate osteotomy described by Steel or one of the technically demanding periacetabular osteotomies described by Wagner, Eppright, or Ganz may be more effective. The triple innominate osteotomy requires osteotomies of the ischium, pubis, and ilium. Concentric hip reduction with hip abduction, flexion, and internal rotation is a prerequisite for the triple innominate osteotomy. This osteotomy surrounds the acetabulum and affords significant mobility of the acetabular fragment, and excessive external rotation of the acetabular fragment must be avoided. The periacetabular osteotomy championed by Ganz is the most technically demanding pelvic osteotomy. It involves osteotomies of the pubis, ilium, and ischium and a vertical osteotomy of the posterior column of the acetabulum approximately 1 cm anterior to the sciatic notch, connecting the iliac and ischial cuts. The osteotomy provides tremendous mobility of the acetabulum, but because the osteotomy does not enter the sciatic notch, it is quite stable. The cuts required for this osteotomy cross the triradiate cartilage; therefore, the periacetabular osteotomy is contraindicated in children in whom this structure is open.

The Pemberton and Dega procedures are reshaping osteotomies. They involve incomplete cuts through the pericapsular portion of the innominate bone. Hinging the periacetabular segment through the triradiate cartilage restores acetabular morphology. Because these osteotomies decrease the volume of the acetabulum, they are most useful for reshaping the capacious or severely misshapen (shallow) acetabulum. They are also appropriate for children between age 2 and 10 years with a concentrically reduced hip and acetabular dysplasia. Because these osteotomies do not enter the sciatic notch, they are inherently stable and do not require internal fixation. In the Pemberton osteotomy, the inner and outer tables of the ilium are divided, beginning laterally about 0.25" above the joint capsule (Fig. 6). By adjusting the orientation of the cuts through the inner and outer tables of the innominate bone, the amount of anterior and lateral augmentation provided by the osteotomy can be modified. The cut through the cancellous portion of the innominate bone is extended to a point just above the ilioischial limb of the triradiate cartilage. The posterior limb ideally is positioned halfway between the sciatic notch and the posterior margin of the acetabulum. In the Dega procedure, the osteotomy is performed only through the outer table of the ilium.

Salvage Procedures A salvage procedure may be indicated if the hip cannot be congruently reduced and does not meet the criteria for a reconstructive osteotomy. Salvage osteotomies reduce point loading at the edge of the acetabulum by increasing the weight-bearing surface of the hip with an extra-articular buttress of bone positioned over the subluxated femoral head. Fibrocartilaginous metaplasia of the interposed joint capsule provides an articulating surface. The Chiari osteotomy is performed by dividing the outer table of the ilium parallel to the insertion of the superior margin of the acetabulum, between the origin of the hip capsule and the reflected head of the rectus

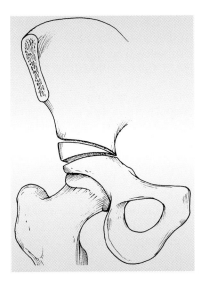

Figure 6 Reshaping osteotomy. *(Reproduced from Gillingham B, Sanchez A, Wenger D: Pelvic osteotomies for the treatment of hip dysplasia in children and young adults. J Am Acad Orthop Surg 1999;7: 325-337.)*

femoris (Fig. 7). The osteotomy is inclined in a slightly cephalad direction (approximately 20°) through the inner table of the ilium. The acetabulum is medially displaced along the plane of the osteotomy by abducting the hip and rotating it through the pubic symphysis. The extent of coverage is determined by the amount of displacement of the acetabulum, which ultimately depends on the width of the ilium at the level of the osteotomy. With stable internal fixation, spica cast immobilization can be avoided. With the shelf procedure, the femoral head is augmented with strips of corticocancellous bone extending over the femoral head that have been placed in a slot created along the rim of the acetabulum. Depending on the stability of the shelf, cast immobilization may or may not be necessary.

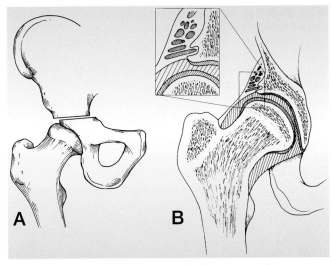

Figure 7 Salvage procedures. **A,** Chiari. **B,** Shelf slotted acetabular augmentation. *(Reproduced from Gillingham B, Sanchez A, Wenger D: Pelvic osteotomies for the treatment of hip dysplasia in children and young adults. J Am Acad Orthop Surg 1999;7:325-337.)*

Complications

Failed Reduction

Redislocation following closed reduction is not uncommon and usually can be managed by repeat closed or open reduction. However, redislocation following open reduction is a more difficult problem to resolve. Factors predisposing to failure of the initial open reduction frequently are the result of surgical technique and include failure to identify the true acetabulum, inadequate inferior capsular release, inadequate capsulorrhaphy, and concurrent femoral or pelvic osteotomy, which can cause posterior subluxation or dislocation. Repeat open reduction and/or revision of the femoral or pelvic osteotomy usually are necessary to address this complication. The rate of ON associated with repeat open reduction is higher, and results of surgery generally worse, than with primary treatment.

Osteonecrosis

ON is a complication associated with treatment of DDH and can occur with every form of treatment, including the Pavlik harness. Causes include excessive pressure on the femoral head and compression of the extrinsic blood supply of the femoral epiphysis. The prevalence of ON is about the same following open or closed reduction. Treatment factors associated with development of ON include immobilization in excessive abduction, failure of prior closed treatment, and repeat surgery for failed reduction. Based on a recent study, nonossification of the femoral head at the time of hip reduction does not increase the risk of ON following either open or closed reduction.

Radiographic evidence of ON includes failure of appearance or growth of the ossific nucleus within 1 year following hip reduction, broadening of the femoral neck over a similar period of time, increased radiographic density and subsequent fragmentation of the epiphysis, and residual deformity of the femoral head and neck after ossification is complete. Various classifications of ON following treatment of DDH have been described. They conceptually are similar in that they attempt to separate mild cases, which affect only a portion of the epiphysis and rarely cause clinical problems, from more severe patterns, which affect the physis, alter growth, and often lead to severe deformity of the femoral head and neck.

Treatment of ON is dictated by the pattern of involvement and resultant deformity of the hip. Acetabular redirection should be considered in young children at the first sign of femoral head subluxation. Proximal femoral varus osteotomy may be indicated to address subluxation associated with coxa valga. Trochanteric epiphysiodesis, performed in children younger than age 8 years, or distal lateral transfer of the greater trochanter, performed in children age 8 years and older, may be necessary to correct coxa breva and the abductor insufficiency associated with elevation of the greater trochanter. Contralateral distal femoral epiphysiodesis occasionally is needed to address limb-length inequality.

Annotated Bibliography

General Knowledge

Guille J, Pizzutillo P, MacEwen G: Developmental dysplasia of the hip from birth to six months. *J Am Acad Orthop Surg* 2000;8:232-242.

This article is an excellent review of the diagnosis and management of DDH in children from birth to age 6 months.

Gillingham B, Sanchez A, Wenger D: Pelvic osteotomies for the treatment of hip dysplasia in children and young adults. *J Am Acad Orthop Surg* 1999;7:325-337.

This article is an excellent overview of the etiology, biomechanics, and principles and techniques of treatment of acetabular dysplasia.

Diagnosis

Lewis K, Jones D, Powell N: Ultrasound and neonatal hip screening: The five-year results of a prospective study in high-risk babies. *J Pediatr Orthop* 1999;9:760-762.

The authors present the 5-year results of an ongoing prospective screening study of DDH using static ultrasound. In 17,792 births, 2,683 infants had risk factors and 354 infants had abnormal scans. Eight cases were missed, two with risk factors. The authors found that selective screening reduced the late rate of DDH per 1,000 births from 2.2 (with simple clinical examination) to 0.34 (with ultrasound) in their region. They concluded that selective screening alone will not eliminate presentation of late DDH, but they indicated the need for a study of ultrasound scanning of a whole population.

Teanby DN, Paton RW: Ultrasound screening for congenital dislocation of the hip: A limited targeted programme. *J Pediatr Orthop* 1997;17:202-204.

The authors report that limited but targeted ultrasound screening (including at-risk groups), either by dynamic methods alone or dynamic and static methods, did not prevent late dislocation that required treatment compared to clinical assessment alone. The authors observed that the rate of surgery for late DDH was reduced from 0.8 per 1,000 births to 0.25 per 1,000 births with ultrasound screening, which they attributed to more accurate assessment of hip pathology and more effective splinting treatment.

Walsh J, Morrissy R: Torticollis and hip dislocation. *J Pediatr Orthop* 1998;18:219-221.

Based on this retrospective review of 70 patients with congenital muscular torticollis, the authors found that the rate of hip disease was approximately 8%, which is lower than the 20% usually quoted.

Imaging

Bond CD, Hennrikus WL, DellaMaggiore ED: Prospective evaluation of newborn soft-tissue hip "clicks" with ultrasound. *J Pediatr Orthop* 1997;17:199-201.

Fifty infants older than age 3 months with soft-tissue hip clicks but stable hip examinations using the Ortolani and Barlow maneuvers, were examined by static and dynamic ultrasound. The average α angle was greater than 60°, femoral head coverage was greater than 50%, and dynamic examinations were normal in all patients. The authors concluded that in the absence of other signs of hip instability, soft-tissue hip clicks are not associated with DDH.

Kim H, Wenger D: The morphology of residual acetabular deficiency in childhood hip dysplasia: Three-dimensional computed tomographic analysis. *J Pediatr Orthop* 1997;17:637-647.

The authors studied 70 hips in 48 patients, using three-dimensional CT and defined four types of acetabular dysplasia: type I, subtle deficiency of the acetabulum with a mild break in Shenton's line (24%); type II, anterosuperior deficiency (29%); type III, midsuperior deficiency (28%); and type IV, global deficiency (9%). Type III deficiency was most common in patients with untreated DDH.

Mandel D, Loder R, Hensinger R: The predictive value of computed tomography in the treatment of developmental dysplasia of the hip. *J Pediatr Orthop* 1998;18:794-798.

Postreduction CT scans were reviewed in 38 children younger than age 24 months. None of the angles measured on the postreduction CT scan was found to predict remodeling potential.

Smith B, Kasser J, Hey L, Jaramillo D, Millis M: Postreduction computed tomography in developmental dislocation of the hip: Part I. Analysis of measurement reliability. *J Pediatr Orthop* 1997;17:626-630.

CT scans were reviewed in 20 infants in spica casts following open or closed reduction of DDH. A new measurement, based on the amount of displacement of the femoral metaphysis from a modified Shenton's line (drawn from the pubic rami), demonstrated high intra- and interobserver reliability in assessing the position of the femoral head.

Smith B, Millis M, Hey L, Jaramillo D, Kasser J: Postreduction computed tomography in developmental dislocation of the hip: Part II. Predictive value for outcome. *J Pediatr Orthop* 1997;17:631-636.

CT was obtained following closed reduction of 68 hips in 53 infants in spica casts. None of 10 measurements made on the CT scans predicted the outcome of residual acetabular dysplasia or the need for additional surgery. Development of ON was statistically associated with hip abduction angles of greater than 55°.

Skaggs D, Kaminsky C, Tolo V, Kay R, Reynolds R: Variability in measurement of acetabular index in normal and dysplastic hips, before and after reduction. *J Pediatr Orthop* 1998;18:799-801.

In this study, the variability in acetabular index (AI) measurement was found to be greater for dysplastic hips than for normal hips and also was greater before reduction than after. The AI proved to be most accurate following closed reduction of a dysplastic hip, supporting its use in monitoring acetabular remodeling.

Sucato D, Johnston C, Birch J, Herring J, Mack P: Outcome of ultrasonographic hip abnormalities in clinically stable hips. *J Pediatr Orthop* 1999;19:754-759.

The authors performed a retrospective review of 192 hips in 112 newborns with normal physical examinations but abnormal ultrasound findings. Forty-three hips were treated with a Pavlik harness (group I), and 149 hips were not treated (group II). None of the hips in group I and only two in group II had radiographic evidence of dysplasia. The authors concluded that a screening ultrasound in children younger than age 1 month for acetabular dysplasia may be too sensitive and does not accurately predict subsequent dysplasia.

Treatment

Hangen D, Kasser J, Emans J: The Pavlik harness and developmental dysplasia of the hip: Has ultrasound changed treatment patterns? *J Pediatr Orthop* 1995;15: 729-735.

Two age-matched groups with DDH were treated with Pavlik harnesses. One group was followed with serial ultrasound in addition to physical examination; the other was not. The ultrasound group had fewer total radiographs and earlier recognition of Pavlik failure.

Harding M, Hons B, Harcke H, Bowen J, Guille J, Glutting J: Management of dislocated hips with Pavlik harness treatment and ultrasound monitoring. *J Pediatr Orthop* 1997;17:189-198.

The authors found that ultrasound was very effective for diagnosing DDH and monitoring attempted reduction of the hip with the Pavlik harness. No anatomic features at the time of initial ultrasound correlated with success or failure of treatment with the Pavlik harness. Diagnosis and initiation of treatment within 3 weeks of birth increased the chances of successful reduction in the harness. Examination by ultrasound at 7 and 14 days after application of the Pavlik harness revealed a clear indication of which hips were likely to be successfully treated.

Huang SC, Wang JH: A comparative study of nonoperative versus operative treatment of developmental dysplasia of the hip in patients of walking age. *J Pediatr Orthop* 1997;17:181-188.

The authors found that open reduction with a Salter osteotomy in 32 patients with no preoperative traction was safe, effective, and shortened treatment time in children of walking age with DDH, compared to closed reduction with or without traction in 17 patients.

Morin C, Rabay G, Morel G: Retrospective review at skeletal maturity of the factors affecting the efficacy of Salter's innominate osteotomy in congenital dislocated, subluxed, and dysplastic hips. *J Pediatr Orthop* 1998;18: 246-253.

The authors reviewed the results of Salter's innominate osteotomy at skeletal maturity in 180 hips in 122 patients. Patients who underwent the osteotomy before age 4 years were most likely to have a satisfactory result. Factors associated with an abnormal result were previous failure of treatment, presence of ON (pre- or postoperatively), inability to achieve a normal acetabular angle, or the need for concomitant open reduction of the hip.

Mostert AK, Tulp NJ, Castelein RM: Results of Pavlik harness treatment for neonatal hip dislocation as related to Graf's sonographic classification. *J Pediatr Orthop* 2000;20:306-310.

Forty-one dislocated hips were prospectively classified according to Graf's sonographic classification prior to treatment in a Pavlik harness. Graf's classification proved to have prognostic significance. Pavlik treatment was successful in 97% of type III hips (cranial displacement) but in only 50% of type IV hips (caudal displacement).

Smith J, Matan A, Coleman S, Stevens P, Scott S: The predictive value of the development of the acetabular teardrop figure in developmental dysplasia of the hip. *J Pediatr Orthop* 1997;17:165-169.

Radiographs of 72 hips in infants were reviewed. In the normal hips (25 hips), the teardrop appeared by age 18 months. In the hips with DDH (47 hips), the teardrop did not appear until the hip was reduced. Statistically, the authors found that the appearance of the acetabular teardrop within 6 months after reduction correlated with a favorable long-term outcome.

Song K, Lapinsky A: Determination of hip position in the Pavlik harness. *J Pediatr Orthop* 2000;20:317-319.

Fourteen children treated with a Pavlik harness for DDH were evaluated at the time of harness application by clinical examination, ultrasound, and plain radiographs. Ultrasound findings correlated with clinical examination for hip position in 100% of hips. Radiographs correlated with ultrasound in only 49% of patients in whom the hip was judged to be dislocated. Ultrasound appears to be a better tool than plain AP radiographs for determining hip position in the Pavlik harness.

Tumer Y, Ward W, Grudziak J: Medial open reduction in the treatment of developmental dislocation of the hip. *J Pediatr Orthop* 1997;17:176-180.

In this retrospective study, medial open reduction (Ferguson's approach) without preliminary traction was performed on 56 developmentally dislocated hips in children younger than age 2 years. Excellent or good outcomes were seen in 98% of the hips; secondary bony procedures were required in 11 hips (19%); and ON developed in five hips (8.9%). The authors concluded that medial open reduction is a safe and effective treatment of DDH in children younger than age 2 years.

Vedantam R, Capelli A, Schoenecker P: Pemberton osteotomy for the treatment of developmental dysplasia of the hip in older children. *J Pediatr Orthop* 1998;18: 254-258.

The authors conducted a retrospective analysis to evaluate the results of Pemberton osteotomies for the treatment of DDH in 14 children (16 hips) older than age 7 years (average age 11 + 6 years). At an average follow-up of 4 + 10 years, the authors found improvement in the status of the hip joint, but they indicated that Pemberton acetabuloplasty might have to be combined with other surgical procedures to achieve a concentric and congruous reduction of the hip joint.

Wood MK, Conboy V, Benson MKD: Does early treatment by abduction splintage improve the development of dysplastic but stable neonatal hips? *J Pediatr Orthop* 2000;20:302-305.

Forty-four patients (63 hips) age 2 to 6 weeks with stable but sonographically dysplastic hips were randomly assigned to one of two treatment groups: abduction splinting or observation. Although changes in percentage acetabular cover were statistically significantly greater for the splinted group, there was no difference between the two groups in acetabular angle measurement on plain radiographs at 3 and 24 months. The authors concluded that stable but dysplastic hips will correct with growth and that there is no added benefit from early splinting.

Complications

Frick S, Kim S, Wenger D: Pre- and postoperative three-dimensional computed tomography analysis of triple innominate osteotomy for hip dysplasia. *J Pediatr Orthop* 2000;20:116-123.

Pre- and postoperative three-dimensional CT was performed in seven patients (eight hips) treated with a triple innominate osteotomy and demonstrated increased external rotation of the acetabulum postoperatively. Associated complications included excessive external rotation of the lower limb, decreased posterior coverage, increased gaps at the pubic and ischial osteotomy sites with resultant nonunion, and lateralization of the joint center. The authors suggested modifications in the surgical technique of this osteotomy to prevent these problems.

Luhmann SJ, Schoenecker PL, Anderson AM, Bassett GS: The prognostic importance of the ossific nucleus in the treatment of congenital dysplasia of the hip. *J Bone Joint Surg Am* 1998;80:1719-1727.

In this retrospective study, 153 hips, with an ossific nucleus present in 90 and absent in 63, were treated with closed or open reduction over a 15-year period and did not show any difference in the development of ON. The data do not support the hypothesis that the presence of an ossific nucleus at the time of reduction of a congenitally dislocated hip is associated with a lower prevalence of ON. The authors concluded that surgical treatment of DDH should be performed when the child can be safely anesthetized and without regard to the status of the ossific nucleus.

Pucher A, Ruszkowski K, Bernardczyk K, Nowicki J: The value of distal greater trochanteric transfer in the treatment of deformity of the proximal femur owing to avascular necrosis. *J Pediatr Orthop* 2000;20:311-316.

Forty-nine patients (55 hips) who underwent a distal greater trochanteric transfer to address deformity of the proximal femur after treatment of DDH were studied retrospectively. Good results were achieved in those who had good range of motion or isolated restriction of abduction. Following surgery, a 22% increase of abductor torque occurred, the Trendelenburg sign disappeared in 30 patients, and gait normalized in 15 patients.

Classic Bibliography

Chiari K: Medial displacement osteotomy of the pelvis. *Clin Orthop* 1974;98:55-71.

Ganz R, Klaue K, Vinh TS, Mast JW: A new periacetabular osteotomy for the treatment of hip dysplasias: Technique and preliminary results. *Clin Orthop* 1988; 232:26-36.

Pemberton PA: Pericapsular osteotomy of the ilium for treatment of congenital subluxation and dislocation of the hip. *J Bone Joint Surg Am* 1965;47:65-86.

Salter RB: Innominate osteotomy in the treatment of congenital hip dislocation and subluxation of the hip. *J Bone Joint Surg Br* 1961;43:518-539.

Staheli LT, Chew DE: Slotted acetabular augmentation in childhood and adolescence. *J Pediatr Orthop* 1992; 12:569-580.

Steel HH: Triple osteotomy of the innominate bone. *J Bone Joint Surg Am* 1973;55:343-350.

Castelein RM, Sauter AJ, de Vlierger M, et al: Natural history of ultrasound hip abnormalities in clinically normal newborns. *J Pediatr Orthop* 1992;12:423-427.

Chapter 18

Congenital and Acquired Tibial Deformity

Deborah F. Stanitski, MD

Congenital Anterolateral Bow and Tibial Pseudarthrosis

Congenital pseudarthrosis of the tibia is a rare condition affecting approximately 1 in 200,000 live births and is quite resistant to conventional treatments to obtain union. An anterolateral bow of the tibia may be the first physical sign of its existence. It has a strong association with neurofibromatosis-1 (NF-1), varying from 50% to 70%. This association initially may be difficult to determine, because other physical signs of NF-1 may be absent at birth. Conversely, however, only approximately 10% of patients with NF-1 have congenital pseudarthrosis of the tibia. In other patients, this condition may be idiopathic in origin; rarely is it associated with fibrous dysplasia.

At birth, the leg has an anterolateral bow and also may be shortened. The apex of the bow is in the distal one third of the leg. The foot and ankle are in the dorsiflexed position. If the pseudarthrosis is associated with neurofibromatosis, café-au-lait spots or cutaneous neurofibromata may be visible, and there may be a fracture at birth.

Isolated congenital fibular pseudarthrosis is extremely rare and is most commonly associated with tibial pseudarthrosis. When present, with or without the tibial component, it may result in fibular shortening and secondary ankle valgus.

Classification

There are a number of classification systems for congenital pseudarthrosis of the tibia. Classification is valuable for analyzing the components of the deformity and predicting the response to treatment. Boyd's system is used most often and describes six types of pseudarthrosis. Type I has anterior bowing and a tibial defect, both of which are present at birth. Type II is characterized by an hourglass constriction and a spontaneous fracture that usually occurs by age 2 years. In type II pseudarthrosis, the tibia classically has a sclerotic, obliterated medullary canal. Type II is the most common type associated with neurofibromatosis, and it has a poor natural history with regard to spontaneous healing. If union is achieved, recurrent fracture is common. Type III has a cystic appearance (Fig. 1). The bowing may not be obvious before the tibia has fractured. Recurrent fracture is less common in type III than in type II, and successful healing occurs more frequently after a single operation. Type IV occurs through a sclerotic tibia of normal diameter (Fig. 2). In this type, the medullary canal is absent, and the fracture often appears transverse and incomplete, similar to a stress fracture. Type V has an associated fibular pseudarthrosis, or it can present as an isolated fibular pseudarthrosis. Type VI has an associated schwannoma or neurofibroma. Very few cases of intraosseous neurofibromata have been documented.

A so-called "congenital" pseudarthrosis may develop after a seemingly innocuous fracture in a leg that previously looked grossly normal or only slightly bowed. This commonly is the scenario in a Boyd type IV pseudarthrosis and usually occurs after age 5 years. Other radiographic features of this condition include a hindfoot positioned in calcaneus, diminished height of the lateral distal tibial epiphysis, and variable shortening of the limb. The differential diagnosis of this condition includes fibrous dysplasia, osteogenesis imperfecta, rickets, and camptomelic dysplasia. One feature that distinguishes congenital pseudarthrosis from the other conditions is that it is rarely bilateral.

Management

Management of congenital pseudarthrosis of the tibia includes bracing, resection of the abnormal tissue, free vascularized fibular graft, intramedullary rodding, Ilizarov bone transport or compression, and distraction. If treatment begins before a fracture occurs, an ankle-foot orthosis (AFO) with an anterior shell or a

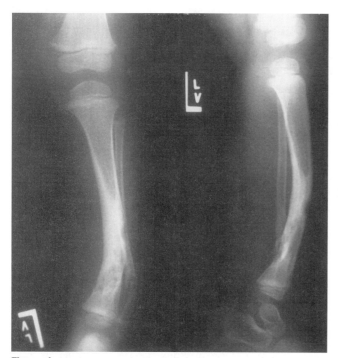

Figure 1 Boyd's type III prepseudarthrotic tibia showing medullary cystic changes. *(Reproduced from Richards BS (ed): Orthopaedic Knowledge Update: Pediatrics. Rosemont, IL, American Academy of Orthopaedic Surgeons, 1996, pp 177-184.)*

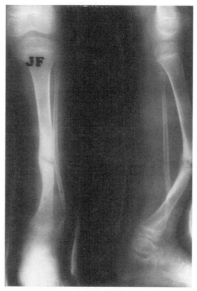

Figure 2 AP and lateral radiographs of a 4-year-old girl with neurofibromatosis and a congenital tibial pseudarthrosis. Boyd's type IV pseudarthrosis occurs through a sclerotic tibia of normal diameter. *(Reproduced from Richards BS (ed): Orthopaedic Knowledge Update: Pediatrics. Rosemont, IL, American Academy of Orthopaedic Surgeons, 1996, pp 177-184.)*

total contact AFO is used in an effort to prevent a fracture. Another preventive step is use of an onlay or bypass bone graft in an attempt to strengthen the prepseudarthrotic tibia. The value of this procedure remains unclear at this time because of conflicting reports. The surgeon should resist the temptation to improve mechanics by performing an osteotomy, which usually results in a failure to heal.

After a fracture has occurred, cast immobilization generally is unsuccessful. Conventional treatment such as bone grafting and plating have reported failure rates approaching 100%. Excellent results have been reported from intramedullary fixation with a Williams nail and a knee-ankle-foot orthosis (KAFO) applied postoperatively (Table 1). In this procedure, the pseudarthrosis is resected and the bow is corrected and protected with a long intramedullary rod. The rod is passed retrograde through the foot and may be left extending into the foot if the distal tibial segment is small. The fracture is surrounded by bone graft. Although the tibia heals more slowly than usual, the rod provides continuous protection. Success rates exceeding 90% have been reported.

Newer treatment modalities, such as free vascularized fibular grafting and the Ilizarov technique of bone transport and/or compression achieve initial union in most patients. Unfortunately, the refracture rate is high after these procedures. In one study, an initial union in 18 of 19 patients using free fibular grafting

was reported. This technique usually can be performed only once because the contralateral normal fibula is used. Usually, the ipsilateral fibula is affected and, therefore, cannot be used. Alternatively, in another recent study, transfer of the ipsilateral fibula with a normal vascular pedicle was successful. Mild weakness of the peroneal muscle and a valgus ankle in the donor limb are possible late complications when the free fibular technique is performed. The Ilizarov technique demonstrates promising (80%) early union rates but an increased risk of refracture. The advantages of this technique are the ability to correct tibial shortening and angulation, even in a small distal segment, and the ability to completely resect dysplastic bone and transport normal bone into the defect. Unfortunately, none of these techniques has completely eliminated the risk of refracture within the first decade. Syme's amputation, which was previously commonplace, does not necessarily result in bony union. However, it decreases the lever arm on the small distal fragment, and the Syme's prosthesis protects the pseudarthrosis. A Syme's amputation currently is recommended only in extreme cases in which the ankle is essentially nonfunctional or the patient has had numerous unsuccessful procedures. Below-knee amputation may be the ultimate solution in some patients once the risk of stump overgrowth has been eliminated. To date, no long-term studies that clarify the issue of bracing in adulthood are available. It is hoped that continued use of the free fibular transfer and/or Ilizarov technique eventually will provide sufficient numbers of mature patients to identify the most effective treatment of this condition.

Congenital Posteromedial Bow

Although congenital posteromedial bow has an equally worrisome visual appearance as anterolateral bow of

TABLE 1 | Treatment Options for Congenital Pseudarthrosis of the Tibia

Procedure	Advantages	Disadvantages	Comments
Intramedullary rod and graft	Excellent alignment Familiar to most surgeons Protects tibia for years	Prolonged healing Ankle stiffness Rod crosses the physis	This is the most commonly used initial procedure
Ilizarov procedure	Corrects angulation May restore length	High refracture rate	This procedure is most useful in children older than age 5 years or in children with hypertrophic pseudarthroses
Ipsilateral fibula transfer	Good local source of normal bone	Requires normal fibula at the level of the pseudarthrosis	This procedure often is not possible to perform
Free vascularized fibula	High rate of union Strong bone graft	Difficult to anchor small distal segment	

the tibia, it is a much more benign condition. There is no known association of this condition with other disorders, and its etiology is unknown. It has been attributed to developmental circumstances, such as intrauterine packing and/or fetal position. The proportionate growth inhibition of the tibia suggests that it is not just a late-gestational osseous deformation.

Clinical findings in the newborn usually include a calcaneovalgus foot position with excessive ankle dorsiflexion. The dorsum of the foot often lies on the anterior surface of the leg and at birth, the infant has a limited ability to plantar flex the foot beyond what appears to be a neutral position. There is apparent or real shortening of the leg, and a posteromedial bow is present at the junction of the middle and distal third of the tibia. Congenital posteromedial bow is always unilateral. Radiographic findings include variable degrees of apex posterior bowing (20° to 60°) and medial angulation of the tibia and fibula (Fig. 3). The bones appear relatively normal with some thickening of the concave cortex, usually as a result of stress concentration. There is no obliteration of the medullary canal as in congenital anterolateral bow.

Differential diagnoses includes the benign and common calcaneovalgus foot, which has a similar foot position but not the palpable tibial bow and corrects itself with no permanent sequelae (Table 2). Other differential diagnoses include fibular hemimelia and distal motor paresis. Fibular hemimelia presents as a valgus limb with some shortening but less dorsiflexion. In addition to the absent fibula, which may be hard to palpate in the newborn, there is often hypoplasia of the lateral rays of the foot. A distal motor paresis, such as that seen in an L5 myelomeningocele, produces a very dorsiflexed foot with slight valgus, although the tibia is straight.

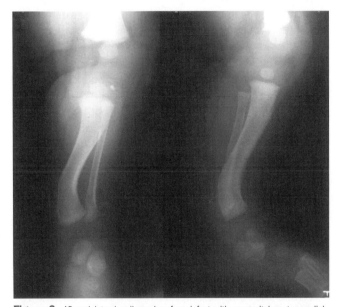

Figure 3 AP and lateral radiographs of an infant with congenital posteromedial tibial bow and concave cortical thickening. *(Reproduced from Richards BS (ed): Orthopaedic Knowledge Update: Pediatrics. Rosemont, IL, American Academy of Orthopaedic Surgeons, 1996, pp 177-184.)*

In many instances, the natural history of this condition is one of spontaneous correction. During the first 2 years of life, approximately 50% of the patients with posteromedial bow of the tibia improve spontaneously. Spontaneous correction of the foot position often occurs before age 9 to 12 months. In general, the severity of the initial deformity is related to the amount of ultimate limb shortening. Spontaneous correction does not occur after age 4 years. The limb-length discrepancy at maturity remains proportionate and varies from 5% to 27%, relative to the contralateral normal tibia. If no corrective procedure has been performed, the mean discrepancy at maturity is 4 cm.

TABLE 2	Differential Diagnosis of Posteromedial Bow of the Tibia	
Differential Diagnosis	**Clinical Findings**	
Calcaneovalgus foot	Similar foot position but rapid resolution, no palpable bony bow	
Fibular hemimelia	No palpable fibula; small foot; possible missing lateral rays	
Neuromuscular calcaneus foot	Spina bifida, L5 level	
Congenital vertical talus	Deformity occurs through midfoot	

Initial treatment of this condition is serial casting or stretching of the ankle and foot deformity in infancy to eliminate the dorsiflexion contracture of the ankle. Clinical and radiographic follow-up is mandatory to determine whether the growth inhibition will require treatment to equalize limb lengths. Generally, if followed appropriately, limb-length inequality can be corrected with an epiphysiodesis of the contralateral side. Because of the persistent tibial bow of 5° to 7° with a posterior and medial apex, limb lengthening with simultaneous deformity correction often is considered. Early osteotomy to correct the bowed tibia does not appear to affect the ultimate growth inhibition.

Blount's Disease

Blount's disease is a developmental condition that affects the medial aspect of the proximal tibial physis, resulting in a varus deformity that worsens with growth. Histologically, disordered endochondral ossification has been identified in the proximal medial tibial physis; however, its cause is not known. Mechanical overload may play a role. Two or three distinct forms of this condition exist and are classified by age at presentation. Infantile Blount's disease affects children younger than age 3 years. The adolescent form affects children older than age 8 years. Some authors describe a middle or juvenile group that falls between these two groups. However, a child in this group should be dis-

tinguished from a 7- or 8-year-old child with unrecognized infantile tibia vara.

The infantile form of tibia vara often is difficult to distinguish from physiologic bowing, particularly in children younger than age 2 years with bilateral bowed legs. Nearly 60% of children with infantile Blount's disease have bilateral involvement. Although not clinically proven, mechanical factors such as early age at ambulation and increased weight are the most commonly proposed theories of the etiology. A familial tendency is sometimes noted, which may be difficult to distinguish from these mechanical factors.

Classification

In 1952, Langenskiöld created his widely used classification system for infantile Blount's disease. It is difficult to apply this classification to the older child. This system consists of six stages with progressively more severe angulation of the medial proximal tibial physis (Fig. 4). In stage VI, the medial segment of the physis is nearly vertical, often with a bar in the region. Stage VI has the poorest prognosis. With increasing weight and increasing varus, the damage to the medial growth plate worsens. Therefore, as soon as a conclusive diagnosis of Blount's disease is made, early intervention appears to be beneficial.

During a child's early years, it often is difficult to differentiate early infantile Blount's disease from the much more common physiologic bowing. Because ossification of the proximal tibial epiphysis is not well developed, the early changes described by Langenskiöld may not be possible to identify with certainty until the child is age 3 or 4 years. Clearly, however, in physiologic bowing, varus occurs almost equally in the distal femur and proximal tibia. For this reason, investigators have subsequently tried to determine a measure that is more reproducible at that age and quantitates the focal bowing in the proximal tibia. Diagnosis often is based on the radiographic metaphyseal-diaphyseal angle (Fig. 5). Radiographs must be carefully obtained to ensure that long views of the limbs include both the hip and the ankle for accurate angle measure-

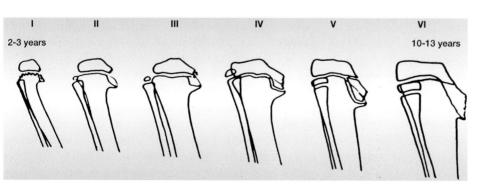

I	II	III	IV	V	VI
2-3 years					10-13 years

Figure 4 Diagrammatic representation of Langenskiöld classification of infantile Blount's disease. *(Reproduced with permission from Langenskiöld A: Tibia vara: A survey of 23 cases. Acta Orthop Scand 1952; 103:1.)*

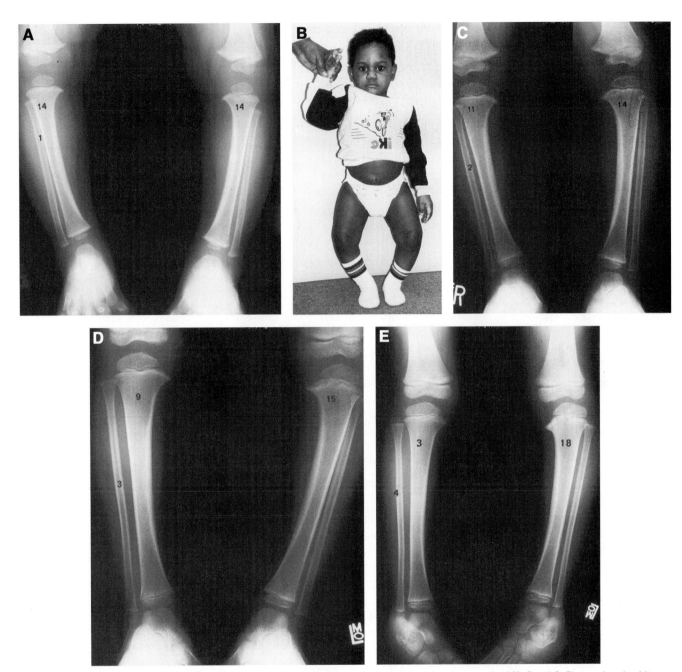

Figure 5 **A,** Radiograph of a 1-year-old boy with moderate bowing and bilateral metaphyseal-diaphyseal angles measuring 14°. **B** and **C,** Photograph and weight-bearing radiograph of the patient at age 2 years. The deformity has subtly resolved on the right; however, the 14° metaphyseal-diaphyseal angle remains on the left. **D** and **E,** At age 3 and 4 years, the physiologic bowing on the right leg has resolved; however, the left leg is clearly affected by Blount's disease. *(Reproduced from Kasser JR (ed): Orthopaedic Knowledge Update 5. Rosemont, IL, American Academy of Orthopaedic Surgeons, 1996, pp 437-451).*

ment. Because many children with Blount's disease also have significant internal tibial torsion, the patellae, rather than the feet, should be pointing forward so that a true AP view of the knee is obtained. Once the patient has reached age 3 to 4 years, weight-bearing radiographs may be obtained. One author has demonstrated that significant inter- and intraobserver error is inherent in measuring the metaphyseal-diaphyseal angle. Although the previously recognized threshold for diagnosing Blount's disease was 11°, it probably is

more accurate at approximately 16° for a clear-cut diagnosis in a young child. Patients with a metaphyseal-diaphyseal angle between 11° and 16° probably should be carefully monitored radiographically approximately every 6 months until progression or regression to normal is noted. If progression is noted, treatment is recommended.

The diagnosis is often easier to make in the adolescent. Usually, the patient has a history of increasing size and/or weight and bowing of one extremity. The

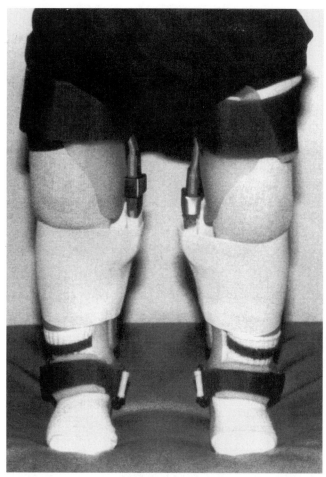

Figure 6 KAFO used for infantile Blount's disease. Valgus is produced by medial thigh and ankle cuffs and an elastic strap around the proximal tibia. The drop-lock knee hinge should be locked during standing but unlocked during sitting. *(Reproduced with permission from Raney EM, Topoleski TA, Yaghoubian R, Guidera KJ, Marshall JG: Orthotic treatment of infantile tibia vara. J Pediatr Orthop 1998; 18:670-674.)*

TABLE 3	Potential Components of Deformity in Blount's Disease

Varus of the proximal tibia

Varus or valgus of the distal femur

Closure of the medial tibial physis

Rotational malalignment

Shortening of the tibia (current and future)

Sagittal deformity

Valgus of the ankle (in severe deformity)

Depression of the tibial plateau (by arthrogram/MRI)

varus deformity in the affected extremity varies markedly from normal, making it clinically apparent. The adolescent form of Blount's disease most often is unilateral. Again, long radiographic views of the extremities should be evaluated for the presence of potential concurrent varus or valgus distal femoral deformities.

Treatment

The treatment of Blount's disease often is age-dependent. In the infantile form, some authors advocate bracing once the diagnosis has been made and before there is significant deformity. Although the role of bracing remains controversial, theoretically, it may be effective. Surgical mechanical realignment can reverse the growth disorder of the proximal tibia. Recent studies suggest that bracing improves the likelihood of resolution of infantile Blount's disease. A definite conclusion concerning the results of bracing has been difficult to reach because of the lack of a precise definition of

the condition and a lack of a controlled prospective study. Bracing should be considered in 2- to 3-year-old children with infantile Blount's disease who have a metaphyseal-diaphyseal angle of greater than 16°. Bracing also should be considered in children with a metaphyseal-diaphyseal angle of greater than 11° who have risk factors such as documented progression, obesity, female gender, or ligamentous laxity. If a brace is used, it should be a KAFO that is worn during weight-bearing hours (Fig. 6). Because infantile Blount's disease may be related to weight bearing, the brace is less effective while the child is sleeping. The brace's knee hinge should be locked during walking to increase the effectiveness of mechanical force distribution and prevent skin irritation during movement. Some braces have a drop-lock to allow knee flexion while the child is seated. These children often have extremely chubby extremities; therefore, it can be difficult to apply corrective pressure to the proper regions with the brace. The proximal-medial (thigh) cuff should be placed as high as is tolerable so that a valgus force is imparted to the limb. At this age, the child is growing quickly, so frequent evaluation with appropriate adjustments of the brace is needed. An elastic or adjustable strap often is used around the proximal tibia at the level of the knee joint to draw the knee out of varus. The ankle joint of the brace should allow free motion. The reported results of bracing are encouraging; bowing resolves in 65% to 90% of treated patients. The prognosis is worse in patients with bilateral varus than in those with unilateral varus.

If progressive deformity is identified, tibial osteotomy is indicated. The best results (the least risk of progressive deformity) have been demonstrated when surgery is performed in children younger than age 4 years. Among the techniques described for correcting the varus and rotational deformity are an

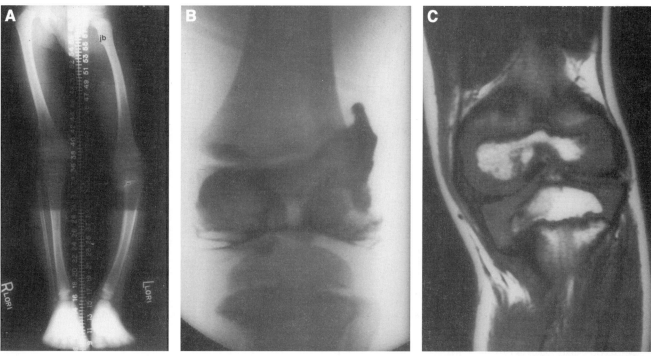

Figure 7   **A,** Radiograph of a 5-year-old boy with Blount's disease. **B** and **C,** Although the epiphysis appears depressed on the radiograph, MRI and arthrography demonstrate a normal shape of the cartilage surface. *(Reproduced with permission from Stanitski DF, Stanitski CL, Trumble S: Depression of the medial tibial plateau in early-onset Blount disease: Myth or reality? J Pediatr Orthop 1999;19:265-269.*

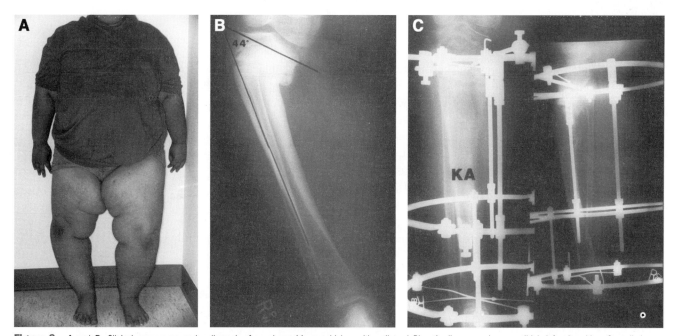

Figure 8   **A** and **B,** Clinical appearance and radiograph of an obese 11-year-old boy with unilateral Blount's disease and severe tibial deformity with a 3-cm limb-length deformity. **C,** Circular external fixation achieved gradual correction of the deformity and restored equal limb lengths. *(Reproduced from Richards BS (ed): Orthopaedic Knowledge Update: Pediatrics. Rosemont, IL, American Academy of Orthopaedic Surgeons, 1996, pp 177-184.)*

oblique metaphyseal osteotomy, focal dome, and others. If osteotomy is performed without adequate fixation, a cast must be used postoperatively with the knee extended to allow assessment of the limb angulation. Postoperatively, patients should be closely monitored for compartment syndrome. The older the patient and the more advanced the deformity, the more difficult it is to analyze and correct the deformity (Table 3). Progression of the disease to a Langenskiöld stage V or VI can be confirmed with MRI. At these stages, recurrent deformity and limb-length inequality are predictable.

In patients with a Langenskiöld stage IV deformity or greater, the medial tibial physis and growth plate must be carefully evaluated for evidence of growth arrest or bar formation. This evaluation is best done using MRI or conventional tomography. In patients with medial physeal closure, the osteotomy must be combined with bar resection or, less commonly, with completion of the epiphysiodesis in an effort to eliminate the risk of recurrent deformity with continued skeletal growth. Attempts also have been made to elevate the medial and often the posterior tibial plateau, although it is not clear whether these efforts are appropriate or eliminate the risk of recurrent deformity. Arthrography or MRI of the cartilaginous joint surface reveals that in most instances in which a depression of the ossified portion of the epiphysis is apparent, cartilaginous material fills the defect (Fig. 7), making a procedure to elevate the joint surface unnecessary. These areas should be carefully assessed before a treatment option is chosen.

Many osteotomy techniques are available to treat adolescent Blount's disease. Current methods of rigid external fixation with acute or gradual correction allow for accurate alignment of the lower extremity. Depending on the presence or absence of femoral deformity, concurrent femoral osteotomy may be indicated. Overcorrection or undercorrection that can occur with osteotomy and internal fixation can be prevented with use of external fixation. Poor outcomes in the treatment of adolescent Blount's disease can be caused by nerve palsy, compartment syndrome, overcorrection, and undercorrection. External fixation, particularly using one of the gradual correction techniques, may prevent many of these potential complications (Fig. 8).

In adolescents who have significant growth remaining, one treatment option is a lateral hemiepiphysiodesis. This procedure causes the least pain and allows the earliest return to function for the patient. Although correction of mild deformities has been reported using this technique, its effectiveness is unpredictable. The assumption that the medial tibial physis can be expected to grow at a "normal" rate when compared to the opposite side may be erroneous. Even with a properly functioning physis, there must be enough growth remaining to correct the deformity. Therefore, a lateral hemiepiphysiodesis should be considered only in adolescents with mild deformity.

Annotated Bibliography

Congenital Anterolateral Bow and Tibial Pseudarthrosis

Boero S, Catagni M, Donzelli O, Facchini R, Frediani PV: Congenital pseudarthrosis of the tibia associated with neurofibromatosis-1: Treatment with Ilizarov's device. *J Pediatr Orthop* 1997;17:675-684.

The authors reexamined 21 patients with congenital pseudarthrosis of the tibia that was associated with NF-1, 2 or more years after treatment with an Ilizarov technique. Good results were achieved in 66.7% of patients. Favorable prognostic factors were age older than 5 years and resection of the dystrophic bone around the pseudarthrosis.

Ghanem I, Damsin JP, Carlioz H: Ilizarov technique in the treatment of congenital pseudarthrosis of the tibia. *J Pediatr Orthop* 1997;17:685-690.

In this retrospective review of 14 patients with congenital pseudarthrosis of the tibia, favorable results following the Ilizarov technique were achieved in two thirds of them. Hypertrophic or normotrophic types of pseudarthrosis, as well as an age older than 5 years were associated with better results.

Blount's Disease

Miller S, Radomisli T, Ulin R: Inverted arcuate osteotomy and external fixation for adolescent tibia vara. *J Pediatr Orthop* 2000;20:450-454.

The authors report that an inverted arcuate osteotomy allows more proximal placement of the osteotomy than a dome osteotomy and is therefore more stable. The procedure is compatible with external fixation. Good results were reported in 13 of 15 osteotomies.

Raney EM, Topoleski T, Yaghoubian R, Guidera KJ, Marshall JG: Orthotic treatment of infantile tibia vara. *J Pediatr Orthop* 1998;18:670-674.

In this article, 60 limbs in 38 children age 2 to 3 years with metaphyseal-diaphyseal angles greater than 16°, (or between 9° and 16° with risk factors for progression) were studied. Resolution of the varus was seen in 90% of patients.

Richards BS, Katz DE, Sims JB: Effectiveness of brace treatment in early infantile Blount's disease. *J Pediatr Orthop* 1998;18:374-380.

The authors report that bracing was successful in 65% of 37 extemities in patients with Langenskiöld stage II Blount's disease. Patients with bilateral disease had poorer results.

Stanitski DF, Stanitski DL, Trumble S: Depression of the medial tibial plateau in early-onset Blount disease: Myth or reality? *J Pediatr Orthop* 1999;19:265-269.

Eleven knees in patients with a mean age of 5.8 years were assessed by MRI and arthrography at the time of surgical correction. Despite an apparent depression of the ossified portion of the proximal medial tibial epiphysis, all studies demonstrated that the space was filled with cartilage-density material with no dye pooling. These results suggest that an osteotomy to elevate the medial plateau should not be performed on the basis of plain radiographic appearance unless such a finding is demonstrated arthrographically.

Classic Bibliography

Anderson DJ, Schoenecker PL, Sheridan JJ, Rich MM: Use of an intramedullary rod for the treatment of congenital pseudarthrosis of the tibia. *J Bone Joint Surg Am* 1992;74:161–168.

Baker JK, Cain TE, Tullos HS: Intramedullary fixation for congenital pseudarthrosis of the tibia. *J Bone Joint Surg Am* 1992;74:169–178.

Boyd HB: Pathology and natural history of congenital pseudarthrosis of the tibia. *Clin Orthop* 1982;166:5–13.

Bradway JK, Klassen RA, Peterson HA: Blount disease: A review of the English literature. *J Pediatr Orthop* 1987;7:472–480.

Coleman SS, Coleman DA: Congenital pseudarthrosis of the tibia: Treatment by transfer of the ipsilateral fibula with vascular pedicle. *J Pediatr Orthop* 1994;14:156–160.

Feldman MD, Schoenecker PL: Use of the metaphyseal-diaphyseal angle in the evaluation of bowed legs. *J Bone Joint Surg Am* 1993;75:1602–1609.

Greene WB: Infantile tibia vara. *J Bone Joint Surg Am* 1993;75:130–143.

Henderson RC, Kemp GJ, Hayes PR: Prevalence of late-onset tibia vara. *J Pediatr Orthop* 1993;13:255–258.

Hofmann A, Wenger DR: Posteromedial bowing of the tibia: Progression of discrepancy in leg lengths. *J Bone Joint Surg Am* 1981;63:384–388.

Johnston CE II: Infantile tibia vara. *Clin Orthop* 1990;255:13–23.

Kline SC, Bostrum M, Griffin PP: Femoral varus: An important component in late-onset Blount's disease. *J Pediatr Orthop* 1992;12:197–206.

Kruse RW, Bowen JR, Heithoff S: Oblique tibial osteotomy in the correction of tibial deformity in children. *J Pediatr Orthop* 1989;9:476–482.

Levine AM, Drennan JC: Physiological bowing and tibia vara: The metaphyseal-diaphyseal angle in the measurement of bowleg deformities. *J Bone Joint Surg Am* 1982;64:1158–1163.

Paley D, Catagni M, Argnani F, Prevot J, Bell D, Armstrong P: Treatment of congenital pseudoarthrosis of the tibia using the Ilizarov technique. *Clin Orthop* 1992;280:81–93.

Pappas AM: Congenital posteromedial bowing of the tibia and fibula. *J Pediatr Orthop* 1984;4:525–531.

Strong ML, Wong-Chung J: Prophylactic bypass grafting of the prepseudarthrotic tibia in neurofibromatosis. *J Pediatr Orthop* 1991;11:757–764.

Thompson GH, Carter JR: Late-onset tibia vara (Blount's disease): Current concepts. *Clin Orthop* 1990;255:24–35.

Tuncay IC, Johnston CE II, Birch JG: Spontaneous resolution of congenital anterolateral bowing of the tibia. *J Pediatr Orthop* 1994;14:599–602.

Weiland AJ, Weiss AP, Moore JR, Tolo VT: Vascularized fibular grafts in the treatment of congenital pseudarthrosis of the tibia. *J Bone Joint Surg Am* 1990;72:654–662.

Chapter 19

Limb-Length Inequality

Deborah F. Stanitski, MD

Limb-length inequality in children usually is the result of an underlying congenital or acquired condition. An accurate diagnosis regarding etiology is mandatory before limb-length discrepancy projections can be made and treatment recommendations provided. The projected limb-length discrepancy at skeletal maturity dictates treatment. Projected discrepancies of 2.0 cm or less do not require treatment. Greater discrepancies usually do require treatment. If these discrepancies are not treated, they may produce an increase in vertical pelvic motion with gait and greater energy expenditure during walking. Although uncompensated limb-length inequality may result in compensatory scoliosis, data do not suggest that limb-length inequality may result in significant back pain or joint pain.

Etiology

Congenital Conditions

The most common causes of limb-length inequality at birth are congenital deficiency disorders, such as proximal (femoral) and distal (tibial and/or fibular) abnormalities. Femoral disorders include proximal femoral focal deficiency (PFFD) (Fig. 1), congenital short femur, and hypoplastic femur. These three disorders may include variable hip dysplasias and proximal femoral deformities, shortening, external rotation (relative femoral retroversion), distal femoral valgus, hypoplasia of the patella and lateral femoral condyle, and AP knee instability.

Fibular hypoplasia (Fig. 2) or aplasia may be associated with shortening of the lower leg and often accompanies congenital shortening of the femur. With fibular hypoplasia, a mild anteromedial bow of the tibia usually is present, which occurs in the middle to distal third of the tibia. The foot may be laterally displaced relative to the tibia, and there may be ankle and/or hindfoot valgus. The foot may have a tarsal coalition and absent lateral rays, in addition to some degree of hindfoot equinus and abnormal ankle motion.

Tibial hypoplasia (Fig. 3) or aplasia is uncommon. If it is present, either partial or complete absence of the tibia with shortening of the limb may exist. The quadriceps mechanism may be absent, and an apparent "clubfoot" often is present. This condition can be hereditary when accompanied by a lobster-claw hand deformity (autosomal recessive).

Hemihypertrophy or hemiatrophy usually is associated with limb-length inequality. Hemihypertrophy is manifested with overgrowth or enlargement of the entire affected side of the body. Hemiatrophy involves underdevelopment of a single extremity while the other extremity remains unaffected. Because of the association between Wilms' tumor and hepatic neoplasms with hemihypertrophy, infants and children with hemihypertrophy should be screened annually with abdominal ultrasound and serum α-fetoprotein levels until age 5 or 6 years. Klippel-Trénaunay-Weber syndrome, Proteus syndrome, and neurofibromatosis occasionally are associated with hemihypertrophy.

Skeletal dysplasias including Ollier's disease, which is not genetic, osteochondromatosis, which are multiple hereditary exostoses, fibrous dysplasia, and chondrodysplasia punctata (Conradi-Hünermann syndrome) may be associated with limb-length inequality.

Acquired Conditions

Inflammation, infection, trauma, and paralytic disorders may result in acquired limb-length inequality. Joint inflammation stimulates longitudinal bone growth, such as with juvenile rheumatoid arthritis and hemophilia, and most commonly occurs around the knee. These inflammatory conditions can cause unpredictable, asymmetric, sporadic growth spurts making prediction of limb-length inequality difficult.

Infection is a relatively common cause of physeal arrest. Physeal arrest may occur as a sequela of systemic sepsis in both neonates and older children. Meningococcal septicemia is the most fulminant of

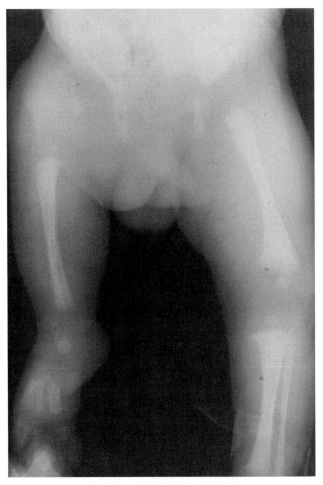

Figure 1 Radiograph of an infant with probable Aitken D PFFD with a subtotal absence of the femur and location of the ankle at the level of the contralateral knee. *(Reproduced from Richards BS (ed): Orthopaedic Knowledge Update: Pediatrics. Rosemont, IL, American Academy of Orthopaedic Surgeons, 1996, pp 185-193.)*

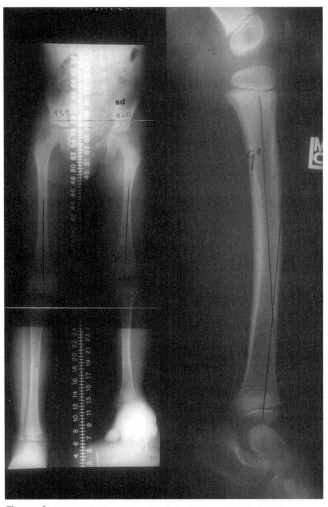

Figure 2 Radiograph of a child with left fibular hypoplasia, limb-length discrepancy, and short femur.

these septic episodes, and injury to multiple physes may result in severe bony deformities and limb-length inequality. Purpura fulminans can cause these types of deformities. Occult septic growth arrests still are common, particularly in premature infants who survive a long course in the neonatal intensive care unit.

The most common cause of trauma-related limb-length inequality is a physeal fracture with subsequent physeal arrest. Diaphyseal and metaphyseal fractures of the tibia and femur that are anatomically reduced in children between age 2 and 10 years may result in "overgrowth" or "regrowth" of the injured extremity with a resultant limb-length discrepancy. Radiation and burns also cause traumatic growth arrest, although radiation is currently much less common than burns. A complete physeal closure may result in limb-length inequality; an incomplete physeal closure may result in a potential limb-length inequality and angular deformity.

Asymmetric neurologic impairment in a growing child can potentially produce limb-length inequality in which the affected extremity is shorter. Common causes include neonatal brachial plexus palsies, congenital hemi- or monoplegic spasticity, as with cerebral palsy, or acquired lesions, as with traumatic injury, tumor, or polio.

Assessment
Manual Methods
Clinical assessment of lower limb-length inequality includes the block method, tape measurement from the anterosuperior iliac spine (ASIS) to the medial malleolus (actual limb length), and tape measurement from the umbilicus to the medial malleolus (apparent limb length). The block method is performed by placing an appropriately sized block under the shorter leg so that the pelvis is clinically level. The block method is more accurate than using either of the tape measurement methods. Limb-length measurements made using a

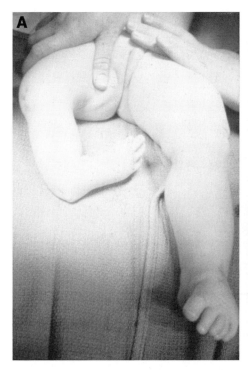

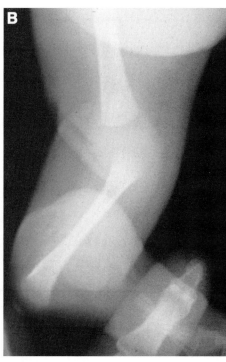

Figure 3 Infant with tibial hemimelia. **A,** Absent tibia causes the foot to assume a varus position, resembling clubfoot. **B,** Radiograph shows absent tibia, hypertrophic fibula, and hypoplastic tarsal bones with no proximal articulation.

tape measure can be altered by abduction, adduction, or flexion of the hip or by flexion of the knee. Furthermore, the ASIS may be difficult to palpate in obese children. Tape measurement from the umbilicus to the medial malleolus may reveal an apparent limb-length discrepancy resulting from pelvic obliquity or scoliosis that may not be revealed when using the actual limb-length method (measuring the ASIS to the medial malleolus). The entire patient must be carefully examined to avoid errors from associated fixed pelvic obliquity, scoliosis, or knee or hip contractures. The standing height of the foot also should be evaluated because it may be shorter than the contralateral foot, particularly in children with congenital conditions.

Imaging
Radiographic assessment of limb-length discrepancy may be performed using either a scanogram or an orthoroentgenogram. Both techniques involve placing a radiopaque ruler under the lower extremities. The scanogram uses an x-ray tube in linear motion with a slit diaphragm. Any movement by the patient is detected by motion on the film. The scanogram's range includes all osseous structures so that any angular deformity can be detected. The orthoroentgenogram is a multiple-exposure radiograph that is designed to obtain a straight projection through each joint of the extremity. However, its range does not show the entire extremity. Therefore, the limb deformity cannot be accurately assessed. The film is 14″ × 17″, so it can easily fit into the standard radiograph folder. The patellae

should point forward to prevent any rotational alteration of limb alignment when using either technique.

Ultrasound techniques have been used in Europe with some success. The advantage of this technique is that no radiation is required. However, a second visit to the office may be necessary to schedule an ultrasound examination, and the technique is not yet considered very accurate. Currently, this technique is not widely used in North America.

CT scanogram is the most accurate technique; it involves little radiation exposure and can be obtained in the lateral projection to eliminate any errors induced by joint contracture. Unfortunately, this is the most expensive technique and, as with an ultrasound examination, may require special scheduling, making it difficult to use in the standard office-hospital setting on a daily basis.

Regardless of what radiographic method is used, serial radiographic examinations over a period of several years are necessary to predict the ultimate limb-length discrepancy and to choose the appropriate treatment. Bone age radiographs must be obtained on each occasion. In addition, weight-bearing AP radiographs of both lower extremities, including the hip, knee, and ankle, help demonstrate angular alignment before surgical intervention is contemplated.

Prediction Methods
The two most widely used methods for predicting limb-length inequality are the Green-Anderson Growth Remaining Chart and the Moseley Straight

Line Graph method. With the latter technique, all of the patient's longitudinal data are recorded on a single sheet of paper. In general, accumulation of radiographic data should begin at age 4 to 5 years. Annual visits that include clinical and radiographic measurements and bone age radiographs are recommended. Bone age radiographs that are based on the Greulich and Pyle atlas may have an inherent error of 12 to 18 months. In addition, neither the Moseley Straight Line Graph nor the Green-Anderson Growth Remaining Chart allow for foot height, which must be added to the final projected limb-length inequality in order to achieve an accurate prediction. To reduce the likelihood of error, all limb-length measurements should be obtained using the same technique and measured by the same individual. Bone age data should probably be collected again because earlier data used in the Greulich and Pyle atlas was obtained during the 1940s and 1950s, and current reports suggest that the tibial and femoral lengths may now be longer. However, in order to obtain more data, radiographs of children with no limb-length inequality would need to be obtained, which currently is not possible because of radiation concerns.

Treatment

Management depends on the extent of the projected limb-length discrepancy (Table 1). In general, for actual or projected discrepancies of less than 2 cm, no treatment is necessary. A 3/8″ insole can be used in patients believed to have symptoms secondary to a small limb-length discrepancy. For larger discrepancies, a lift must be added to the sole of the shoe and tapered toward the toe to allow a more normal gait pattern. Any lift added to the sole will render the shoe "stiff," which makes this treatment option very unpopular in children because they are unable to run and jump normally. In addition, lifts on the sole are conspicuous and may attract unwanted attention from peers. Lifts that exceed 8 to 10 cm may be unstable and require additional support, such as an ankle-foot orthosis, to prevent the child from falling off of the shoe. In children with severe limb-length discrepancy, extension prostheses often are used. These put the child's foot into extension so that it fits into the prosthesis. The prosthetic foot is attached distally. Extension prostheses should be discouraged in any child who is likely to undergo attempts at limb-length equalization because these prostheses eventually result in deformity of the foot and ankle. Such deformities make it extremely difficult to obtain a plantigrade foot position with a mobile ankle joint. Prostheses may be necessary in severe forms of PFFD. A through-knee type prosthesis may be necessary in patients with

| TABLE 1 | Projected Limb-Length Discrepancy and Management |

Size of Discrepancy	Management
0 to 2 cm	No treatment
	Shoe lift if symptomatic
2 to 5 cm	Epiphysiodesis
	Gradual distraction lengthening if angular deformity is present
	Acute shortening in skeletally mature patient
>5 cm	Gradual distraction lengthening
>18 cm	Multiple gradual distraction lengthening procedures, 3 to 5 years apart
	Contralateral epiphysiodesis
	Amputation for unsalvageable deformities

tibial hemimelia who have undergone a through-knee amputation.

Epiphysiodesis is appropriate for children who have a predicted limb-length inequality in the range of 2 to 5 cm. Adequate longitudinal data must be available so that the timing of the epiphysiodesis can be accurately predicted. Contraindications to an epiphysiodesis include inadequate data or inadequate time remaining until the end of growth. A relative contraindication is short stature. If there is significant axial or angular deformity within the short limb, an osteotomy to correct the axial or angular deformity should follow the epiphysiodesis.

The selected site or sites of the epiphysiodesis should not result in significant knee height difference. Either a percutaneous or open (Phemister) technique may be used. The percutaneous technique can be done through small incisions (less than 1.5 cm) or with screws. The physis is drilled and curetted, and the wounds are irrigated to eliminate any bony or cartilaginous debris. A soft bulky dressing or removable splint may be applied postoperatively. Weight bearing as tolerated is allowed. Sports or physical contact may be resumed following radiographic evidence of physeal closure. The older open technique of the Phemister epiphysiodesis is being used less frequently now than in the past. Complications from the percutaneous techniques are less common than those from the Phemister epiphysiodesis. Physeal stapling also may be used for epiphysiodesis; however, the staples may require removal. Staples also may migrate or cause soft-tissue impingement or catching.

Acute shortening may be indicated in patients who are either skeletally mature or in whom the existing data are inaccurate or confusing. Acute shortening usually is performed through the femur because of the increased complications observed when performed through the tibia. Complications of acute tibial shortening include neurovascular compromise, compartment syndrome, chronic muscle weakness, and severe edema. Acute shortening is reserved for patients with a limb-length discrepancy of 2 to 5 cm. Acute shortening should be performed only when the child is at or near skeletal maturity in order to ensure limb-length equalization.

Femoral shortening may be performed using either the open or closed technique. The open technique uses plate fixation in the proximal subtrochanteric region to maximize the efficiency of the quadriceps mechanism. The closed technique employs intramedullary shortening as first described by Winquist and Hansen in which a specialized intramedullary saw is used with an intramedullary nail that is interlocked both proximally and distally to avoid rotational malunion. All acute shortenings are accompanied by temporary loss of strength in the thigh muscle, which must be regained to ensure normal limb function.

Indications for limb lengthening include predicted limb-length inequality exceeding 5 cm or limb-length inequality of less than 5 cm in a patient with significant concurrent deformity. An acute lengthening method or gradual distraction may be used to lengthen the limb. Acute lengthening is performed by removing a segment of cortical bone from one side and inserting it in the other side of the bone after a femoral distractor or similar device has been used. Unfortunately, because sciatic palsy can be a complication of an acute lengthening, the procedure probably should be performed only for lengthenings of less than 3 cm. Currently, gradual incremental distraction techniques are used that avoid the need for bone graft and plate fixation. Lengthening can be achieved using these techniques with correction of any concurrent deformity. The rate of lengthening should not exceed 1 mm per day, in 3 or 4 increments, and the distraction rate should depend on the radiographic appearance of the bone formation.

Gradual incremental lengthening techniques involve using either circular external fixation or monolateral fixation. Monolateral cantilever-type fixators require half-pin fixation of the bone. Slide-type lengtheners are the most commonly used cantilever fixators in North America (Fig. 4). At least three half pins should be placed proximal to the lengthening site and two or three placed distal to the lengthening site to prevent potential pin bending. The advantages of monolateral fixation include its ease of application, fewer pin sites, less bulk than circular fixation, and more limited muscle transfixion. Recent modifications to monolateral fixation devices allow correction of angular and axial

deformities. A ball-joint type of monolateral fixator should not be used for lengthening because it is unstable to the forces encountered during limb lengthening and may result in angulation.

The most commonly applied circular external fixation technique in North America is the Ilizarov technique, in which small tensioned transosseous wires traditionally are affixed to rings to achieve bony stability (Fig. 5). Currently, the advantages of this technique include the ability to control the position of adjacent joints to prevent subluxation or dislocation, absence of patient and bone size limitations, and the ease of correcting any deformity that may develop during lengthening, without the need for anesthesia. Disadvantages include its bulk, steep learning curve, increased soft-tissue transfixion, and the need for more pin sites.

Patients with Aitken grade C or D PFFD present the most difficult challenge for limb lengthening. Not only must the limb-length discrepancy be addressed, but the angular deformity, hip instability, ankle instability, and foot deformity must be addressed as well. A stable relationship between the femur and pelvis must exist so that significant lengthening is achieved. Limbs with Aitken grades A and B PFFD may be salvageable but also may require pelvic osteotomy prior to lengthening. Extension of circular fixation to the pelvis may protect the hip joint during lengthening. Staged lengthenings are always required so that complications associated with extensive limb lengthening are minimized.

Large projected discrepancies can be managed if a functional plantigrade ankle and foot can be produced in the presence of fibular hemimelia and femoral hypoplasia. Discrepancies of greater than 18 to 20 cm are correctable, using two or three lengthening procedures with or without a contralateral epiphysiodesis. During each procedure, lengthening should be limited to less than 30% of the affected bone's length to avoid significant effects on the associated joints and muscles. The lengthening should be staged at least 3 to 5 years apart so that in the intervening period, the child can lead a normal life. Enough time before skeletal maturity should be available after the final lengthening for a contralateral epiphysiodesis to make up any remaining difference.

Physeal bar resection may be performed for partial physeal arrest if there is significant longitudinal limb growth remaining. The involved physis must be assessed radiographically with combined AP and lateral plain tomography, CT, or MRI using relatively small (2-mm) cuts to determine the area of the physis that is involved with the bar. However, MRI may be too sensitive and show a larger zone of abnormal physis than actually is included in the bar. Generally, physeal bar resection should be considered only if the

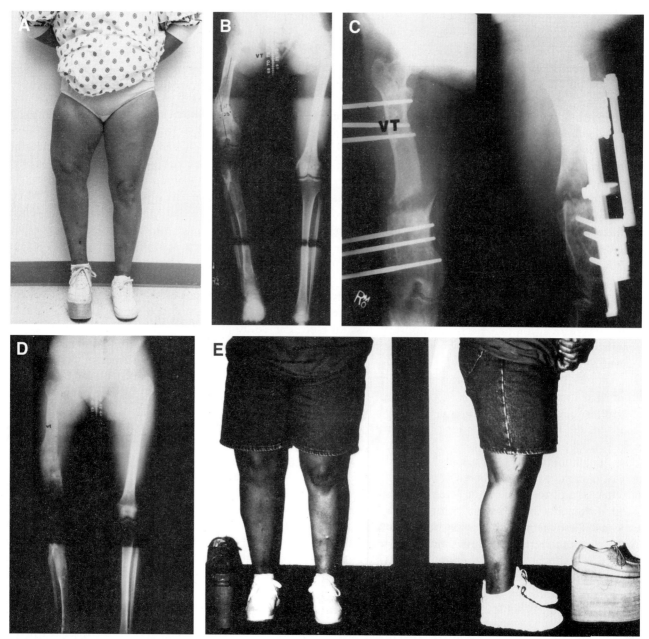

Figure 4 **A**, Preoperative clinical appearance and **B**, radiograph of a patient with Ollier's disease and a 13-cm limb-length discrepancy following tibial lengthening and prior to femoral lengthening. **C**, Radiograph of femur during distraction using a slide lengthener. **D**, Radiograph and **E**, clinical appearance at the end of treatment. *(Reproduced from Richards BS (ed): Orthopaedic Knowledge Update: Pediatrics. Rosemont, IL, American Academy of Orthopaedic Surgeons, 1996, pp 185-193.)*

physeal bar involves less than 50% of the total area of the physis. Otherwise, longitudinal growth following bar resection is unlikely.

Peripheral physeal bars can be surgically resected; however, they have a higher recurrence rate following resection than central physeal bars do. Central bar resection technically is more difficult. Bar resection is carried out via a metaphyseal window. A dental mirror can be used for circumferential vision of the central bar. Fat often is interposed to prevent bar reformation, and a marker is useful to monitor subsequent growth. Generally, physeal bar resection is not useful in

patients with less than 2 to 3 years of growth remaining. Additionally, subsequently normal longitudinal growth might not be achieved, and angular deformity might not spontaneously correct with growth. Osteotomy may be needed following physeal bar resection if any angular deformity does not spontaneously resolve.

Amputation occasionally is recommended in children with congenital limb-length discrepancy. Patients with Aitken grade C or D PFFD may be treated with either an ankle disarticulation with placement into an above-knee prosthesis or a Van Ness femoral rotationplasty with placement into a below-knee prosthesis. Patients

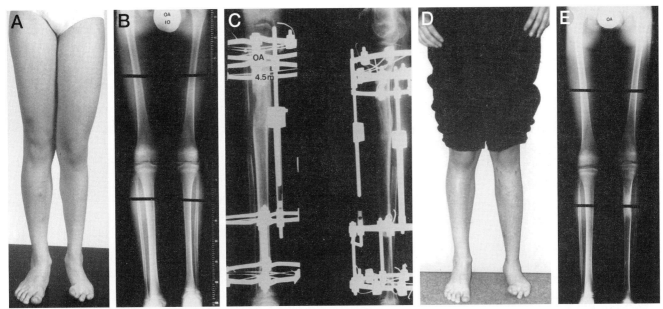

Figure 5 **A,** Preoperative clinical appearance and **B,** radiograph of a boy with type IA fibular hemimelia and a projected 9-cm limb-length discrepancy. **C,** AP and lateral radiographs of the tibia during the consolidation phase. **D,** Clinical appearance and **E,** radiograph at the conclusion of treatment. *(Reproduced from Kasser JR (ed): Orthopaedic Knowledge Update 5. Rosemont, IL American Academy of Orthopaedic Surgeons, 1996, pp 437-451.)*

with tibial hemimelia and absent knee extension are best treated with early through-knee amputation that may be converted to an above-knee through-bone amputation in the older individual. If the proximal tibia has good active knee extension, differential lengthening of the tibia may be considered in an effort to match the fibular length. A formal ankle arthrodesis can stabilize the distal foot-leg relationship.

Current Controversies in Limb Lengthening

Lengthening for Stature

Limb lengthening may be considered for patients with short stature. Activities of daily living, such as use of public transportation, toilet facilities, and drinking fountains, are compromised in individuals with significant short stature. Lengthening for stature should be avoided in those patients with a natural history of degenerative joint disease and in those who have unstable joints such as diastrophic dysplasia, pseudoachondroplasia, and the epiphyseal dysplasias. Patients with short stature who have normal joints and disproportionate short limb dwarfism (achondroplasia, hypochondroplasia, or mesomelic dysplasia) or those with familial short stature may benefit from limb lengthening, provided that excessive lengthening is avoided. Bilateral tibial lengthening may provide an adequate increase in height while avoiding the complications associated with femoral lengthening.

Devices

Currently, controversy exists about whether a circular-type external fixator or a cantilever-type of fixator should be used. In the past, a circular fixator allowed rotational and angular correction. Modifications to current cantilever fixators have allowed rotational and angular corrections to be built into the device. As mentioned before, some disadvantages of circular fixation include its bulk, steep learning curve, increased soft-tissue transfixion, and added pin sites. Often, circular fixation is initially chosen because of the patient's small size, and is followed by subsequent lengthenings with the monolateral device.

Annotated Bibliography

Assessment

Beumer A, Heijboer RP, Fontijne WP, Swierstra BA: Late reconstruction of the anterior distal tibiofibular syndesmosis: Good outcome in 9 patients. *Acta Orthop Scand* 2000;71:519-521.

The authors discussed some of the potential difficulties involved with the use of the Moseley Straight Line Graph, which is based on data obtained in the 1940s and 1950s. They used data collected between 1979 and 1994 to determine that in both boys and girls the mean femur and tibia length had increased and with the new data, final limb length could be better predicted.

Treatment

Coppola C, Maffulli N: Limb shortening for the management of leg length discrepancy. *J R Coll Surg Edinb* 1999;44:46-54.

In this article, the necessity of exact timing in performing an epiphysiodesis was discussed as well as when shortening and lengthening procedures should be performed.

Guichet JM, Casar RS: Mechanical characterization of a totally intramedullary gradual elongation nail. *Clin Orthop* 1997;337:281-290.

In this article, the intramedullary gradual elongation nail (Albizzia) was compared with other intramedullary nails for bending stiffness, torsional stiffness, ultimate bending strength, and torsional strength.

Noonan KJ, Leyes M, Forriol F, Canadell J: Distraction osteogenesis of the lower extremity with use of monolateral external fixation: A study of two hundred and sixty-one femora and tibiae. *J Bone Joint Surg Am* 1998;80:793-806.

The authors reviewed the results of monolateral lengthening and discussed the complications associated with limb lengthening for stature, especially in patients with congenital and familial short stature and Turner's syndrome.

Scott AC, Urquhart BA, Cain TE: Percutaneous vs modified Phemister epiphysiodesis of the lower extremity. *Orthopedics* 1996;19:857-861.

In this article, the percutaneous and modified Phemister approaches for epiphysiodesis of the lower extremity for limb-length discrepancy were compared. The authors determined that the percutaneous method was preferred because of the ease of the procedure, fewer incisions, and limited disability to the normal extremity.

Classic Bibliography

Achterman C, Kalamchi A: Congenital deficiency of the fibula. *J Bone Joint Surg Br* 1979;61:133-137.

Blair VP III, Schoenecker PL, Sheridan JJ, Capelli AM: Closed shortening of the femur. *J Bone Joint Surg Am* 1989;71:1440-1447.

Gabriel KR, Crawford AH, Roy DR, True MS, Sauntry S: Percutaneous epiphyseodesis. *J Pediatr Orthop* 1994;14:358-362.

Hope PG, Crawfurd EJ, Catterall A: Bone growth following lengthening for congenital shortening of the lower limb. *J Pediatr Orthop* 1994;14:339-342.

Loder RT, Herring JA: Fibular transfer for congenital absence of the tibia: A reassessment. *J Pediatr Orthop* 1987;7:8-13.

Moseley CF: Assessment and prediction in leg-length discrepancy. *Instr Course Lect* 1989;38:325-330.

Pirani S, Beauchamp RD, Li D, Sawatzky B: Soft tissue anatomy of proximal femoral focal deficiency. *J Pediatr Orthop* 1991;11:563-570.

Sasso RC, Urquhart BA, Cain TE: Closed femoral shortening. *J Pediatr Orthop* 1993;13:51-56.

Schoenecker PL, Capelli AM, Millar, et al: Congenital longitudinal deficiency of the tibia. *J Bone Joint Surg Am* 1989;71:278-287.

Shapiro F: Developmental patterns in lower-extremity length discrepancies. *J Bone Joint Surg Am* 1982;64:639-651.

Snyder M, Harcke HT, Bowen JR, Caro PA: Evaluation of physeal behavior in response to epiphyseodesis with the use of serial magnetic resonance imaging. *J Bone Joint Surg Am* 1994;76:224-229.

Stanitski DF, Bullard M, Armstrong P, Stanitski CL: Results of femoral lengthening using the Ilizarov technique. *J Pediatr Orthop* 1995;15:224-231.

Steel HH, Lin PS, Betz RR, Kalamchi A, Clancy M: Iliofemoral fusion for proximal femoral focal deficiency. *J Bone Joint Surg Am* 1987;69:837-843.

Suzuki S, Kasahara Y, Seto Y, Futami T, Furukawa K, Nishino Y: Dislocation and subluxation during femoral lengthening. *J Pediatr Orthop* 1994;14:343-346.

Timperlake RW, Bowen JR, Guille JT, Choi IH: Prospective evaluation of fifty-three consecutive percutaneous epiphysiodeses of the distal femur and proximal tibia and fibula. *J Pediatr Orthop* 1991;11:350-357.

Chapter 20

Knee Disorders

Carl L. Stanitski, MD

Basic Considerations

During the embryonic period, the knee begins as a mesenchymal condensation with cleft formation and converts to a cartilage model that undergoes endochondral ossification. By the end of the embryonic period (8 weeks), the components of the knee have been formed. Active motion has begun, and the quadriceps-patella-femoral complex and menisci and cruciate ligaments are well developed. In the full-term infant, the distal femoral epiphysis can be seen on radiographs. Postnatally, the distal femoral and proximal tibial secondary ossification centers accommodate longitudinal and latitudinal growth to provide adult morphology at skeletal maturity.

The two epiphyses contribute two thirds of the lower extremity's longitudinal growth; tibial growth is approximately 80% of femoral growth. The patella ossifies at age 3 to 5 years.

Imaging

Weight-bearing AP, tunnel, lateral, and skyline views may be helpful in assessing the pediatric knee. The skyline view should be done in less than 25° of flexion. These views allow assessment of femoral, tibial, fibular, and patellar morphology and relationships and disorders such as osteochondritis dissecans. Ratios to determine patella alta in children must be calculated with caution because of the significant amount of nonossified cartilage present in the patella and proximal tibia. In patients with acute patellar dislocations, a significant number of osteochondral injuries are not recognized radiographically when compared to findings at surgery. Fewer than 30% of osteochondral lesions have been identified on initial postinjury radiographs, and fewer than 30% of loose bodies, ranging in size from 2 mm to 20 mm, have been documented on initial postdislocation radiographs. The lack of recognition of osteochondral injury may account for poor outcomes following acute patellar dislocations.

Ultrasound examinations help to assess congenital knee dislocations and popliteal cysts. CT, especially with the quadriceps contracted and relaxed, helps to differentiate patellar tilt from translation. Dynamic CT scanning is becoming available and should prove quite useful to evaluate chronic patellar instability.

MRI has replaced arthrography as a tool to assess intra-articular knee conditions. Unfortunately, MRI has come to be considered as a screening test. An 80% false-positive grade 3 signal (an intrameniscal change that extends through the meniscal surface) was seen in the medial meniscus of asymptomatic normal children younger than age 10 years. Grade 3 medial meniscal signals were reported in 65% of asymptomatic normal children from age 10 to 13 years. Similar findings were seen in one third of asymptomatic normal teenagers age 14 and 15 years, which is a value similar to the 29% false-positive rate reported for asymptomatic normal adults. In studies that correlated arthroscopic findings with MRI reports, a 55% false-positive meniscal tear rate was seen in patients younger than age 15 years. MRI accuracy was 35%, positive and negative predictive indices were 50%, sensitivity was 50%, and specificity was 45% in a group of young adolescents. A significant number of false-positive and false-negative MRI findings were noted for menisci and anterior cruciate ligament (ACL) evaluations. Because of the high error rate that occurs with MRI in children and adolescents, MRI should be used as an adjunct, when indicated, to an expert clinical examination and not as a screening study.

Congenital Disorders

Many congenital abnormalities, such as patellar or knee dislocations, formation of discoid menisci or patellar variations, and cruciate ligament absence occur either in isolation (rare) or in association with femoral, tibial, or fibular anomalies. Syndromes such as Down, Larsen's, nail-patella, thrombocytopenia,

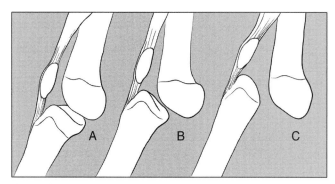

Figure 1 Classification of congenital knee hyperextension and dislocation. **A,** Type I, hyperextended knee. **B,** Type II, tibial subluxation. Tibial plateau and femoral condyle deformity with continuity. **C,** Type III, tibial dislocation. Further changes of the tibial plateau and femoral condyle contours have occurred with loss of suprapatellar space, progressive quadriceps-patellar tendon shortening, and lack of contact between the femoral and tibial articulation.

and absent radius or conditions such as multiple epiphyseal dysplasia and arthrogryposis often have knee abnormalities.

Congenital Knee Dislocation

Congenital knee hyperextension or dislocation presents as knee recurvatum that is evident at birth. It can occur in isolation or in association with hip dislocation, clubfoot, myelodysplasia, Larsen's syndrome, or arthrogryposis. Involvement ranges from mild (type I) to severe (type III) (Fig. 1). Lateral radiographs identify the femorotibial relationship. Ultrasound or MRI defines the magnitude of joint incongruity and associated problems, such as quadriceps fibrosis or absence of a suprapatellar pouch in patients with severe conditions (Fig. 2). Type I (hyperextended knee) dislocations resolve spontaneously in most patients. Patients with type II (tibial subluxation) dislocations respond rapidly to serial casting. A Pavlik harness may be used once 90° of flexion is attained. In patients who are unresponsive to nonsurgical management and in most patients with type III dislocation (tibial dislocation), early open reduction and quadricepsplasty are required to prevent abnormal joint development and articular cartilage deformation. Knee dislocation should be resolved prior to treatment of concurrent hip instability. Outcome is better for less involved knees, especially those classified as type I dislocations, and in patients with isolated dislocations, ie, without associated syndromes.

Congenital Patellar Dislocation

Congenital patellar dislocation cannot be reduced at birth. It usually is an isolated entity but may occur with conditions such as myelodysplasia or arthrogryposis. Hypoplasia of the patella, lateral femoral condyle, and quadriceps mechanism are seen in addition to

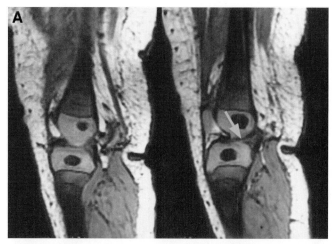

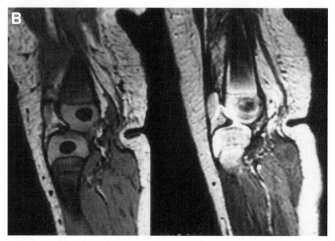

Figure 2 MRI scans of a 5-month-old girl with type II congenital dislocated knees. **A,** Note presence of the ACL (*arrow*) and **B,** absence of the ACL.

fixed lateral displacement of the patella. Knee flexion contracture, genu valgum, and external tibial rotation deformities are present. Surgical correction is required during infancy and consists of complete iliotibial band release, lateral and medial quadriceps mechanism stabilization, and patellar tendon centralization. Injury to the tibial tubercle apophysis must be avoided. Outcome depends on the time of treatment and the presence of associated syndromes.

Bipartite Patella

Bipartite patella is the most common of the multipartite patellae conditions and is typically an incidental finding on radiographs. It appears in 1% to 6% of children with a boy-to-girl ratio of occurrence of 8:1. Bilaterality is common, and the etiology is unknown. The Saupe classification is based on fragment location: type I occurs at the inferior patellar pole (5%); type II affects the entire lateral patellar margin (20%); and type III occurs at the superior lateral patellar corner (75%) (Fig. 3).

Symptoms occur at the patella-fragment junction following direct acute trauma or repetitive microtrauma

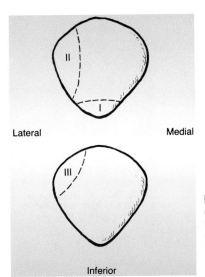

Figure 3 Saupe classification of bipartite patella. *(Reproduced with permission from Stanitski CL, DeLee AB, Drez CD (eds): Pediatric and Adolescent Sports Medicine. Philadelphia, PA, WB Saunders, 1994, p 312.)*

that causes separation. Following an acute fracture, focal tenderness and radiographic evidence of fragment margin irregularity are seen. Acute trauma may cause separation of a preexisting bipartite fragment, but junction irregularity is not as apparent radiographically. In chronic cases, patients report localized pain and tenderness at the fragment junction with the main patella. Radiographs reflect the type and junction morphology. Type I lesions may be confused with patellar sleeve fractures or Sinding-Larsen-Johansson disease.

Acute injuries are immobilized if the fragment is minimally displaced. In patients with chronic conditions and in whom overuse is a factor, management consists of activity modification or brief periods of immobilization. Fragment excision produces excellent results if symptoms persist. Partial excision of the lateral quadriceps retinaculum fragments promotes union of type III fragments.

Discoid Meniscus

The incidence of lateral discoid meniscus is estimated to be 1% to 3% of the pediatric population, with a higher frequency in Asian populations. The condition is bilateral in 10% to 20% of patients. Medial discoid menisci are extremely rare. At no time during normal human knee development is the meniscus disk-shaped. The etiology appears to be an error of the meniscal genetic template with superimposed changes from abnormal joint mechanics. The Watanabe classification presents three types of lateral discoid menisci: types I and II are stable, thickened disks and are considered to be complete or incomplete, depending on the amount of the tibial articular surface covered. Type III discoid menisci are shaped normally except for a thickened posterior horn and are unstable as a result of congenital absence of the meniscotibial ligament (Fig. 4).

Symptoms of painless snapping and popping occur in children between age 3 and 6 years. Onset of pain occurs between age 9 and 12 years and usually results from a meniscal tear in types I and II menisci. Patients with type III menisci often report knee instability. Clinical examination findings mirror the meniscus type with snapping in mid to full flexion in types I and II menisci. Symptoms can be reproduced in full flexion or extension in patients with type III menisci. The presence of an effusion usually indicates a meniscal tear. Occasionally, routine radiographs reveal a widened lateral joint space and tibial eminence flattening. MRI confirms the diagnosis. Treatment is indicated when the patient is symptomatic, usually from meniscal instability or a tear, and depends on the meniscal type, continuity, and stability. Sculpting of the meniscus to a more normal configuration is attempted for types I and II menisci. If a peripheral tear is present, the meniscus is sculpted and the tear repaired, if possible. If repair is not possible, a partial meniscectomy is recommended. Type III menisci are stabilized with a capsular suture. Total meniscectomy should be avoided, if possible. Although the overall short-term clinical results of total meniscectomy are favorable, a disturbingly high rate of radiographically evident premature osteoarthrosis in patients who are often asymptomatic after total meniscectomy warrants concern.

Congenital Short Femur and Fibular Hemimelia

Congenital short femur and fibular hemimelia cases demonstrate sagittal plane instability resulting from associated hypoplastic or absent ACLs. Functional instability is infrequent. The varied degree of sagittal plane translation is independent of the amount of femoral or tibial shortening. Femoral and tibial lengthenings must be performed with caution because of the proclivity for knee subluxation during the procedure in patients with inherent sagittal plane instability.

Nail-Patella Syndrome

Nail-patella syndrome is a clinical tetrad of nail dysplasia, absent or hypoplastic patellae, radial head instability, and iliac horns. Diminished development of the patella and quadriceps mechanism occasionally results in symptomatic patellar instability. Generally, favorable outcomes follow surgical reconstruction, usually lateral release and medial vector augmentation. Nephrotic syndrome is common in patients with nail-patella syndrome.

Larsen's Syndrome

Patients with this syndrome usually have bilateral congenital knee dislocations. Associated hip and elbow

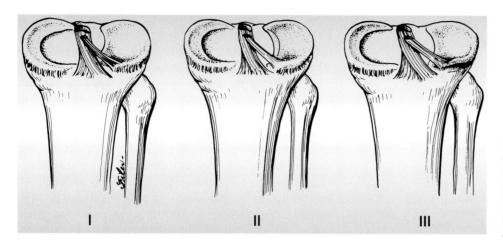

Figure 4 Watanabe classification of discoid menisci. Type I, stable complete; type II, stable, incomplete; type III, unstable due to lack of a meniscotibial ligament. (*Reproduced with permission from Stanitski CL, DeLee AB, Drez CD (eds): Pediatric and Adolescent Sports Medicine. Philadelphia, PA, WB Saunders, 1994, p 383.*)

dislocations, clubfoot, and cervical kyphosis also are common. Deformities of the extremity usually are of the teratogenic, rigid types that require early surgical intervention. Tracheal and laryngeal flaccidity may increase anesthetic and respiratory risks during infancy.

Thrombocytopenia Absent Radius Syndrome

Thrombocytopenia absent radius (TAR) syndrome is a combination of thrombocytopenia and absent radius in which the upper extremity deformity is obvious at birth. The thrombocytopenia, which may be part of a pancytopenia, may be unrecognized. Knee involvement also is common and includes asymmetric knee laxity with varus instability, patellar abnormalities, and hypoplastic or absent menisci. Knee deformity is complicated by ball-and-socket medial compartment femorotibial joint formation. Femoral and tibial osteotomies may be required as well as soft-tissue reconstructions. The recurrence rate of deformities is high.

Overuse Disorders

The patellofemoral joint is the site of numerous junctional tissues, including the patella-quadriceps retinaculum, patella-patellar tendon, and patellar tendon-tibial tubercle unions. Overuse symptoms occur when abnormal demands are placed on normal tissue without adequate time provided for repair. Submaximal persistent trauma results in a secondary inflammatory response at these junctions. Causative factors, including overzealous training programs, anatomic malalignment, environmental problems such as faulty training surfaces or equipment, or a combination of these factors, usually can be identified by clinical examination. A five-step treatment protocol includes factor identification, factor modification, pain control after the diagnosis, progressive rehabilitation, and a maintenance program to prevent recurrence.

Adolescent Anterior Knee Pain

During adolescence, the knee is a common site of pain resulting from major acute and/or repetitive minor trauma. In the skeletally immature patient, knee pain must be considered to be referred hip pain until proven otherwise. A thorough hip examination is part of the evaluation of knee pain.

The term chondromalacia patella has evolved from a gross pathologic description of articular cartilage change seen in adults at autopsy or surgery to an ill-defined, nonspecific clinical term to account for anterior knee pain. The natural history of nonstructural adolescent anterior knee pain suggests a self-resolving, benign course without sequelae. There is no evidence that adolescent anterior knee pain is associated with premature aging of the patellofemoral joint. Chondromalacia is a nonspecific clinical term and should not be used. The articular surfaces in this condition are pristine. Efforts should focus on precise identification of the causes of the pain, which can include Sinding-Larsen-Johansson disease, pathologic plica, reflex sympathetic dystrophy, patellar instability, osteochondritis dissecans, saphenous nerve entrapment, and patellar tendinitis. Diagnosis usually can be made by clinical evaluation.

Patients with idiopathic adolescent anterior knee pain have poorly localized pain that may be related to activity and aggravated by sitting or climbing stairs. When asked to identify the site of the pain, the patient typically grasps the entire anterior knee (grab sign) instead of pinpointing a specific area. In athletes, overuse related to training should be considered. One must be cautious of a teenage patient whose parent complains more about the child's condition than the child does. Knee pain complaints may be a mechanism the child uses to avoid participating in sport or other activities.

Physical examination includes assessment of gait; lower extremity alignment; range of motion of the hips, knees, ankles, and feet; knee stability; and patellar tracking. Normative values for patellar tilt and glide in children and adolescents have not been published. Quadriceps and hamstring strength and flexibility should be evaluated as well. Patella alta is commonly seen during the adolescent growth spurt when soft-tissue adjustment has not kept pace with the osseous growth rate. Diffuse tenderness about the patella, patellar tendon, and anterior joint lines may be present. Routine radiographs usually are normal.

After other sources of anterior knee pain have been ruled out, more than 80% of patients with this idiopathic condition respond well to nonsurgical, often nonspecific treatment that emphasizes normalization of quadriceps and hamstring flexibility and strength. Minor lower extremity malalignments may require use of a shoe orthotic. Although a variety of patellar braces has been advocated, no objective data relative to their mechanism of action or outcomes have been documented. Placebo effect and possibly proprioceptive feedback from use of the brace or taping techniques may account for their reported efficacy. If pain persists following a well-monitored rehabilitation program, the accuracy of the diagnosis should be questioned and other causes of pain, including nonorthopaedic and psychosocial causes, should be sought. The patient and parents should be reassured of the benign nature of the condition to allay concerns of a perceived serious problem. Arthroscopic patellofemoral procedures have a high surgical complication rate and should be avoided as treatment of nonspecific knee pain.

Reports of adolescent anterior knee pain are common. The correct diagnosis allows specific treatment. Most chronic painful knee conditions are diagnosed by clinical examination rather than MRI or arthroscopy and managed without surgery. Modification, not elimination, of activity usually is possible, and continued participation is encouraged.

Osgood-Schlatter Disease

This condition involves the immature junction of the patellar tendon and tibial tubercle and is seen in athletic boys and girls early in adolescence during a period of rapid growth. The condition rarely is seen in nonathletic individuals. Bilateral symptoms occur in 20% of affected patients. Bilateral tibial tubercle enlargement commonly occurs with only one symptomatic side. The lesion in this disorder is caused by unresolved submaximal avulsion fractures at the immature junction. The classic presentation is swelling at the tibial tubercle and intermittent, activity-related symptoms

during a rapid growth spurt, which makes the diagnosis straightforward. Patients and parents often are concerned about a tumor because of the increased tubercle size. Clinical examination shows varying degrees of tibial tubercle prominence and tenderness. Radiographs rule out rare conditions such as tumors or infections. Ossicle formation occurs within the patellar tendon in up to 40% of patients. Symptoms resolve as the child matures and rarely persist into adulthood despite the prominent tubercle. Treatment is symptomatic and includes ice massage, nonsteroidal anti-inflammatory drugs (NSAIDs), quadriceps and hamstring flexibility exercises, and the use of knee pads. The patient and family must understand that the undulating symptom pattern may persist for 18 to 24 months. Activities must be balanced with symptoms. Immobilizing the limb in a cylinder cast or splint for brief periods usually is not needed unless pain interferes with routine daily activity. The ossicle is enucleated if focal symptoms persist. The tubercle may be debulked at the time of ossicle excision in skeletally mature patients.

Sinding-Larsen-Johansson Condition

Sinding-Larsen-Johansson condition is the proximal counterpart of Osgood-Schlatter disease and occurs at the inferior patella-patellar tendon junction resulting from sequelae of chronic tensile stress on the immature tissues. The condition is seen primarily in preteen-age boys, and symptoms are activity related. Focal tenderness occurs at the inferior patellar pole. In athletic older adolescents, signs and symptoms occur within the patellar tendon, the so-called "jumper's knee." In Sinding-Larsen-Johansson condition, lateral radiographs reveal changes of inferior patellar pole ossification. Differential diagnosis includes type I bipartite patella and patellar sleeve fracture. Treatment is symptomatic and similar to that of Osgood-Schlatter disease.

Pathologic Synovial Plica

Plicae are normal synovial folds in which pathologic changes may occur from direct or indirect trauma with subsequent intraplical hemorrhage, hyalinization, and fibrosis. Patients report a painful snapping in midknee flexion at 40° to 70° and have local tenderness over the medial plica. If the etiology is from overuse, treatment begins with identification and modification of causative factors. In patients who do not respond to treatment, arthroscopic resection is helpful. Appropriate history and clinical examination findings should correlate with a thickened, fibrotic plica and concomitant articular erosion of the medial femoral condyle seen during arthroscopy. Indiscriminate resection of normal plicae should be avoided.

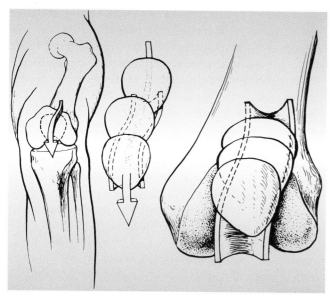

Figure 5 Toroidal path of the patella through the femoral sulcus. *(Reproduced with permission from Stanitski CL, DeLee JC, Drez D (eds) Pediatric and Adolescent Sports Medicine. Philadelphia, PA, WB Saunders, 1994, p 307.)*

Reflex Sympathetic Dystrophy

Reflex sympathetic dystrophy (RSD) is seen with increasing frequency in children. It often is not considered in the differential diagnosis of knee pain in this age group, which delays treatment. With RSD, negative secondary effects of disuse such as atrophy, loss of motion, and strength may be advanced. The hallmark of RSD is pain that is out of proportion to any precipitating injury. Extreme pain accompanies even the slightest touch. Signs of autonomic dysfunction, such as changes in skin color and sweating, may be absent in the early phase but appear as the condition progresses. Underlying psychosocial and family problems, including divorce, loss of parent or sibling, family illness, or school difficulties, are common in this condition and must be ruled out. Radiographs usually are normal, but effects of disuse, such as osteoporosis, become apparent as the disease progresses. Bone scan findings reflect the stages of the disease. Treatment includes NSAIDs; active, functional rehabilitation; and, where required, psychological services. If this treatment plan is unsuccessful, sympathetic nerve blocks may be necessary. Generally, RSD is seen more often in the lower extremities of children, compared with the upper extremities in adults, and the prognosis is better in children than in adults.

Patellar Instability

The patella follows a toroidal path with flexion/extension, rotation, and translation via three axes through the femoral sulcus (Fig. 5). Normal motion is the result of a complex interaction of static and dynamic stabiliz-

ers that produce four-quadrant equilibrium in three planes. The quadriceps complex, patella, and femur must be thought of as a unit. Patellofemoral sulcus incongruity is a result of consequences of anatomic maldevelopment based on the genetic template and effects of use.

Patellar instability covers a wide spectrum of patterns from a minor tracking abnormality to subluxation and dislocation. A multifactorial etiology is usually present. The definition of instability is imprecise because the terms malalignment, maltracking, and instability are often used interchangeably. Malalignment is an abnormal static relationship between the patella and femur and may result from congenital, developmental, or posttraumatic causes. Maltracking refers to dynamic aberrations of tracking that range from mild to severe. This abnormal motion can be related to malalignment and may or may not be symptomatic. Classic instabilities are subluxation and dislocation with loss of articular congruence during patellar excursion, usually at 10° to 25° of knee flexion. Acute instability is produced by direct contact or, more commonly, by noncontact mechanisms such as deceleration or rotation.

During the clinical examination, evaluation of the mechanism of injury, acuity, previous episodes and treatment, and opposite knee status is essential. Generalized laxity, the presence of a hemarthrosis, tenderness, and attenuation or gap in the quadriceps mechanism at the immediate peripatellar zone or medial patellofemoral ligament should be assessed. The integrity of the ACL should be tested because noncontact mechanisms that cause patellar instability also can cause injury to the ACL. Four-view radiographs of the knee should be obtained; the tangential (sunrise) view should be taken in no more than 30° of flexion. Marginal patellar avulsion fractures in the nonarticular zone often are seen in patients with recurrent instability. In reported series, 20% to 70% of osteochondral injuries associated with an acute patellar dislocation were not evident on routine radiographs.

Treatment is individualized, based on the alignment of the lower extremity, joint motion, ligamentous laxity, muscle strength, and quadriceps mechanism competence. The goal of treatment is to prevent recurrence. In the absence of an osteochondral fragment on radiographs, limb immobilization for 7 to 10 days followed by a rehabilitation program to restore motion and strength are indicated. A multitude of surgical reconstructions are proposed to treat recurrent patellar instability. These procedures use one or a combination of three techniques: lateral retinacular release, medial vector augmentation, and patellar tendon realignment. Surgical treatment includes arthroscopic evaluation of the articular injury with removal or replacement of osteochondral fragments. Quadriceps transfers, particularly of the vastus medialis obliquus with its attendant patellofemoral ligament, restore medial vector balance. Medial hamstring transfer (Galeazzi technique) may be needed to provide an additional medial tenodesis effect. Distal realignment by tibial tubercle medial transposition is performed in skeletally mature patients. Creation of a patella infera by distal and posterior tubercle transfer must be avoided. Tubercle rotational transposition successfully restores distal patellar mechanism alignment. A combination of tubercle rotation, proximal lateral release, medial capsulorrhaphy, and tendon transfer may be needed to establish appropriate static and dynamic alignment.

Patellar instability associated with abnormal ligamentous laxity in patients with Down, Ehlers-Danlos, or Marfan's syndromes presents a significant challenge. Approximately 10% of patients with Down syndrome have patellar instability, usually bilaterally. Despite chronic patellar displacement from a combination of increased laxity, genu valgum, and hypotonia, these patients usually are asymptomatic and function well, and they rarely require surgical intervention. Patients with Ehlers-Danlos syndrome, especially those with type III, have increased joint laxity and symptoms of patellar instability, which cause diminished function and pain in early adulthood. The heterogeneous connective tissue disorder in Marfan's syndrome, secondary to fibrillin abnormality, may present as hypermobility with patella alta, hypotonia, and patellar instability. Patients with these syndromes must be advised of the abnormal nature of their collagen biology and must be aware that, given their abnormal tissue, surgical treatment may not overcome their genetic predisposition for instability.

Osteochondritis Dissecans

Osteochondritis dissecans (OCD) is a lesion of subchondral bone and articular cartilage that may either heal or result in nonunion of the fragment with instability of the subchondral bone, sequestrum, and/or articular cartilage. Its etiology is unknown. Following acute trauma, an acute osteochondral fracture must be considered as a differential diagnosis. Bilaterality occurs in 20% to 30% of patients. Previous reports often combined data from juvenile and adult types of OCD, which caused confusion about outcome and treatment requirements because of the markedly different natural history and prognosis for each type. Symptoms are related to the acuity of the condition and may be present only with activity. Symptoms may be associated with recurrent effusions. Locking is rare. Physical examination findings often are nonspecific, such as effusion and generalized tenderness. Focal ten-

derness may be present with direct pressure on an unstable lesion. Routine radiographs, particularly the tunnel view, demonstrate the lesion. In 70% of patients, the classic site of the condition is in the non–weight-bearing, posterior lateral aspect of the medial femoral condyle. The lateral femoral condyle is involved in 20% of patients, and the patella is involved in 10% of patients. MRI helps assess the viability of the fragment's subchondral bone. Improvement in MRI software techniques may allow better definition of the articular segment. A computerized bone scan can assess the circulation between the fragment and its bed. If a child younger than age 13 years has increased blood flow is this area, the prognosis for healing is good. None of these techniques directly assesses the subchondral bone-articular composite stability. Lesions are classified as open or closed, based on articular cartilage integrity, and stable or unstable according to the underlying stability of the subchondral bone and its bed. A loose body is an example of an open, unstable lesion (Fig. 6).

The natural history of OCD is age dependent. Patients with completely open distal femoral physes have the juvenile type of OCD, and the prognosis is excellent if the lesion is closed and stable. In patients with partial physeal closure (adolescent type), the prognosis is less well defined because the lesion may act as either the juvenile or adult type. The adult type (closed physes) has a poor prognosis because of the lesion's limited healing potential. Treatment recommendations are based on the patient's physiologic stage and the status of the fragment. If lesions are closed and stable, healing potential is high. Conversely, instability and/or loss of continuity of the articular surface compromise healing. Nonsurgical management is recommended for patients with closed, stable lesions. Activity modification may be required and brief immobilization is occasionally necessary for episodes of discomfort or effusion. In patients with an unstable subchondral junction, surgery is suggested for closed lesions. Fragment fixation or drilling allows subchondral union and prevents conversion to an open, unstable lesion. In the event of a loose body, restitution is recommended if the fragment can be anatomically reduced and has an adequate amount of subchondral bone for fixation and a congruent articular surface following replantation. If there is minimal or no subchondral bone or the fit is incongruous or the articular surface is damaged, fragment excision is recommended. Elective osteochondral grafting should be considered for large, irreparable lesions in a weight-bearing zone, often in the lateral femur. Associated meniscal and tibial articular surface damage should be assessed and meniscal repair or partial meniscectomy performed as indicated by the

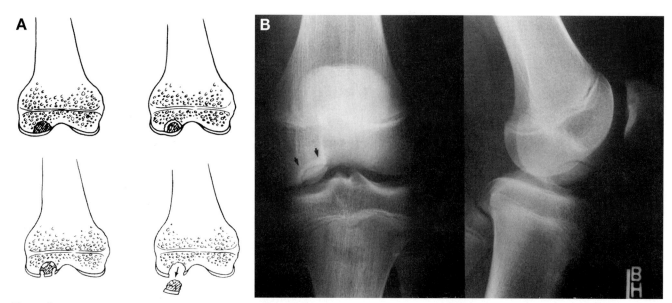

Figure 6 **A,** OCD classification based on articular continuity and subchondral stability. *(Reproduced with permission from Stanitski CL, DeLee AB, Drez CD (eds): Pediatric and Adolescent Sports Medicine. Philadelphia, PA, WB Saunders, 1994, p 396.)* **B,** Symptomatic OCD in a 15-year-old boy. Note classic location at lateral portion of medial femoral condyle. *(Reproduced from Richards BS (ed): Orthopaedic Knowledge Update: Pediatrics. Rosemont, IL, American Academy of Orthopaedic Surgeons, 1996, pp 195-202.)*

meniscal injury pattern. Patellar OCD is uncommon and occurs in the distal half of the patella. In patellar OCD, 20% to 30% of the lesions are bilateral. The differential diagnosis should include bipartite patella, dorsal patellar defect, infection, and tumor. The prognosis for patellar OCD is less clear than for femoral OCD. Subchondral bed sclerosis denotes a poor prognosis, as occurs with femoral lesions. Treatment principles are similar to those for femoral OCD.

Popliteal Cyst

The so-called "Baker's" cyst is located at the posteromedial aspect of the knee at the level of the popliteal crease. This unilateral mass is commonly seen in children age 4 to 8 years and usually is asymptomatic. Parents are concerned that the mass is a tumor. Cysts vary in size and firmness, depending on the amount of fluid within and are positioned between the semimembranosus and medial gastrocnemius muscles. Clinical examination reveals that the cyst is more prominent with full knee extension and is transilluminated in contrast to a solid mass. The remainder of the knee and extremity is normal. Imaging is used to rule out other conditions. Routine radiographs often demonstrate the cyst, especially if soft-tissue exposure techniques are used. Ultrasound is an inexpensive, noninvasive means of documentation.

Aspiration of the cyst aids in diagnosis but does not result in cyst ablation. Steroid injection into the cyst is not indicated. In contrast with popliteal cysts in adults with chronic intra-articular knee pathology, popliteal cysts in children rarely communicate with the knee joint and no intra-articular pathology exists. The natural history of pediatric popliteal cysts is spontaneous resolution in more than 70% of patients within 12 to 24 months. Surgery should be reserved for the highly uncommon situation in which the cyst's encroachment on local tissues causes persistent symptoms. Parents must understand that the cyst recurs in 30% to 40% of patients following surgery.

Annotated Bibliography

Basic Considerations

Dimeglio A: Growth in pediatric orthopaedics. *J Pediatr Orthop* 2001;21:549-555.
This excellent review of growth includes data to predict growth-remaining contributions from the distal femoral and proximal tibial physes.

Imaging

Andrish JT: Meniscal injuries in children and adolescents: Diagnosis and management. *J Am Acad Orthop Surg* 1996;4:231-237.
In this article, lesions of normal and pathologic menisci and their clinical and imaging diagnoses and surgical treatment are reviewed.

Lonner JH, Parisien JS: Arthroscopic treatment of meniscal cysts. *Op Tech Orthop* 1995;5:72-77.
The authors reviewed arthroscopic management of meniscal lesions and associated cysts and noted that both the cyst and any meniscal tear or instability must be addressed to prevent recurrence of the cyst.

McDermott MJ, Bathgate B, Gillingham BL, Hennrikus WL: Correlation of MRI and arthroscopic diagnosis of knee pathology in children and adolescents. *J Pediatr Orthop* 1998;18:675-678.

The arthroscopic findings in 59 knees in 51 patients with suspected ACL or meniscal pathology were compared with MRI findings in 20 patients younger than age 15 years and in 39 patients between age 15 and 17 years. In the older age group, the MRI's accuracy, predictability, specificity, and sensitivity were high for ACL and meniscal pathology and were similar to adult data. In the younger age group, false-positive meniscal findings were reported in 11 patients, and an ACL tear was noted arthroscopically following a negative MRI report in two patients. The authors emphasized caution in interpreting MRI findings in younger patients, especially concerning meniscal pathology.

Stanitski CL: Correlation of arthroscopic and clinical examinations with magnetic resonance imaging findings of injured knees in children and adolescents. *Am J Sports Med* 1998;26:2-6.

The author reviewed clinical diagnosis, MRI readings, and arthroscopic evaluations in 28 patients. Findings relative to meniscal, cruciate ligament, and articular injury were correlated with MRI findings. Poor correlation was seen between the clinical and arthroscopic findings and the MRI findings. MRI accuracy was only 35%, positive and negative predictive indexes were 50%, sensitivity was 50%, and specificity was 45%. Significant numbers of false-positive and negative results for meniscal and ACL injuries were noted on MRI. The author emphasized that MRI should not be used as a screening test but should be ordered for specific indications following expert clinical evaluation.

Stanitski CL, Paletta GA Jr: Articular cartilage injury with acute patellar dislocation in adolescents: Arthroscopic and radiographic correlation. *Am J Sports Med* 1998;26:52-55.

In 48 adolescents with initial acute patellar dislocations, major disparity was noted between osteochondral injury seen on initial radiographs and findings at arthroscopy. Radiographic evidence of articular injury was seen in only 21% of patients, in contrast with 71% seen arthroscopically. Only 29% of osteochondral loose bodies, ranging in size from 2 mm to 20 mm were identified radiographically. The authors cautioned that if articular injury is not properly diagnosed at the time of an acute patellar dislocation, unrecognized intra-articular damage may be the cause of a poor outcome.

Takeda Y, Ikata T, Yoshida S, Takai H, Kashiwaguchi S: MRI high-signal intensity in the menisci of asymptomatic children. *J Bone Joint Surg Br* 1998;80: 463-467.

MRI scans of 108 knees in 80 normal, asymptomatic children between age 8 and 15 years (average age, 12 years) were reviewed for meniscal findings. In children younger than age 10 years, 80% had grade III signals. In children between age 10 and 13 years, 65% had grade III signals, and in children between age 14 and 15 years, 33% had grade III signals that approached the 29% false-positive rate reported for asymptomatic adults. The authors suggested that the change in medial meniscal signal intensity was proportional to meniscal vascularity, especially in the posterior horn, and was not caused by meniscal degeneration. Caution is needed in interpretation of MRI findings in the knee in young patients. Clinical correlation is mandatory.

Congenital Disorders

Gordon JE, Schoenecker PL: Surgical treatment of congenital dislocation of the patella. *J Pediatr Orthop* 1999;19:260-264.

In this retrospective review of 17 knees in 11 patients, follow-up occurred in 10 patients (13 knees) more than 2 years after surgery, and four of these 10 patients had associated syndromes. All patients had fixed lateral dislocations at an average of 7 to 9 years at surgery. The authors emphasized the need for a major quadriceps mechanism realignment, including lateral and tensor fascia release, medial vector quadriceps reconstruction, and patellar tendon alignment to provide a lasting result. Diagnosis in this group often was delayed. Until proven otherwise, a child with a valgus, flexed knee with associated tibial external rotation should be considered to have a congenital patellar dislocation.

Mori Y, Okumo H, Iketani H, Kuroki Y: Efficacy of lateral retinacular release for painful bipartite patella. *Am J Sports Med* 1995;23:13-18.

Sixteen knees in 15 patients were retrospectively reviewed following resection of a strip of the lateral quadriceps retinaculum for treatment of type III symptomatic bipartite patellae. Excellent outcomes were achieved in 15 knees, with fragment union in 69% within 4 months, and all but one by 8 months postoperatively. The authors hypothesized that reduced tensile force of the quadriceps allowed union.

Raber DA, Friederich NF, Hefti F: Discoid lateral meniscus in children: Long-term follow-up after total meniscectomy. *J Bone Joint Surg Am* 1998;80: 1579-1586.

This was a retrospective review of 17 knees in 14 patients who were treated by complete removal of a discoid meniscus with an average follow-up of 19.8 years. Although clinical evaluation revealed good functional results, two thirds of the knees showed radiographic evidence of significant osteoarthritic changes. The authors recommended avoidance of total meniscectomy if possible.

Roux MO, Carlioz H: Clinical examination and investigation of the cruciate ligaments in children with fibular hemimelia. *J Pediatr Orthop* 1999;19:247-251.

During the clinical examinations of 66 patients (69 knees) with fibular hemimelia, 20 patients were examined with arthroscopy and 14 with MRI. Eleven patients reported knee instability and two had limitations resulting from instability. Results were positive in 84% of patients following Lachman and anterior drawer tests and in 45% of patients following a pivot shift test. An absent ACL was documented by MRI or arthroscopy in 80% of patients. In this subgroup, normal lateral menisci were seen in 75% of patients, and discoid menisci were seen in 10%. An absent ACL or hypoplasia did not correlate with the type of hemimelia. The authors cautioned that the potential for dislocation or subluxation of the knee increases with femoral lengthening. Whether these children will continue to have asymptomatic knees following limb equalization and increase in activity demands remains to be seen.

Sanpera I Jr, Fixsen JA, Sparks LT, Hill RA: Knee in congenital short femur. *J Pediatr Orthop B* 1995;4: 159-163.

The authors reviewed 24 patients (25 knees) with associated degrees of fibular hemimelia. Sagittal plane instability was quite variable and independent of mean amount of shortening. The authors suggested caution in patients with positive Lachman and anterior drawer test results during femoral lengthening because of tibial subluxation/dislocation potential. The variability of ACL deficiencies in these patients is discussed, as well as the infrequent symptoms that accompany hypoplastic or absent ACLs in this patient group, all of whom do not have low-activity demands. With current limb reconstruction and equalization techniques, whether restoring these genetically unique knees to normalcy will allow major sports demands to be placed on them is uncertain.

Washington ER III, Root L, Liener UC: Discoid lateral meniscus in children: Long-term follow up after excision. *J Bone Joint Surg Am* 1995;77:1357-1361.

In this retrospective review of 18 knees in 15 patients who were treated for symptomatic discoid menisci with total meniscectomy by various surgeons over a 28-year period, clinical outcomes showed good results. Final radiographs were obtained in only eight patients, and three of these patients had radiographic evidence of early osteoarthrosis. The average age of these patients was in the late third or early fourth decade.

Adolescent Anterior Knee Pain

Kowall MG, Kolk G, Nuber GW, Cassisi JE, Stern SH: Patellar taping in the treatment of patellofemoral pain: A prospective randomized study. *Am J Sports Med* 1996;24:61-66.

Two groups of patients with patellofemoral nonstructural pain were treated, one with conventional therapy measures and one with conventional therapy measures plus patellar taping. Both groups demonstrated similar improvement in pain relief and quadriceps strength. The authors found that taping in this group of patients provided no additional benefits.

Nimon G, Murray D, Sandow M, Goodfellow J: Natural history of anterior knee pain: A 14 to 20 year follow-up of nonoperative management. *J Pediatr Orthop* 1998;18: 118-122.

This article is a sequel of a report made by the authors in 1985. A consecutive series of adolescent girls who had anterior knee pain with no structural cause was treated by reassurance that the nature of the condition was benign and the potential of spontaneous recovery was high. Symptoms improved in 71% of patients, and 88% of patients had little or no need for analgesics. In addition, 90% of patients were regular active sports participants. At follow-up, patients with symptoms had no identifying features when compared with patients with no symptoms. Although 82% of patients noted crepitus, there was no correlation between crepitus and pain. Crepitus and no pain was reported by 45% of patients. There was no evidence of significant structural disease in patients who did not improve.

Osgood-Schlatter Disease

Flowers MJ, Bhadreshwar DR: Tibial tuberosity excision for symptomatic Osgood-Schlatter disease. *J Pediatr Orthop* 1995;15:292-297.

Thirty-five patients (42 knees) with symptomatic Osgood-Schlatter disease who were unresponsive to conservative management were treated by tibial tubercle ossicle and prominence excision. At follow-up 5 years later, 95% reported pain relief and 86% were pleased with the morphology of the tubercle. All 35 patients reported a rapid return to work and sport. Although surgery rarely is required for patients with Osgood-Schlatter disease, patients with persistent symptoms from nonunion of an ossicle and associated tubercle prominence sustain lasting relief and minimal morbidity from surgery.

Patellar Instability

Desio SM, Burks RT, Bachus KN: Soft tissue restraints to lateral patellar translation in the human knee. *Am J Sports Med* 1998;26:59-65.

In this article, a cadaveric, serial cutting model was used to demonstrate that the patellofemoral ligament provides 60% of resistance to lateral patellar translation with the knee in 20° of flexion. The medial patellomeniscal ligament provided an additional 13% of medial vector restraining force. These medial ligamentous structures are the primary static restraints to lateral patellar instability. Attenuation of these structures at the time of dislocation results in persistent medial vector incompetence.

Sallay PI, Poggi J, Speer KP, Garrett WE: Acute dislocation of the patella: A correlative pathoanatomic study. *Am J Sports Med* 1996;24:52-60.

Results of routine radiographs and MRI obtained for 23 patients with acute patellar dislocation indicated that 87% of the patients had tears at the origin of the medial patellofemoral ligament. At arthroscopy and open exploration of the medial patellar area, 68% of the patients had an osteochondral lesion of the patella or lateral femoral condyle and 94% had an avulsion of the medial patellofemoral ligament from the femur. Direct repair of the avulsion resulted in no recurrent dislocations.

Stanitski CL: Patellar instability in the school age athlete. *Instr Course Lect* 1998;47:345-350.

In this review of factors that predispose the patient to patellar instability, treatment options are discussed in view of clinical and imaging findings. The author emphasizes that pathoanatomy predisposes the patient to recurrence and a poor outcome.

Osteochondritis Dissecans

Hefti F, Beguiristain J, Krauspe R, et al: Osteochondritis dissecans: A multicenter study of the European Pediatric Orthopedic Society. *J Pediatr Orthop B* 1999;8:231-245.

Data from 452 patients with 509 affected knees in 12 centers were analyzed. Follow-up occurred at a minimum of 1 year; the mean follow-up was at 3.2 years. Skeletally immature patients with lesions in the classical site and no sign of fragment dissection had a predictable good outcome. With signs of dissection, results were better with surgery than without. If a loose fragment was excised from a weight-bearing area with no other surgical intervention, results were poor.

Paletta GA Jr, Bednarz PA, Stanitski CL, Sandman GA, Stanitski DF, Kottamasu S: The prognostic value of quantitative bone scan in knee osteochondritis dissecans: A preliminary experience. *Am J Sports Med* 1998;26:7-14.

In this article, six skeletally immature and six skeletally mature patients with OCD at the classical site underwent quantitative bone scans to determine whether increased fragment uptake could predict eventual outcome. None of the patients was treated with surgery. The lesion healed in four of six patients age 9 to 12 years who had increased uptake. Of the patients with decreased uptake, two of six patients required surgery for nonunion of the fragment. In the skeletally mature group, all patients showed an increase in fragment uptake, but fragments united in only two of the six patients, a 67% failed predictive value.

Schenck RC Jr, Goodnight JM: Osteochondritis dissecans. *J Bone Joint Surg Am* 1996;78;439-456.

This extensive review of literature focuses on OCD of the knee, although OCD of the elbow and ankle is included. Theories of etiology, clinical and imaging diagnosis methods and treatment, and outcome data in both skeletally immature and mature patients are included in this report.

Popliteal Cyst

Curl WW: Popliteal cysts: Historical background and current knowledge. *J Am Acad Orthop Surg* 1996;4:129-133.

In this article, the author reviewed the literature for diagnosis and management of adult and childhood popliteal cysts. The author emphasized the caveat that surgical treatment of childhood cysts should be avoided because of their usual spontaneous resolution and extremely high rate of recurrence following surgery.

Classic Bibliography

Bourne MH, Bianco AJ Jr: Bipartite patella in the adolescent: Results of surgical excision. *J Pediatr Orthop* 1990;10:69-73.

Clark CR, Ogden JA: Development of the menisci of the human knee joint: Morphological changes and their potential role in childhood meniscal injury. *J Bone Joint Surg Am* 1983;65:538-547.

Crawfurd EJ, Emery RJ, Aichroth PM: Stable osteochondritis dissecans: Does the lesion unite? *J Bone Joint Surg Br* 1990;72:320.

Gao GX, Lee EH, Bose K: Surgical management of congenital and habitual dislocation of the patella. *J Pediatr Orthop* 1990;10:255-260.

Guidera KJ, Satterwhite Y, Ogden JA, Pugh L, Ganey T: Nail patella syndrome: A review of 44 orthopaedic patients. *J Pediatr Orthop* 1991;11:737-742.

Guzzanti V, Gigante A, DiLazzaro A, et al: Patellofemoral malalignment in adolescents: Computerized tomographic assessment with or without quadriceps contraction. *Am J Sports Med* 1994;22:55-60.

Laville JM: Knee deformities in Larsen's syndrome. *J Pediatr Orthop* 1994;3:180-184.

Parsch K, Schulz R: Ultrasonography in congenital dislocation of the knee. *J Pediatr Orthop* 1994;3:76-81.

Schoenecker PL, Cohn AK, Sedgwick WG, Manske PR, Salafsky I, Millar EA: Dysplasia of the knee associated with the syndrome of thrombocytopenia and absent radius. *J Bone Joint Surg Am* 1984;66:421-427.

Stanitski CL: Anterior knee pain syndromes in the adolescent. *Instr Course Lect* 1994;43:211-220.

Wilder RT, Berde CB, Wolohan M, et al: Reflex sympathetic dystrophy in children: Clinical characteristics and follow-up of seventy patients. *J Bone Joint Surg Am* 1992;74:910-919.

Chapter 21

Clubfoot

Alvin Crawford, MD

Atiq Durrani, MD

Introduction

Antonio Scarpa's 18th century definition of clubfoot as "a twisting of the scaphoid, os calcis and cuboid around the astragalus" was made almost two centuries ago. Since then, we have learned much about this condition. Clubfoot, or more technically congenital talipes equinovarus, is a syndrome comprising an in utero malalignment of talocalcaneonavicular and calcaneocuboid axes of the child's foot, and atrophy of the calf with a concomitant variable decrease in the foot size and tibial length.

Epidemiology

Congenital clubfoot is one of the most common birth defects, occurring in 1 in 1,000 live births. A male to female preponderance of 2.5:1 has been reported. A positive family history, with at least one other family member affected, has been reported in one fourth to one third of patients. Data on occurrence among siblings of an affected child show that the presence of an affected male child increases the risk to 1 in 42 for a subsequent male sibling but there is no additional risk for a female sibling. Conversely, the presence of an affected female child increases the risk for siblings of both genders (males 1:16, females 1:40). A family with both an affected parent and child increases the risk for the disorder in the subsequent siblings to 1 in 4.

Etiology

Etiology of clubfoot can at best be described as multifactorial. To the previous theories have been added a neurogenic theory, a myogenic theory, and a vascular theory. Some researchers suggest a partial intrauterine loss of innervation followed by a subsequent reinnervation is responsible. Others have reported an increased activity of myofibroblast-like cells in the medial ligaments of the ankle prior to the third trimester, resulting in severe clubfeet. The focus in recent years has shifted toward identifying a possible gene locus; results of segregation analysis in 186 families concluded that a multifactorial inheritance pattern was most likely at work. A study of 190 Caucasian probands implicated a single incompletely dominant gene as the mode of inheritance. In this study, researchers concluded that 94% of cases could be explained by a single Mendelian gene theory. Other studies identified a major autosomal locus controlling clubfoot with an additional polygenic component. Most authors would agree that clubfoot results from a combination of unidentified environmental factors acting on a genetically susceptible host.

Pathoanatomy

Two concepts are basic to understanding the pathoanatomy of clubfoot. First is osseous deformity of the talus itself. Second is the concept of abnormal rotatory malalignment of the talocalcaneal joint in the sagittal, coronal, and horizontal planes (ie, medial spin) of the calcaneus. A deformed talus in which the anterior aspect is plantar flexed and medially deviated results in contracture of the posterior ankle structures, including the posterior ankle capsule, and a talonavicular subluxation with the navicular often articulating with the medial malleolus; these deformities result in shortening of the posteromedial structures. The plantar flexed talus forces the calcaneus into plantar flexion. There is contracture of the Achilles tendon. The calcaneus rotates in the horizontal plane and pivots on the interosseous ligament; it is abnormally positioned under the head and neck of the talus anterior to the ankle joint, and the calcaneal tuberosity moves toward the fibular malleolus posterior to the ankle joint. Shortening of the posterolateral structures occurs. The varus appearance of the heel results from the rotation of the calcaneus in the coronal plane. This deformity of the calcaneus leads to medial displacement of the cuboid on the long axes of the os calcis, which with the medial displacement of the navicular leads to adduction of the midfoot. The varus and adduction deformities of the heel and midfoot cause the supination of the forefoot. Radiographically, this supination gives the appearance of "stacking" of the cuneiforms and metatarsal bases.

The direction of talar rotation in the mortise remains controversial. Findings in a recent assessment of the hindfoot deformity in which three-dimensional MRI was used concurred with earlier findings of external rotation of the talus in the mortise; the authors recommended medial derotation of the talus at the time of surgery. The report of another three-dimensional analysis of clubfoot deformities described the talus to be in pronation (intorsion). Other investigators, using CT to investigate tibial torsional deformities in clubfeet, found no appreciable difference in the amount of femoral or tibial torsion in limbs with and without clubfeet. A 67% prevalence of ankle valgus was recently reported in long-term follow-up. This condition could ameliorate the effects of hindfoot varus or give a spurious impression of an overcorrected clubfoot after surgical correction.

Prenatal Diagnosis

Improvements in obstetrical ultrasound (US) have led to an increase in prenatal sonographic diagnosis of clubfoot. During prenatal US evaluation of 14,013 patients, 61 were found to have clubfeet, for a prevalence of 0.43%. Associated anomalies were found in 67% of these 61 patients, while 33% had isolated clubfeet. The false-positive rate for isolated clubfoot was 40%, all diagnosed in the third trimester of pregnancy. In another study, associated anomalies occurred in 28 of 35 patients with clubfeet detected on prenatal screening of 23,863 patients. Over 50% of the patients prenatally diagnosed with isolated clubfeet were later found to have additional severe abnormalities that were detected during the neonatal period. Prenatal diagnosis of clubfoot adds parental counseling to the responsibilities of the orthopaedic surgeon, who must keep in mind the limitations of US diagnosis of clubfoot and associated anomalies indicated by the studies described.

Neonatal Diagnosis

In the characteristic clinical picture of clubfoot, the foot points plantarward with the small calcaneus drawn up and rolled under the talus in an inverted position, leaving the heel pad empty. There is a deep crease at the posterior aspect of the ankle. The midfoot and forefoot are adducted and supinated. The anterior end of the talus is prominent on the dorsolateral aspect of the foot. The skin creases are deep on the concave medial and plantar aspects of the foot. The navicular abuts the anterior aspect of the medial malleolus, and the fibular malleolus lies posterior to the medial malleolus. There may be varying degrees of calf atrophy and shortening of the affected foot.

Congenital clubfoot must be differentiated from a postural clubfoot, which results from an intrauterine malposture. The latter type is flexible and may have slight forefoot varus but the hindfoot equinus and varus deformities of true clubfoot are absent.

Clubfoot can be associated with other anomalies or is part of a generalized developmental syndrome. The incidence of associated anomalies ranges from 14% to 67%, making it important to perform a multisystem physical examination on the child. Some of the common pathologic conditions associated with clubfoot include proximal femoral focal deficiency, arthrogryposis, amniotic band syndrome, myelodysplasia, diastrophic dwarfism, Pierre Robin syndrome, Larsen's syndrome, Möbius' syndrome, and Freeman-Sheldon syndrome.

Clinical Grading of Clubfoot

A standardized, widely accepted system of clubfoot grading does not exist. However, two grading systems, those of Pirani and associates and Dimeglio and associates, have recently been proposed. In a recent study of 55 feet, the interobserver variation of these two grading systems was analyzed. Each foot was graded independently by a staff pediatric orthopaedic surgeon, a pediatric orthopaedic fellow, and a physical therapist. The mean difference between the scores assigned by the examiners was 0.6 points using the Pirani system and 1.4 points using the Dimeglio system, correlation coefficients of 0.90 and 0.83, respectively. Lower correlation coefficients were reported for classification of the first 15 feet, indicating the presence of a learning curve.

Diagnostic Imaging of Clubfoot
Radiography

An AP view of the foot and a lateral view of the foot and ankle at rest and at maximum dorsiflexion provide the most complete radiographic picture. A talocalcaneal angle of less than 20° on an AP view indicates a hindfoot varus, and an angle of less than 35° on a lateral view indicates a hindfoot equinus and varus. A talo-first metatarsal angle of more than 0 on an AP view indicates a medial deviation of the foot. Inability of the long axes of the talus and calcaneus to converge on a forced dorsiflexion lateral view indicates an equinus contracture. A tibiocalcaneal angle of greater than

90° confirms the equinus contracture. The use of analytic radiography in clubfoot has limitations because the bones are small, and ossification centers in these bones lie eccentrically. A number of experts treat only the clinical, rather than the radiographic, parameters of clubfoot.

Ultrasound

A standard technique for postnatal US in assessment of clubfoot has been described. With US, one can visualize the talonavicular articulation and perform a dynamic assessment of clubfoot by visualizing the nonossified talar cartilage. A standard technique for the US assessment of clubfoot is needed because it would help the development of a standard grading system.

Treatment

Both nonsurgical and surgical treatment is based on the concept of congenital subluxation of the talocalcaneonavicular complex. The arrangement of these anatomic structures, which are called the acetabulum pedis, is similar to that around the hip joint. The talar head corresponds to the femoral head, and the medially displaced navicular, distal end of the calcaneus, cuboid, and Y-bifurcate ligament correspond to the acetabulum. In clubfoot, the socket is medially displaced on the talar head, which is fixed in the ankle mortise, and the structures of the socket that move in unison must be rotated laterally on the talar head.

Nonsurgical Treatment

Most orthopaedists agree that initial treatment of clubfoot should be nonsurgical and should be instituted soon after birth. The three goals of nonsurgical treatment are providing manipulative correction, restoring movement, and maintaining the correction. Three methods are available to achieve these goals: taping and strapping, functional treatment, and manipulation and sequential cast changes.

Taping and Strapping

This method currently is most appropriate in premature infants in neonatal intensive care units whose feet need to be available for blood draws. Taping and strapping is ineffective in correcting a stiff forefoot deformity and in most cases simply acts as an adhesive strapping between the knee and the convex outer border of the foot. One review of the results of this technique described a 94% successful result in patients treated at birth.

Functional Treatment

Functional treatment of the clubfoot, commonly known as the French technique, has recently become popular.

The basic concept of this treatment is to align the foot while retaining active mobility and suppleness. Functional treatment consists of gentle manipulations, active physiotherapy, and splinting. Correction of the deformity is attempted in a sequential manner. The first step consists of unlocking the Chopart joint by reducing the talonavicular joint. The second step is correction of forefoot adduction by stabilizing the global adduction of the calcaneo-forefoot block. A progressive reduction of the heel varus is attempted in the third step, and heel equinus is corrected last. Each session lasts 30 minutes per foot. These manipulations are followed by active physiotherapy and splint fixation. Below-knee splints of elastic tape are made at the end of each session to maintain the foot in a slightly undercorrected position. Treatment is performed daily from birth until the infant is 4 to 12 weeks old. At this time, patients are reassessed, and if they show improvement, the manipulations are decreased to three sessions per week, which continue throughout infancy. In a 10-year follow-up of 350 feet treated using this technique, 63% of feet treated by well-trained physical therapists avoided surgery compared with only 30% of feet treated by less-trained physical therapists. The authors noted a decrease in the severity of clubfeet in their patient population, with a significant difference between the results achieved by well-trained versus less-trained physical therapists.

In a recent report of 201 clubfeet treated between 1991 and 1997 using a multiplanar continuous passive motion machine on the child's foot during sleeping periods in addition to functional treatment, 74% did not require surgery. In this series, 46% of the severe clubfeet and 30% of the moderate clubfeet required surgical correction. The authors believed that even in those patients who required surgical correction, the surgeries were less extensive as a result of the functional treatment.

Although functional treatment looks promising, longterm results from this technique are not yet available. Both proponents of this technique have their own rating systems, based on clinical examination, but no radiographic parameters exist to objectively support the clinical rating. Recurrence of the deformity, especially in the severe to moderate clubfeet that improved only one or two clinical grades in their series, is a legitimate concern. Longer follow-up may reveal that more of these feet require subsequent surgical correction. Functional treatment requires a very well-trained physical therapist and an extensive commitment from the family. In the present system of managed care, this treatment protocol may not be cost effective, especially if 46% of the severe cases eventually require surgical correction, even in the best hands.

Manipulation and Sequential Cast Changes

The sequential manipulative correction of the deformity followed by retentive casts is based on sound biomechanical principles. However, controversy still exists concerning whether to correct all components of the deformity except equinus simultaneously or to correct them sequentially beginning with forefoot adduction followed by hindfoot varus and finally the equinus.

With the first option, the manipulation begins with the correction of cavus by supinating the forefoot and dorsiflexing the first metatarsal to align the forefoot and midfoot in one plane. This manipulation creates an effective lever arm necessary for correction of hindfoot varus by abducting the forefoot while applying a counterpressure with the thumb against the head of the talus. The calcaneus abducts and simultaneously extends and everts by rotating and sliding under the talus, leading to the correction of hindfoot varus. Correction of equinus is not attempted until the foot can be fully abducted on the talus past neutral.

Above-knee casts control eversion better than below-knee casts and are less likely to slide off. Casts are changed at weekly intervals for the first month, and the foot is manipulated at each cast change. Crawford and Gupta follow a simple rule of 70, 20, 10, manipulating forefoot adduction 70 times, manipulating hindfoot varus 20 times, and stretching the heel 10 times at each visit. Casts are changed every 2 weeks during the second month and once during the third month. At this time, the foot is reassessed clinically and radiographically, and a decision as to the future course is made. A lateral maximum dorsiflexion view is analyzed for correction of equinus. If the equinus is corrected, the child is placed in reverse-last shoes; if the equinus still persists, a percutaneous heel cord release is indicated followed by use of corrective shoes until the child begins walking.

The results of sequential manipulation and retentive casts have varied. One group reported an 89% satisfactory functional outcome with serial casting and limited surgical intervention. Another reported a 35% long-term success and cautioned that recurrence can be seen up to age 6 years, and a third had success in only 10% of severe clubfeet. There are a number of pitfalls of cast treatment of clubfoot. If the foot is pronated in the cast, the adducted calcaneus is locked under the talus and the cavus deformity is increased. External rotation of the foot to correct adduction while the calcaneus is in varus results in external rotation of the talus in the mortise and posterior displacement of the lateral malleolus. If the forefoot is abducted with the thumb at the calcaneocuboid joint, correction of the heel varus is blocked; the thumb should be on the talar head laterally instead. Attempts to correct equinus before supination and varus

are corrected result in a rocker bottom deformity. Eversion of the hindfoot before the midfoot varus is corrected results in a horizontal breach and a bean-shaped foot.

In the event of a rocker bottom deformity that results from casting, further manipulations of the foot should be stopped and the foot should be maneuvered to its original deformity and an early heel cord release planned. A horizontal breach, or bean-shaped foot, should be treated with an early posterior release for mild deformities. A Dillwyn-Evans operation, in which the first cuneiform is opened and a closing wedge cuboid osteotomy is combined with a soft-tissue release, should be performed in children older than age 4 years with a severe horizontal breach. Prolonged casting in maximum dorsiflexion results in anterior ankle contracture, which should be treated with plantar flexion stretching exercises in infants younger than age 6 months. After age 6 months, an anterior ankle capsulotomy generally is required. In 28% to 83% of children treated with casting, a flat top talus occurs, which is believed to result from the nutcracker effect of forced dorsiflexion against tight posterior structures. This condition can only be diagnosed with a lateral ankle radiograph in which the fibula overlaps the tibia. Studies have shown that a flat top talus can remain asymptomatic at a 30-year follow-up.

Casts should be used only as retaining devices. If casts are used as corrective instruments, compression fractures of the distal tibial anterior metaphysis and epiphysis and fracture of the distal fibula can occur.

Response to Nonsurgical Treatment

As the child gets older, the response to nonsurgical treatment is assessed clinically and radiographically. Clinical assessment could involve using grading systems of either Dimeglio and associates or Pirani and associates to obtain some objectivity regarding the response to treatment. Standing AP, lateral, and stress dorsiflexion lateral views remain the gold standard for evaluation of the residual deformity. The stress dorsiflexion view will show three signs of a fixed equinovarus deformity: lack of dorsiflexion of the calcaneus (tibiocalcaneal angle of greater than 90°), failure of the long axes of the talus and calcaneus to intersect, and lack of overlap between the distal end of the calcaneus and talus (ie, an open sinus tarsi).

If the evaluation reveals that the deformity is yielding to nonsurgical treatment and the radiographic parameters are within the normal limits, it is prudent to continue with a further cast change at a month followed by straight or reverse-last shoes. The use of a Denis Browne bar has recently lost popularity. Full-time corrective shoe wear is gradually weaned to night-time use only, at which time the shoe heels can be tied

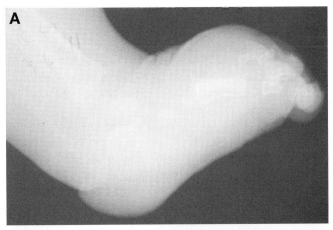

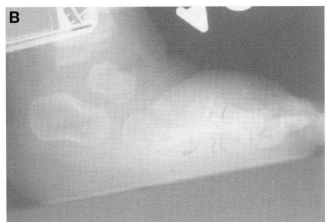

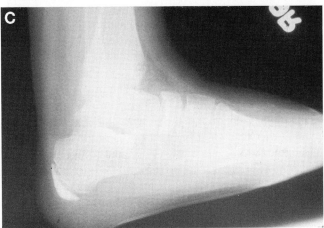

Figure 1 Nine-year follow-up of a child treated by manipulation, retention cast, and percutaneous heel cord release. **A,** True lateral view of the foot showing the equinus position of the calcaneus. The soft-tissue thickness of the heel fat pad would give the clinical appearance of a corrected foot as opposed to the radiographic appearance showing persistent equinus. **B,** Lateral maximum dorsiflexion view of this foot at 1 year showing a tendency to a rocker bottom configuration. A percutaneous Achilles tenotomy was performed. **C,** Forced lateral maximum dorsiflexion view 9 years later showing the foot to be well aligned with a normal talocalcaneal angle.

to keep the feet externally rotated. According to the literature, the duration for the use of corrective shoes in an attempt to rebalance the musculotendinous units varies from 1 year to 6 years, with no objective data supporting any one approach.

If the deformity persists and the radiographic parameters show residual deformity, the options are limited surgical correction or immediate or delayed definitive surgical correction.

Limited Surgical Correction

Percutaneous Heel Cord Release

One author strongly advocates outpatient heel cord tenotomy under lidocaine or prilocaine analgesia for patients with persistent equinus despite improvements in the cavus and adduction deformities. Following tenotomy, the foot is placed in a cast for 3 weeks, after which time lateral radiographs are obtained to confirm the convergence of talocalcaneal axes. Following a successful heel cord release, the foot is placed in a corrective shoe full-time for 3 months followed by gradual weaning to nighttime use only, which is maintained for a variable period (Fig. 1). A review of the long-term results of this method indicated that 27 of the 71 feet initially treated by serial casting required a heel cord tenotomy, and 38 feet required a subsequent anterior tibial tendon transfer. Functional outcome was excellent in 78% of these patients. In another review of calcaneal tendon lengthening, six of 25 feet required additional surgery.

Limited Posterior Release

In one study, a limited posterior release, consisting of a sagittal plane z-lengthening of the Achilles tendon, a posterior tibiotalar capsulotomy, and a posterior talocalcaneal capsulotomy was performed on 100 feet in children age 1 to 8 months. Results were good in 71% of feet with mild deformities but only 34% in those with severe deformities. Thus, this approach should be limited to mild deformities. In a subsequent study, 100 patients with clubfoot who had a posterior release were compared to 100 patients who had a posteromedial release. The authors concluded that feet with more severe deformities required a posteromedial release.

Limited Posterolateral Release

A study evaluating the effectiveness of a posterolateral release along with z-lengthening of the invertors and reefing of the peroneus longus as a one-stage procedure was performed on 125 feet in children approximately 6 weeks of age. Of these feet, 66 required a second-stage operation for correction of forefoot deformity.

Definitive Surgical Correction

The need for surgery should not be regarded as a failure of the treating physician to achieve correction by nonsurgical means. Rather, it is a mere recognition of the fact that the deformity requires more than manipulations to yield.

Timing

One thing on which an apparent consensus seems to be evolving is the timing of clubfoot surgery. Early surgical intervention bears the promise of an immediate start in the process of remodeling but also predisposes the foot to iatrogenic scarring of the cartilage and physeal damage. One report on the results of surgical correction when the patient was younger than age 3 months indicated that about half of the feet required further surgical intervention. Subsequent surgery was required in 11 of 28 patients in another series who underwent a subtalar realignment at age 6 weeks.

Most surgeons will recommend the surgical correction when the child is between age 9 and 12 months because of decreased anesthetic risk, the ease of handling larger tissues, and the desire to give the child a plantigrade foot before ambulation to provide dynamic assistance in dorsiflexion with weight bearing.

Type and Extent of Surgical Release

Considerable controversy and variation exist in the type and extent of the surgical correction of clubfoot. The technique of posteromedial release with pin fixation was described in 1971, and follow-up occurred in both 1979 and 1994. However, the release of the talocalcaneal interosseous ligament and the deltoid ligament remains controversial because these structures are the primary restraints to valgus overcorrection. An important addition to the surgical correction of clubfoot is the recent recognition of the calcaneocuboid deformity. Simons emphasized the importance of evaluating the calcaneocuboid articulation while planning the surgical release of clubfoot. He graded the calcaneocuboid joint deformity and reported that grade 1 deformity does not require correction, grade 2 requires an extensive soft-tissue release, and grade 3 requires a bony procedure in addition to the release. He cautioned against doing a partial release because it may lead to a rotatory hindfoot valgus when the talonavicular articulation is restored.

A different approach to the surgical management of clubfoot, termed "á la carte surgery," has been advocated by Seringe. This approach assumes that not all clubfeet are alike; therefore, a single recipe does not serve them all. This technique tailors surgery to the need of the foot and consequently avoids overcorrection.

Type of Incision

Use of a single posteromedial incision made release of the posterolateral structures very tedious. This problem has been circumvented by the use of the circumferential Cincinnati incision or a two-incision approach. The Cincinnati incision allows excellent circumferential access to all facets of the deformity (Fig. 2). Its benefit for visualization of the pathology and for training residents has been well documented. However, skin necrosis is a potential concern with this approach. In a series of 31 feet in which the medial wound of the Cincinnati incision was left open to gap about 10 mm (Fig. 3), all but one wound healed in 6 weeks. In addition, the appearance of the incision was similar to those in which primary closure was performed. The authors concluded that correction of the deformity should not be compromised to approximate the skin because primary skin closure is not essential. In another study, no difference was found in the quality of scar in patients undergoing primary healing compared to that in healing by secondary intention. The twin incision approach tends to avoid potential skin necrosis, and because it is a limited approach, it may limit scarring.

Use of Intraoperative Pin Fixation and Casts

Turco advocated the use of pin fixation following surgical correction. Most surgeons advocate one, two, or three pins to hold the correction. Traditionally, a single smooth pin is used to hold the talonavicular articulation in a reduced position. Other surgeons use a smooth pin to hold both the talocalcaneal and the calcaneocuboid articulations.

Secondary Procedures

Residual deformities after surgical correction of clubfoot that require secondary surgical procedures have been reported with varying frequencies. Some surgeons believe that residual deformities result when either full correction is not obtained nor maintained long enough for the tarsal bones to remodel. Others agree that recurrence will not occur after a foot is completely corrected and maintained and that a neurologic cause should be considered if recurrence occurs after an initial procedure is deemed successful. The authors who evaluated 159 feet that required a second procedure

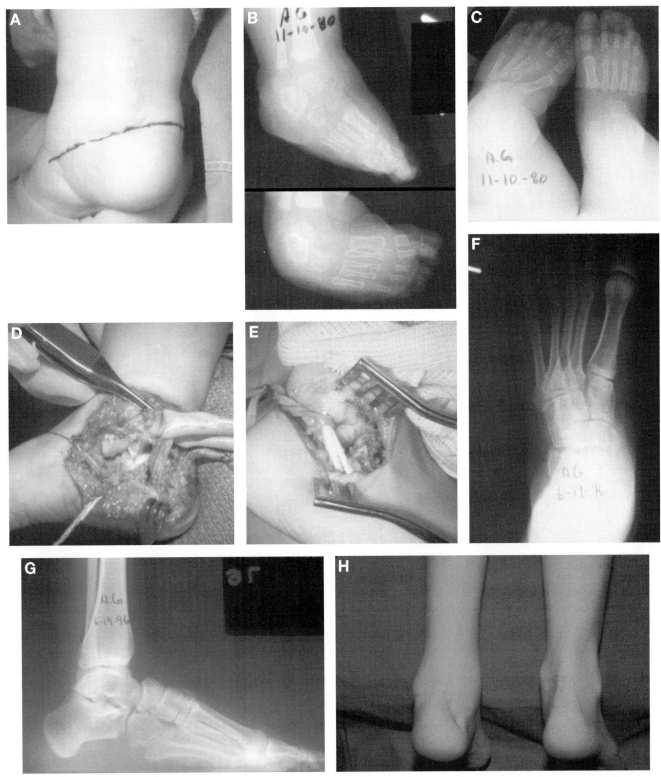

Figure 2 Sixteen-year follow-up on a child with recurrent clubfoot after posterior medial release with a J-type incision. A mediolateral release was performed through the Cincinnati incision. **A,** Posterior medial view of a child outlining the Cincinnati incision with a felt tip marker. **B,** True lateral and maximum dorsiflexion view at age 1 year. Note the apparent varus position. Also note there is no convergence of talar and calcaneal axes on the forced dorsiflexion view. **C,** Comparison views of both feet showing the forefoot adduction and hindfoot varus. **D,** Surgical view of the medial side of the foot illustrating the talocalcaneal interosseous ligament in the foreground. The neurovascular bundle is being retracted with a Penrose drain, and the forceps is attached to the proximal posterior tibialis tendon. **E,** Surgical view of the lateral side of the foot illustrating the peroneus longus and brevis tendon are bound by an elastic. The subtalar joint is just superior to the peroneal tendons just below the incised Y-bifurcate ligament. **F,** True AP view of the foot 16 years later. There is correction of the forefoot; however, there is still some residual or superimposition of the talocalcaneal bones. **G,** True weight-bearing lateral view of the foot 16 years later. **H,** At follow-up 16 years later, the skin at the area of the initial J-incision, which was done before the child was age 1 year, remains indented. The transverse Cincinnati incision is barely seen.

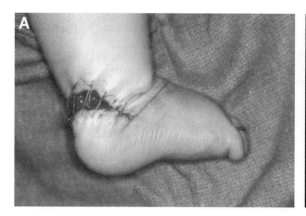
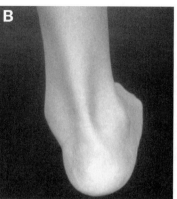

Figure 3 Postoperative clinical photograph of a clubfoot treated by the Cincinnati incision, which was allowed to remain open in the initial postoperative period because of the tension of the skin and followed for 3.8 years. **A,** Posterior lateral view of the foot showing some retention sutures over the transverse incision, but the wound is not completely closed. The child was returned to the operating room within 2 weeks at which time Steri-Strip™ closure was achieved. **B,** Posterior view of the foot 3.8 years after surgery. The patient had no postoperative complications.

reported an 81% incidence of adduction, 49% supination, 38% heel varus, 29% cavus, and 24% equinus.

Forefoot supination and adduction leading to internal foot progression angle are reportedly the most common residual deformities postoperatively. In one report, the main cause of the deformity in 21 of 28 clinically adducted feet was metatarsus adductus. Failure to release the calcaneocuboid joint was believed to be significant in producing a residual forefoot adduction. An imbalance between a strong tibialis anterior and weak peronei results in a supination deformity.

The use of gait analysis in surgically treated clubfeet showed that all except one patient with intoeing had increased activity of the tibialis anterior during stance phase. Another study using gait analysis of patients with internal foot progression angle following clubfoot release showed that the most common cause of deformity was a persistent internal tibial torsion; in this study, only a minority of patients had increased activity of the tibialis anterior during stance phase. Various procedures have been described to correct this deformity.

Lateral transfer of the tibialis anterior to the third cuneiform is the most commonly used procedure. In one series, 38 of 71 feet required a transfer of the tibialis anterior tendon, with six of these patients requiring additional surgery. Others have advocated a split transfer of the tibialis anterior muscle. A biomechanical study indicated that the axis of the fourth metatarsal for split transfer and that of the third metatarsal for the whole tendon transfer were ideal sites for insertion of the tendon. No difference was found between the maximum dorsiflexion achieved by split versus whole tibialis anterior tendon transfer.

Fowler's opening wedge osteotomy of the first cuneiform has been used to correct residual forefoot adduction. Use of this procedure was justified in later studies that showed that most forefoot adduction was attributed to metatarsus adductus. In a report of the results of Fowler's osteotomy along with radical plantar release, there was a 72% correction of adduction and a 47% correction of equinus deformity.

Dillwyn-Evans wedge resection and fusion of the calcaneocuboid joint has been used widely to correct relapse of clubfoot. The premise is to reduce the navicular on the head of the talus by shortening the lateral column. The results of this procedure were evaluated in 60 feet in patients at a mean age of 29 years. Function was deemed satisfactory in 68% of the patients, and 90% of the patients were able to perform all desired activities. Evaluation of the results of a modified Evans procedure in 45 feet indicated results were satisfactory in 30 feet, with most patients able to participate in recreational activities.

An opening wedge medial cuneiform osteotomy and a closing wedge cuboid osteotomy (flip-flop procedure) has been proposed to correct forefoot adduction with supination (a so-called bean-shaped foot). This approach combines forefoot correction with midfoot correction. One cadaveric experiment showed that although forefoot adduction changed in direct proportion to the width of the wedge used in Fowler's procedure, and a cuboid wedge resection corrected the midfoot, as evidenced by a decrease in Meary's angle. Short-term results of the cuboid resection indicated that six of seven feet showed a correction of forefoot adductus and in the "bean" shape of the foot. However, there was still some foot dragging during the swing phase, which probably represents the dynamic component of the deformity. Finally, a medial rotational osteotomy of the tibia was proposed for correction of severe residual deformities in clubfoot with satisfactory results.

Analysis of Treatment Results

Surgical correction of clubfoot aims to provide patients with a near anatomically normal, pain-free plantigrade foot with reasonable mobility that fits in a normal shoe and maintains lasting correction. Unfortunately, comparing the results of various surgical techniques is often difficult because no two clubfeet are alike, and there is no universal grading and evaluation system for clubfoot. One study compared the results of postero-medial release with those of a complete circumferential release performed by the same surgeon. Both patient groups had similar radiographic presentations and 2 years postoperatively there was no difference between groups in the radiographic and clinical results. Another study compared the long-term results of posterior release with those of a Carroll comprehensive release performed at the same institution. Although the two patient groups did not differ on the function weighted Ponseti scale, those undergoing the Carroll procedure had fewer complications, more complete correction of heel varus, and improved subtalar motion. In another comparison of the results of the Carroll, McKay, and Turco procedures, results were excellent in 11% of feet in the Carroll group, 12.5% of feet in the McKay group, and 12.5% of feet in the Turco group.

Meta-analysis of Results

A meta-analysis of the literature focusing on results of various surgical techniques for clubfoot showed excellent results in 42% of patients undergoing posterior release only, 56% of those undergoing posterior and partial medial release, 64% of patients undergoing posteromediolateral release, and 65% of those undergoing a Turco procedure. In 29 patients with unilateral deformity, the treated foot was compared with the contralateral normal foot. The most significant limitations in the treated feet averaged a 65% decrease in normal dorsiflexion, a 24% decrease in plantar flexion strength, which correlated directly to the number of heel cord lengthenings, and a 10% decrease in calf girth unrelated to the total time spent in the cast. In a review of the radiographic appearance of 24 feet undergoing a Turco procedure at a mean follow-up of 7 years, there was wedging of the navicular with dorsal displacement in 16 feet and flattening of the trochlear surface of the talus in 13 feet, with relative shortening of the talar neck and head in nine feet. Investigators who reported a 7.1% incidence of dorsal subluxation of the tarsal navicular created an anatomic model to explain that this radiographic appearance is the result of a rotatory subluxation of the navicular in the coronal plane. They stressed the need for checking the rotation of the navicular at the time of internal fixation.

Dorsal navicular subluxation may, in some cases, be iatrogenic. Special attention should be directed toward assessing anatomic positioning and pinning of the navicular with radiographic confirmation. Recently, the ankle valgus in clubfeet has received much attention, with one study reporting a 67% prevalence of ankle valgus in a long-term follow-up of surgically treated clubfeet. This ankle valgus could ameliorate the effects of a residual hindfoot varus or give a spurious impression of an overcorrected clubfoot after surgical correction.

Gait Analysis

Gait analysis is being used more and more to study the effects of treatment of clubfoot. In one study that followed patients an average of 10 years after unilateral clubfoot surgery, ankle sagittal plane mechanics were disturbed in 20 of 23 clubfeet. Initial contact during the first rocker occurred in a position of increased plantar flexion, with a decrease in dorsiflexion during the second rocker and limited plantar flexion during push-off. Both knees showed abnormal kinematics. Children with limited dorsiflexion during the second rocker hyperextended their knees to prevent early heel rise during the stance phase, whereas children with a foot drop showed a decrease in ipsilateral knee loading response. In the coronal plane, there was a trend toward increased knee valgus. Fixed pelvic obliquity was seen in 17 of 23 patients, with the surgically treated side depressed by an average of 7°. This pelvic obliquity was independent of limb-length difference. Internal foot progression was seen in 14 of 23 patients with internal tibial torsion, the major contribution in half of these patients. Kinetically, the power generated by the ankle at push-off was significantly decreased with an average gastrocnemius-soleus weakness of 27%. This weakness was not seen in patients who had undergone casting alone and also did not correlate with calf atrophy. Six patients showed more than 10% relative weakness of the tibialis anterior compared to the control limb. These abnormal knee and hip mechanics are of concern in the long run because they may predispose patients to early arthritic changes at these joints.

Recent investigations have hinted at the possibility of predicting the final results of surgical treatment of clubfoot based on histopathologic abnormalities in the muscles of the foot. The postoperative functional result was poor after posteromedial release in patients with diminished type 1 to type 2 fiber area ratios in the triceps surae. Incidence of recurrent equinovarus deformity was increased after following a posteromediolateral release in patients with type 1 fiber atrophy in the ipsilateral peroneus brevis muscle.

Overcorrection

A severe, unacceptable flatfoot deformity increasingly is being recognized as a complication of aggressive surgical treatment of clubfoot. A reported 3.8% incidence of overcorrection at first reoperation increased to 17.5% and 18.2% for second and third reoperations, respectively. An increasing incidence of this complication, which initially was attributed to release of talo-calcaneal interosseous ligament and early patient age at surgery, has been reported in series without these variables. In a long-term follow-up study of posteromedial release, 75% of unsatisfactory outcomes were attributed to overcorrection. Clinically, this deformity is characterized by a contracted tibialis anterior tendon, limited plantar flexion, severe flatfoot with heel valgus, concavity of the sinus tarsi, and hallux flexus with a dorsiflexed first ray. Patients also may have a dorsal bunion. These feet are functionally and cosmetically worse than undercorrected feet. A subgroup of patients with idiopathic clubfeet prone to postoperative overcorrection was identified retrospectively. This group had hypotonia, loose jointedness, fine transverse skin crease around the heel, lateral insertion of the heel cord, and a higher incidence of gestational diabetes. Once these problems are recognized, extreme caution should be taken to avoid extensive release and especially dorsal subluxation of the navicular on the talus.

Annotated Bibliography

Etiology

van der Sluijs JA, Pruys JE: Normal collagen structure in the posterior ankle capsule in different types of clubfeet. *J Pediatr Orthop B* 1999;8:261-263.

The authors analyzed modifications and cross-links in collagen in 21 feet in 17 children with different types of clubfoot. Possible relationships with clinical stiffness of the clubfoot deformity were measured using the Dimeglio/Bensahel method. Results were normal, despite the variety of types of clubfoot, indicating that collagen molecules are processed normally and alignment of collagen molecules within fibrils is normal.

Pathoanatomy

Hootnick DR, Packard DS Jr, Levinsohn EM, Crider RJ Jr: Confirmation of arterial deficiencies in a limb with necrosis following clubfoot surgery. *J Pediatr Orthop B* 1999;8:187-193.

The authors described postoperative necrosis of the hallux and first ray in children following surgery to correct clubfoot. Arteriography demonstrated hypoplasia of both the anterior and posterior tibial arteries and failure of the dorsalis pedis to traverse the tarsus and complete the deep plantar arch. These findings confirm an association between congenital vascular deficiency in clubfoot and necrosis following surgery. The authors concluded that the metabolic demands of wound healing were sufficient to cause localized distal hypoperfusion that resulted in necrosis in a limb with congenital vascular deficiency.

Diagnostic Imaging of Clubfoot

Treadwell MC, Stanitski CL, King M: Prenatal sonographic diagnosis of clubfoot: Implications for patient counseling. *J Pediatr Orthop* 1999;19:8-10.

Authors studied the incidence of prenatally, sonographically diagnosed clubfoot; the incidence of associated anomalies; and the correlation with postnatal findings. The incidence of prenatally diagnosed clubfoot was 0.43%. This was isolated in 33% of the patients and associated with other anomalies in 67%. There was a 40% false-positive rate for isolated clubfoot, all diagnosed in the third trimester of pregnancy. The correct identification of associated anomalies facilitates prenatal counseling, but limitations of prenatal US must be remembered.

Nonsurgical Treatment

Dimeglio A, Bonnet F, Mazeau P, De Rosa V: Orthopaedic treatment and passive motion machine: Consequences for the surgical treatment of clubfoot. *J Pediatr Orthop B* 1996;5:173-180.

The authors reported that this treatment can noticeably reduce the rate of surgery and, when surgery still is required, reduce its extent. In grade II soft > stiff feet, surgery is required in only 32% of cases, and posterior surgery often is sufficient. In grade III stiff > soft feet, surgery most often includes posterior and medial release, variably associated with plantar release. Lateral release is exceptional (15%), and surgery is necessary in 75% of cases. In grade IV stiff = stiff feet, surgery is necessary in 90% of cases. Lateral release is performed in 50%.

Limited Surgical Correction

Cooper DM, Dietz FR: Treatment of idiopathic clubfoot: A thirty-year follow-up note. *J Bone Joint Surg Am* 1995;77:1477-1489.

Authors evaluated 45 patients who had 71 congenital clubfeet at an average age of 34 years. With the use of pain and functional limitation as the outcome criteria, 35 of the 45 patients (78%) had an excellent or good outcome. The patient's occupation, passive dorsiflexion as measured with a hand-held goniometer, the AP calcaneus-fifth metatarsal angle, the total foot pressure time integral, and the number of rapid single-limb toe-ups that could be performed were the only variables that differed significantly between the feet that had an excellent or good result and those that had a poor result (P < 0.05). The data suggest that a sedentary occupation and avoidance of excessive weight gain may improve the over-all long-term result. Excessive weakening of the triceps surae may predispose patients to a poor result. The outcome could not be predicted from the radiographic result.

Haasbeek JF, Wright JG: A comparison of the long-term results of posterior and comprehensive release in the treatment of clubfoot. *J Pediatr Orthop* 1997;17:29-35.

In this study, the long-term results of posterior and comprehensive release in the treatment of clubfoot were compared. Eligibility was based on an idiopathic clubfoot and treatment before age 2 years. The posterior releases had been performed prior to 1971; comprehensive releases were performed after 1972. Patients in the posterior release group were evaluated at an average of 28 years postoperatively. Patients in the comprehensive release were evaluated at an average of 16 years postoperatively. Although Ponseti scores were higher in the comprehensive release group (mean, 86 versus 81), they were not statistically different ($P = 0.13$). The patients in the comprehensive release group had fewer operations, more complete correction of heel varus, and improved subtalar motion.

Analysis of Treatment Results

Ferlic RJ, Breed AL, Mann DC, Cherney JJ: Partial wound closure after surgical correction of equinovarus foot deformity. *J Pediatr Orthop* 1997;17:486-489.

This is a retrospective review of 31 feet in 22 patients whose medial skin incisions were left open (typically 10 mm) to heal by secondary intention. One or two cast changes were performed under outpatient anesthesia at 7- to 14-day intervals for wound care. All wounds except one were healed by week 6 at the time of outpatient clinic cast removal. The appearance of the incisions is similar to those in feet in which primary closure is possible. One foot required split-thickness skin grafting at 3 weeks postoperatively to achieve wound coverage. There were no infections.

Johnston CE II, Hobatho MC, Baker KJ, Baunin C: Three-dimensional analysis of clubfoot deformity by computed tomography. *J Pediatr Orthop B* 1995;4:39-48.

Three-dimensional reconstruction of transverse CT images of 27 feet in children age 3 to 10 years was assessed. This technique allows visualization of deformities that otherwise cannot be visualized on plain radiographs and shows that a variety of interosseous relations comprise the entity known as clubfoot. Abnormal talar pronation was an unexpected finding of the three-dimensional analysis.

Karol LA, Concha MC, Johnston CE II: Gait analysis and muscle strength in children with surgically treated clubfeet. *J Pediatr Orthop* 1997;17:790-795.

Twenty-three children who had unilateral surgery for idiopathic clubfeet underwent gait analysis and isokinetic muscle-strength testing at an average of 10 years after surgical release. Ankle sagittal-plane kinematics were disturbed in 20 clubfeet. Fifteen children had an internal foot-progression angle. Genu valgum and knee hyperextension were common. Plantar flexion power was decreased by 23% on the side of surgery. Quadriceps weakness was seen in nine of 22 surgically treated limbs and hamstring weakness in eight of 22.

Classic Bibliography

Carroll NC: Pathoanatomy and surgical treatment of the resistant clubfoot. *Instr Course Lect* 1988;37:93-106.

Carroll NC, McMurtry R, Leete SF: The pathoanatomy of congenital clubfoot. *Orthop Clin North Am* 1978;9:225-232.

Crawford AH, Marxen JL, Osterfeld DL: The Cincinnati incision: A comprehensive approach for surgical procedures of the foot and ankle in childhood. *J Bone Joint Surg Am* 1982;64:1355-1358.

Dunn HK, Samuelson KM: Flat-top talus: A long-term report of twenty club feet. *J Bone Joint Surg Am* 1974;56:57-62.

Evans D: Treatment of the unreduced or 'relapsed' club foot in older children. *Proc R Soc Med* 1968;61:782-783.

McKay DW: New concept of and approach to clubfoot treatment: Section I. Principles and morbid anatomy. *J Pediatr Orthop* 1982;2:347-356.

McKay DW: New concept of and approach to clubfoot treatment: Section II. Correction of the clubfoot. *J Pediatr Orthop* 1983;3:10-21.

McKay DW: New concept of and approach to clubfoot treatment: Section III. Evaluation and results. *J Pediatr Orthop* 1983;3:141-148.

Ponseti IV: Treatment of congenital club foot. *J Bone Joint Surg Am* 1992;74:448-454.

Ponseti IV, Campos J: Observations on pathogenesis and treatment of congenital clubfoot. *Clin Orthop* 1972;84:50-60.

Simons GW: Complete subtalar release in club feet: Part I. A preliminary report. *J Bone Joint Surg Am* 1985;67:1044-1055.

Simons GW: Complete subtalar release in club feet: Part II. Comparison with less extensive procedures. *J Bone Joint Surg Am* 1985;67:1056-1065.

Turco VJ: Surgical correction of the resistant club foot: One-stage posteromedial release with internal fixation. A preliminary report. *J Bone Joint Surg Am* 1971;53:477-497.

Turco VJ: Resistant congenital club foot: One-stage posteromedial release with internal fixation. A follow-up report of a fifteen-year experience. *J Bone Joint Surg Am* 1979;61:805-814.

Chapter 22

Flexible Flatfoot and Tarsal Coalition

Vincent S. Mosca, MD

Flexible Flatfoot

Flexible flatfoot is the term used to describe a specific foot shape that is defined not only by its structure (flat), but also by its function (flexible). It is ubiquitous in children and common in adults. Although flexible flatfoot has been recognized and studied extensively for decades, controversy surrounds its definition, incidence, natural history, and management.

There are no universally accepted clinical or radiographic definitions of the average height, or the normal range of heights, of the longitudinal arch of the foot. Therefore, the point at which a low normal arch becomes a flatfoot is unknown. One radiographic study of the foot in adults and one study in children reported the average values and normal ranges of values for various interosseous angular measurements. It would be scientifically justified to define a flatfoot as a foot in which the radiographic measurements that relate to arch height are more than two standard deviations from the mean, but the medical community has not embraced this approach.

Flatfoot is the term that is applied to a foot shape that results from a number of altered relationships between several bones of the foot and ankle. It is not a single deformity at a single joint. The most obvious deformities are the valgus alignment of the hindfoot and the sag of the midfoot, both of which are caused by malalignment of the subtalar joint complex. The subtalar joint complex comprises the talus, calcaneus, spring ligament, and navicular. Historically, this unique articulation has been likened to the hip joint by comparing the head of the talus with the head of the femur and then comparing combined calcaneus, spring ligament, and navicular (the so-called pes acetabulum) with the acetabulum. However, unlike the hip joint, the oblique axis and unusual anatomy of the subtalar complex create constrained motions of the pes acetabulum around the talus that defy application of the terminology used at other joints in the body. The terms

inversion and eversion apply to the constrained multiplanar motions in this location. A weight-bearing flatfoot (Fig. 1) has excessive eversion of the subtalar complex, which is characterized by valgus, external rotation, and dorsiflexion of the calcaneus in relation to the talus. In addition, the navicular is dorsiflexed and abducted on the head of a plantar flexed talus. The midfoot sags with lowering of the longitudinal arch. There is a real or apparent shortening of the lateral border, or column, of the foot in relation to the medial border. The forefoot in a flatfoot deformity is supinated in relation to the hindfoot with dorsiflexion of the first metatarsal, creating a deformity in the opposite direction from that in the hindfoot, as if the foot was wrung out.

As previously stated, there is no consensus regarding what magnitude of these deformities is necessary for a foot to be defined as flat. Nevertheless, there is no question that certain feet have excessive flattening of the longitudinal arch. According to their definition, Harris and Beath found flatfoot in approximately 23% of the adult population they studied. They found that the flatness of the arch in weight bearing was less important than the mobility of the joints and tendons. Therefore, they documented three types of flatfoot based on the functional mobility of the subtalar joint complex and the ankle joint. Two thirds of the group had a flatfoot that was flexible, or hypermobile, with good mobility and excursion of the subtalar complex and ankle joint. They documented this type as of little or no clinical concern as a potential cause of disability. An additional 25% of the total group had a flexible flatfoot with good mobility of the subtalar complex but with contracture of the Achilles tendon with restriction of ankle dorsiflexion. This group tended to have pain and disability. The final 9% of the group had a rigid flatfoot with restriction of subtalar motion, which tended to cause disability more commonly than a simple flexible flatfoot.

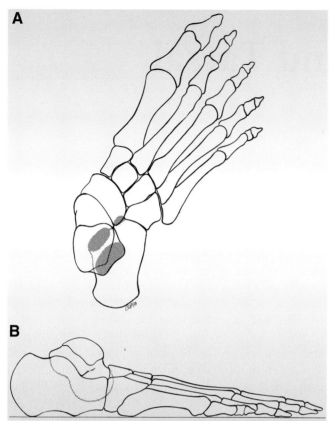

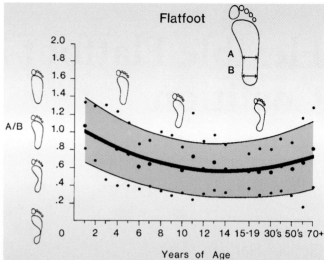

Figure 2 The height of the longitudinal arch as determined by evaluation of the footprint. The ratio of midfoot-to-heel width (A/B) is plotted against age in untreated individuals. The average value and two standard deviation ranges change spontaneously with age. A higher ratio, which is higher on the chart, represents a flatter foot. *(Reproduced with permission from Staheli LT, Chew DE, Corbett M: The longitudinal arch: A survey of eight hundred and eighty-two feet in normal children and adults. J Bone Joint Surg Am 1987;69:426-428.)*

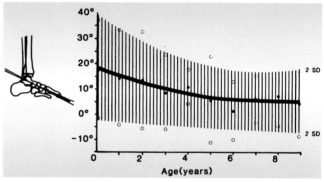

Figure 3 The lateral talo-first metatarsal angle plotted against age in untreated individuals. A larger angle signifies a greater sag of the midfoot and a flatter longitudinal arch. *(Reproduced with permission from Vanderwilde R, Staheli LT, Chew DE, et al: Measurement on radiographs of the foot in normal infants and children. J Bone Joint Surg Am 1988;70:407-415.)*

Figure 1 Flatfoot. **A,** A flatfoot is characterized by excessive eversion of the subtalar complex, which includes external rotation of the calcaneus in relation to the talus and abduction of the navicular on the talar head. The lateral column of the foot is short relative to the medial column. **B,** Although the calcaneus is dorsiflexed in relation to the talus (increased lateral talocalcaneal angle), the calcaneus and talus are both plantar flexed in relation to the tibia. The navicular is dorsiflexed on the head of the talus, creating a sag at the talonavicular joint with lowering of the longitudinal arch. The hindfoot is in valgus, yet all metatarsal heads touch the ground. The forefoot, therefore, must be supinated in relation to the hindfoot. *(Reproduced with permission from Mosca VS: Calcaneal lengthening for valgus deformity of the hindfoot: Results in children who had severe, symptomatic flatfoot and skewfoot. J Bone Joint Surg Am 1995;77:500-512.)*

Manual testing determines flexibility, or mobility, of the subtalar complex. Creating the longitudinal arch with toe standing and the Jack toe-raising test confirms flexibility. The Achilles tendon is considered to be of normal length if it allows at least 10° of ankle dorsiflexion when tested with the subtalar joint held in neutral alignment and the knee fully extended.

Flexible flatfoot is present from birth and has normal muscle function. Bone shape and ligament laxity in the foot determine the height of the longitudinal arch. Muscles are important for balance and function, but not for structure.

Footprint (Fig. 2) and radiographic (Fig. 3) studies on the child's foot have confirmed that most babies are flatfooted, the height of the longitudinal arch increases spontaneously during the first decade of life in most children, and there is a wide range of normal arch

heights skewed toward flatness at all ages, particularly in young children.

Unfortunately, there are no long-term prospective studies on the natural history of untreated flexible flatfoot with regard to pain and disability. Based on the available cross-sectional data that have been presented, the flexible flatfoot is a normal variation of shape that is not known to cause disability. Even the authors of the radiographic studies on feet clearly stated that, in both adults and children, radiographic values are descriptive and, even if beyond the normal ranges, should not be used to determine clinical management.

Furthermore, there are no controlled prospective studies that document that prophylactic surgical or nonsurgical treatment prevents long-term pain or disability. Therefore, recommendations to "treat" asymptomatic flexible flatfoot by any means are unfounded.

Research from developing countries suggests that shoes may have a detrimental effect on the development of the longitudinal arch. Results of one study indicated a higher prevalence of flatfoot, some of which was painful and restricted mobility, among shoe-wearing Chinese individuals who were compared with individuals who never wore shoes. In another study, a greater prevalence of flatfoot was discovered in shod children than in unshod children in India. And most recently, in a study from India, a higher prevalence of flatfoot was reported in adults who began wearing shoes at a young age.

Results of two well-controlled and prospective studies did not show any benefit from shoe modifications or inserts over spontaneous natural improvement in the height of the longitudinal arch in children. All other studies that have reported such a beneficial effect did not use controls.

Some children with flexible flatfoot have activity-related pain in the leg or foot that is not well localized, may also be experienced at night, and is believed to represent an overuse syndrome. Inexpensive, over-the-counter shoe inserts can improve symptoms and increase the useful life of shoes that would otherwise be worn unevenly by children with severe flatfoot. These effects are achieved without a simultaneous permanent increase in the height of the arch.

Some children with flexible flatfoot have pain with weight bearing and callosities under the head of the plantar flexed talus. In these children, contracture of the Achilles tendon prevents normal dorsiflexion of the talus in the ankle joint during the midstance phase of the gait cycle. The dorsiflexion stress is shifted to the subtalar joint complex, which has the ability to dorsiflex around the talus as a component of the motion known as eversion. The symptoms are created by excessive direct axial loading and shear stress on the soft tissues under the head of the talus. Firm arch supports placed beneath the unyielding plantar flexed talar head may exaggerate these pressures. An aggressive Achilles tendon stretching program performed with the subtalar complex inverted may relieve the symptoms.

Surgery is rarely, if ever, indicated for flexible flatfoot. The flexible flatfoot with a short, or contracted, Achilles tendon might benefit from surgery, but only after prolonged conservative treatment has failed to relieve the pain and callosities under the head of the talus. Many surgical procedures to correct the flatfoot were proposed during the last century and include osseous excisions, osteotomies, arthrodesis of one or more joints, and interposition of bone or synthetic materials into the sinus tarsi. Most of these procedures

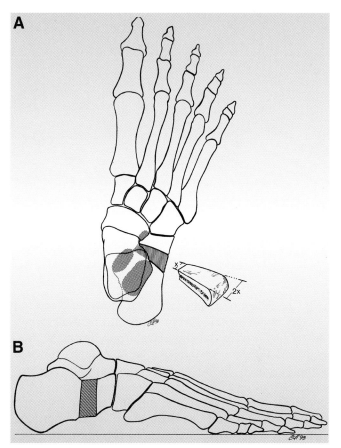

Figure 4 Calcaneal lengthening osteotomy. All components of the subtalar complex deformity have been corrected by insertion of a trapezoid-shaped, tricortical iliac crest graft into the osteotomy that was made between the anterior and middle facets of the calcaneus. Lengthening of the gastrocnemius or the triceps surae is required in most cases. **A,** Dorsal view. **B,** Lateral view. *(Reproduced with permission from Mosca VS: Calcaneal lengthening for valgus deformity of the hindfoot: Results in children who had severe, symptomatic flatfoot and skewfoot. J Bone Joint Surg Am 1995;77:500-512.)*

have been abandoned because of failure to relieve symptoms or to achieve or maintain correction of the deformity. Results of all long-term studies on procedures that involve arthrodesis of the midtarsal joints, such as the Hoke procedure and its many modifications, reveal degenerative arthrosis at the adjacent unfused joints. Furthermore, because these procedures address the secondary deformity, the supination of the forefoot, and not the primary deformity, the valgus/eversion deformity of the hindfoot, they should be expected to fail. Most orthopaedic surgeons have not embraced the technique of interpositioning a synthetic spacer into the sinus tarsi to block eversion motion. The implants are foreign bodies that can cause infection as well as pain. Although the posterior calcaneal displacement osteotomy can improve the clinical appearance of the valgus hindfoot, it does not correct the malalignment at the talonavicular joint or the lateral rotation of the foot through the subtalar complex. The calcaneal lengthening osteotomy (Fig. 4), origi-

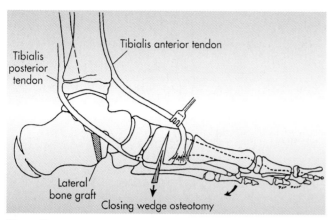

Figure 5 Supination deformity of the forefoot, if present, must be corrected by a separate procedure, such as a medial cuneiform plantar-based closing wedge osteotomy. (*Reproduced with permission from Anderson A, Fowler S: Anterior calcaneal osteotomy for symptomatic juvenile pes planus. Foot Ankle 1984;4:274-283.*)

nally described by Evans, has been shown to correct all components of even severe eversion/valgus deformity of the hindfoot at the site of deformity in the subtalar complex. Function of the subtalar complex is restored, symptoms are relieved, and the adjacent joints are protected from developing early degenerative arthrosis by avoiding arthrodesis. If present, supination deformity of the forefoot must be recognized as an additional deformity and managed concurrently with a procedure such as a plantar flexion osteotomy of the medial cuneiform (Fig. 5). The final deformity that must be treated concurrently is the one that created the disability, the contracture of the Achilles tendon. Intraoperative assessment after correction of the hindfoot will confirm the need for lengthening the Achilles tendon or the gastrocnemius alone.

Tarsal Coalition

Tarsal coalition, which is a fibrous, cartilaginous, or bony connection between two or more tarsal bones that results from a congenital failure of differentiation and segmentation of primitive mesenchyme, is the most common cause of a rigid flatfoot. The tarsal coalition may be large or small, present at birth or developmental, an incidental finding, or a cause of disability. When associated with other congenital disorders, such as fibular hemimelia, Apert's syndrome, or Nievergelt-Pearlman syndrome, the tarsal coalition is usually large, present at birth, and asymptomatic. This discussion will focus on the autosomal dominant variety (with nearly full penetrance) that affects approximately 1% of the general population. This type is usually small, developmental, and may cause pain and disability.

Tarsal coalitions were first recognized in 1750. The first detailed clinical description of a peroneal spastic flatfoot was presented in 1897. In 1921, the peroneal

spastic flatfoot was linked with calcaneonavicular coalition and, in 1948, the peroneal spastic flatfoot was linked with talocalcaneal coalition. Since 1965, tarsal coalition has also been linked to the infrequently occurring tibialis spastic varus foot.

The most common sites of coalitions are between the talus and the calcaneus at the middle facet joint and between the calcaneus and the navicular. Review of the literature indicates that talocalcaneal and calcaneonavicular coalitions occur with about equal frequency and together account for approximately 90% of the total number of coalitions. In recent study, a 20% incidence of multiple coalitions in the same foot was demonstrated, which is a higher incidence than had previously been reported. The incidence of bilaterality is believed to be between 50% and 80%. Because many individuals with tarsal coalition are asymptomatic and never evaluated, the true relative incidence of the different types of coalitions, the true incidence of bilaterality, and the true incidence of tarsal coalitions in general is unknown.

The pathophysiology is one of gradual metaplasia from a syndesmosis (fibrous coalition) to a synchondrosis (cartilage) to a synostosis (bone) between the affected bones. A coincident progressive restriction of subtalar motion with flattening of the longitudinal arch and valgus deformity of the hindfoot occurs. With calcaneonavicular coalitions, these changes generally take place between age 8 and 12 years, and they take place with talocalcaneal coalitions between age 12 and 16 years. These changes occur in almost all affected feet, but only approximately 25% of feet with tarsal coalition become symptomatic. The onset of symptoms usually coincides with metaplasia of the coalition from cartilage to bone; however, symptoms may occur while the coalition is still in the fibrous stage.

The pain has been attributed to ligament strain, peroneal muscle spasm, irritation or impingement in the sinus tarsi, subtalar joint irritation, fracture through the synchondrosis, stress shift to the adjacent mobile joints, and degenerative arthrosis. There may, in fact, be multiple sites and sources of pain in a foot with a coalition, depending on the location of the coalition, the age of the patient, the mobility of the Achilles tendon, and other factors. Results of a recent histologic evaluation of nonosseous talocalcaneal coalitions suggested that repetitive mechanical stress seemed to induce pain via free nerve endings in the periosteum and the articular capsules surrounding the coalition. There was evidence of microfracture, repair, and remodeling in the boundary between the coalition site and the bone. In that study, no nerve elements were observed in the fibrocartilaginous tissue at the coalition.

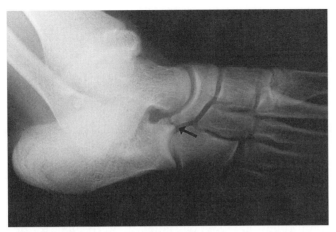

Figure 6 Oblique radiograph of a foot with a cartilaginous calcaneonavicular coalition (arrow). *(Reproduced from Richards BS (ed): Orthopaedic Knowledge Update: Pediatrics. Rosemont, IL, American Academy of Orthopaedic Surgeons, 1996, pp 211-218.)*

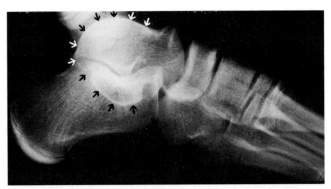

Figure 7 The C sign (*arrows*) is formed by the medial outline of the talar dome and the inferior outline of the sustentaculum tali. The C sign is a very reliable indicator of a talocalcaneal coalition.

The onset of pain is often insidious, but may be precipitated by some unusual activity or injury. Pain is usually aggravated by activity and relieved by rest. Deep aching pain of mild to moderate severity is usually experienced in the sinus tarsi area, particularly with calcaneonavicular coalitions. Pain may also be experienced along the medial aspect of the hindfoot, particularly with talocalcaneal coalitions. Occasionally, children report recurrent ankle sprains with anterolateral ankle pain. Pain under the head of the plantar flexed talus that is induced by weight bearing, as occurs in a flexible flatfoot with a short Achilles tendon, is often reported in feet with the most severe valgus deformities. There is usually tenderness at the site of the coalition, and there may be tenderness on the dorsal aspect of the talonavicular joint.

The flatfoot deformity in tarsal coalition has variously been described as rigid and peroneal spastic. Rigidity refers to the restriction of subtalar joint motion, which can be assessed in several ways. The subtalar joint must be isolated and manipulated with the ankle joint held in neutral alignment. With a talocalcaneal coalition, the subtalar joint will not invert and the arch will not elevate during toe standing and the Jack toe-raising test. With a calcaneonavicular coalition the foot is generally less rigid and less flat than with a talocalcaneal coalition, which makes inherent sense because a calcaneonavicular coalition does not cross the subtalar joint and a talocalcaneal coalition does. The concept of peroneal spasm has been questioned. There certainly appears to be adaptive shortening of the peroneal tendons associated with tarsal coalition, but most authors question whether the muscles are actually in spasm.

Radiographic evaluation should include weight-bearing AP, lateral, oblique, and axial (Harris)

views. An oblique radiograph of the foot (Fig. 6) provides the best view of a calcaneonavicular coalition. A cartilaginous coalition appears as an articulation with somewhat undulating subchondral bone surfaces. An osseous coalition is obvious and is seen on the weight-bearing lateral radiograph as an elongated process of the anterior calcaneus, called the anteater nose sign.

Other radiographic findings that are best seen on the lateral view may include dorsal beaking on the talar head, broadening and rounding of the lateral process of the talus, and narrowing of the posterior talocalcaneal facet joint. The C sign (Fig. 7), a C-shaped line formed by the medial outline of the talar dome and the inferior outline of the sustentaculum tali, is a very reliable indicator of a talocalcaneal coalition.

The normal subtalar joint complex is the shock absorber of the foot and has both gliding and rotatory motions during walking. Excessive stress is applied to the other joints of the foot when these motions are restricted. The talar beak, which often forms on the dorsal surface of the talar head in feet with tarsal coalitions, most likely represents a traction spur caused by stress on the dorsal talonavicular ligament. The talar beak likely does not indicate early degenerative arthrosis of the talonavicular joint; however, if actual degeneration of the articular surfaces occurs, a talar beak will be present eventually. Other indications of unusual stresses created by restricted subtalar motion include flattening and broadening of the lateral talar process, which result from impingement of the talus on the lateral aspect of the calcaneal sulcus and are seen on lateral radiographs.

An AP radiograph of the ankle should also be obtained, which may reveal a ball-and-socket ankle in patients with longstanding tarsal coalition, particularly with large nonidiopathic types of coalitions.

Although a talocalcaneal coalition can be seen on an axial, or Harris, radiograph, the best way to assess a coalition in this location is with a CT scan (Fig. 8). The

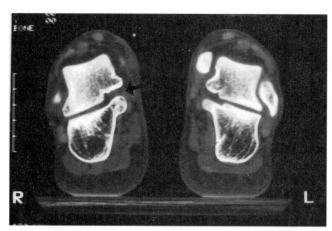

Figure 8 CT image of a talocalcaneal coalition of the middle facet of the subtalar joint (*arrow*). The facet joint is narrow, irregular, and down-sloping. (*Reproduced from Richards BS (ed): Orthopaedic Knowledge Update: Pediatrics. Rosemont, IL, American Academy of Orthopaedic Surgeons, 1996, pp 211-218.*)

images must be obtained in the coronal plane using 3- to 5-mm thick slices. Prior to resection of a tarsal coalition, a CT scan in the transaxial and coronal planes should be obtained because of the known risk of multiple coalitions in the same foot.

If the plain radiograph and CT scan are nondiagnostic, an MRI study can be used to identify a symptomatic tarsal coalition that is still in the fibrous stage of differentiation. The MRI should not be a first-line study. A bone scan can help to identify the true cause of pain in a foot with radiographic evidence of a tarsal coalition but an atypical history or pain pattern.

Other causes of a rigid flatfoot include juvenile rheumatoid arthritis, septic arthritis, and osteomyelitis. If evaluation fails to confirm a suspected tarsal coalition, a complete blood count with differential, erythrocyte sedimentation rate, C-reactive protein, antinuclear antibody, and rheumatoid factor may be warranted.

Treatment is indicated only for symptomatic tarsal coalitions. It is not clear what causes some coalitions to become painful, but injury underlies the pain. Symptom relief should be attempted by nonsurgical means such as activity modification, nonsteroidal anti-inflammatory drugs, over-the-counter shoe inserts, and immobilization in a cast-type walking boot or a below-the-knee walking cast. Pain is generally relieved completely within 24 to 48 hours of cast application, although the cast should remain in place for 4 to 6 weeks. Lasting pain relief has been reported in 30% to 68% of patients with talocalcaneal coalitions and in 58% of patients with calcaneonavicular coalitions who were treated by nonsurgical means.

Surgery is indicated for patients with recurrent and disabling symptoms following legitimate attempts at nonsurgical management. The goal of nonsurgical treatment is pain relief, not the elimination of the coalition or the reestablishment of the longitudinal arch.

The goal of surgery is pain relief with elimination of the coalition and reestablishment of subtalar motion and the longitudinal arch. If elimination of the coalition and reestablishment of motion are not possible, then pain relief may be achieved by arthrodesis. Surgical options, therefore, include resection of the coalition, osteotomy, and arthrodesis. Resection of calcaneonavicular coalitions was first reported in 1927. Interposition of the extensor digitorum brevis into the resection cavity was added to the procedure and reported on in 1970. When compared with resection alone, the combined procedure decreases the incidence of recurrence and increases the incidence of long-term pain relief in 77% of patients. According to one report, resection of a calcaneonavicular coalition with muscle interposition is indicated in a patient younger than age 16 years who has a cartilaginous bar with no other coalitions present, no evidence of degenerative arthrosis, and who has undergone unsuccessful nonsurgical treatment. However, the age limit, the coalition tissue type, and the influence of coexisting coalitions have not been established scientifically. The presence of a talar beak does not indicate degenerative arthrosis and is not, by itself, a contraindication for resection.

The role of surgical resection of a talocalcaneal coalition is less clear. This coalition is located on the tension side of the valgus deformity of the hindfoot, and further progressive flattening of the arch may occur following resection. Investigation has only recently focused on a frequently quoted, but unproven, statement in the literature that a talocalcaneal coalition should not be resected if it occupies more than one half of the width of the subtalar joint. Unsatisfactory results of resection in feet in which the ratio of the surface area of the coalition to the surface area of the posterior facet was greater than 50% (as determined by CT scan mapping of the entire joint) were reported. There was excessive valgus deformity of the hindfoot in all of these feet. Many of the feet with poor outcomes also had narrowing of the posterior facet and impingement of the lateral process of the talus on the calcaneus. Neither this study nor any other to date has determined the independent influence of the size of the coalition.

Successful resection and interposition grafting of talocalcaneal coalitions have been reported in up to 89% of patients at 10 years' follow-up; however, most published and unpublished studies have documented a lower success rate at a shorter follow-up. The poor results have been attributed to poor surgical indications, which include resection of large coalitions in feet with excessive hindfoot valgus, and in the presence of degenerative arthrosis. Interposition can be with fat or a split portion of the flexor hallucis longus tendon.

Documented degenerative arthrosis, particularly in adults, and persistent or recurrent pain following resection of a coalition are reasonable indications for a triple arthrodesis; however, establishing which joint or joints are arthritic is important. If the talocalcaneal joint is the only degenerative joint, an isolated subtalar arthrodesis can reasonably be performed while avoiding arthrodesis of the talonavicular and calcaneocuboid joints. Motion in those transverse tarsal joints will be diminished by 40%. Maintaining some motion, however, can help compensate for the loss of subtalar joint mobility and provide some stress relief for the ankle joint. The talonavicular and calcaneocuboid joints can be fused at a later time if degeneration and pain occur.

As an alternative to arthrodesis, osteotomy may play a role in treating symptomatic tarsal coalitions. A medial closing wedge osteotomy of the posterior portion of the calcaneus has been shown to relieve symptoms and improve foot shape in certain feet with severe valgus deformity of the hindfoot for which arthrodesis is being considered. The Evans calcaneal lengthening osteotomy completely corrects valgus deformity of the hindfoot at the site of deformity with or without resection of the coalition. However, the respective roles of these procedures in the management of tarsal coalitions remain uncertain. These two procedures should be considered for the painful rigid flatfoot with severe valgus deformity, minimal degenerative arthrosis, pain under the talar head, an unresectable coalition, or a coalition with recurrent pain or deformity following resection.

Annotated Bibliography

Flexible Flatfoot

Cowan DN, Robinson JR, Jones BH, Polly DW Jr, Berrey BH: Consistency of visual assessments of arch height among clinicians. *Foot Ankle Int* 1994;15: 213-217.

Four-plane photographs of the weight-bearing right foot of 246 young male army trainees were independently evaluated by six clinicians and rated on a five-category scale that ranged from clearly flatfooted to clearly high arched. The clinicians' assessments varied, even for extremes of foot type.

Sachithanandam V, Joseph B: The influence of footwear on the prevalence of flat foot: A survey of 1846 skeletally mature persons. *J Bone Joint Surg Br* 1995;77: 254-257.

Static footprints of 1,846 skeletally mature individuals were analyzed. A 3.24% incidence of flatfoot among those who started to wear shoes before age 6 years, a 3.27% incidence in those who began to wear shoes between age 6 and 15 years, and a 1.75% incidence in those who first wore shoes at age of 16 years were noted. This was statistically significant and suggested an association between the wearing of shoes in early childhood and the incidence of flatfoot.

Sekiya JK, Saltzman CL: Long term follow-up of medial column fusion and tibialis anterior transposition for adolescent flatfoot deformity. *Iowa Orthop J* 1997;17: 121-129.

This is a report on flatfoot in four feet in three adolescent patients that were corrected surgically more than 50 years previously. The surgery involved medial column stabilization with fusion procedures and tibialis anterior transposition to the navicular. The authors reported a high rate of painful arthrosis that developed over time in the contiguous joints of the foot.

Verheyden F, Vanlommel E, Van Der Bauwhede J, Fabry G, Molenaers G: The sinus tarsi spacer in the operative treatment of flexible flat feet. *Acta Orthop Belg* 1997;63:305-309.

A sinus tarsi spacer was inserted in 45 feet in 29 patients with flexible flatfoot. Although there was radiographic improvement in the height of the arch, the patients had pain and functional impairment for an average of 5 months, as well as a high rate of spacer dislocation. In consideration of these results and the known natural history of spontaneous arch development in children, the authors no longer advise using this procedure as a routine treatment for flexible flatfoot.

Tarsal Coalition

Clarke DM: Multiple tarsal coalitions in the same foot. *J Pediatr Orthop* 1997;17:777-780.

With the use of CT scans, 6 of 30 children with symptomatic tarsal coalition were found to have multiple coalitions in the same foot, which is a higher percentage than had previously been reported. The author recommended that CT evaluation of both feet in transaxial and coronal planes be obtained in patients with suspected tarsal coalition.

Cohen BE, Davis WH, Anderson RB: Success of calcaneonavicular coalition resection in the adult population. *Foot Ankle Int* 1996;17:569-572.

Following failure of conservative treatment, 10 of 12 adult patients, age 19 to 48 years, achieved subjective pain relief at an average of 36 months after resection of calcaneonavicular coalitions. Preoperative radiographs showed evidence of degenerative arthrosis in 10 feet and talar beaking in seven feet.

Emery KH, Bisset GS III, Johnson ND, Nunan PJ: Tarsal coalition: A blinded comparison of MRI and CT. *Pediatr Radiol* 1998;28:612-616.

Coronal and axial CT and MRI studies were obtained for 40 feet in 20 patients with symptoms suggesting tarsal coalition. Both modalities correctly identified 15 coalitions and missed one calcaneonavicular coalition. The MRI study resulted in only one false-negative result, an atypical incomplete talocalcaneal coalition that was seen on the CT scan. The authors concluded that CT is the gold standard and the more cost-effective imaging study for detecting tarsal coalition. MRI is also very good for detecting tarsal coalition, particularly if other causes for ankle or foot pain are being considered.

Kumai T, Takakura Y, Akiyama K, Higashiyama I, Tamai S: Histopathological study of nonosseous tarsal coalition. *Foot Ankle Int* 1998;19:525-531.

Thirty-one talocalcaneal, nine calcaneonavicular, and 15 naviculocuneiform nonosseous tarsal coalitions were resected in 48 patients at an average age of 19.8 years (range 5 to 61 years), and the specimens were subjected to histopathologic study. The histology of the fibrocartilaginous tissue in the coalition was similar to that seen in the tendinous attachment site of Osgood-Schlatter disease, accessory navicular, and bipartite patellae. The histologic features were consistent with a process of destruction, repair, and remodeling of osteochondral damage and with chronic degenerative changes of the interface between the cartilage and bone tissue.

Lateur LM, Van Hoe LR, Van Ghillewe KV, Gryspeerdt SS, Baert AL, Dereymaeker GE: Subtalar coalition: Diagnosis with the C sign on lateral radiographs of the ankle. *Radiology* 1994;193:847-851.

The authors describe the C sign as a C-shaped line that is formed by the medial outline of the talar dome and the inferior outline of the sustentaculum tali on lateral radiographs of the ankle. In the retrospective portion of the study, surgery confirmed the C sign's reliability as an indicator of subtalar coalition; in the prospective portion of the study, CT or MRI confirmed its reliability.

Mann RA, Beaman DN, Horton GA: Isolated subtalar arthrodesis. *Foot Ankle Int* 1998;19:511-519.

Isolated subtalar arthrodesis was performed on 44 feet with hindfoot pathology on which 10 of the feet had a talocalcaneal coalition. The average age at surgery for this subgroup was 26 years. At an average follow-up of 91 months, the AOFAS score was 93 of a possible 100 points, and 88% of the patients were satisfied or very satisfied with their results. Six patients had radiographic evidence of mild talonavicular arthrosis, but all were asymptomatic. Sixty percent of transverse tarsal motion was preserved.

Raikin S, Cooperman DR, Thompson GH: Interposition of the split flexor hallucis longus tendon after resection of a coalition of the middle facet of the talocalcaneal joint. *J Bone Joint Surg Am* 1999;81:11-19.

Fourteen feet in 10 patients with painful middle facet talocalcaneal coalitions that had failed conservative management underwent resection of the coalition and interposition of a split portion of the flexor hallucis longus tendon. At a mean follow-up of 51 months (range 32 to 60 months), 12 of the feet were rated as excellent and good using the AOFAS rating system. None of the patients had symptoms or functional impairment of the great toe.

Wechsler RJ, Schweitzer ME, Deely DM, Horn BD, Pizzutillo PD: Tarsal coalition: Depiction and characterization with CT and MR imaging. *Radiology* 1994;193:447-452.

Preoperative CT and MRI were obtained for 10 feet in nine patients, age 11 to 18 years, who had not responded to nonsurgical treatment of suspected tarsal coalition. All nine coalitions found at surgery were correctly depicted on MRI; however, MRI incorrectly characterized a case of proliferative synovitis as a fibrous coalition. Six coalitions were depicted on CT; however, the fibrous coalitions were not correctly characterized.

Classic Bibliography

Evans D: Calcaneo-valgus deformity. *J Bone Joint Surg Br* 1975;57:270-278.

Harris RI, Beath T: *Army Foot Survey: An Investigation of Foot Ailments in Canadian Soldiers.* Ottawa, Ontario, Canada, National Research Council of Canada, 1947.

Harris RI, Beath T: Etiology of peroneal spastic flat foot. *J Bone Joint Surg Br* 1948;30:624-634.

Mosca VS: Calcaneal lengthening for valgus deformity of the hindfoot: Results in children who had severe, symptomatic flatfoot and skewfoot. *J Bone Joint Surg Am* 1995;77:500-512.

Simmons EH: Tibialis spastic varus foot with tarsal coalition. *J Bone Joint Surg Br* 1965;47:533-536.

Slomann HC: On coalitio calcaneo-navicularis. *J Orthop Surg* 1921;3:586-602.

Wilde PH, Torode IP, Dickens DR, Cole WG: Resection for symptomatic talocalcaneal coalition. *J Bone Joint Surg Br* 1994;76:797-801.

Chapter 23

Miscellaneous Foot Disorders

Richard S. Davidson, MD

Bunions

A bunion is an enlargement of the first metatarsophalangeal (MTP) joint at the medial aspect and often is associated with hallux valgus. Although bunions generally are considered an adult or geriatric condition, they may occur in early adolescence or before. Onset often coincides with the wearing of stylish shoes that are too narrow. Progression of the deformity through adolescence may be related to persistent ligamentous laxity and continued angular growth of the foot.

The etiology of the bunion is multifactorial and may include improperly fitting shoes, genetics, ligamentous laxity, pes planus, pronation of the hallux, and spasticity, as with cerebral palsy. Often, a varus angulation of the first metatarsocuneiform joint exists, which may predispose the patient to hallux valgus if tight-fitting shoes are worn. No gender predilection has been documented, although women undergo surgical correction more often than men.

Patients usually are concerned about the appearance of the foot and also report difficulty with shoe fit and pain in the region of the bunion or first MTP joint. Additional causes of pain such as plantar fasciitis, hammer toe, stress fracture, ingrown toenail, accessory tarsal navicular, or sesamoiditis should be ruled out. Pes planus, foot pronation, and hallux pronation often are present, and the tibia may be externally rotated. The patient should be observed walking without shoes, and the angular and rotational alignment of the lower extremities should be clinically assessed. Hindfoot and forefoot valgus should be evaluated, as well as ankle, subtalar, and toe range of motion. Often, ankle dorsiflexion is limited as a result of a tight heel cord. Limited hindfoot inversion with excessive eversion or a stiff hindfoot should be ruled out, as well as hallux rigidus and limited dorsiflexion of the first MTP joint. The foot should be palpated for areas of tenderness and callus formation.

Radiographic evaluation includes weight-bearing AP and lateral views of both feet. The shape, congruity, and orientation of the first MTP joint and the cuneiform-first metatarsal joint should be evaluated. The intermetatarsal and hallux valgus angles should be measured. The intermetatarsal angle, which is the angle between the first and second metatarsal, normally is 6° to 10°, and the hallux valgus angle normally is 10° to 20° (Fig. 1). Oblique and Harris radiographic views or CT may be indicated if a tarsal coalition is suspected. Bone scan or MRI should be obtained if a stress fracture is suspected.

Treatment of bunions in the child or adolescent begins with a complete understanding of the patient's and parent's concerns. Usually, the patient is asymptomatic but wants to know if the bunion should be prophylactically repaired to prevent later problems. In these circumstances, reassurance usually is all that is necessary. Pain with shoe wear may be treated successfully with patient education and shoe modifications. The patient and parents should be instructed on proper shoe fit and the need to avoid shoes with high heels and narrow toe boxes. Occasionally, shoe modifications such as bunion lasts, soft uppers, metatarsal bars, and heel cups to accommodate a narrow heel are necessary. The benefit of night splints is controversial; in a recent study, no benefits from the use of orthotics were reported.

Surgery may be considered in patients who experience pain that interferes with normal activities and has not been relieved with shoe modifications. A pain-free foot should not be treated surgically because of the risk of postoperative pain and stiffness. In addition, surgical correction generally should be postponed until skeletal maturity because of the high recurrence rate of bunions in young adolescent patients. Surgical options include soft-tissue balancing procedures of the first MTP joint, distal first metatarsal osteotomy, proximal first metatarsal osteotomy, and double first meta-

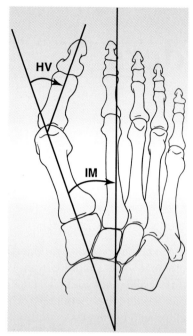

Figure 1 Drawing demonstrates method of measuring the intermetatarsal angle (IM) and the hallux valgus angle (HV).

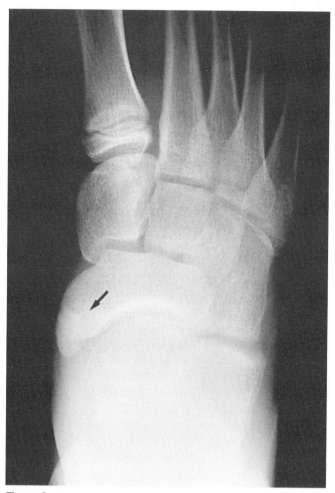

Figure 2 Accessory tarsal navicular. (Reproduced from Richards BS (ed): Orthopaedic Knowledge Update: Pediatrics. Rosemont, IL, American Academy of Orthopaedic Surgeons, 1996, pp 219-225.)

tarsal osteotomies. Mild bunion deformities (intermetatarsal angle of less than 25°) may be treated with a distal first metatarsal osteotomy or the McBride procedure. Moderate and severe bunion deformities (intermetatarsal angle of greater than 25°) with subluxation of the MTP joint may be treated with a proximal first metatarsal osteotomy and distal soft-tissue balancing. Distal osteotomies combined with soft-tissue balancing of the first MTP joint should be avoided to prevent osteonecrosis of the first metatarsal head. An abnormal distal metatarsal articular angle may be treated with a double osteotomy of the first metatarsal. Excessive varus of the first metatarsocuneiform joint may be treated with an opening wedge osteotomy of the first cuneiform.

Accessory Tarsal Navicular

An accessory tarsal navicular is an accessory bone that is located at the medial tuberosity of the navicular bone. It may be either a separate small bone within the posterior tibial tendon at its insertion or a large bone at the tendon insertion that is separated from the navicular by a thin fibrocartilaginous plate (Fig. 2). Approximately 10% to 14% of adolescents have accessory tarsal navicular bones. Most patients are asymptomatic and diagnosed serendipitously on radiograph. If symptoms do occur, they usually develop between age 8 and 14 years, when the ossicle first begins to ossify. A history of minor trauma or shoe pressure on the affected area is common. Generally, the area over the navicular tuberosity prominence is tender. Pes planus is apparent in

many patients as the prominent navicular tuberosity creates a convexity along the medial longitudinal arch. Careful examination can differentiate a painful accessory tarsal navicular from other painful conditions, such as sesamoiditis, stress fractures of the first metatarsal or tarsal, posterior tibial tendinitis, tarsal coalition, tarsal tunnel syndrome, plantar fasciitis, synovitis, arthritis, or tumors.

The accessory tarsal navicular is best viewed on oblique radiographs of the foot. Weight-bearing AP and lateral views also should be obtained to rule out other conditions and provide additional information about the navicular. In the very young child, a palpable mass may not be seen on radiographs because of a lack of ossification, although MRI may reveal an accessory tarsal navicular before it is ossified enough to be seen on radiographs. MRI of a patient with a symptomatic accessory navicular may show a bone marrow edema pattern. Scintigraphy also may be used to identify a symptomatic accessory navicular.

Almost all children and adolescents with symptomatic accessory navicular bones become asymptomatic as they reach skeletal maturity and the medial tuberosity of the navicular is completely ossified. Therefore, patients and parents should be reassured of the self-limiting nature of this problem. Initial treatment of symptoms includes non-narcotic analgesics, restriction of activity, and shoe modification to avoid pressure on the tender prominence. Orthotics (arches) may support the foot and relieve tension on the posterior tendon and prevent the prominence from pushing against the medial aspect of the shoe or from bearing weight. Below-knee casts and the judicious use of steroid injections may help resolve the condition. Several weeks of nonsurgical treatment should be attempted before surgery is considered.

Surgery should be considered in patients in whom an extended period of nonsurgical treatment was unsuccessful and who continue to have symptoms that interfere with activities. Simple excision of the accessory tarsal navicular is recommended, as is repair of the roughened posterior tibialis tendon to the cancellous bed of the excised accessory tarsal navicular. Advancement of the tibialis posterior tendon does not improve the results. Removal of the accessory tarsal navicular and complete removal of the medial prominence are recommended because symptoms may persist in patients who have a residual medial prominence. Surgical removal of an asymptomatic accessory tarsal navicular is not necessary.

Congenital Vertical Talus

A vertical talus is a fixed congenital dorsolateral dislocation of the talonavicular joint with hindfoot equinus. The talus is plantar flexed in a vertical posture with the dorsally dislocated navicular pressing down on the talar neck. Clinically, the patient has a rocker bottom flatfoot (also called congenital convex pes valgus) in which the heel is fixed in an equinovalgus position, the midfoot is fixed in valgus, and the forefoot is dorsiflexed on the midfoot (Fig. 3). In addition, there are contractures of the Achilles tendon, peroneal tendons, and anterior ankle tendons. The talar head is prominent in the plantar medial aspect of the foot and is easily palpated but is not reducible.

Congenital vertical talus is uncommon. Approximately 60% of cases are idiopathic; the remaining 40% are associated with conditions such as arthrogryposis multiplex congenita syndrome, Larsen's syndrome, neurofibromatosis, nail-patella syndrome, chromosomal anomalies (trisomy 13 to 15 and 19), and certain neurologic conditions (myelomeningocele, tethered cord, lipoma of the cord, and sacral agenesis). Dysplasia of the hip and contralateral

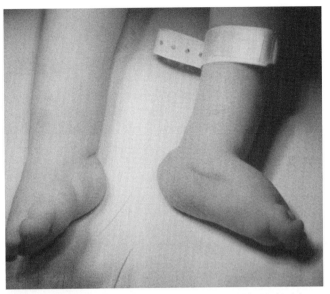

Figure 3 Photograph of an infant's feet showing a right clubfoot and a left congenital vertical talus.

clubfoot may occur with increased frequency in patients with this disorder.

In many patients, a neuromuscular imbalance results in contracture of the posterior muscles (the gastrocnemius-soleus muscles), lateral muscles (the peroneus longus and brevis muscles), and anterior muscles (the tibialis anterior, extensor digitorum longus, extensor hallucis, and possibly the peroneus tertius muscles). The talonavicular joint dislocates dorsolaterally, forcing the navicular to rest on the dorsolateral talar neck and subsequently plantar flexes the talus in the mortise. The os calcis laterally rotates from under the talus. The lateral column of the foot is deformed into valgus.

The differential diagnosis includes oblique talus (the talonavicular joint is subluxated but reduces with plantar flexion), calcaneovalgus foot, flexible flatfoot with midfoot sag and short Achilles tendon, rigid flatfoot associated with tarsal coalition, and peroneal spastic flatfoot. In the young child, hypermobility and a flexible valgus flatfoot are included as well.

AP, dorsiflexed lateral, and plantar flexed lateral radiographs (Fig. 4) should be obtained to confirm the diagnosis. The AP view demonstrates the midfoot valgus and increased talocalcaneal angle. The dorsiflexed lateral view demonstrates the dislocation of the navicular on the talar neck, as well as the fixed equinus position of the hindfoot. The increased talocalcaneal angle confirms the hindfoot valgus. The plantar flexed lateral view demonstrates that the talonavicular dislocation is not reducible. A line drawn on the radiograph through the long axis of the talus and another drawn through the first metatarsal will not converge in front of the talar head. In the infant, only the metatarsals,

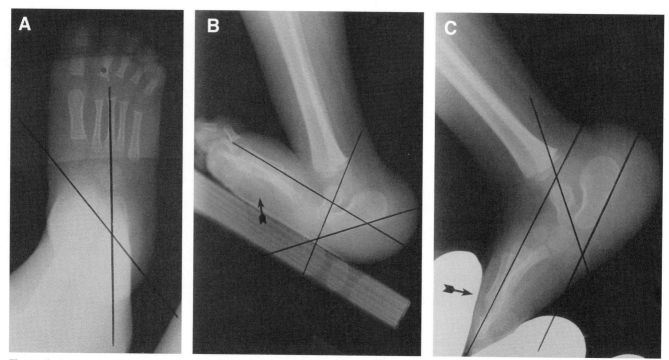

Figure 4 Congenital vertical talus. **A,** AP radiograph reveals that the angle between the talus and calcaneus is increased. **B,** The dorsiflexion stressed lateral radiograph shows that the calcaneus remains in the equinus position. **C,** The plantar flexion-stressed lateral radiograph reveals that the forefoot remains dorsally dislocated on the talus. The talar line and first metatarsal line should parallel each other. *(Reproduced from Richards BS (ed): Orthopaedic Knowledge Update: Pediatrics. Rosemont, IL, American Academy of Orthopaedic Surgeons, 1996, pp 219-225.)*

talus, and calcaneus are likely to be ossified. Drawing lines through these three bones on the radiograph confirms the diagnosis.

Congenital vertical talus produces few problems in shoe wear or ambulation in the very young child. However, a painful callus over the weight-bearing talar head develops in the older child, resulting in difficulty with shoe fit. Ultimately, degenerative arthritis and pain at the dislocated talonavicular joint develop.

Initial treatment includes stretching exercises and/or serial casting with the forefoot plantar flexed on the hindfoot. Although these techniques are unlikely to reduce the dislocated talonavicular joint, they will stretch the contracted tendons and facilitate reduction at the time of surgery. During surgery, the talonavicular dislocation must be reduced, the subtalar joint derotated, and the contracted posterior, lateral, and dorsal muscles and tendons lengthened. In addition, the posterior ankle and subtalar (talocalcaneal and talonavicular) capsules and ligaments must be lengthened as needed. The Cincinnati incision allows sufficient exposure to accomplish a complete release. Kirschner wire (K-wire) fixation holds the reduction in place. Postoperative casting for 3 months is recommended. Residual or untreated deformity of the vertical talus in the older child may be salvaged by arthrodesis or talectomy.

Sever's Disease

Sever's disease is an apophysitis of the calcaneus. It is the most common cause of heel pain in the adolescent. Patients typically have a history of sports participation and intermittent heel pain. The heel pain tends to occur after physical activity or with the first few steps taken after awakening. A history of trauma is conspicuously absent. The patient may limp; however, swelling and discoloration usually are absent. The calcaneal tuberosity is tender. Other conditions, such as Achilles tendinitis, stress fracture of the os calcis, plantar fasciitis, entrapment of the plantar or calcaneal nerves (tarsal tunnel syndrome), medial facet talocalcaneal coalition, accessory tarsal navicular, Salter-Harris type I fracture of the calcaneal apophysis, cysts, and tumors, also may result in foot pain near the heel and should be ruled out.

Weight-bearing AP, lateral, oblique, and Harris view radiographs should be obtained to rule out other abnormalities, such as bone cyst or stress fracture, particularly if unilateral. Sever's disease, however, is not diagnosed on radiographs. Sclerosis and irregularities of the calcaneal apophysis are common in both the symptomatic and asymptomatic heel.

Treatment of calcaneal apophysitis begins with a period of rest, ice massage, and activity restrictions. Heel cord stretching exercises are initiated when acute inflammation resolves. Footwear can be modified to include a heel cushion and, when appropriate, arch supports to limit hindfoot valgus. Cast immobilization, with or without weight bearing, may be considered to relieve symptoms. Fortunately, calcaneal apophysitis affects only skeletally immature patients. Surgery is not indicated.

Freiberg's Infraction

Freiberg's infraction is an osteochondrosis of the second or, less commonly, third metatarsal head and may occur bilaterally. It typically is seen in healthy, athletic, adolescent girls age 10 to 18 years. Typically, the patient reports vague pain, swelling, and loss of motion in the involved MTP joint.

Potential causes include acute trauma, repetitive trauma, and osteonecrosis. Synovitis, inflammation, loose bodies of cartilage and bone, and osteophytes may be present. Histologically, necrotic bone often is observed. Clinically, the differential diagnosis includes metatarsalgia and stress fracture.

An AP radiograph of the forefoot may demonstrate varying degrees of involvement. In the earliest stages, radiographs usually are normal. In more advanced stages, a subchondral fracture may be evident with joint widening, sclerosis, and flattening of the metatarsal head (Fig. 5). Collapse, fragmentation, osteophytes, revascularization, and healing may be evident with further disease progression, followed by degenerative arthrosis. An early diagnosis may be made using bone scan and MRI.

Nonsurgical treatment is most effective in the early stages of Freiberg's infraction and includes activity restriction, shoe modifications using stiff rocker soles or metatarsal bars, cast immobilization, avoiding weight bearing, and judicious use of corticosteroids. Return to regular sports activities should be gradual. It may be months or years before pain-free activity can be resumed.

Surgery occasionally is necessary and may include joint débridement, subchondral bone grafting, shortening osteotomy of the metatarsal, partial or complete metatarsal head excision, joint replacement, excision of the proximal portion of the proximal phalanx, replacement and pinning of large fragments, and metatarsal neck osteotomy to redirect the articular surface. Most authors report success with these treatments; however, studies have been small and not comparative.

Cavus Foot

A cavus foot has an excessively high arch, which can be the result of plantar flexion of the first metatarsal, pronation of the forefoot, contracture of the plantar fascia, plantar flexion of the talonavicular or naviculocuneiform joints, hindfoot varus, or calcaneus defor-

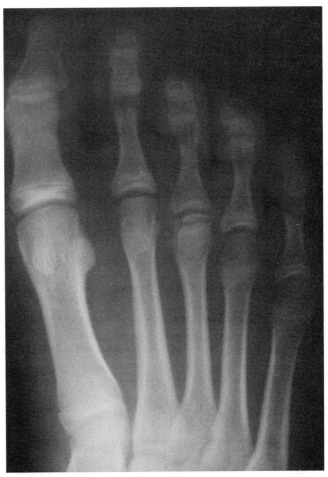

Figure 5 Freiberg's infraction. AP radiograph demonstrates a subchondral fracture and flattening of the third metatarsal head.

mity. Many of these deformities occur in combination. The anatomic deformity may be idiopathic or the result of a neurologic abnormality. Neurologic causes include Charcot-Marie-Tooth disease, Dejerine-Sottas disease, Refsum's disease, spina bifida, tethered cord, and polio. Because of the numerous neurologic causes of cavus foot, every patient with cavus foot should undergo a thorough neurologic exam.

Patients generally report foot deformity or pain, or difficulty with shoe wear. A known underlying neurologic condition may be present. Evaluation includes observation of the foot during walking, in stance, and while suspended, and ankle and subtalar range of motion. Particular attention should be paid to any fixed hindfoot varus. The lateral block test is used to differentiate rigid from flexible hindfoot varus and calcaneus varus. The forefoot is evaluated for supination and the toes for clawing.

Weight-bearing AP and lateral radiographs demonstrate the skeletal deformity. Hindfoot talocalcaneal and first metatarsal-talus angles are measured on the lateral projection. The first metatarsal-talus angle is normally 0° and increases (apex dorsal) as a cavus deformity worsens.

Any underlying neurologic conditions must be ruled out prior to initiating treatment. Conditions that can be treated with surgery, such as tethered cord, should be corrected prior to surgery for the cavus foot. Progressive neurologic diseases, such as Charcot-Marie-Tooth disease, may result in a progressive foot deformity that can recur after surgical correction. Treatment of cavus foot is indicated when the patient has pain, difficulty with shoe wear, and progressive foot deformity. Many patients with mild cavus foot deformities have no pain and participate in essentially unlimited activities. These patients need no specific treatment. Shoe modifications accommodate claw toes, forefoot pronation, metatarsalgia, high instep, and heel varus in patients with mild symptoms. Stretching exercises may help these patients, and molded ankle-foot orthoses may allow them to participate in recreational sports throughout the school years. However, many patients do not return to sports after undergoing an osteotomy or arthrodesis.

Soft-tissue releases of the plantar fascia, intrinsic muscles, and peroneus longus and tendon transfer of the posterior tibialis to the dorsum of the foot may improve the flexible foot. The disease process eventually may weaken the transferred posterior tibialis tendon, limiting the benefit of the transfer.

Osteotomy and/or arthrodesis may be required to correct rigid deformities in skeletally mature patients. Osteotomies that are commonly used include dorsal closing wedge osteotomies of the first, or infrequently, all of the metatarsals; tarsometatarsal wedge osteotomies; and valgus, posterior, and/or lateral sliding osteotomies of the os calcis. Soft-tissue release prior to osteotomy and arthrodesis reduces the amount of bony correction that is required. Arthrodesis should be used only to correct severe deformity, because loss of joint motion may transfer stresses to adjacent joints, resulting in subsequent degenerative arthritis. Persistent neuromuscular imbalance and/or progression of the disease process may result in a recurrence of the deformity despite surgery performed early in the course of the disease.

Curly Toe

A curly toe is clinically manifested by excessive flexion of the MTP and interphalangeal (IP) joints with medial deviation of the involved toe under the adjacent uninvolved toe (Fig. 6). The third toe most often is involved. The etiology is unknown but an autosomal dominant inheritance pattern is suspected. The deformity itself is caused by a contracture of the flexor digitorum longus. Generally, the deformity improves with time, and many completely resolve. Curly toe does not interfere with a toddler's ability to walk, and buddy taping or splinting

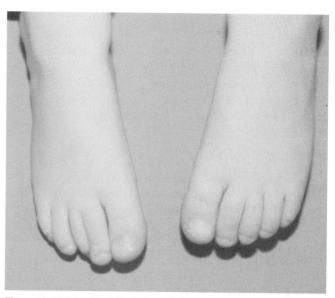

Figure 6 Curly toe. The right middle toe is plantar flexed and deviated medially.

the toe in an attempt to correct the deformity is not necessary. Curly toe deformities rarely produce pain. Tenotomy of the flexor digitorum at the distal IP joint corrects the deformity in 90% of infants and young children.

Annotated Bibliography

Bunions

Coughlin MJ: Juvenile hallux valgus: Etiology and treatment. *Foot Ankle Int* 1995;16:682-697.

In this article, the author recommended a multiprocedural approach to treatment rather than using one standard method because of the high recurrence rate and the variety of associated anatomic deformities. For mild deformity, a Chevron osteotomy or a McBride procedure was recommended. For moderate to severe deformities with subluxation of the MTP joint, a distal soft-tissue procedure with proximal metatarsal osteotomy was recommended. For moderate to severe deformities with an increased metatarsal articular angle, a double osteotomy, including Chevron osteotomy, Aitkin osteotomy, first metatarsal osteotomy, and cuneiform osteotomy, were recommended. Of 60 feet treated with this method, there were six recurrences and eight complications, including six hallux varus, one wire breakage, and one undercorrection.

McDonald MG, Stevens DB: Modified Mitchell bunionectomy for management of adolescent hallux valgus. *Clin Orthop* 1996;332:163-169.

In this article, the authors reported that the modified Mitchell procedure was successful in 81% of 17 adolescent feet with hallux valgus.

Weiner BK, Weiner DS, Mirkopulos N: Mitchell osteotomy for adolescent hallux valgus. *J Pediatr Orthop* 1997;17:781-784.

A modified Mitchell osteotomy with a trapezoid step-off osteotomy to maintain length was performed in 69 adolescent feet with hallux valgus. A success rate of 91% was reported over an average 6-year follow-up. Complications included stiffness.

Accessory Tarsal Navicular

Miller TT, Staron RB, Feldman F, Parisien M, Glucksman WJ, Gandolfo LH: The symptomatic accessory tarsal navicular bone: Assessment with MR imaging. *Radiology* 1995;195:849-853.

The authors reported that increased bone marrow edema was demonstrated on MRI of symptomatic accessory navicular tarsal bones.

Congenital Vertical Talus

Kodros SA, Dias LS: Single-stage surgical correction of congenital vertical talus. *J Pediatr Orthop* 1999;19:42-48.

A single-stage surgical correction procedure, using the Cincinnati incision to release and realign the foot, was performed on 41 patients with 55 congenital vertical tali. At follow-up (average 7 years), the authors found no wound complications and 31 good and 11 fair results. The authors cautioned that underlying diagnoses are common and should be identified to minimize the risk of recurrence.

Stricker SJ, Rosen E: Early one-stage reconstruction of congenital vertical talus. *Foot Ankle Int* 1997;18: 535-543.

The method of Simeon, in which tendons of the anterior ankle are lengthened through an anterior longitudinal incision, was used to treat 20 feet with vertical talus. During this procedure, the talonavicular capsule was released to reduce the talonavicular joint, which was then held with a K-wire. The authors reported no excellent results, but 17 good and 3 fair results. Most patients demonstrated midfoot sag.

Sever's Disease

Liberson A, Lieberson S, Mendes DG, Shajrawi I, Ben Haim Y, Boss JH: Remodeling of the calcaneus apophysis in the growing child. *J Pediatr Orthop* 1995;4:74-79.

The authors used radiographs and CT scans to compare the heels of 35 children with symptoms of calcaneal apophysis and 52 control children. On lateral radiographs, increased density of the calcaneal apophysis was noted in all heels. One or two radiolucent lines (fragmentation) were noted in all of the painful heels but in only 27% of the heels in the control group. CT demonstrated normal increased density with growth.

Cavus Foot

Helliwell TR, Tynan M, Hayward M, Klenerman L, Whitehouse G, Edwards RH: The pathology of the lower leg muscles in pure forefoot pes cavus. *Acta Neuropathol* 1995;89:552-559.

The authors studied up to five muscles in each of 17 patients with cavus foot and evaluated the muscles histologically. Pathology was described for several diseases. The peroneus longus muscle was hypertrophied in diseases of unknown cause as compared to diseases of other causes.

Classic Bibliography

Canale PB, Aronsson DD, Lamont RL, Manoli A II: The Mitchell procedure for the treatment of adolescent hallux valgus: A long-term study. *J Bone Joint Surg Am* 1993;75:1610-1618.

Carpintero P, Entrenas R, Gonzalez I, Garcia E, Mesa M: The relationship between pes cavus and idiopathic scoliosis. *Spine* 1994;19:1260-1263.

Kilmartin TE, Barrington RL, Wallace WA: A controlled prospective trial of a foot orthosis for juvenile hallux valgus. *J Bone Joint Surg Br* 1994;76:210-214.

Peterson HA, Newman SR: Adolescent bunion deformity treated with double osteotomy and longitudinal fixation of the first ray. *J Pediatr Orthop* 1993;13:80-84.

Sproul J, Klaaren H, Mannarino F: Surgical treatment of Freiberg's infraction in athletes. *Am J Sports Med* 1993;21:381-384.

Tynan MC, Klenerman L: The modified Robert Jones tendon transfer in cases of pes cavus and clawed hallux. *Foot Ankle Int* 1994;15:68-71.

Section 4

Neuromuscular Disorders

Section Editor:
Mark F. Abel, MD

Section 4

Neuromuscular Disorders

Overview

The chapters in this section provide updated information on the pathophysiology of the conditions as well as current treatments. Classifications of muscular dystrophies, hereditary-sensory-motor neuropathies, and other neurodegenerative disorders have been recently modified based on new genetic information regarding the specific defects involved. New techniques for management of spasticity in patients with cerebral palsy are described. Because these conditions are incurable and amelioration is the primary goal, analysis of treatments has shifted to include more objective, outcome-based evidence, using tools such as gait analysis.

Mark F. Abel, MD
Section Editor

Chapter 24

Cerebral Palsy

Mark F. Abel, MD

Diane L. Damiano, PhD, PT

Epidemiology and Etiology

Cerebral palsy (CP) is a heterogeneous condition resulting from a static brain lesion that occurs prior to birth (prenatal) or for a variable amount of time after birth (perinatal or postnatal). The brain lesion is permanent and has deleterious effects on subsequent development and aging. The etiology of cerebral palsy includes embolic, hemorrhagic, and hypoxic brain injuries, as well as insults resulting from brain malformations and infections. Patients with genetic syndromes, metabolic derangements (enzyme deficiencies), progressive neuromuscular conditions, and brain injury acquired after childhood are excluded from this group.

The incidence of CP is 1 to 3 per 1,000 live births, making it the most prevalent physical disability originating in childhood. It is well recognized that premature infants, especially those born before 32 weeks' gestation, are at increased risk for CP, and improved survival rates of premature infants means that this incidence has not declined over the last decade. Other risk factors include maternal chorioamnionitis, placental bleeding, multiple pregnancies, hypotension, hypoventilation, hypoxia, and pulmonary insufficiency. In 35% of patients, no etiology can be determined, which underscores the limitations of current brain imaging and other diagnostic techniques. Approximately 750,000 individuals in the United States are believed to have CP.

Theories on the pathophysiology of CP are still evolving, but preterm infants appear to be selectively vulnerable to periventricular white matter injury or periventricular leukomalacia (PVL). Signs of PVL or hemorrhage are found in 50% of patients with CP who were born preterm and in 10% to 20% of those who were full-term infants, especially those with bilateral lower extremity spasticity (diplegia).

Although preterm infants are more susceptible to periventricular injury, full-term infants appear to be more susceptible to thrombotic injury. Thrombotic lesions usually are located in the distribution of the middle cerebral artery and are identified in approximately 30% of patients with congenital spastic hemiplegia.

Severe brain dysfunction results from prolonged hypoxia (hypoxic-ischemic encephalopathy), infections (viral and bacterial), brain malformations (dysgenesis of the corpus callosum and neuronal migration), and large hemorrhagic lesions. Hypoxic-ischemic encephalopathy (HIE) secondary to obstetric complications is quite rare; however, nuchal cords, prolonged extractions from the birth canal, and severe placental hemorrhage are documented in some cases. In most patients with HIE, a precise cause is not identified.

In summary, CP is a group of entities that have in common a static lesion of the immature brain. Generally, prenatal or perinatal causes are evident in 50% to 60% of patients, postnatal causes are evident in 5%, and no obvious etiology is evident in 35%. Although motor impairments are orthopaedists' primary concern, functional prognosis in CP is related to the time and extent of brain injury and the associated comorbidities. Table 1 shows the conditions that are associated with CP. As the extent of brain injury increases, seizures, mental retardation, visual impairment, hydrocephalus, malnutrition, and complex movement disorders are more likely to occur.

Management of CP is palliative, and many treatments have similar indications. Unfortunately, most studies focusing on treatment of CP are retrospective, uncontrolled cohort studies, in which the impact on function and disability are not measured. This chapter will review the classifications and management of CP.

Classifications

Classifications of CP are based on the type of movement abnormality (physiologic classification) and the affected region of the body (anatomic classification). These time-honored classifications are relevant to treatment options and prognosis (Table 2).

TABLE 1	Conditions That May Be Associated With Cerebral Palsy

Condition	% of Patients
Mental impairment or severe learning disability	40
Seizures	30
Complex movement disorders	20
Visual impairment	16
Malnutrition (gastroesophageal reflux, obesity, undernutrition)	15
Hydrocephalus	14

TABLE 2	Classifications of Cerebral Palsy

Physiologic Type	% Prevalence
Spastic	80
Extrapyramidal (dystonic)	20
Athetosis	
Chorea	
Ataxia	
Hypotonic	

Anatomic Type	% Prevalence
Diplegia	50
Hemiplegia	30
Quadriplegia (total body involvement)	20

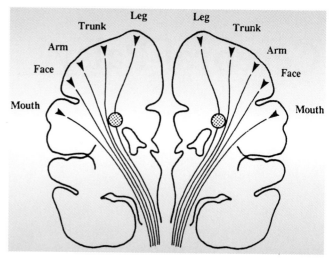

Figure 1 Diagram showing the radiation of the corticospinal tracts from the motor cortex, passing by the lateral ventricles. The proximity of the leg tracts to the ventricles is believed to be the reason for frequent leg impairment with periventricular lesions. The tight clustering of the tracts means that hemorrhagic lesions could affect the leg, trunk, and arm. *(Reproduced with permission from Gage JR (ed): Gait Analysis in Cerebral Palsy. London, England, MacKeith Press, 1991, p 9.)* •

The physiologic classification divides patients into two groups, those with spasticity and those with extrapyramidal or dyskinetic movements, based on the manifested muscle tone and movement disorder. The descriptive terms used for these classifications relate to clinical signs and movement patterns. Hyperreflexia, clonus, and velocity-dependent resistance to joint motion characterize spasticity. Spasticity is not specific for a particular brain lesion, but is a hallmark of upper motor neuron lesions in general. Nonetheless, within the context of CP, spasticity suggests injury to the pyramidal or corticospinal tract. Athetosis (writhing or jerking movements of the extremity), chorea, and ballismus indicate extrapyramidal motor damage, such as to the basal ganglia. Ataxia (impaired balance) suggests injury to the cerebellum. Hypotonia (decreased muscle tone) is another form of motor dysfunction

attributed to extrapyramidal damage. Dystonia is a general term applied to extrapyramidal movement pathology. The neuroanatomic foci that underlie these movement patterns are less specific. Generally, spasticity responds best to current interventions, while extrapyramidal movement patterns are less predictably controlled.

Treatment objectives also are related to the severity of the palsy, which in turn is related to the extent that the body is affected. The anatomic classification divides patients based on the extent of body involvement. Hemiplegia refers to involvement on one side, diplegia to involvement of the legs primarily with relative sparing of the upper extremities, and quadriplegia to involvement of all four extremities. Patients with quadriplegia are described as having 'total-body-involved' CP and are totally dependent on others for their daily needs because they lack selective movement of all extremities and truncal balance. Triplegia refers to impairment of three extremities; however, total sparing of the fourth extremity (generally an arm) is unusual (Fig. 1). Monoplegia is sparing of all extremities except one, but is rare.

In reality, neither classification system adequately conveys the heterogeneity of the population with cerebral palsy. Within each subcategory, patients have a variety of brain lesions, with a range of associated conditions and functional capacities. For example, to most clinicians familiar with CP, diplegia renders a mental image of a child born prematurely who has spasticity and poor motor control of the legs. However, the symmetry of involvement, extent of trunk and arm involvement, and need for walking aids vary with each patient

TABLE 3	Clinical Signs of Cerebral Palsy and Treatment Options

Positive Signs	Treatment Options
Hypertonicity (spasticity)	Selective dorsal rhizotomy
	Muscle-tendon surgery
	Intrathecal baclofen
	BTX-A injection
	Bracing treatment
Static contractures	Muscle-tendon surgery
Torsional deformities/joint deformity	Osteotomy
	Arthrodesis

Negative Signs	Treatment Options
Weakness	Physical therapy
Poor balance	Walking aids, bracing treatment

with diplegia. In addition, the positive signs associated with CP (spasticity) are emphasized in the two classification systems, and the other motor impairments such as weakness and impaired balance are neglected (Table 3). The negative signs are poorly measured and relatively neglected in treatment regimens.

Diagnosis and Evaluation

The history and physical examination remain the fundamental tools of diagnosis and assessment. These are complemented by three-dimensional motion analysis for detailed assessment of dynamic movement, radiographs for assessing the skeleton, and brain imaging modalities for documenting the pathologic lesion and diagnosis. The clinician must ascertain that CP is the correct diagnosis by establishing that the deficits result from a brain injury and are not progressive. Associated impairments, which are common in CP, negatively impact treatment outcomes and must be enumerated.

A thorough history of the pregnancy and delivery may shed light on the etiology and prognosis. An Apgar score of less than 5 at 10 minutes after birth and neonatal seizures often indicate significant anoxia. The ages at which motor milestones are achieved has prognostic implications as well. Prognosis for independent ambulation is guarded if sitting balance is not achieved by age 2 years. Poor ambulation can be predicted if primitive reflexes, including the Moro reflex, extensor thrust, and tonic neck reflexes, or absence of stepping and protective parachute responses are

retained beyond age 24 months. Hand dominance determined before age 18 months suggests contralateral brain injury. Combat crawling or lack of reciprocal lower extremity movements is often seen in patients with diplegia. Finally, numerous researchers have shown that the acquisition of major gross motor skills, such as the ability to walk, plateaus at approximately age 7 years.

The physical assessment should include inspection of the body habitus, sitting and trunk balance, and walking pattern. Motor tone must be determined and spasticity differentiated from extrapyramidal signs. The physical examination should include a careful assessment of joint motion to establish if contractures are interfering with limb position or function.

Pathophysiology of Contractures

Orthopaedists often differentiate between dynamic deformity, which is present during an action such as walking, and static deformity, which is always present. The implication is that dynamic deformities are the result of abnormal muscle activation, whereas static deformities are the result of contracture of the muscle-tendon unit and are reflected by reduced joint motion on physical examination. Chronic muscle hypertonicity inhibits muscle-tendon growth so that joint contractures eventually occur (Fig. 2). Generally, muscle-tendon lengthening procedures are needed to overcome static contractures, whereas bracing treatment or techniques of tone reduction can alter dynamic deformities. In reality, muscle-tendon contractures exist in a continuum with hypertonicity, resulting in reduced joint excursion and, ultimately, shortening of muscle and tendon. Usually, children younger than age 4 years with spastic CP have near full range of joint motion when relaxed. The orthopaedist must recognize that the patient's anxiety or discomfort can increase tone throughout the body and influence examination findings. Repeat examinations are important to corroborate the original findings. Assessing joint motion under anesthesia establishes the true passive range of motion.

Treatment Priorities

A range of specialists, including orthopaedists, physical therapists, neurologists, developmental pediatricians, neurosurgeons, physiatrists, and orthotists, participate in the management of patients with CP. Treatment alters limb posture and/or muscle tone with the intent of improving function. Ankle-foot orthoses (AFOs) and walkers control posture and enhance balance. Neurotoxins, particularly botulinum, temporarily weaken selected muscles directly or by chemical neurolysis using alcohol and phenol. Oral medications,

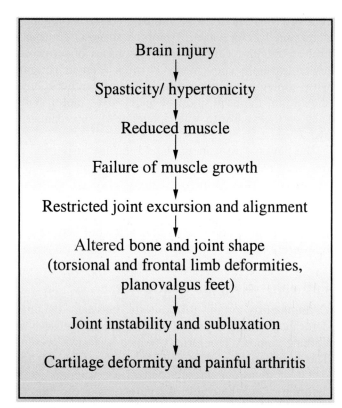

Brain injury
↓
Spasticity/ hypertonicity
↓
Reduced muscle
↓
Failure of muscle growth
↓
Restricted joint excursion and alignment
↓
Altered bone and joint shape
(torsional and frontal limb deformities,
planovalgus feet)
↓
Joint instability and subluxation
↓
Cartilage deformity and painful arthritis

Figure 2 Theoretical pathophysiology of spasticity-induced contractures and osseous deformities.

selective dorsal rhizotomy, and intrathecal baclofen reduce muscle tone and spasticity. Physical therapy maintains joint mobility and enhances function.

It is convenient to consider treatment objectives for patients with spasticity based on the extent of body involvement. For the patient, enhancing walking ability usually is the orthopaedist's primary concern. Most patients with spastic diplegia wear braces, undergo physical therapy, and have some musculoskeletal surgery within their lifetime. Furthermore, within the last decade, botulinum toxin and selective rhizotomy have been used with greater frequency.

For patients with spastic hemiplegia, treatments also are focused on enhancing walking, although these patients compensate well with the sound side and do not require handheld aids. AFOs are prescribed and muscle-tendon procedures and osteotomies performed primarily to improve foot and ankle position. Significant deficits in gross and fine motor function of the upper extremity are common, and tendon transfers occasionally are performed to improve extremity position. Botulism also is used to reduce tone in specific muscles of the leg, foot, or upper extremity in patients with spastic hemiplegia.

Patients with total body involvement have the greatest number of impairments and place the largest demand on the health care system. They are dependent on others for their daily needs and have little capacity for functional improvement. The orthopaedic objectives are to improve trunk and limb position for seating, prevent painful joint dislocations, and prevent contractures from interfering with hygiene. AFOs, spinal and hip bracing treatment, adaptive seating, orthopaedic procedures (osteotomies and contracture releases), intrathecal baclofen, oral medications, and physical therapy are used in this group of patients.

The Role of Gait Analysis in Patients With Ambulatory Cerebral Palsy

Gait laboratories are equipped with cameras linked to computers, in-floor force plates, and dynamic electromyography. The data from these laboratories are assimilated to characterize the pathologic gait and evaluate treatment effects. Through pre- and postintervention assessments, the indications for and effects of a number of orthopaedic, neurosurgical, and orthotic procedures have been refined. For surgery of the muscle-tendon unit in particular, the data are used in conjunction with physical assessments to determine which specific procedure provides appropriate balance of muscle activity, not only across a joint, but between adjacent joints. However, data are used differently among surgeons, and prospective clinical trials are needed to establish the link between passive joint motion, specific kinematic characteristics, treatments, and outcomes.

Orthopaedic Procedures
Muscle-Tendon Procedures

Muscle-tendon procedures, such as lengthening, releases, or transfers, are performed in patients with CP to alter agonist-antagonist balance, overcome static contractures, and enhance dynamic limb alignment when function, hygiene, and joint stability are believed to be compromised. Muscle-tendon surgery is recommended when less invasive methods such as casting and bracing are ineffective. The rationale for muscle-tendon surgery in patients with spastic diplegia is based on the belief that the shortening of the muscle-tendon units and restriction of joint motion caused by CP produces postural abnormalities that result in abnormal joint loading and, ultimately, premature degenerative arthritis.

To achieve functional gains following muscle-tendon surgery, iatrogenic deformities resulting from weakness and the unmasking of spastic antagonists must be avoided. Overlengthening of the hamstrings can precipitate knee hyperextension, excessive pelvic flexion in stance, and/or poor knee flexion in swing, hampering foot clearance (stiff-knee gait). Overlengthening of the

Achilles tendon can result in reduced push-off and excessive knee 'crouch.' To minimize these adverse effects, most surgeons have adopted conservative methods of surgery. The muscle-tendon unit may be released from its origin or insertion (tenotomy), virtually eliminating its function at the spanned joint. This approach usually is performed for smaller muscles within a group that span a joint such as the semitendinosus, adductor longus, and gracilis muscles. A tendon Z-lengthening technique, as opposed to release, frequently is performed; however, the surgeon must determine the correct length at which to reconnect. If too much slack is introduced, weakness and new deformities will ensue. Excessive lengthening of the muscle-tendon unit is virtually impossible to reverse.

Muscle-tendon units with a broad, fibrous aponeurotic expanse at the muscle-tendon junction can be lengthened by transection of the aponeurosis (recession), followed by manual stretching until the desired joint position is achieved. Typically a 1.0- to 3.0-cm gap in the aponeurosis is produced while continuity of the underlying muscle is maintained. The total amount of lengthening may be less with a recession technique than with a Z-lengthening technique, but the muscle fibers that become exposed can elongate further through stretch from day-to-day activities and bracing treatment. As with releases and tenotomies, the recession technique is simple to perform in a uniform manner. Muscle-tendon structures conducive to aponeurotic lengthening include the semimembranosus, biceps femoris, gastrocnemius-soleus complex, and iliopsoas muscles.

Despite the popularity of muscle-tendon surgery as a treatment of spastic diplegia, no randomized trials evaluating its efficacy have been conducted to date. An uncontrolled, prospective study was conducted on 30 patients to evaluate the functional impact of muscle-tendon surgery on patients with spastic diplegia. A standard approach to this surgery that consisted of recessions or releases was employed. The mean age at surgery was 8.7 years (4 to 20 years), and 3.5 muscle tendon units per extremity were recessed or released at surgery. The most common muscles addressed were the hamstrings and gastrocnemius-soleus complex, which were lengthened in 21 of the 30 patients. Hip adductors were lengthened in 13 patients. Rectus femoris transfers were performed in five patients, all of whom had undergone previous distal hamstring lengthening.

Passive ankle, knee, and hip motion increased following muscle-tendon surgery. The primary dynamic or kinematic change in hip and knee motion was a shift in the sagittal joint position to provide a more erect posture with minimal effects on overall excursion.

Gastrocnemius-soleus muscle recessions reduced the marked plantar flexion or equinus position and shifted the timing of maximum ankle dorsiflexion to later in the stance, thus restoring more normal ankle mechanics. These kinematic changes were associated with functional improvements in walking velocity and stride length that were evident by 6 months postoperatively.

By 9 months postoperatively, patients demonstrated a 25% increase in velocity and an 18% increase in stride length, but changes in total Gross Motor Function Measure scores were smaller (2.2% change), occurring primarily in the standing dimension and the walking, running, and jumping dimensions. Further improvements in gait speed were seen at 2 years postoperatively, but the magnitude of change was smaller.

Muscle-tendon surgery is the only technique available to correct static shortening of the tendinous portion of the muscle-tendon unit; however, specific indications and outcomes have yet to be ascertained through clinical trials. Consequently, the role of specific muscle-tendon procedures, such as iliopsoas lengthening and rectus femoris surgery (transfers or releases) remains to be determined. Other problems with muscle-tendon surgery that continue to be reported in clinical series include iatrogenic deformities such as stiff-knee gait, recurvatum, crouch, and excessive lordosis, as well as the 20% incidence of repeat surgery on hamstrings and gastrocnemius-soleus muscles.

Osteotomies and Arthrodesis

Rotational osteotomies ameliorate severe intoeing or outtoeing. The skeleton functions as a series of levers over which the muscles work, and, theoretically, the torsional deformities commonly seen in patients with CP reduce muscle efficiency and function. For example, the posterior calf muscles normally restrain the tibia so that the ground reaction force remains in front of or near the knee center, thus reducing quadriceps demand. In patients with spastic diplegia, internal femoral rotation, external tibial torsion, and midfoot abduction (pes planovalgus) combine to move the ground reaction force external to the knee, reducing the effectiveness of the foot lever and promoting crouch gait (stance phase knee flexion) (Fig. 3). Rotational osteotomies and subtalar corrections restore alignment and enhance muscle function. Osteotomies frequently are combined with muscle-tendon surgery to correct the accompanying contractures.

Excessive femoral anteversion is associated with increased passive internal hip rotation relative to external rotation. The thigh-foot angle, measured with the subtalar joint in neutral position, is used to assess tibial torsion that can either be inward (internal torsion) or

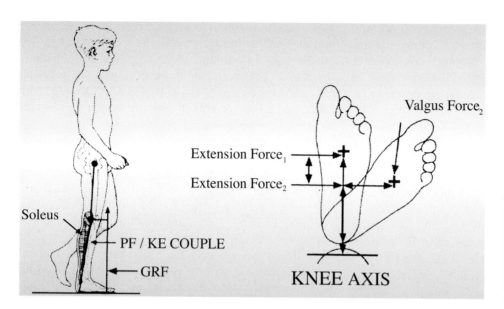

Figure 3 An example of the effects of "lever arm dysfunction" produced by torsional deformities. In this patient, external tibial torsion reduces the plantar flexion/ knee extension (PF/KE) couple by shifting foot center of pressure laterally and proximally. *(Reproduced with permission from Gage JR (ed): Gait Analysis in Cerebral Palsy. London, England, MacKeith Press, 1991, p 106.)*

outward (external torsion). Excessive forefoot adduction and/or plantar flexion during walking produces dynamic internal rotation, while midfoot and subtalar abduction produce an external foot progression angle.

Femoral rotation osteotomies can be performed at the subtrochanteric level or supracondylar level of the femur. The advantage of performing the osteotomy in the distal femur is that percutaneous techniques with pins and casts can be used in lieu of the plates that would be necessary proximally. However, the impact on patellofemoral mechanics may be deleterious. Tibial rotation osteotomies are performed at the supramalleolar level of the tibia, with or without concomitant fibular osteotomy. Following rotational osteotomies, muscle length and tension may be altered.

Osteotomies for paralytic hip dysplasia also are commonly performed, again in association with soft-tissue procedures. Varus femoral osteotomies, with or without external rotation, are combined with acetabular osteotomies to improve femoral head coverage.

As with other conditions, arthrodesis in patients with CP is reserved for treatment of pain associated with end-stage joint deterioration in which ligamentous and muscle constraints cannot be reconstructed and/or articular cartilage is severely damaged. Common sites for arthrodesis include the subtalar and midfoot joints for planovalgus foot deformity, the first metatarsophalangeal joint for dorsal bunions or hallux valgus, the wrist for severe flexion deformities, and the thumb interphalangeal joint or metacarpophalangeal joint for thumb-in-palm contractures.

Medical Management

Botulinum Toxin

The neurotoxin produced by the *Clostridium botulinum* has achieved widespread use during the last decade to selectively weaken spastic muscles in patients with CP. The botulinum toxin-A serotype (BTX-A) has been marketed under the name Botox® in the United States. Other new serotypes of the toxin exist and currently are in development. One problem with this type of substance is that potency and dosing is unique to each serotype. In this section, the use of BTX-A is discussed. Botox has been approved by the Federal Drug Administration (FDA) for the treatment of strabismus, focal cervical and facial spasm, and blepharospasm. However, despite the lack of FDA approval for use in children with CP, extensive use of BTX-A in children with CP has shown that adverse reactions are rare and many state Medicaid programs cover the drug for this indication.

BTX-A's mechanism of action and means of reversibility currently are being clarified. It is known that when Botox is injected into muscle, it enters the nerve terminal to block release of acetylcholine. With time, new nerve terminals are believed to develop and reattach to the muscle end plate to reverse weakening effects. Weakness is evident within 24 to 72 hours and lasts from 2 to 6 months. Systemic spread after local injection does occur, but, thus far, total body doses of 10 to 12 units/kg do not seem to have significant short-term deleterious effects. The LD_{50} (lethal dose) for monkeys is approximately 40 units/kg.

Because of dosing limitations and the short duration of action, BTX-A is most commonly used for localized treatment of a few muscles in young children before significant muscle-tendon contractures have developed. For example, a 3-year-old, 15-kg child with congenital hemiplegia could reasonably be treated with BTX-A to address the dynamic contracture of the gastrocnemius-soleus complex, wrist flexion contracture, and thumb-in-palm deformity. However, dosage restrictions may prevent a similarly sized child with total body involvement from receiving injections in all involved muscles bilaterally. Furthermore, the end point of treatment is not always clear in chronic conditions such as CP. Therefore, the drug typically is used in children younger than age 6 or 7 years prior to muscle-tendon surgery or rhizotomy. The drug also may be useful to simulate surgical effects; however, the changes do not seem to be as dramatic. Finally, BTX-A may be useful as an adjunct to serial casting by reducing the stretch response and eliminating some tonic muscle activity.

Transient pain from the injection is the most frequent complaint, and serious adverse reactions are rare following BTX-A injections. However, bladder incontinence, seizures, constipation, and difficulty with swallowing and breathing have been reported. In addition, safety is less certain in patients with muscle weakness such as myasthenia gravis or muscular dystrophy. Aminoglycosides such as gentamicin may potentiate the neuromuscular blockade and should not be used concomitantly. Antibodies can form and reduce the effectiveness of subsequent injections; therefore, the interval between injections must be at least 3 months. Finally, long-term effects and chronic usage have not been adequately studied so that multiple repeat injections must be performed cautiously and only when alternative, safer methods fail.

Chemical Neurolysis: Alcohol and Phenol

Both ethyl alcohol and phenol have been injected epidurally, perineurally, and intramuscularly to reduce spasticity in patients with CP. Alcohol and phenol denature proteins and induce axon degeneration, thus disrupting nerve conduction for several months until myelin regenerates. Phenol causes more tissue destruction than alcohol; therefore, it is applied perineurally to the motor branches using an open technique. Local pain at the injection site, dysesthesia, and possible permanent neuronal loss are not infrequent side effects. Because experience with these agents is limited, questions regarding safety and efficacy remain unanswered.

Oral Medications

Muscle relaxants are commonly used to ameliorate diffuse spasticity, but the potential for adverse side effects has resulted in restriction of their use to patients with severe spasticity and total body involvement or in the postoperative setting to treat patients with spasms associated with healing. Baclofen and diazepam are the most frequently used muscle relaxants in patients with CP.

Gamma aminobutyric acid (GABA) is an inhibitory neurotransmitter that is ubiquitous, both peripherally and centrally. Baclofen mimics GABA's action, and diazepam potentiates it. Therefore, both drugs produce sedation in conjunction with peripheral spasticity reduction. Furthermore, cessation of either drug following prolonged use can produce adverse effects that include seizures, muscle irritability, and hallucinations.

Intrathecal Baclofen

In addition to mimicking GABA's action, baclofen reduces monosynaptic and polysynaptic spinal reflexes and motor neuron drive. Oral baclofen does not readily pass through the blood-brain barrier; consequently, high concentrations in the blood are often required before spasticity is reduced. With these concentrations, sedation frequently is difficult. Administration of intrathecal baclofen (ITB) drastically reduces the dose requirements needed to affect lower extremity spasticity so that central sedation is less of a problem. A reservoir and programmable pump has been designed that delivers baclofen at a rate commensurate with the desired spasticity reduction. The pump is placed subcutaneously over the abdomen and a catheter leading from the pump is positioned at the thoracolumbar junction. The drug diffuses into the spinal cord and, based on its concentration, variable distances up the cord. Thus, higher infusion rates are more likely to reduce trunk tone, exacerbate weakness, and produce sedation.

The standard pump is approximately the size of a hockey puck, and a thinner pediatric version also exists. However, bulkiness of the pumps precludes implantation in small patients. Adjusting the dose takes several months, and refills are required approximately every 3 months. Complications include catheter and pump malfunctions, serious drug reactions such as respiratory depression, and infections. In 10% to 20% of patients, complications require surgery or pump removal. Furthermore, drug tolerance and withdrawal reactions are significant concerns, and long-term results in patients with CP are limited. Thus, ITB should be reserved for patients with spasticity whose tone is compromising their quality of life and who have not benefited from less risky methods. Finally, because the ITB is new, the risks and benefits should be explained and the treatment should be closely supervised.

Selective Dorsal Rhizotomy

Over the last 15 years, selective dorsal rhizotomy (SDR) has been used across the United States for management of spasticity in patients with diplegia. Although SDR also has been used in nonambulatory patients, experience is less extensive and outcomes are less well documented than in ambulatory patients.

Technical aspects of the procedure and patient selection criteria vary; consequently, conclusions regarding its effectiveness are still being debated. As it is currently performed, SDR techniques essentially have one common element: a percentage of the dorsal rootlets from the L2-S1 levels are transected. Variations exist in the level of exposure, criteria for rootlet transection, inclusion of L1 rootlet transection, and postoperative management. Therefore, generalizations about the procedure are difficult to make. Some surgeons perform laminectomies throughout the lumbar spine and identify the dorsal root at the level of the foramen. Limited exposure through an L1-2 laminectomy is a popular approach. Decreased postoperative pain and a smaller risk of late spinal deformity are advantages of this technique.

The concept of SDR is based on the belief that in patients with spastic diplegia, heightened responses to afferent impulses, whether from the muscle spindle or skin, spread to adjacent levels, thus interfering with function. In fact, after SDR is performed, reflexes and resistance to passive limb movement generally are reduced in the lower extremities, but the functional gains are variable. Thus, the relationship between the reduction in spasticity and observed functional gains are still debatable. Complications are rare, but can include bowel and bladder incontinence if sacral rootlets are not properly identified, lower extremity dysesthesia, and dural leaks. Furthermore, following SDR, musculoskeletal complications, including spinal deformities, hip subluxation, midfoot subluxation, and muscle-tendon contractures, still can develop.

Physical Therapy

For decades, physical therapy (PT) has been a mainstay of nonsurgical management of motor dysfunction in CP, as a stand-alone intervention or a supplement to other treatments. Physical therapists are involved with direct administration of exercise programs, family education about handling and positioning the patient, and as consultants for the medical team managing children with CP. Although the evidence is limited, the value of PT in promoting and maintaining inherent functional capacity and augmenting surgical outcomes is well recognized.

Recent trends in PT have begun to specifically address muscle weakness, and results of studies suggest that strength and endurance training can have pronounced positive effects on gait and motor function. Strengthening may be especially effective when combined with other interventions that alleviate spasticity or muscle tightness. Finally, a greater focus on functional goals in PT, rather than merely addressing movement quality or developmental milestones, has

been shown to produce positive measurable outcomes. For example, if surgery is performed to improve gait, physical therapy should focus on maximizing attainment of that goal. Therefore, PT programs often incorporate manual stretching of shortened muscles supplemented with bracing treatment; strengthening of weak muscles to improve posture, stability, and skill development; and gait training to achieve maximum independence in the home and community. PT goals differ in nonambulatory patients with total body involvement and tend to center around preventing secondary musculoskeletal deformities that could interfere with optimal positioning, patient comfort, or ease of care.

Casting, Bracing, and Seating

In addition to providing postoperative protection, casts stretch muscle-tendon units and reverse contractures. In young patients, casting may be effective and, once completed, allow bracing in AFOs. However, in the absence of further treatment, recurrent contractures are common following stretch casting. BTX-A injection may be useful as an adjunct to casting.

Bracing the lower extremities in AFOs is extremely common for patients with CP. The goals of bracing treatment are to correct or control limb alignment, enhance stability, and prevent contracture development. Most studies are uncontrolled, but in several, a functional benefit from AFOs prescribed for patients with crouch and equinus was found when AFOs were compared to barefoot walking. AFOs usually are made of polypropylene and can cause skin irritation, hamper shoe fitting, and interfere with transitional movements such as sit-to-stand movements. However, there also is evidence of loss of joint motion within weeks when use of AFOs was discontinued. Therefore, for patients with pronounced equinus, weakness, crouch, and midfoot collapse, bracing treatment should be offered if its use is not precluded by static contractures. Nonambulatory patients can also use AFOs to support the foot and prevent deformities that may preclude shoe wear.

For children with total body involvement, seating systems play an integral part in providing trunk support and allowing mobility. Several components currently are available, including cushioning, molded seats, propulsion controls, and supports for the head, trunk, and upper extremities. Because seating systems improve quality of life, the patient should be referred to a tertiary care facility staffed by physical therapists and seating technicians.

Postoperative Management

Early mobilization is an important goal in postoperative management of patients with CP because contractures, stiffness, osteopenia, and weakness tend to develop. However, casting and periods of restricted weight bearing often are required because of a lack of stable bone fixation and the need for muscle-tendon units to heal and pain to be controlled. For ambulatory patients, evidence from animal studies and clinical series suggests that muscle-tendon units heal sufficiently to allow unprotected weight bearing in 3 to 4 weeks. Braces and splints can be used to stretch the extremity and muscle-tendon units during periods of inactivity. Medications such as codeine and diazepam can be used to control postoperative pain and muscle spasms. More recently, BTX-A has been administered to patients 2 weeks prior to hip adductor surgery to reduce postoperative spasm, pain, and the need for abduction splinting. Finally, physical therapy is crucial to assist the patient during postoperative rehabilitation.

Management of Specific Anatomic Regions

Spine

The prevalence of scoliosis in patients with spastic CP is related to the severity of functional impairment; it may be as high as 65% in patients with total body involvement and only slightly higher than in the normal population for the most functional patients. The characteristics of scoliosis in patients with CP differ in several respects from those of idiopathic scoliosis. In patients with CP, the curves tend to be longer and often include the pelvis. Progression in adult life is more common, especially for patients with curves greater than 40°. Factors such as increased and asymmetric muscle tone and poor trunk balance are believed to be underlying causes of this deformity. Consequently, patients with total body involvement should be regularly monitored for scoliosis and treatment considered for children and adolescents with curves greater than 50°. Bracing treatment can provide trunk support, but effects on curve progression are unpredictable.

The goals of surgery are to stop curve progression and ultimately correct the curve to enhance sitting posture, pulmonary function, and digestion and thus ease the care burden. Most patients with severe scoliosis tend to be totally dependent on others for all their needs; many are mentally retarded and have seizures, impaired swallowing, and a propensity for respiratory infections. These associated comorbid conditions and the rigidity of the curves increase the risks and expense of correction. Infection rates have been reported to be as high as 15% following surgery, and other complications, which include pneumonia, ileus, pseudarthrosis, and neurologic injury, raise the overall complication rate to approximately 20%. Given the risks and the fact that quality of life and pain are dif-

ficult to measure in patients with total body involvement, some authors have questioned the wisdom of surgery to correct scoliosis in this population. Clearly, these patients require detailed preoperative assessments of nutrition and cardiopulmonary function. Ideally, the surgery should be performed before the curves become severe, even if patients are skeletally immature. With these factors in mind, discussion about the appropriateness of surgery should begin when curves exceed 50°.

The surgical technique usually entails long fusions from the upper thoracic spine (T2) to the pelvis to correct scoliosis and pelvic obliquity (Fig. 4). An anterior release is performed if curves are rigid and crankshafting is expected because of significant residual growth potential. Segmental fixation with sublaminar wires, hooks, and pedicle screws is the most popular technique because it exerts excellent correction forces and produces stability without the need for postoperative bracing. Fixation to the pelvis is commonly achieved using the Galveston technique with rod insertion between the iliac cortical tables at the level of the posterior iliac spine. More recently, screws directed into S1 have been used to avoid crossing the sacroiliac joint. Progressive kyphosis, pelvic obliquity, crankshafting, and trunk decompensation are more likely to occur when the proximal extent of the fusion is not above the apex of the thoracic kyphosis and the distal extent is above the pelvis. Grafting is performed using autogenous bone, if possible, but supplemental allogenic cancellous bone often is needed because of the long exposure.

Hip

Hip instability with progressive subluxation occurs in approximately 15% of patients with spastic CP. Most of these patients have total body involvement and severe spasticity (Fig. 5). Therefore, the incidence of subluxation in patients with spastic quadriparesis ranges from 25% to 50%, and perhaps one third to one half of these patients experience hip pain. Furthermore, the adduction and other contractures that accompany hip subluxation make sitting and perineal hygiene difficult. Orthopaedic procedures or tone reduction techniques are performed in an attempt to prevent the adverse consequences of hip subluxation.

Hip subluxation in patients with CP results from chronic muscle hypertonicity, especially in the adductor group. Constant high muscular tension pulls the femoral head to the edge of the acetabulum so that the lateral margin erodes with time and the head progressively migrates from the acetabulum. At birth, the hip joint usually is normal in patients with CP, and radiographic dysplasia with subluxation becomes apparent

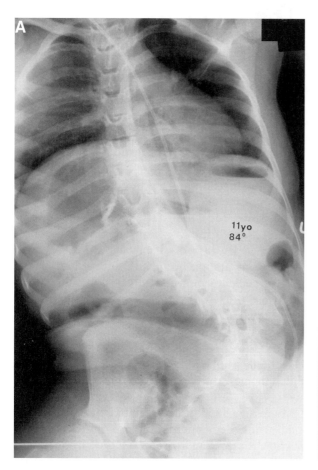

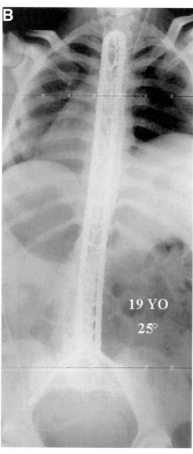

Figure 4 A, Typical neuromuscular scoliosis in a patient with CP with total body involvement. Scoliosis frequently involves the entire spine and can result in pelvic obliquity. Sagittal plane deformities (not shown) frequently include excessive lumbar lordosis and/or thoracic or thoracolumbar kyphosis. **B,** Radiographs 8 years following posterior instrumentation with segmental fixation from T2 to the pelvis. Fusion was promoted by the addition of autograft combined with allograft.

between age 2 and 4 years. Without intervention, complete dislocation is evident by approximately age 7 years. Bony architecture also is distorted, the acetabula become globally deficient, and the femora have increased neck-shaft angles and frequently are excessively anteverted. In the chronic case, not only does the acetabular roof become eroded, but the femoral head becomes steeple-shaped from the combined pressure of the acetabulum medially and the labrum and gluteal muscles laterally.

Subluxation in CP typically is measured using the Migration Index of Reimers (Fig. 6) to quantify the percentage of the femoral head that lies outside the bounds of the lateral acetabulum. However, the patho-anatomy, acetabular index, neck-shaft angle, femoral version, and muscle contractures must be considered when treatment plans are developed. Traditionally, muscle releases are performed in children younger than age 4 years who have restricted hip motion, hypertonicity, and minimal bony pathology (less than 30% migration index). One common approach has been to release muscles of the adductor group, particularly the adductor longus muscle. Although anterior branch obturator neurectomy is detrimental to ambulatory function, in nonambulatory patients with hip subluxation, the benefits of neurectomy as an adjunct

to muscle releases are unclear. Other muscles that often are released to manage hip subluxation include the iliopsoas and the proximal hamstrings. Early soft-tissue releases can successfully prevent progressive subluxation in approximately 60% of patients, but chronic hypertonicity, pelvic obliquity, and scoliosis combine to produce recurrent subluxation in the remainder. Some authors suggest long-term, postoperative hip abduction bracing to reduce the incidence of recurrent subluxation.

Osteotomies (acetabular, femoral, or both types) are performed to correct later stages of subluxation (Fig. 7). In the absence of controlled studies, indications and success rates vary considerably. As a general guideline, for children between age 4 and 8 years with migration percentages between 30% and 50%, soft-tissue releases should be combined with femoral varus, shortening, or acetabular osteotomies. On the acetabular side, equivalent results have been reported with a variety of osteotomies, including hinging acetabuloplasties, rotational acetabular osteotomies, and augmentation acetabuloplasties. External rotation of the femoral shaft often is performed in conjunction with varus and shortening to reduce the femoral anteversion. Combined acetabular and femoral osteotomies are recom-

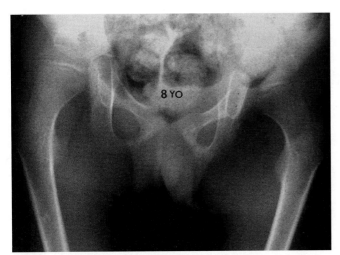

Figure 5 Characteristic hip deformities in a patient with CP with total body involvement. Contractures are evident with the hips held in flexion and adduction. Subluxation is posterior and superior, the acetabula are shallow, and the femoral heads have lateral erosions secondary to pressure from the gluteal muscles and labrum. Femoral neck-shaft angle and anteversion are increased in this patient. *(Reproduced with permission from Abel MF, Wenger DR, Mubarak SJ, Sutherland DH: Quantitative analysis of hip dysplasia in cerebral palsy: A study of radiographs and 3-D reformatted images. J Pediatr Orthop 1994;14:283-289.)*

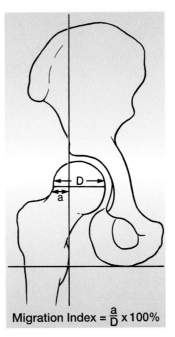

$$\text{Migration Index} = \frac{a}{D} \times 100\%$$

Figure 6 The Migration Index (MI) of Reimers is commonly used as a measure of hip subluxation for patients with CP. The MI is the percentage of the femoral head diameter that is outside of the lateral boundary of the acetabulum. *(Reproduced with permission from Abel MF, Wenger DR, Mubarak SJ, Sutherland DH: Quantitative analysis of hip dysplasia in cerebral palsy: A study of radiographs and 3-D reformatted images. J Pediatr Orthop 1994;14:283-289.)*

mended for patients older than age 8 years with a migration percentage of greater than 50%.

Using these guidelines, success as determined by radiographic measures of migration percentage can be achieved in 70% to 80% of patients. Patients with severe spasticity, especially those with asymmetric hypertonicity, are at high risk for repeat subluxation. In addition, the poor baseline health of many patients increases the rate of complications, such as hip stiffness, hypersensitivity, skin breakdown, recurrent subluxation, pneumonia, urinary tract infections, and ileus. The high rate of adverse outcomes, which are especially prevalent in patients with the most severe spasticity, has encouraged physicians to treat the hypertonicity with ITB or oral antispasmodic medications, either as preventive or adjunctive treatments. Once tone has been reduced, contractures and bony pathology are addressed. Prospective, controlled studies are necessary to identify an approach for managing subsets of the population with spastic quadriparesis.

Salvage operations for older patients with chronically subluxated or dislocated and painful hips include proximal femoral resection or valgus osteotomy. Proximal femoral resections have been reported in retrospective analysis to improve pain in 70% of patients. Valgus procedures are performed to realign the adducted femur when this position adversely affects pelvic alignment and sitting. Total hip replacement for patients with spastic CP has been described, but experience and follow-up are limited.

Knee

Chronic knee flexion deformities are common in patients with spastic CP and often are addressed differently for ambulatory and nonambulatory patients. For ambulatory patients, stance-phase knee crouch increases the load on the patella, resulting in patella alta, fragmentation of the inferior patellar pole, and patellofemoral arthritis. Early in the ambulatory course of progressive crouch, patients with sufficient motor control can attempt quadriceps strengthening. Bracing treatment can be used to restrain anterior tibial translation. Hamstring lengthening commonly is performed to overcome contractures and promote knee extension during stance. However, if swing-phase spasticity of the quadriceps is not recognized, the resulting 'stiff-knee' may impede foot clearance. Consequently, hamstring lengthening often is combined with rectus femoris transfer.

Hamstring lengthening in nonambulatory patients can be performed distally if knee flexion deformities interfere with sitting or dressing. Alternatively, proximal release of the hamstring increases hip flexion, abduction, and knee extension if both hip and knee deformities impede sitting.

Foot

Foot deformities are extremely common in patients with spastic CP and, as with hip and knee deformities, they may produce functional deficits or interfere with normal shoe wear. In addition to equinus, other related deformities include pes planovalgus (spastic flatfoot), equinovarus, hallux valgus, and dorsal bunions.

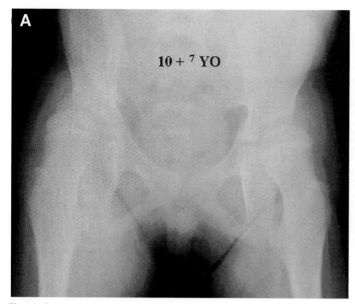
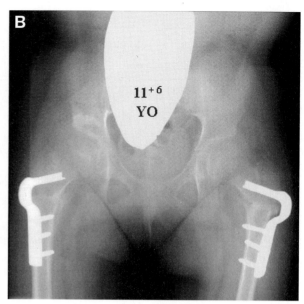

Figure 7 **A,** Hip deformities in this ambulatory patient with CP include bilateral coxa valga and globally deficient acetabula with hip subluxation. Deformities are worse on the right side than on the left. CT (not shown) also confirmed that femoral anteversion was excessive in this patient. **B,** Radiographs of the same patient following bilateral femoral varus and external rotation osteotomies plus hinging acetabuloplasty on the right side that was designed to improve anterior and lateral coverage. In many nonambulatory patients, the osteotomies must be designed to improve posterolateral acetabular deficiencies.

The pathogenesis of pes planovalgus involves ambulation in a crouch position, while posterior calf muscle contracture limits ankle dorsiflexion. The ground reaction force line and body weight pass through the midtarsal joints so that, with time, the ligaments stretch and the forefoot rolls into abduction.

Despite the common occurrence of pes planovalgus, prospective trials have not been conducted to determine the effectiveness of treatment. As with other skeletal deformities in CP, in younger children with pes planovalgus, braces may stabilize the leg and foot and delay or prevent development of static deformity. For static planovalgus deformities, however, soft-tissue contractures and bony deformities must be addressed. Surgery frequently entails lengthening the posterior calf musculature, particularly the gastrocnemius-soleus complex and possibly the peroneus brevis, followed by subtalar realignment procedures. These procedures typically involve extra-articular fusions, but, more recently, lateral calcaneal lengthening osteotomies have become popular.

The pes planovalgus deformity commonly is associated with hallux valgus, external tibial torsion, femoral adduction, and femoral internal rotation. The dynamic relationships among limb segments should be considered if surgery is planned at any one segment. If surgery is not planned, deformities would seem likely to recur. Adjunctive procedures include dorsiflexion osteotomies of the first metatarsal or rotational osteotomies of the tibia and/or the femur. Long-term postoperative bracing with AFOs may provide protection against recurrence.

Bunions, either hallux valgus or dorsal bunions, commonly are seen in patients with spastic CP. Hallux valgus is a common component of the spastic flatfoot. Surgical treatment typically involves metatarsal osteotomies and soft-tissue realignments. The long-term effectiveness of these procedures in patients with spasticity is not known; however, the associated proximal bony deformities and persistently high muscle tone increase the chance of recurrent deformities. For this reason, surgery is indicated to relieve pain that has not been managed with orthotics and shoe adaptations.

Dorsal bunions most commonly affect nonambulatory patients with severe spastic overpull of the ankle dorsiflexors, which in turn creates a flexion deformity of the great toe metatarsophalangeal (MTP) joint. The deformity often is associated with callus and pain over the dorsal MTP joint. McKay's procedure, dorsal transfer of the flexor hallucis brevis, and reefing of the dorsal capsule are surgical options if nonsurgical measures such as braces and shoe adaptations fail. MTP fusion is another technique that can be used to treat severe and chronic MTP subluxation. However, MTP fusion may hamper crawling and walking in some patients.

Upper Extremity

As with the lower extremity, upper extremity contractures frequently occur in spastic CP. Resulting deformities include thumb-in-palm contractures, wrist and finger flexion contractures, elbow flexion contractures, forearm pronation deformities, and shoulder rotational and abduction deformities. As a consequence of some of these deformities, the patient might have difficulties with hygiene and functional deficits from impaired grasp, release, and reach. However, unlike the lower extremity, the hand must be used for fine motor skills. Therefore, functional gains from various treatments such as BTX-A injections, bracing, and surgery have been difficult to quantify. It has been suggested that enhancement of hygiene is a more achievable goal of surgery.

Conclusion

Cerebral palsy is a chronic condition for which there is no cure. Many treatment options have become available over the years; however, data on their effectiveness are still being collected. The motor impairments produced by CP include spasticity, weakness, lack of selective muscle control, and impaired balance. Management should include a meticulous evaluation with stated treatment objectives. Medications, rhizotomy, BTX-A injection, orthopaedic procedures, bracing, and physical therapy often are used in complimentary combinations to address impairment. Because of the limited amount of efficacy data, parents and patients must be informed of options and risks. Follow-up documentation is important to establish whether objectives were achieved and the patient and parent are satisfied with the outcome.

Annotated Bibliography

Epidemiology and Etiology

Badawi N, Watson L, Petterson B, et al: What constitutes cerebral palsy? *Dev Med Child Neurol* 1998;40:520-527.

The authors describe the types of CP and etiologic relationships. Descriptions of syndromes are included.

Kuban KC: White-matter disease of prematurity, periventricular leukomalacia, and ischemic lesions. *Dev Med Child Neurol* 1998;40:571-573.

In this article, causes and relationships of white matter lesions are reviewed, especially of periventricular leukomalacia to CP.

Classifications

Blair E, Stanley FJ: Issues in the classification and epidemiology of cerebral palsy. *Mental Retard Devel Disab Res Rev* 1997;3:184-193.

The authors present an excellent review of epidemiology and classification. The discussion includes definitions, prevalence of subtypes, and information on risk factors and etiologies.

Role of Gait Analysis

Gage JR, Deluca PA, Renshaw TS: Gait analysis: Principle and applications. Emphasis on its use in cerebral palsy. *J Bone Joint Surg Am* 1995;77:1607-1623.

In this article, the authors reviewed the principles of normal gait and gait in patients with CP, as defined with three-dimensional gait analysis.

Muscle-Tendon Surgery

Abel MF, Damiano DL, Pannunzio M, Bush J: Muscle-tendon surgery in diplegic cerebral palsy: Functional and mechanical changes. *J Pediatr Orthop* 1999;19:366-375.

The authors reviewed the effects of muscle-tendon surgery performed as an isolated procedure in 30 patients with spastic diplegia.

Delp SL, Zajac FE: Force- and moment-generating capacity of lower-extremity muscles before and after tendon lengthening. *Clin Orthop* 1992;284:247-259.

In this article, the authors discuss the mechanical effects of muscle-tendon surgery based on the location of the lengthening and the muscle architecture. Muscles with shorter fibers were more sensitive to weakening effects of tendon lengthening as compared with muscles with longer fibers. For example, the soleus is weakened more by lengthening of the Achilles tendon than the gastrocnemius because its fibers are shorter.

Botulinum Toxin

Auff E, Poewe W: The clinical applications of botulinum toxin type A. *Eur J Neurol* 1999;6:1-125.

The entire supplement to this journal was funded by Allergan, the manufacturer of Botox®, and focused on reports on the use of botulinum toxin.

Brin MF: Botulinum toxin: Chemistry, pharmacology, toxicity, and immunology. *Muscle Nerve* 1997;(suppl 6):S146-S168.

In this article, the author describes the mechanisms of action of botulinum toxin.

Intrathecal Baclofen

Albright AL: Baclofen in the treatment of cerebral palsy. *J Child Neurol* 1996;11:77-83.

Baclofen is a γ-aminobutyric acid agonist that acts at the spinal cord level to impede the release of excitatory neurotransmitters that cause spasticity. The author reviewed the uses of baclofen administered intrathecally, including doses, effects, and complications.

Selective Dorsal Rhizotomy

McLaughlin JF, Bjornson KF, Astley SJ, et al: Selective dorsal rhizotomy: Efficacy and safety in an investigator-masked randomized clinical trial. *Dev Med Child Neurol* 1998;40:220-232.

The authors evaluated the functional impact of selective dorsal rhizotomy in one of three randomized, single institutional trials. Findings show that selective dorsal rhizotomy is safe and reduces spasticity in children with spastic diplegia. However, at 24 months, physical therapy alone resulted in equal improvements in independent mobility as PT plus rhizotomy.

Physical Therapy

Damiano DL, Abel MF: Functional outcomes of strength training in spastic cerebral palsy. *Arch Phys Med Rehabil* 1998;79:119-125.

The authors describe the functional impact of a rigorously defined program of isotonic strengthening on patients with spastic CP.

Spine

Bulman WA, Dormans JP, Ecker ML, Drummond DS: Posterior spinal fusion for scoliosis in patients with cerebral palsy: A comparison of Luque rod and Unit Rod instrumentation. *J Pediatr Orthop* 1996;16:314-323.

In this article, the U-shaped unit rod for posterior spinal arthrodesis is compared to conventional Luque constructs with two rods. Two groups of 15 patients had long fusions to the pelvis. The authors determined that the unit rod instrumentation allowed significantly greater correction of both the major curve and pelvic obliquity than the conventional construct.

Comstock CP, Leach J, Wenger DR: Scoliosis in total-body-involvement cerebral palsy: Analysis of surgical treatment and patient and caregiver satisfaction. *Spine* 1998;23:1412-1425.

The authors analyzed spinal fusions in patients with total body involvement and determined that progressive deformity and complications from surgery were common. They concluded that anterior releases with end plate excision might prevent late deformities in the skeletally immature patient. Although the study design did not allow definitive conclusions, the review and discussion emphasized many pertinent issues related to spinal deformity correction in patients with total body involvement.

Saito N, Ebara S, Ohotsuka K, Kumeta H, Takaoka K: Natural history of scoliosis in spastic cerebral palsy. *Lancet* 1998;351:1687-1692.

During a 17-year follow-up of patients with spasticity, the authors determined that with onset of deformity before age 10 years, progression was most rapid during puberty with continued progression into the adult years. Curves greater than 40° in patients younger than age 15 years had particularly high rates of progression.

Yazici M, Asher MA, Hardacker JW: The safety and efficacy of Isola-Galveston instrumentation and arthrodesis in treatment of neuromuscular spinal deformities. *J Bone Joint Surg Am* 2000;82:524-543.

The latest techniques of segmental fixation were illustrated in this article. The procedure provided excellent technical correction; however, repeat surgery was necessary in 11% of patients because of complications.

Hip

Abel MF, Blanco JS, Pavlovich L, Damiano DL: Asymmetric hip deformity and subluxation in cerebral palsy: An analysis of surgical treatment. *J Pediatr Orthop* 1999;19:479-485.

In this retrospective study that took place over 7 years, the authors studied the onset of hip subluxation and scoliosis in patients with spastic CP with total body involvement. A mean of two surgical procedures was performed per patient in an attempt to prevent hips from subluxating. Despite aggressive management, one third of this group with high and asymmetric tone still had at least one hip with greater than 30% migration.

Abel MF, Wenger DR, Mubarak SJ, Sutherland DH: Quantitative analysis of hip dysplasia in cerebral palsy: A study of radiographs and 3-D reformatted images. *J Pediatr Orthop* 1995;14:283-289.

In this extensively referenced article, the authors showed the characteristic hip deformities in patients with spastic quadriplegia using three-dimensional reformatted images.

Cabanela ME, Weber M: Total hip arthroplasty in patients with neuromuscular diseases. *J Bone Joint Surg Am* 2000;82:426-432.

The authors reported on a Mayo Clinic experience in treating patients with spasticity with total hip arthroplasty. Results were good in 15 ambulatory patients who had undergone hip replacement. The greatest benefit appeared to be pain relief rather than functional increases. However, a relatively high number of complications occurred.

McNerney NP; Mubarak SJ; Wenger DR: One-stage correction of the dysplastic hip in cerebral palsy with the San Diego acetabuloplasty: Results and complications in 104 hips. *J Pediatr Orthop* 2000;20:93-103.

The authors retrospectively reviewed 92 patients with CP who underwent extensive hip reconstruction with acetabular and femoral osteotomies, soft-tissue release, and, in some cases, capsulorrhaphy. Details of the acetabuloplasty are illustrated well. This series reveals that high complication rates can be expected, but ultimate radiographic success in terms of stable positions can be achieved in a high percentage of patients. Effects on pain reduction and seating were less obvious. This article provides guidelines for reconstruction of chronic deformities.

Miller F, Bagg MR: Age and migration percentage as risk factors for progression in spastic hip disease. *Dev Med Child Neurol* 1995;37:449-455.

In this retrospective review, the long-term changes in hip development in patients with spastic CP are studied. The authors confirm that, in general, subluxation increases with age and the greater the amount of spasticity, the more likely severe subluxation will occur.

Knee

Chambers H, Lauer A, Kaufman K, Cardelia JM, Sutherland D: Prediction of outcome after rectus femoris surgery in cerebral palsy: The role of cocontraction of the rectus femoris and vastus lateralis. *J Pediatr Orthop* 1998;18:703-711.

The authors discuss the role and effects of rectus femoris transfer surgery. Although preoperative selection criteria were not ascertained, rectus femoris transfer appears to provide better swing phase knee motion than release.

Classic Bibliography

Bagg MR, Farber J, Miller F: Long-term follow-up of hip subluxation in cerebral palsy patients. *J Pediatr Orthop* 1993;13:32-36.

Bleck EE (ed): *Orthopaedic Management in Cerebral Palsy*. London, England, MacKeith Press, 1987.

Elmer EB, Wenger DR, Mubarak SJ, Sutherland DH: Proximal hamstring lengthening in the sitting cerebral palsy patient. *J Pediatr Orthop* 1992;12:329-336.

Gage JR (ed): *Gait Analysis in Cerebral Palsy*. London, England, MacKeith Press, 1991.

Kitchens DL, Park TS: Dorsal rhizotomy for spastic diplegia: Operative indications and techniques. *Contemp Neurosurg* 1994;16:1-7.

Lonstein JE, Akbarnia A: Operative treatment of spinal deformities in patients with cerebral palsy or mental retardation: An analysis of one hundred and seven cases. *J Bone Joint Surg Am* 1983;65:43-55.

Chapter 25

Myelomeningocele and Intraspinal Lipoma

Luciano Dias, MD

Introduction

Myelomeningocele, also referred to as spina bifida, is a fluid-filled cystic swelling, formed by dura and arachnoid. It protrudes through a defect in the vertebral arches and contains spinal nerve roots that are carried into the sac. A true myelomeningocele is believed to result from failure of fusion of the neural folds during neurulation. In the United States, the incidence of myelomeningocele is from 0.6:1,000 to 0.9:1,000 births. Recent studies suggest that sibling recurrence is approximately 2% to 7%. Prenatal diagnosis can be made by biochemical and enzyme evaluation as well as by ultrasound examination. The least invasive method is maternal serum α-fetal protein screening, which has an accuracy rate of 60% to 95%. With improvement in ultrasonographic techniques, prenatal diagnosis using ultrasound is also quite accurate. Cesarean section is the preferred method of delivery for affected neonates because it avoids trauma to the large myelomeningocele sac. Other abnormalities of the spinal cord and vertebral column often are associated with myelomeningocele, including duplication of the cord, diastematomyelia, and congenital scoliosis, kyphosis, and kyphoscoliosis.

The use of periconceptional vitamin supplementation has been suggested as a method of preventing neural tube defects. Recent studies have established that the daily ingestion of 4 mg of folic acid supplement, before and during early pregnancy, reduced the risk of neural tube defects by 60% to 72%. A relatively high dietary intake of folate also may reduce the risk.

The orthopaedist is only one member of a multidisciplinary team of physicians involved in the care of children with myelomeningocele, and often medical, neurosurgical, or urologic treatment is of primary concern. The goal of orthopaedic treatment is to make the musculoskeletal system as functional as possible. Ambulation is not the goal for every child with myelomeningocele. Walking ability, which will be discussed later in this chapter, is highly dependent on the neuromuscular level of the lesion. Before aggressive orthopaedic treatment is initiated, consideration must be given to the lifetime prognosis for these patients. If a child with myelomeningocele is not a community ambulator by age 6 years, community walking as an adult is unlikely. More important than the use of the lower extremities, however, is the child's total development. Emphasis on the intellectual and personality development of children with myelomeningocele, including emphasis on wheelchair mobility, wheelchair sports programs beginning in preschool, and educational mainstreaming, has dramatically increased the independence of these patients. The overall mortality rate in the first 25 years is approximately 25%. Mortality is higher for infants with the Arnold-Chiari malformation.

Associated Neurologic Conditions

Hydrocephalus

Of children with myelomeningocele, 80% to 90% have hydrocephalus that requires cerebrospinal fluid shunting. The incidence of hydrocephalus is related to the neurologic level of the lesion; it is 83% in high lesions (thoracic and upper lumbar) and 60% in low lesions (lower lumbar and sacral). Infection and obstruction are the most serious late complications of cerebrospinal fluid shunts because they affect the child's motor and intellectual development. In terms of upper extremity function and trunk balance, as well as lower incidences of hydromyelia and tethered cord, children who do not require shunting may have a better prognosis than children who require shunting.

Arnold-Chiari Malformation

The Arnold-Chiari malformation (Chiari II) is a consistent clinical and pathologic finding in patients with myelomeningocele. The basic lesion is caudal displacement of the posterior lobe of the cerebellum. The clinical manifestation of Arnold-Chiari malformation is dysfunction of the lower cranial nerves, causing weakness or paralysis of the vocal cords and difficulty in feeding, crying, and breathing. Respiratory difficulties, such as apnea, cyanotic attacks, and associated brachycardia, are not uncommon. Ocular manifestations also are typical of this condition.

Tethered Spinal Cord

The spinal cord ascends during fetal development until at birth it is at the L3 level and by the second month of life has reached the adult L1-3 level. Most children with myelomeningocele show signs of tethering on MRI, but the clinical manifestations of tethered cord are present in only approximately 30% of these children. The clinical signs of tethering are variable, but the most consistent are (1) loss of motor function; (2) development of spasticity in the lower extremities, mainly in the medial hamstrings and ankle dorsiflexors and evertors (rarely, spastic paralysis is present at birth); (3) development of scoliosis (before age 6 years) in the absence of congenital anomalies of the vertebral bodies; (4) back pain and increased lumbar lordosis in the older child; and (5) changes in urologic function. It is not uncommon for a child to have more than one clinical sign of tethered cord. All children with suspected tethered cord syndrome should be evaluated by MRI or CT-myelography. When tethered cord is suspected, it is important to rule out shunt malfunction.

Surgical treatment is indicated to prevent further deterioration of motor function and to decrease the progress of spasticity and scoliosis when clinical signs are documented. The best response to untethering of the spinal cord is seen in patients with sacral-level lesions. Improvement in motor strength and decreased spasticity have been seen in this patient population. Some improvement in scoliosis and its management has been documented when the cord is untethered, if the curvature is less than 45°. In children who have high lumbar or thoracic lesions with spasticity, anterior selective rhizotomy may improve the result of tethered cord release.

Hydromyelia

Hydromyelia is an accumulation of fluid in the enlarged central canal of the spinal cord. It occurs frequently in children with myelomeningocele and may manifest as scoliosis. Progressive scoliosis ranging from 30° to 85° and hydromyelia have been reported in 12 patients. After surgical treatment of the hydromyelia, there may be some improvement in the scoliosis. Eval-

uation of hydromyelia should include CT of the head and MRI of the entire spine.

Classification

The best known classification of myelomeningocele is based on the neurologic level of the lesion (Table 1).

Orthopaedic Evaluation

Serial Muscle Test

This test, which is used to evaluate the neurologic level of function, should be done at birth, before closure, 10 to 14 days after closure, and then annually. If possible, the manual muscle test for the lower extremity should always be performed by the same physical therapist. It is important to recognize that the motor level should remain the same throughout the child's life. Any change in the muscle strength, which sometimes can be very subtle, is very frequently a sign of tethering of the spinal cord. Children may be 3 to 4 years old before a neurologic level is absolutely defined. Usually the gluteus medius and maximus strength can be accurately determined only around this age.

Sitting Balance

The ability to sit without hand support is a good indication of nearly normal central nervous system function. If one- or two-handed support is required for sitting, walking ability with an orthosis and external support is likely to be severely impaired.

Upper Extremity Function

Decreased grip strength and atrophy of the thenar musculature are reliable signs of hydromyelia. Impaired hand function is found in 82% of children with myelomeningocele, with differences in hand function between children with high-level lesions and those with low-level lesions.

Spinal Examination

Spinal radiographs are indicated on an annual basis in the child with a high-level lesion to evaluate any abnormal curvature. The incidences of scoliosis are quite low in the child with a low lumbar- or sacral-level lesion. Any abnormal spine curvature in children with lesions at these two levels is highly suggestive of tethering of the spinal cord.

Hip Range of Motion

Contractures at the hip, especially flexion contractures, are quite common in children with high-level lesions and low lumbar-level lesions. Either adduction or abduction contractures can cause infrapelvic obliquity

TABLE 1 | Classification of Myelomeningocele

Group	Lesion Level	Function	Ambulation*
1	Thoracic and high lumbar	No quadriceps function	Some degree to age 13 years with use of an HKAFO or RGO; 95% to 99% are wheelchair-dependent as adults, although exceptions are seen
2	Low lumbar	Quadriceps and medial hamstring function; no gluteus medius and maximus function	Require AFO and crutches; 79% retain community ambulation as adults; most use wheelchair for long-distance mobility; significant difference in ability to walk between children with L4 and L3 level lesions; medial hamstring function needed for community ambulation; children with L4 lesions have the most to gain from proper care of musculoskeletal deformities
3	Sacral	Quadriceps and gluteus medius function	94% retain walking ability as adults
	High sacral	No gastrocnemius-soleus strength	Walk without support but use AFO braces; have characteristic gluteus lurch with excessive pelvic obliquity and rotation during gait
	Low sacral	Good gastrocnemius-soleus strength Normal gluteus medius and maximus function	Walk without need for AFO braces; gait is close to normal

*HKAFO, hip-knee-ankle-foot orthosis; RGO, reciprocating gait orthosis; AFO, ankle-foot orthosis

that interferes with bracing and ambulation. Internal rotation deformity during gait, especially when associated with an external tibial torsion, is a frequent source of increased valgus stress at the knee joint.

Knee Alignment and Range of Motion

Knee flexion contractures are common; when this deformity exceeds 20° it can lead to problems with bracing and to a severely crouched gait. Knee extension contractures are usually congenital. An external tibial torsion is common in children with low lumbar-level lesions and often is associated with a valgus stress at the knee joint when the thigh-foot angle (TFA) is more than 20°. An internal tibial torsion is frequently associated with congenital clubfoot deformities.

Ankle Valgus Deformity

Valgus deformity at the ankle may interfere with orthotic wear or cause pressure sores at the medial malleolus.

Foot Deformities

It is important to have an accurate record of the foot alignment, hindfoot and forefoot, as well as an accurate record of the ankle range of motion. Approximately 90% of patients with myelomeningocele have some type of foot deformity. The use of a myelomeningocele orthopaedic data base is very helpful in maintaining accurate records. The subtle changes that occur with tethered cord can be recognized at an early

stage. When this is done, early neurosurgical intervention may prevent further loss of muscle function.

Gait Analysis
Clinical Application

Much attention has been devoted to the application of clinical gait analysis in the treatment of children with cerebral palsy. Gait analysis also has proved to be helpful in two main groups of patients with myelomeningocele: (1) the patient with a low lumbar-level lesion who walks with a below-knee orthosis and external support and (2) the patient with a sacral-level lesion who walks with ankle-foot orthoses (AFOs) and no support. The average walking velocity for the child with a low lumbar-level lesion is 54% of normal. The child with a high sacral-level lesion walks with a velocity of about 70% of normal.

Kinetic Pattern

Because of gluteus medius and maximus weakness, compensatory movements occur at the pelvis and hip to facilitate forward progression and maintain independent ambulation. Such characteristics include increased active pelvic rotation and stance phase hip abduction. The lower the motor level, the less pronounced these movements are. All children with low lumbar-level lesions show increased anterior pelvic tilt.

Gait analysis has been helpful in the decision-making process for treatment of orthopaedic deformities such as hip flexion-adduction contracture, unilateral dislocation, or subluxation in the child with a low lumbar-level lesion and unilateral dislocation of the hip in a child with a sacral-level lesion. Gait analysis has been found to be particularly helpful in the treatment of rotational malalignments of the lower extremity, especially external tibial torsion that leads to a quite significant increased valgus stress at the knee joint. The use of gait analysis in the patient with low lumbar- and sacral-level myelomeningocele has the same value as the use of gait analysis in the patient with spastic cerebral palsy. Understanding the effects of the hip deformities on walking leads to intervention at an early stage. Further understanding of the quality of gait in the crutch-walking child has led to a more conservative approach to the hip subluxation and dislocation. The high valgus stress at the knee joint found with gait analysis has led to correction of rotational malalignment, as will be discussed further.

Principles of Orthopaedic Management

Orthotic Management

Approximately 95% of children with myelomeningocele will require orthotic support to achieve ambulation. The goal of orthotic treatment is to achieve effective mobility with minimal restriction. Bracing and splinting vary with the degree of motor deficit and trunk balance. Night splints are frequently indicated to prevent orthopaedic deformities. For the child with a high-level lesion and complete paralysis of the lower extremity, the use of a nighttime total body splint can help to prevent hip flexion-external rotation deformities, knee flexion contractures, and equinus. The lower extremity is aligned with the hips in 15° of abduction, the knee in extension, and the ankle in a neutral position. The AFO is helpful in preventing the development of an equinus deformity. It also is believed that night splints should be used after surgical correction of some foot deformities. Careful fitting is essential, and the parents should be provided with detailed explanation of skin care to prevent pressure sores.

The A-frame, a prefabricated trunk-hip-lower extremity brace, allows the child to stand without hand support and should be used up to 3 hours a day, divided into periods of 20 to 30 minutes. It is recommended for children age 12 to 18 months and is easily fitted. Similar braces that allow trunk mobility include the parapodium and reciprocating gait orthosis (RGO). The RGO is indicated for the child with a high-level lesion who has good sitting balance and good upper extremity function. This brace usually is introduced at approximately age 2 years. Most children will use a walker and some, those with excellent coordination, will be able to achieve effective mobility with crutches.

The contraindications for the RGO include poor trunk balance (requires the use of hand support when sitting), severe upper extremity involvement, mental retardation, severe visual defects, scoliosis of more than 50°, and hip flexion contracture of more than 30° to 40°. The parapodium is indicated for children older than age 2 years with poor trunk balance and/or spastic upper extremity. Accurate fitting of the orthosis is mandatory.

The hip-knee-ankle-foot orthosis is indicated for the child with a high lumbar-level lesion who has achieved a swing-through ambulation with crutches. The knee-ankle-foot orthosis is used on occasion for the child with low lumbar-level paralysis to reduce excessive valgus stress at the knee joint when too young for osteotomies (see later discussion). AFOs are used for children with low lumbar- or high sacral-level lesions, and they are designed to be rigid enough to provide ankle and foot stabilization while maintaining the shank-ankle angle at 90° to minimize knee crouch. In the older child, carbon reinforcement is recommended. Some special padding may be required over the medial malleolus, the head of the talus, and the navicular to prevent pressure sores.

AFOs with twister cables are useful for rotational malalignment, either intoeing or outtoeing, that is seen frequently in patients with low lumbar-level and high sacral-level lesions. Most of these children eventually require surgery, but outcomes seem more effective when surgery is performed in children older than age 6 years. The AFO with twister cables may be introduced as early as age 2 years.

A wheelchair may become an important part of the life of the child with spina bifida as the main means for achieving independent mobility. An important consideration in the design of the wheelchair is the seat. Special wheelchair cushions may be necessary to avoid the development of decubitus ulcers in the ischium and sacrum. The back rest should be equipped with trunk supports when needed for children with high-level lesions. The arm rests should be detachable to facilitate transfer in and out of the chair. When a new wheelchair is delivered, it should be evaluated carefully by the prescribing physician and physical therapist.

Physical Therapy Intervention

Overall development depends largely on the child's ability to move, explore, and experience his or her environment. In a vast number of children with myelomeningocele, this ability is hampered by an abnormal central nervous system as well as by lower extremity paralysis. Ninety percent of these children are hypotonic. The proprioceptive stimuli to their heads and bodies are abnormal. They are deprived of the movement and sensation provided by their legs as a result of the paralysis and anesthesia. Physical therapy has a primary role in maintaining a good range of motion of the lower extremity, preventing the development of contractures, and gait training with orthoses and crutches. A strengthening exercise program and instruction in physical fitness and aerobic types of sports activities also play important roles. Another goal is to carefully monitor development so that neurologic deterrioration is avoided and the child's final ability more consistently matches the prognosis given at birth based on the level of the lesion. Providing an intensive, multifaceted therapy program should lessen the child's disability.

Fractures and Physeal Injuries

Children with spina bifida are especially susceptible to fractures of the long bones, particularly after the paralyzed limb has been further immobilized by casting. Most fractures occur in the femur and tibia (supracondylar area, proximal tibial metaphysis) and generally occur with no history of trauma. The physical findings include an erythematous, warm, and swollen extremity. Low fever, elevated white blood cell count, and erythrocyte sedimentation rate also occasionally are present. The fractures have a remarkable ability to heal rapidly; therefore, most can be treated nonsurgically. The goal should always be to try to maintain functional alignment and rotation so that the child eventually may stand and walk with braces. Short periods of immobilization in well-padded casts are sufficient to provide enough stability for ambulation with the orthosis.

Physeal injuries are not as common as fractures and usually occur at the distal femur, proximal tibia, or distal tibial physis. Physeal injuries often are caused by repetitive overuse, similar to the Charcot joints of patients with neuropathy, and they sometimes can be complicated by delayed union or premature fusion of the physis. Consequently, for treatment of physeal injuries of the distal femur, and proximal and distal tibia, immobilization without weight bearing until there is clinical and radiographic healing has been recommended. Union can be difficult to determine in the child with spina bifida who has a physeal injury. The absence of swelling with return to a normal anatomic contour as compared with the opposite side is a useful clinical determinant.

In summary, most of the diaphyseal and metaphyseal fractures will show early callus formation, allowing for a short period of immobilization, early motion, and weight bearing to prevent further osteopenia. The incidence of fracture is much higher in the child with a high-level lesion and occurs only rarely in the child with a sacral-level lesion.

Treatment of Foot Deformities

Most children with myelomeningocele have deformities of the foot. Despite the presence of muscle weakness, children with myelomeningocele require a plantigrade foot and maximal range of motion. The following principles apply to surgery: (1) Tendon excisions are more reliable than tendon transfer or tendon lengthenings; and (2) arthrodesis should be avoided whenever possible because of the stiffness that results. Instead, correction of bony deformities should be obtained by appropriate osteotomies that preserve joint motion. A mobile, flail foot is safer to brace than a rigid foot. Studies have shown that arthritic changes in the ankle joint frequently develop after a subtalar fusion. Pressure sores and ulcerations have been reported to be more frequent after triple arthrodesis than after soft-tissue procedures and osteotomies. Deformities resulting from muscle imbalance are gradually progressive and if not treated early, bony deformities will occur, which require osteotomies to achieve full correction. Even subtle muscle imbalance can lead to more significant deformities. Recognition of these muscle imbalances by serial manual muscle testing coupled with early intervention may prevent fixed bony deformities. Bracing with an AFO is recommended postoperatively to maintain the correction and prevent recurrence.

Clubfoot

Approximately 30% of children with myelomeningocele have a clubfoot at birth. There is a marked difference between the idiopathic clubfoot and the equinovarus deformity in children with spina bifida that resembles the deformity seen in arthrogryposis. In spina bifida, the clubfoot deformity often is characterized by a severely rigid foot. Frequently, there also is a supination deformity caused by the unopposed action of an active anterior tibial muscle. Rotational malalignment of the calcaneus and talus and calcaneocuboid joints are present as well as talonavicular subluxation with a cavus component. Many patients also have a severe internal tibial torsion. Rarely, if ever, is correction achieved by nonsurgical management. Serial casting most likely will improve some of the deformity, but surgical treatment is indicated in most patients. Serial casting should be used initially to achieve partial correction, especially of the forefoot deformity. It also will help to stretch the soft tissue and the skin, permitting better closure of the incision at the time of surgery. Experience demonstrates that the best time for surgical treatment of clubfoot is at approximately age 10 to 12 months.

The surgical treatment consists of a radical posteromedial-lateral release. A Cincinnati incision, with a wide exposure of all the anatomic structures

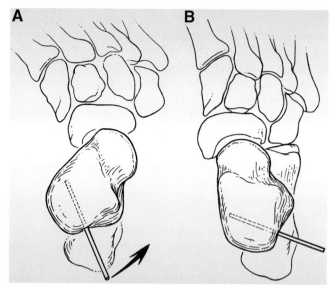

Figure 1 **A,** The abnormal rotation of the talus is seen. The K-wire is used to derotate the talus to its normal position. **B,** With the talus in a normal alignment and the talonavicular joint reduced, a second K-wire is then used to maintain this correction.

medially, posteriorly, and laterally, is preferred. At surgery, all tendons are excised rather than lengthened. A tenotomy of the anterior tibial tendon with excision always should be performed to correct the supination deformity and prevent its recurrence. The subtalar joint, including the interosseous ligament, is released completely. The calcaneocuboid joint is then released circumferentially. In some instances, a plantar release is also performed through a separate plantar incision. The talonavicular joint is released superiorly, medially, and inferiorly. To correct the external rotation of the talus, a temporary Kirschner wire (K-wire) is placed into the posterolateral aspect of the talus to rotate the talus medially in the ankle mortise (Fig. 1). With the talus rotation maintained by this K-wire, the navicular is reduced in front of the talar head, and the reduction is held by a second K-wire driven through the body of the talus, catching the navicular and exiting anteriorly in the foot. The temporary talus K-wire is then removed. The calcaneus is then reduced under the talus in a normal position and another K-wire is placed through the talocalcaneal joint to maintain its proper alignment. If necessary, a third K-wire can be used for the calcaneocuboid joint. Correction of the rotational malalignment of the talus and os calcis is very important. Postoperatively, a long leg splint is used with the foot in mild equinus to decrease any tension at the suture line for the first 2 weeks. The cast is then changed for a long leg cast applied with the foot in the corrected position for another 6 weeks. At the time of final cast removal, the K-wires also are removed, and an AFO splint is fitted for night

use for an indefinite period, as well as an AFO brace for daytime use.

In one report of experience with this approach, poor results were reported in 30% of 42 feet in which the K-wire derotation technique was not used. However, in 21 feet in which the derotation of the talus was performed, poor results were seen in only 10%. The outcome of clubfoot surgery was found to be better in children with low lumbar- and sacral-level lesions. When combining these two groups, only 11% had a poor result. For children with thoracic and high lumbar-level lesions, poor results were reported in 50% of feet. It is important to emphasize that at the time of cast removal, when the child is approximately age 12 to 13 months, the use of a standing A-frame is advised as is the use of the AFO brace and splint.

The most common residual deformity after clubfoot surgery in children with spina bifida is an adduction deformity of the forefoot, which is frequently secondary to the growth imbalance between the lateral and medial columns. Bracing is the first line of treatment; however, if the adduction deformity is rigid and interferes with brace wear, then surgical correction can be achieved by a closing wedge osteotomy of the cuboid with an opening wedge osteotomy of the medial cuneiform. The surgery should be performed after the medial cuneiform is well ossified, which is usually when the child is age 4 to 5 years.

If, after the clubfoot surgery, there is a complete recurrence of the deformity, a second posteromedial-lateral release could be quite difficult in view of the extensive scar tissue surrounding the neurovascular bundle. The best procedure for achieving a plantigrade foot in these patients is a talectomy. In a review of 28 feet that underwent talectomy, 82% had a good result. To avoid a residual adduction deformity, it is important to recognize that the talus is part of the medial column of the foot. A closing wedge osteotomy of the cuboid, balancing the medial and lateral column, is done while performing the talectomy, in hope of avoiding the need to perform a lateral column shortening later.

Equinus Deformity

Equinus deformity occurs more frequently in children with a high lumbar- and thoracic-level lesion. Prevention is attempted by bracing (AFO). Surgical treatment is indicated to achieve a plantigrade, braceable foot. If the deformity is mild, a simple Achilles tendon excision can be performed. The Achilles tendon is exposed through a short longitudinal incision, and about 2 cm of the tendon and tendon sheath are excised. A short leg cast is applied with the foot in a neutral position;

the cast is worn for approximately 10 to 14 days, followed by an AFO brace and night splint.

For the more severe equinus deformity in which there is a contracture of the posterior tibiotalar and talocalcaneal joints, a radical posterior release is necessary. One group uses a limited Cincinnati incision in which all tendons are excised, and an extensive capsulotomy of the ankle and subtalar joint is performed. It is very important to divide the calcaneofibular ligament to achieve full correction. On occasion, a talocalcaneal K-wire may be used to maintain the hindfoot in the proper alignment. A short leg cast is used for at least 6 weeks followed by an AFO splint at night and brace during the day. If the equinus is very severe, problems with skin closure may be encountered when using the Cincinnati incision. In such instances, a longitudinal incision can be made, medial to the Achilles tendon, but a short posterolateral incision may be needed for complete access and release of the calcaneofibular ligament.

Vertical Talus

Approximately 10% of children with spina bifida have a vertical talus deformity at birth that is characterized by malalignment of the hindfoot and midfoot. The talus is in an almost vertical position, the calcaneus is in equinus and valgus, the navicular is dislocated dorsally and laterally on the talus, and at times the cuboid may be dorsally subluxated in relation to the calcaneus. Vertical talus typically is congenital but may be developmental. For the vertical talus, manipulation and serial casting may partially correct the soft-tissue contractures, but ultimately a complete posteromedial-lateral and dorsal release should be performed when the child is approximately age 10 to 12 months. In a review of their experience with 21 patients with spina bifida and vertical talus feet, one group considered that 18 patients had good and three had fair results, based on clinical evaluation. An equinovarus deformity secondary to a tethered cord problem developed in one patient, requiring a posteromedial release. One patient who had a significant heel valgus subsequently underwent a calcaneus osteotomy.

Calcaneus and Calcaneovalgus Deformities

Calcaneus deformity occurs in approximately 30% of children with spina bifida and is caused by relative strength in or spasticity of the ankle dorsiflexors. It is most commonly seen in children with an L5 level lesion. Calcaneus with valgus (calcaneovalgus) is most typically caused by associated imbalance between the evertors and the invertors. This valgus may be either at the subtalar joint alone or at the ankle joint. If the

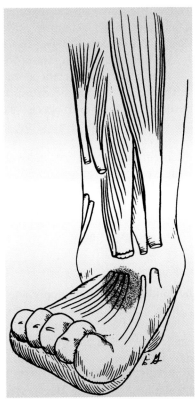

Figure 2 Tenotomy with tendon excision.

deformity is not rigid, the foot usually can be brought to a neutral position by an AFO. If the deformity is rigid, then serial casting is indicated followed by an AFO splint. If untreated, persistent weight bearing on a calcaneus deformity produces a bulbous heel that is prone to cracking of the skin or pressure sores. External tibial torsion frequently is associated with the calcaneovalgus deformity but this and other deformities may be avoided by early correction of the muscle imbalance. Anterolateral release by simple tenotomy of all ankle dorsiflexors and a tenotomy of the peroneus brevis and longus tendon can achieve a braceable, supple, plantigrade foot (Fig. 2).

Results of the anterolateral release for correction of the calcaneus deformity in 76 patients with spina bifida were reported in 1992. In 82% of feet, there was a good result, with a braceable, supple, plantigrade foot. However, 18% had either a recurrence of the deformity requiring a second release or an equinus deformity that required an Achilles tendon release. Most of those requiring a second surgery achieved a good result. The anterolateral release is a simpler procedure than the anterior tibial tendon transfer to the os calcis. It can be performed on an outpatient basis, requires a very short time in a cast (2 weeks), and can be performed on a child as young as age 18 months.

In the older child, in whom there is a significant bony deformity with the os calcis in a vertical position, surgical correction is directed toward the os calcis deformity. A closing wedge osteotomy of the os calcis in association with a plantar release can improve the alignment of the os calcis and hindfoot, allowing more effective bracing and avoiding the development of pressure sores on the heel area. It is important at the same time to proceed with a release of all the extensor tendons, and if the peroneus longus and brevis are also active or spastic, their release and resection is indicated.

In summary, early intervention for the calcaneovalgus deformity, before the vertical position of the os calcis is well established, is recommended. Then, through a simple anterolateral release, it is possible to achieve a very braceable foot that will not have problems with pressure sores later on in life.

Ankle Valgus–Hindfoot Valgus

Valgus deformity of the ankle joint is commonly seen in the child with L4-L5 level spina bifida, and its presence can hamper brace fitting and can lead to pressure sores over the medial malleolus. These children usually have associated external tibial torsion. In the normal ankle joint, the fibula usually extends more distally than the tibia, and the relationship among the medial malleolus, the lateral malleolus, and the talus is important for the normal biomechanics of the ankle joint. The calcaneovalgus position of the foot and ankle can be associated with abnormal shortening of the fibula, which promotes further valgus tilt of the talus in the ankle mortise. Relative shortening of the fibula has been found to be quite common, but a clinically significant valgus deformity of the ankle is not as frequent; it is present mainly in the child with a L4-L5 level lesion.

Radiologic Evaluation

A radiologic method has been devised to estimate the degree of fibular shortening. The fibular growth plate is more sharply defined than the tip of the lateral malleolus in the AP ankle radiograph, so the relationship between the distal fibular growth plate and the dome of the talus can be used as a measure of fibular length. In a normal ankle, the distal fibular growth plate is located approximately 2 to 3 mm proximal to the dome of the talus during the first 4 years of life. After age 6 years, the distal fibular growth plate will gradually become distal to the dome of the talus, and when the child is older than age 8 years, the fibular growth plate is approximately 2 to 3 mm distal to the dome of the talus.

Surgical Treatment

Surgical treatment of ankle valgus is indicated when the deformity causes problems with orthotic fitting and cannot be alleviated with orthotic changes. Three dif-

ferent methods of surgical treatment have been described. The Achilles tendon tenodesis to the fibula was first described for patients with poliomyelitis and more recently described for patients with spina bifida. Long-term follow-up has shown unpredictable results; in approximately 30% of patients, stretching of the tenodesis led to minimal stimulation of fibular growth. This treatment presently is not advised. A hemiepiphysiodesis is indicated for mild deformities; experience with this technique when using a cannulated AO screw has been described recently. It is important to place the screw in a most medial position, quite vertical. This procedure can be performed on an outpatient basis. To avoid a permanent closure of the physis, the screw should be removed within 2 years of its insertion. With the temporary growth arrest of the medial aspect of the physis and continued growth of the lateral aspect, there is a gradual correction of the lateral wedging of the tibial epiphysis, which corrects the valgus tilt. If overcorrection occurs, or there is a permanent arrest of the medial part of the physis, the epiphysiodesis should be completed laterally.

In the more severe ankle valgus deformity in the older child with no growth potential remaining, a supramalleolar varus internal rotation osteotomy is indicated. Osteotomies of the distal tibia have a high incidence of complications, such as delayed union, nonunion, wound infection, wound dehiscence, and loss of correction. To prevent some of the complications, multiple holes should be drilled, and the osteotomy should be completed with an osteotome, rather than with power instruments. If external tibial torsion is present, then an internal rotation of the distal fragment should be performed concurrently.

It also is important, when analyzing the valgus deformity, to recognize that frequently there may be an associated valgus of the hindfoot. In this situation, a medial sliding osteotomy of the os calcis is indicated. The amount of displacement of the distal fragment is generally 50% of the width of the fragment. A threaded K-wire is used for internal fixation. After surgery, a well-padded, short leg non–weight-bearing cast is applied. The K-wire is removed at 2 weeks, and a short leg walking cast is applied for another 4 weeks. The results of this procedure have recently been described. The authors reviewed 38 feet in 27 patients; 63% of the patients had low lumbar-level lesions. There were no delayed unions or nonunions, and 82% of patients had a good result while only 13% had a poor result. Three of the poor results were secondary to a supramalleolar valgus component that was not recognized preoperatively.

Supination and Forefoot Adduction Deformities

A supination deformity, which frequently is associated with an adduction deformity of the forefoot, is produced by the unopposed action of the tibialis anterior when the peroneus brevis and longus are paralyzed. This deformity occurs most often in children with an L5 or S1 lesion, but also can be seen after a clubfoot surgery if the anterior tibial tendon was not excised. If the muscle imbalance persists, the deformity can become fixed. If the foot is supple, a simple tenotomy of the anterior tibial tendon is indicated. In certain patients, especially those with very low-level lesions, with gastrocnemius-soleus strength, and the ability to walk with no orthosis, the anterior tibial tendon can be transferred to the midfoot (lateral cuneiform) in line with the third metatarsal. In general, the split transfer of the anterior tibial tendon in spina bifida is not recommended. When the deformity is fixed, in addition to the tenotomy or transfer of the anterior tibial tendon, a plantar closing wedge osteotomy of the medial cuneiform is performed to plantar flex the first ray and realign the forefoot. In the more severe supination deformity, including the entire forefoot, a midtarsal osteotomy is done.

After the posteromedial-lateral release, one of the most common residual deformities that may interfere with bracing is the forefoot adduction deformity. Most of these deformities are secondary to the growth imbalance between the medial and lateral column. On occasion, this adduction deformity is related to a persistent medial subluxation of the navicular. Surgical correction can be achieved by a closing wedge osteotomy of the cuboid and, if necessary, an opening wedge osteotomy of the medial cuneiform (Fig. 3). The abductor hallucis brevis and/or the plantar fascia can be released at the same time. If the residual adduction deformity is secondary to subluxation of the navicular, then a medial release with reduction of the navicular in association with a lateral column shortening (closing wedge osteotomy of the cuboid) is indicated.

Varus and Cavovarus Deformities

A cavovarus deformity occurs mainly in children with sacral-level lesions. Cavus is the primary deformity, and the varus is caused by the muscle imbalance between the posterior tibialis and peronei. The degree of rigidity of the varus deformity determines the treatment. If the varus is supple, a radical plantar release should be performed without hindfoot surgery. If the varus is rigid, then after the plantar release, with or without midtarsal or first metatarsal osteotomy, the varus deformity of the hindfoot should be corrected by a closing wedge osteotomy of the calcaneus. Any muscle imbalance must be corrected at the same time.

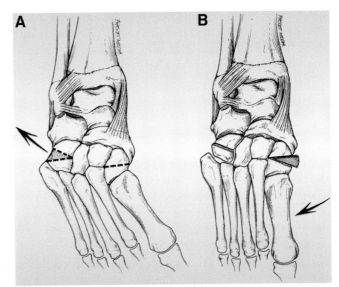

Figure 3 A, Foot showing the wedge to be removed from the cuboid and the osteotomy of the medial cuneiform. **B,** Foot with the wedge inserted at the medial cuneiform and the cuboid osteotomy being closed.

Internal fixation, either with staples or a K-wire, is indicated. Usually the K-wire can be removed 2 to 3 weeks after surgery, and a new short leg walking cast should be applied. Total time in the cast will be approximately 6 weeks.

A supple, plantigrade, braceable foot is the final goal of orthopaedic treatment. Early recognition of muscle imbalance and prompt treatment may prevent bony deformities. Tendon excisions are preferable to tendon lengthenings or tendon transfers. After any surgery, the use of day braces and nighttime splinting will help to prevent recurrence of the deformities. The surgeon should avoid any arthrodesis (subtalar or triple) and use osteotomies with preservation of joint motion if possible.

Treatment of Knee Deformities

The two most common deformities are (1) knee flexion contracture and (2) knee extension contracture. Two other less common deformities are a valgus or a varus deformity.

Flexion Contracture

A flexed position of the knee at birth is common and generally corrects spontaneously. The factors that lead to a fixed knee flexion contracture are: (1) the typical position assumed in the supine position, hips in abduction, flexion, and external rotation, knees in flexion, and feet in equinus; (2) a gradual contracture of the hamstrings and biceps, also with contracture of the posterior knee capsule secondary to the quadriceps weakness and prolonged sitting; (3) spasticity and contracture of the hamstrings as a result of tethered cord syndrome; and (4) quadriceps weakness and the paralysis of the gastrocnemius-soleus and gluteus medius and maximus. In the child with a high-level lesion, a knee flexion contracture can be prevented with the use of early splinting.

A crouched gait has a high energy cost. Studies have shown that if there is an increased knee flexion of more than 40° during gait, the energy of walking is increased. Recent studies have shown that in children with external tibial torsion of more than 20°, despite the absence of a fixed knee flexion contracture, a crouched gait is present because of the inability of the AFO brace to improve the extension of the knee joint during the stance phase. In this particular situation, correction of the external tibial torsion by an internal rotation osteotomy will improve knee extension during the stance phase. Gait analysis studies also have shown, for instance, that a patient with a knee flexion contracture of 15° on the examining table will show a flexed position of 30° during gait. Because of the increased energy use with a crouched gait, correction of a knee flexion contracture of 20° or more is indicated. A radical flexor release is indicated for the child with a high-level lesion, and a knee flexor lengthening is indicated for the child with a low lumbar- and sacral-level lesion.

For a flexion deformity of less than 45°, a transverse incision, extending from medial to lateral approximately 1 cm above the flexor crease is advised. In the child with a high-level lesion, all the medial and lateral hamstring tendons are divided and resected. In the child with a low lumbar- or sacral-level lesion, tendons are lengthened to preserve some flexor power. The hamstrings are helpful in achieving extension of the hip joint. Next, the origin of the gastrocnemius is freed from the medial and lateral femoral condyles, exposing the posterior knee capsule, and an extensive capsulectomy is performed. The posterior cruciate ligament should be left intact. It should be possible to achieve either full extension of the knee joint at the end of the surgery or −10° of full extension. A long leg cast is applied for 3 weeks followed by a long leg splint or a total body splint. During the same surgical procedure, it is important to correct any hip flexion contracture, if present.

A supracondylar extension osteotomy of the femur rarely is indicated; it is used primarily in older community ambulators with fixed knee flexion deformities of more than 20° in whom a radical knee flexor release was unsuccessful. In the older child who is not a community ambulator, no surgical treatment is indicated because the knee flexion contracture is not interfering with mobility. This supracondylar extension osteotomy can be performed through a multiple drill hole technique and a greenstick type of extension without the need for rigid fixation. It recently was suggested that for flexion deformities of 20° or less, an anterior stapling of the distal femoral physis be used in a growing child, leading to a gradual correction of the flexion deformity.

Extension Contracture

An extension contracture of the knee is much less common than a flexion deformity. The deformity is usually bilateral and frequently is associated with other congenital anomalies such as dislocation of the ipsilateral hip, external rotation contracture of the hip, equinovarus deformity of the foot, and, occasionally, a valgus deformity of the knee. Treatment with serial casting, attempting to achieve at least 90° of knee flexion, is successful in most patients. If nonsurgical treatment does not correct the deformity, lengthening of the quadriceps mechanism is indicated. The use of the V-Y quadriceps lengthening procedure is favored. Ninety degrees of knee flexion should be obtained at the time of surgery. After surgery, the knee is immobilized in a cast at 45° for approximately 2 to 3 weeks.

Treatment of Hip Deformities
Hip Contractures

Several factors lead to hip contractures in children with spina bifida: (1) muscle imbalance, as is commonly seen in the child with a low lumbar-level lesion; (2) spasticity of the hip musculature commonly seen in patients with a tethered cord, especially those with high-level lesions; and (3) habitual posture such as in wheelchair-dependent children with high-level lesions or in those who lie supine for prolonged periods.

The presence of hip contractures and restricted motion can be more deleterious than hip subluxation or dislocation. The use of gait analysis has documented that hip adduction or abduction contractures cause an increase in pelvic obliquity, leading to an asymmetric gait and compensatory scoliosis. Also, recent gait analysis studies have shown that in children with a low lumbar lesion who walk with AFOs and crutches, a hip flexion contracture of more than 20° can cause a significant anterior pelvic tilt and is associated with a decrease in walking velocity and an increased demand on the upper extremities.

The amount of hip flexion contracture should be measured using the Thomas test. In the first 2 years of life, the deformity decreases, except in patients with high-level lesions. Because of this tendency to decrease, a hip flexion deformity rarely requires surgical treatment in patients younger than age 24 months. Furthermore, the treatment of a hip flexion contracture varies according to the child's functional level. In the child with a high-level lesion, a flexion contracture of up to 30° to 40° may be tolerated if it is not interfering with the child's bracing and walking. Frequently, when the contracture is greater than 30° to 40° in a child walking with an RGO, the flexion contracture will result in a very short stride length and an increased lumbar lordosis, indicating that surgical treatment is needed for this degree of contracture. However, for the child with a low lumbar-level lesion, a flexion deformity of as little as 20°, as stated before, can result in a major impairment in walking ability and walking velocity. For the child with a high-level lesion, surgery for a hip flexion contracture is performed through an anterior approach and involves the release of the sartorius, rectus femoris, iliopsoas, and tensor fascia latae. On occasion, the anterior hip capsule also can be divided. In the child with a low lumbar-level lesion, preservation of the hip flexor power must be attempted. In these patients, the tensor fascia latae is released, and the sartorius is detached from the antero-superior iliac spine and reattached to the anteroinferior iliac spine. The rectus is released proximally, if necessary, and the iliopsoas is lengthened inside the pelvis (above the brim lengthening). After surgery, a hip splint should be used maintaining the hips in extension for the first 10 to 14 days, followed by early mobilization and use of the splint at night for a prolonged period of time.

An adduction deformity is treated by an adductor myotomy and includes the adductor longus, gracilis, and, if necessary, the adductor brevis. In the more severe cases, it may be necessary to add a subtrochanteric valgus osteotomy of the proximal femur to achieve enough abduction to correct the pelvic obliquity. Abduction contractures are usually mild, and the well-known Ober-Yount procedure should correct the deformity. For either the adductor release or the Ober-Yount procedure, there is no need for immobilization in a spica cast. The use of a hip splint, full time for the first 10 days, followed by early mobilization, is adequate.

Hip Subluxation and Dislocation

Nearly half of the children with myelomeningocele will show some degree of hip instability during the first 10 years of life. Muscle imbalance between hip flexors and extensors and the hip abductors and adductors accounts for this tendency. The lack of muscle force also is a main cause of hip instability. The treatment of an unstable hip in myelomeningocele remains a controversial issue. Over the years, the treatment pendulum has swung from benign neglect to extensive surgical reconstruction. This has occurred without clear indications, consistent patient

selection criteria, or standardized evaluation or outcome measures. Although most reconstructions in the past were offered to ambulatory patients, nonambulators also have had hip reconstruction that offered little benefit and frequently led to stiff hips that often remained dislocated. Treatment decisions were, and often still are, based mainly on the radiographs rather than on functional consequences of the unstable hip. There is general agreement, however, that ambulatory ability per se is not predicated on reduced stable hips. Classification based on neurologic levels alone can be misleading and inaccurate. Frequently, lower extremity function differs considerably between the two sides. Instead, the functional group classification outlined in Table 1 can be used to guide treatment of the unstable hip.

For patients in group 1, the stability of the hip has little clinical effect. However, the presence of hip contractures can result in difficulty with bracing and the production of functional spinal deformities. Treatment of hips in this group should be limited to release of contractures and/or realignment osteotomies. Such treatment allows for proper sitting posture, facilitates perineal care, and provides normalized alignment for the application of orthoses. There appears to be no convincing evidence to support hip reduction in this group.

Patients in group 2 have a high incidence of unstable hips. In the past, hip reconstruction, with or without muscle transfers, had inconsistent results. One group reported that reducing the hip into the acetabulum did not improve hip range of motion, reduce pain, or reduce the amount of bracing needed, and that a few children had increased hip stiffness after surgery. They stressed that maintaining a level pelvis and flexible hips was more important than reduction of the hips. Modern gait analysis has shown that the gait of children in this group can be improved without hip reduction by simply repositioning the leg with soft-tissue releases with or without realignment osteotomies to normalize the functional range of motion.

Patients classified as group 3 typically have gluteus medius or medius and maximus function, and the degree of excessive pelvic obliquity and rotation is related to the strength of the gluteus musculature. Because these children place high demand on the hip, the hip instability should be approached aggressively in this group to achieve concentric reduction, adequate acetabular coverage, and supplementary muscle augmentation, if necessary. In addition to a pelvis radiograph for preoperative evaluation, the use of CT with three-dimensional reconstruction is advised to study the type of pelvic osteotomy required to improve the femoral head coverage. Most of these patients will do well with a Dega or Pemberton pelvic osteotomy. If the degree of acetabular dysplasia is severe, a Chiari pelvic osteotomy or a shelf procedure, as described by Staheli, is indicated. If there is capsular laxity, a capsular plication is indicated and concomitant correction of the rotational malalignment of the femur (femoral antetorsion) is indicated. The surgeon should avoid excessive varus because these patients require good hip abduction function for stance stability and to improve their foot clearance during the swing phase. The Sharrard iliopsoas transfer also should be avoided because this procedure will eliminate the iliopsoas, a major power-generating force for swing phase. If there is a need for tendon transfers for augmentation of the hip abductor power, the external oblique transfer is the procedure of choice. It is important to remember that the incidence of hip dislocation in group 3 is not common. The fact that the gluteus medius is present to a certain degree will ensure a high surgical success rate.

Proximal Femoral Resection With Interposition Arthroplasty

One of the most serious problems in hip surgery in spina bifida is severe stiffness of the joint. Very little has been written about the management of this complication, but resection of the femoral head and neck is not effective. The proximal femoral resection and interposition arthroplasty can be used for this extremely serious complication in patients with spina bifida. With experience limited to approximately six hips in the last 25 years, good range of flexion, extension, abduction, and adduction has been achieved, facilitating the patient's sitting ability and perineal care.

Rotational Deformities
External Tibial Torsion

The susceptibility of paralyzed limbs to angular deformities is well known. Rotational deformities of the paralyzed lower limbs, however, have received scant attention until recently. The external rotation deformity of the hip has been described as being secondary to contracture to the posterior part of the capsule and the short external rotator muscles. Other authors noted the external rotation deformity of the leg associated with the shortened fibula and valgus deformity of the ankle. One group reported a 24% incidence of late knee pain in patients with lumbosacral-level lesions and described a knee valgus and flexion deformity. Most often, this appear-

ance of the knee valgus results from a combination of lateral pelvic and hip internal rotation, external tibial torsion, and stance-phase knee flexion. Over time, the constant proximal swivel movement of the pelvis and hip over the planted stance foot induces rotational deformities (external tibial torsion).

The possible sources of the high incidence of knee pain were demonstrated by showing an excessively high internal knee varus moment related to the magnitude of external tibial torsion in association with increased pelvic rotation and lateral trunk sway. It was concluded that increased external tibial torsion is likely to result in an abnormal varus knee stress, a TFA of greater than 20° appears to increase this stress significantly, and knee flexion is an important related parameter. It is believed that this abnormal stress may predispose the knee to late arthrosis and that internal rotational osteotomies to normalize the TFA may improve long-term outcome. The decrease of this abnormal internal varus moment after internal rotation osteotomy of the tibia has been documented with preoperative and postoperative gait analysis. An improvement in knee extension during the stance phase was found after correction of this rotational malalignment.

The other components of this abnormal stress at the knee can be recognized through gait analysis. It is not uncommon for an increased internal rotation of the hip to be associated with excessive external tibial torsion. In these patients, correction of the excessive hip internal rotation by an intertrochanteric external rotation osteotomy of the femur and correction of the abnormal external tibial torsion by a supramalleolar internal rotation osteotomy are indicated. Improving external tibial torsion will improve the effectiveness of the AFO brace in achieving better extension of the knee joint during stance phase. The excessive pelvic rotation, which is also one of the components of the abnormal knee stress, can be decreased only by the use of external support (crutches).

Rotational osteotomies of the tibia are known to have a high rate of complications (delayed union). The osteotomy should be performed just above the distal tibial physis. An osteotomy of the distal fibula is performed through a separate incision. It is important to avoid use of a power saw when performing the tibial osteotomy. Multiple drill holes and a corticotomy with an osteotome are indicated. An AO plate is preferred for internal fixation, either a 4-hole or 5-hole plate. A long leg cast is applied after surgery, and no weight bearing is allowed for the first 3 weeks. After that, a short leg walking cast is used until the osteotomy is well healed. A recent review of 39 rotational osteotomies of the tibia using this approach has shown only two patients with delayed union.

Internal Tibial Torsion

Internal tibial torsion is not an acquired deformity in spina bifida. It is present from birth and usually is associated with patients who are born with a talipes equinovarus. An internal tibial torsion can result in quite significant intoeing, with the patients tripping and falling. The initial treatment in the first 5 years should be a twister cable attached to the AFO brace, but if the problem is significant after age 5 years, an external rotation osteotomy of the tibia should be performed distally as was described for external tibial torsion. Recent studies conducted with the use of gait analysis have shown that internal tibial torsion does not lead to an abnormal internal valgus or varus moment of the knee joint. It is important to recognize at the time of surgery that if there is any muscle imbalance, such as an active or spastic anterior tibial tendon associated with the tibial torsion, a tenotomy with tendon excision should be performed simultaneously with the osteotomy.

Hip External and Internal Rotation

Both excessive hip external and internal rotation in gait can occur in spina bifida. As mentioned previously, the hip internal rotation can be associated with an external tibial torsion, leading to a quite severe valgus stress of the knee joint. However, on occasion, significant external rotation may occur at the hip joint itself. These patients can have severe outtoeing when this hip external rotation is associated with an external tibial torsion. Physical examination and gait analysis help to define the site and degree of rotational deformity. Some of these rotational problems at the hip are not really related to fixed deformities of excessive femoral antetorsion or retroversion; they seem to be more of a proprioceptive deficit that can improve. Therefore, the initial treatment is with a twister cable attached to the AFOs, and if the problem persists beyond age 5 to 6 years, an osteotomy is performed. The femoral osteotomy is done proximally and held with an AO plate.

Treatment of Spinal Deformities

Scoliosis

Paralytic spinal deformities have been reported in up to 100% of children with high-level lesions, approximately 40% to 60% of those with low lumbar-level lesions, and approximately 5% to 10% of children with sacral-level lesions. The curves develop gradually before the child reaches age 10 years and increase rapidly with the adolescent growth spurt. Scoliosis in spina bifida can be divided into two types, developmental or congenital. In one study, congenital curves that involve the structure of the vertebral bodies were present in 48% of patients, and developmental curvatures were present in 52%.

A number of reports have suggested that developmental scoliosis may be caused by hydromyelia or tethered cord syndrome. A tethered cord should be considered the most common etiology in a child with a sacral-level lesion. The early onset of scoliosis (in a child younger than age 6 years) frequently is related to these pathologies. Curves developing late in the child with a high-level lesion are most likely developmental paralytic curves.

Because of the frequency of scoliosis in patients with myelomeningocele, spinal radiographs should be obtained periodically beginning at approximately age 5 years. If scoliosis is found in the child with low lumbar- and sacral-level involvement, MRI is indicated to determine if hydromyelia or a tethered cord is present. Orthotic treatment is advised when the curvature is greater than 25°, and the thoracolumbosacral orthotic brace should be used only during the day. Although most curvatures will progress despite bracing, bracing slows progression and delays surgical intervention. Untethering of the spinal cord in patients with low lumbar- and sacral-level lesions has also shown positive benefits in controlling curvature. Indications for spinal fusion are a progressive increase in angular deformity that cannot be controlled by nonsurgical treatment. For a severe curve, anterior and posterior spinal fusion is indicated.

Kyphosis

Congenital kyphosis, the most severe spinal deformity in patients with myelomeningocele, occurs in approximately 10% of the patients. The kyphosis is usually present at birth, is progressive throughout life, and is usually greater than 90° by the time the child is age 2 to 3 years. Congenital kyphosis is completely unresponsive to bracing, and unless the deformity is mild, it must be corrected surgically. Techniques for surgical correction of the kyphosis have been reported, and more recently, a decancellation procedure has been shown to provide excellent correction of the deformity with decreased morbidity.

Surgical treatment of spinal deformities in spina bifida has a high incidence of complications, and appropriate preoperative and postoperative care is imperative. Infection rate can be as high as 10%.

Intraspinal Lipoma

Lipomeningocele, first described in 1857 by Johnson, is a subcutaneous lipoma that may present as a lumbosacral mass connected to the neural elements through a spina bifida defect and result in a tethered spinal cord. The spinal cord lipoma is the second most common form of occult spinal dysraphism, occurring in 1:4,000 births. There are two types of intraspinal lipomas. The most common type is intramedullary; the second, lipomas of the filum terminale. Most patients with lipomeningocele are not born with deformities, but neurologic deterioration can occur at any age, even into adulthood, producing severe lower extremity dysfunction. Symptoms of spinal cord tethering often appear during periods of rapid gains in height or weight. The symptoms are caused by the intramedullary lipoma compressing the spinal cord, resulting in cord stretching and ischemia. The muscle imbalance caused by tethering of the spinal cord leads to deformities, especially at the foot level. These deformities usually are asymmetric.

Patients with an intraspinal lipoma are quite different from patients with spina bifida. First, they do not have hydrocephalus; second, their involvement usually is asymmetric; third, most will have foot deformities that can be corrected by surgery; fourth, most are community ambulators and require AFO braces. When tethering of the spinal cord causes muscle imbalance, complete recovery is not seen, even after surgical excision of the lipoma and untethering. For this reason, early aggressive treatment by the neurosurgeon, in the first 6 to 8 weeks of the child's life, with resection of the lipoma and untethering of the spinal cord is indicated. Rarely do patients, if treated properly, lose quadriceps function. A lifetime of follow-up is indicated with serial annual muscle testing to detect retethering.

Retethering of the spinal cord occurs in approximately 30% of patients with intraspinal lipoma. In a recent review of 101 patients with intraspinal lipoma, 56% had a foot deformity. Of these, most were acquired, but some, such as equinovarus, were congenital. Of the foot deformities, the most common was a cavus, cavovarus, and equinovarus deformity. Soft-tissue procedures such as a plantar release and/or tendon transfers, if done early, will improve the foot alignment. In older patients with fixed deformities, the soft-tissue procedures, in association with bony procedures, were needed.

The second most common orthopaedic deformity in this patient population was scoliosis, either paralytic or congenital. Approximately 20% of patients present with scoliosis. In approximately half of these patients, scoliosis was related to tethering of the spinal cord; in the other half it was congenital, associated with hemivertebrae, unilateral bar, or sacral agenesis.

Adult Spina Bifida: Prognosis for Long-Term Walking Ability

The walking ability of the child with spina bifida is highly dependent on the motor level affected. Other factors that influence walking ability are sitting balance, upper extremity spasticity, mental retardation, obesity, and availability of braces. There are three distinct functional motor levels. The child with a high-level lesion with no quadriceps function is able to achieve some degree of ambulation during the first 13 years of life. In a review of 32 adults with high-level lesions, only one retained the level of community ambulation. The inability to retain walking as an adult is related primarily to the high energy cost required to achieve meaningful ambulation. In this particular group of patients with spina bifida, there is a high incidence of spinal deformities requiring surgical treatment. The incidence of hip and knee flexion contractures is high, and, despite aggressive treatment during childhood, some degree of recurrence is always present as an adult.

In a review of 26 patients with low lumbar lesions, 79% retained a degree of community ambulation as adults. Frequently, these patients use a wheelchair for long-distance mobility. Aggressive treatment of hip contractures rather than reduced hips, and treatment of rotational malalignment of the tibia and deformities of the knee, ankle, and foot are essential for patients with a good trunk balance and normal upper extremity function. The incidence of spinal deformities is much lower than in those with high level lesions, and these deformities are related either to congenital scoliosis or to tethered cord syndrome.

Of the patients with sacral-level lesions, 94% retained community ambulation as adults. Aggressive treatment of tethered cord syndrome; avoidance of fusion at the foot level; aggressive treatment of deformities at the knee, ankle, and foot; and correction of rotational malalignment are important if patients in this group are to retain their level of ambulation as adults.

In summary, walking ability as an adult for patients with involvement at the following functional levels is as follows: (1) thoracic-high lumbar level, 1% to 5% community ambulators, 10% to 15% household ambulators, and 80% nonambulators; (2) low lumbar level, 80% community ambulators, and 20% either household or nonambulators; (3) sacral level, 94% community ambulators and 6% either household or nonambulators.

Annotated Bibliography

Introduction

Shaw GM, Rozen R, Finnell RH, Wasserman CR, Lammer EJ: Maternal vitamin use, genetic variation of infant methylenetetrahydrofolate reductase, and risk for spina bifida. *Am J Epidemiol* 1998;148:30-37.

The authors discuss whether the maternal periconceptional use of vitamin supplements containing folic acid substantially reduces the risk of neural tube defects in the offspring.

Principles of Orthopaedic Management

Vankoski S, Moore C, Statler KD, Sarwark JF, Dias L: The influence of forearm crutches on pelvic and hip kinematics in children with myelomeningocele: Don't throw away the crutches. *Dev Med Child Neurol* 1997;39:614-619.

Patients with higher sacral-level spina bifida have a significant gluteus lurch with excessive pelvic rotation and abnormal valgus stress at the knee joint. The use of forearm crutches decreases the pelvic motion and the stress at the joints.

Treatment of Foot Deformities

de Carvalho Neto J, Dias LS, Gabrieli AP: Congenital talipes equinovarus in spina bifida: Treatment and results. *J Pediatr Orthop* 1996;16:782-785.

The authors reviewed the results of clubfoot surgical treatment using the Cincinnati incision, a radical posteromedial-lateral release with excision of the tendons, and derotation of the talus and os calcis. In patients with low lumbar- and sacral-level lesions, good results were seen in 76%. In patients with a high-level lesion, only 50% had good results.

Selber P, Dias L: Sacral-level myelomeningocele: Long-term outcome in adults. *J Pediatr Orthop* 1998;18:423-427.

The authors reviewed 46 adult patients with sacral-level lesions. At follow-up, 89.13% were community ambulators. Twelve patients underwent surgical release of a tethered cord. They concluded that in the sacral level, aggressive management of tethered cord, surgical correction of musculoskeletal deformities, and avoidance of arthrodesis at the foot level, are the main factors in accounting for these results.

Stevens PM, Belle RM: Screw epiphysiodesis for ankle valgus. *J Pediatr Orthop* 1997;17:9-12.

The authors report the results of treatment of ankle valgus with a single cannulated 4.5-mm vertical screw to retard the growth of the medial part of the distal tibial physis.

Torosian CM, Dias LS: Surgical treatment of severe hindfoot valgus by medial displacement osteotomy of the os calcis in children with myelomeningocele. *J Pediatr Orthop* 2000;20:226-229.

This is a retrospective review of 27 patients with severe hindfoot valgus who were treated with a medial sliding osteotomy of the os calcis. The group consisted of 38 feet in 27 patients with myelomeningocele ranging in age from 7 to 17 years. Eighty-two percent of the patients had good results. Most had complete correction of the hindfoot deformity.

Treatment of Knee Deformities

Lim R, Dias L, Vankoski S, Moore C, Marinello M, Sarwark J: Valgus knee stress in lumbosacral myelomeningocele: A gait analysis evaluation. *J Pediatr Orthop* 1998;18:428-433.

Valgus stress at the knee joint is multifactorial. More than 20° of external tibial torsion is one of the most common causes. The excessive external tibial torsion also can cause a crouched gait.

Treatment of Hip Deformities

Frawley PA, Broughton NS, Menelaus MB: Anterior release for fixed flexion deformity of the hip in spina bifida. *J Bone Joint Surg Br* 1996;78:299-302.

The authors review the results of anterior hip release for contractures of greater than 30°. Forty-three of the 57 hips had a good outcome. Successful surgery correlated with the walking ability of the child at the latest follow-up.

Classic Bibliography

Beaty JH, Canale ST: Orthopaedic aspects of myelomeningocele. *J Bone Joint Surg Am* 1990;72:626-630.

Brinker MR, Rosenfield SR, Feiwell E, Granger SP, Mitchell DC, Rice JC: Myelomeningocele at the sacral level: Long-term outcomes in adults. *J Bone Joint Surg Am* 1994;76:1293-1300.

Burke SW, Weiner LS, Maynard MJ: Neuropathic foot ulcers in myelodysplasia. *Orthop Trans* 1991;15:102.

Dias LS: Surgical management of knee contractures in myelomeningocele. *J Pediatr Orthop* 1982;1:127-131.

Fraser RK, Hoffman EB, Sparks LT, Buccimazza SS: The unstable hip and mid-lumbar myelomeningocele. *J Bone Joint Surg Br* 1992;74:143-146.

Litner SA, Lindseth RE: Kyphotic deformity in patients who have a myelomeningocele: Operative treatment and long-term follow-up. *J Bone Joint Surg Am* 1994;76:1301-1307.

Mazur JM, Shurtleff D, Menelaus M, Colliver J: Orthopaedic management of high-level spina bifida: Early walking compared with early use of a wheelchair. *J Bone Joint Surg Am* 1989;71:56-61.

Rodrigues RC, Dias LS: Calcaneus deformity in spina bifida: Results of anterolateral release. *J Pediatr Orthop* 1992;12:461-464.

Swank M, Dias L: Myelomeningocele: A review of the orthopaedic aspects of 206 patients treated from birth with no selection criteria. *Dev Med Child Neurol* 1992; 34:1047-1052.

Tosi LL, Slater JE, Shaer C, Mostello LA: Latex allergy in spina bifida patients: Prevalance and surgical implications. *J Pediatr Orthop* 1993;13:709-712.

Ward WT, Wenger DR, Roach JW: Surgical correction of myelomeningocele scoliosis: A critical appraisal of various spinal instrumentation systems. *J Pediatr Orthop* 1989;9:262-268.

Williams JJ, Graham GP, Dunne KB, Menelaus MB: Late knee problems in myelomeningocele. *J Pediatr Orthop* 1993;13:701-703.

Chapter 26

Muscular Dystrophies and Other Neurodegenerative Disorders

R. Tracy Ballock, MD

Stephen R. Skinner, MD

Mark F. Abel, MD

Introduction

This chapter describes a group of disorders in which there is progressive functional decline secondary to muscle or neurologic degeneration. In the muscular dystrophies, the primary defect is in the muscle; in the hereditary motor and sensory neuropathies (Charcot-Marie-Tooth polyneuropathies), the primary site is the peripheral nervous system; in Friedreich's ataxia, degeneration is primarily in the spinocerebellar system; and in the spinal muscular atrophy syndromes, anterior horn cell function is defective.

Modern Molecular Genetics

Traditional classification of neurodegenerative diseases has been based on clinical observations of phenotype; however, such classifications change continually in the light of new molecular genetic knowledge. The gene loci for many of the diseases described in this chapter are known, and new discoveries occur daily. Consequently, most names applied to these conditions describe a group of disorders that have a common defect at the gene level or a defect in a common biochemical path that produces similar phenotypic features.

The nomenclature for describing a gene locus begins with a number, which is the number of the chromosome. By convention, human autosomes (chromosomes other than sex chromosomes) are numbered with the largest as number 1 and the smallest as number 22. Following the chromosome number, the letter p (for petite) indicates the short arm or the letter q indicates the long arm of the chromosome. The last numbers indicate the gene's position on the chromosome arm, based on the bands observed with special stains.

Diagnostic Evaluation

Important aspects of the clinical history for children with neurodegenerative diseases include recollections of intrauterine fetal movements, neonatal history, time of achievement of gross motor milestones, and family history of similar problems. The key point is to distinguish whether the child's disability is static or progressive. Physical examination must include assessment of posture and gait. Careful manual muscle testing is essential, as is a complete neurologic examination, including assessment of vibration and position sense, deep tendon reflexes, and cerebellar function. Clinical laboratory testing frequently includes measurements of serum creatine phosphokinase (CPK) and aldolase enzymes. These substances often are elevated in dystrophic muscle diseases. Electrodiagnostic testing with electromyograms (EMGs) and nerve conduction velocity tests often can distinguish between primary disease of muscle (myopathy) and primary disease of nerve (neuropathy) (Table 1). In myopathy, EMGs show low amplitude, often polyphasic potentials with decreased duration of response. Nerve conduction velocity should be normal in myopathy but decreased in demyelinating neuropathies. Axonal diseases are characterized by decreased compound muscle action potentials. In chronic neuropathy, EMGs show increases in the amplitude and duration of the potentials, although fibrillation potentials of low amplitude can be seen early in the disease.

Muscle and nerve biopsies commonly are required in the diagnostic workup. In general, weak muscles are selected for biopsy, but they must not be so atrophied that the muscle tissue has been replaced by fibrous tissue and fat. The vastus lateralis and tibialis anterior often are selected in the lower extremity, whereas the triceps and biceps commonly are chosen in the upper extremity. It is important not to distort the biopsy specimen with injection of local anesthetics. Traditionally, open biopsies have been performed using special clamps to maintain muscle length and fiber orientation. However, less invasive techniques with needles and trocars seem to provide adequate sampling in larger patients. Muscle biopsy specimens are examined using

TABLE 1 | Electrodiagnostic Criteria for Neuromuscular Disorders

Disorder	Nerve Conduction Velocities	Electromyography
Myopathies	Normal	Short-duration motor unit potentials; spontaneous fibrillations (myositis); myotonic discharges (myotonia)
Demyelinating neuropathies (HSMN I & III)	Decreased	Decreased muscle action potential
Axonopathy (HSMN II)	Varies from slight decrease to normal	Decreased compound muscle action potential
Motor neuron disease (spinal muscular atrophy)	Normal	Denervation, fasciculation

both traditional light microscopy with special stains, such as dystrophin stain, and electron microscopy. Nerve biopsy specimens almost always are obtained from the sural nerve behind the distal fibula. Preoperative consultation with the pathologist is advisable to coordinate effort and maximize the yield of specimens for diagnosis.

Anesthesia Considerations

Malignant hyperthermia induced by general anesthetics has been associated with primary muscle diseases, particularly central core disease. Potentially lethal malignant hyperthermia associated with rhabdomyolysis and myoglobinuria can occur as a result of an unknown interaction with halogenated inhalational agents or depolarizing neuromuscular blocking agents such as succinylcholine.

Patients with neuromuscular diseases often have cardiomyopathy or cardiac conduction defects, which may be relatively asymptomatic until a patient is stressed by anesthetics and large fluid volume shifts. Pulmonary function studies should be performed routinely before spinal surgery, and if the vital capacity is less than 30% to 40% of predicted volumes, the patient needs prolonged ventilatory support and possible tracheostomy. Weakness of pharyngeal muscles can predispose to aspiration. Joint contractures and muscle atrophy can make positioning on the operating table difficult.

Common Musculoskeletal Problems

Musculoskeletal deformities frequently occur in patients with neurodegenerative diseases. Casting and bracing may help prevent progression of deformity or partially compensate for muscle weakness, but surgery frequently is required for amelioration. Soft-tissue surgery, such as tendon lengthening or tendon transfer, can weaken deforming forces in the early stages. Later, osteotomies are required to correct fixed deformities. Fusions such as the triple arthrodesis commonly were

used as a definitive treatment for progressive foot deformity in these neurodegenerative conditions. Recent reports on long-term follow-up of triple arthrodesis suggest that initial good results deteriorate with time as degenerative arthritic changes develop in proximal joints. Nonetheless, patients queried after many years were satisfied with the outcome. However, no long-term studies have been conducted comparing triple arthrodesis to the natural history of the foot deformity or to other surgical approaches.

Progressive hip subluxation and spinal deformity are more common in neurodegenerative conditions and often are treated surgically. Bracing may serve to provide temporary support for the spine or hip but is unlikely to arrest the progressive deformity. For hip subluxation, soft-tissue procedures are less likely to provide long-term stability than they would in developmental dysplasia. Spinal orthoses can compromise breathing, cause pressure sores, or interfere with function. Progressive spinal deformities are best treated with segmental instrumentation and posterior fusion when pulmonary function is relatively preserved. Outcomes are compromised when anterior fusion is required, pulmonary function is severely impaired, or the curves are so large and stiff that a balanced spine cannot be achieved. Spinal fusion done while patients are still ambulatory may result in loss of walking ability, because the patients may use trunk position to compensate for weak pelvic girdle muscles in walking. The goal of the instrumentation is to provide for curve correction without the need for postoperative orthotic support.

The ability of vigorous exercise to maintain muscle strength has not been studied adequately, but stretching and splinting are offered to prevent or ameliorate joint contractures. Patients with neurodegenerative diseases usually lose the ability to walk as a result of progression of the disease itself, rather than as a result of joint contractures.

Muscular Dystrophies and Myopathies

Muscular dystrophy is a general term used to describe a heterogeneous group of inherited and progressively disabling disorders of muscle weakness. The identification of a series of sarcolemmal membrane proteins that link the actin cytoskeleton to the surrounding extracellular matrix, combined with the discovery that mutations in genes encoding these key sarcolemmal membrane proteins cause many forms of muscular dystrophy, has resulted in a hypothesis that muscle membrane instability is the cause of many forms of muscular dystrophy. When present, this membrane instability leads to fiber damage with muscle contractions and to increases in serum CPK and adolase. When this occurs, repair does not continue as expected, and muscles are replaced by fibrosis and, finally, fatty infiltration.

The Dystroglycan and Sarcoglycan Complexes

The gene coding for dystrophin is the largest cloned mammalian gene, carrying 2.5 million bases. Because of its size, defects in this gene account for 70% of those with muscular dystrophy. The identification of mutations in this gene as the cause of Duchenne muscular dystrophy (DMD) heralded a new era in the molecular genetics of skeletal muscle diseases. Dystrophin is a rod-shaped cytoskeletal protein found on the inner surface of muscle fibers. It originally was believed to provide structural support to the muscle membrane during forceful contractions. Recent advances have revealed that dystrophin actually is part of a large and elaborate protein complex that links the actin cytoskeleton to the extracellular matrix. This protein complex is organized into two functionally related components, the dystroglycan complex and the sarcoglycan complex.

The dystroglycan complex consists of dystrophin and two dystrophin-associated proteins, α-dystroglycan and β-dystroglycan. The link between the actin cytoskeleton of the muscle cell and its surrounding extracellular matrix originates with one end of the dystrophin molecule binding to the actin filaments in the cytoplasm, while the other end of the dystrophin molecule binds to the transmembrane protein β-dystroglycan. The β-dystroglycan, in turn, associates with the extracellular protein α-dystroglycan, which binds to laminin molecules in the extracellular matrix to complete the connection.

The sarcoglycan complex is closely associated with the dystroglycan complex and consists of four transmembrane proteins, α-sarcoglycan, β-sarcoglycan, γ-sarcoglycan, and δ-sarcoglycan. Mutations in dystrophin or in any of the sarcoglycan proteins result in deficiency of the entire sarcoglycan complex, suggesting that the biologic function of the sarcoglycan complex is to stabilize the dystrophin-dystroglycan-laminin connection.

Recent studies have linked mutations in the genes encoding for several proteins, including those of the dystroglycan and sarcoglycan complexes, to muscular dystrophies and myopathies (Table 2). This new information not only has permitted molecular distinction between clinically similar forms of muscular dystrophy, but also has forced a reclassification of these muscle diseases.

The Dystrophinopathies

Duchenne and Becker muscular dystrophies are both caused by mutations in the gene encoding dystrophin; therefore, these two disorders are collectively referred to as dystrophinopathies.

Duchenne Muscular Dystrophy

DMD is a fatal X-linked recessive condition resulting in a complete absence of dystrophin and progressive axial and appendicular muscle weakness. DMD is the most common inherited muscle disease, affecting 1:3,500 boys. It is caused by a frameshift mutation in the dystrophin gene located on the short arm of the X chromosome (Xp21.2). This gene mutation results in the synthesis of an unstable protein that is degraded rapidly. In the absence of dystrophin, the sarcolemma no longer is protected from acute injury during a forceful muscle contraction, resulting in muscle fiber necrosis, inflammation, and replacement by fat and fibrous tissue.

Progressive proximal muscle weakness and contractures of the joints of the upper and lower extremities commonly develop in boys with DMD; they eventually become wheelchair-dependent. The clinical features often become apparent between age 3 and 6 years. Patients with DMD may initally have delayed independent ambulation, toe walking, frequent episodes of tripping and falling, or difficulty with running or climbing stairs. With time, gluteal weakness leads to excessive lumbar lordosis and a circumducting gait to compensate for weak hip flexors. In addition, weakness in the pelvic girdle and proximal thigh muscles makes it difficult for patients with DMD to rise from a sitting position on the floor without using their upper extremities to force the knees and hips into extension (Gowers' sign). Pseudohypertrophy of the calf muscles is common in the ambulatory phase. Cardiac muscle is involved in most patients, resulting in sinus tachycardia and right ventricular hypertrophy. Mild mental retardation commonly is present. Most patients stop walking by age 12 years and often die of pulmonary insufficiency by age 20 years if they are not provided ventilatory support.

TABLE 2 | Neuromuscular Diseases

Type of Muscle Disease	Inheritance Pattern*	Molecular Defect	Common Phenotype
Dystrophinopathies			
Duchenne muscular dystrophy	XR	Dystrophin (frameshift mutation)	Male; severe proximal and axial weakness; progressive (dystrophin absent); later contractures and spinal deformity; some mental retardation
Becker muscular dystrophy	XR	Dystrophin (in-frame mutation)	Male; less severe than DMD; proximal weakness (dystrophin deficient)
Limb-Girdle Muscular Dystrophies			
LGMD 1A	AD	5q22-34 region	Poorly described
LGMD 1B	AD	Calveolin-3	Poorly described
LGMD 2A	AD	Calpain 3	Usually leads to early wheelchair dependency
LGMD 2B	AD	Dysferlin	Adolescent or early adult onset
LGMD 2C-F	AR	Mutations in sarcoglycan genes	Both genders; mild to severe muscle weakness; similar to DMD and BMD; distal muscle weakness in severely involved patients
Congenital Muscular Dystrophies			
Merosin-deficient form	AR	Mutation in laminin-α2 gene	Onset in utero or in infancy; variably progressive; diffuse weakness; contractures in feet, hands; arthrogrypotic; facial muscles; peripheral neuropathy occasionally; cerebral hypomyelination
Fukuyama form	AR	Mutation in gene encoding fukutin; protein in heart, muscle, brain, pancreas	Onset in infancy; mental retardation; ocular deficits; diffuse weakness; seizures; most die by age 20 years; orthopaedic problems similar to merosin-deficient form
Facioscapulohumeral Muscular Dystrophy			
FSHMD	AD	4q35 region (deletion of tandem repeats)	Weakness proximal to distal, difficulty whistling, closing eyes; orthopaedic problems include winged scapula, hand, leg, and axial weakness
Myotonic Dystrophy	AD	MDPK (repeat in 3' untranslated region)	Most common adult-onset type, but also a more severe congenital form; associated with mild mental retardation, frontal baldness, weakness of throat muscles, myotonia; distal muscle weakness first, then proximal; cardiac conduction and other organ abnormalities
Emery-Dreifuss Muscular Dystrophy			
EDMD	XR	Mutation in gene encoding emerin	Fibrosis common of elbows, Achilles tendon, and posterior cervical muscles; cardiac abnormalities common
Congenital Myopathies			
Central core	AD (19q13.1)	Ryanodine receptor for central core, other gene products unknown	Infants hypotonic; weakness leads to developmental delay; reports of malignant hyperthermia
Nemaline core	AD (1q42.1, 1q22-23) and AR (2q22, 1q42.1)		Long faces; high-pitched voices
Myotubular	AD, AR, and XR		Scapular winging; arachnodactyly; joint contractures, clubfeet; dislocated hips

*XR, X-linked recessive; AD, autosomal dominant; AR, autosomal recessive

TABLE 2 | Continued

Type of Muscle Disease	Inheritance Pattern*	Molecular Defect	Common Phenotype
Charcot-Marie-Tooth Polyneuropathies			
Hereditary Motor and Sensory Neuropathy			
Type I: Hypertrophic, demyelinating	Most AD, some recessive varieties (more severe)	Deficient peripheral myelin protein; myelin protein zero	Sensory defects and distal weakness of clawing hands and feet; equinovarus, scoliosis, hip dysplasia; decreased reflexes; weakness usually slowly progressive, with onset in childhood except Dejerine-Sottas (type III) variety has onset in infancy
Type II: Axonal (neuronal)	AD and XR		Rarer, with normal reflexes, neuronal loss, leading to sensory and motor defects; variable severity
Type III: Dejerine-Sottas			Same as type I with onset in infancy
Types IV-VII: Others	Variable		Phytanic acid excess; familial spastic paresis; optic atrophy and retinitis pigmentosa
Friedreich's Ataxia			
Spinocerebellar degeneration	AR	Frataxin: unstable GAA trinucleotide repeat at 9q21	Adolescent onset; ataxia, dysarthria, and progressive loss of motor function; decreased reflexes; scoliosis; cardiomyopathy
Spinal Muscular Atrophy			
Type I: Werdnig-Hoffman disease	AR	Survival motor neuron gene defect leads to early death of anterior horn and brain neurons (linked to 5q13)	Onset birth to 6 months; severe and diffuse weakness; early death
Type II: Intermediate	AR		Onset before 18 months; life expectancy into fourth and fifth decades
Type 3: Kugelberg-Welander syndrome	AR		Onset in childhood with normal life expectancy; osteopenia with fractures, contractures, and scoliosis

*XR, X-linked recessive; AD, autosomal dominant; AR, autosomal recessive

Serum CPK levels in patients with DMD may be elevated over 100 times normal. Immunohistochemical staining of muscle biopsy specimens with dystrophin-specific antibodies reveals a complete absence of dystrophin and distinguishes DMD from Becker muscular dystrophy (BMD) in which dystrophin levels are diminished.

Although prednisone may offer a beneficial short-term effect in preventing progressive weakness, the lack of a specific medical treatment has focused therapeutic efforts on myoblast transplantation and gene therapy approaches. To date, however, new genetic manipulations have not been successful clinically.

Orthopaedic treatment of DMD consists primarily of physical therapy and bracing to prevent contractures, surgery to release the contractures that develop despite therapy, and spinal fusion for the scoliosis that develops once the patient has become wheelchair-dependent. The contractures that develop in patients with DMD result from asymmetric weakness in the balance of muscle forces across a joint. These contractures are manifested primarily as flexion and abduction contractures of the hips, flexion contractures of the knee, and equinus or equinovarus contractures of the ankles. The goals of the orthopaedic surgeon are to maintain a plantigrade foot and normal alignment of the limb to facilitate bracing and enhance ambulatory potential.

Results of several retrospective studies have suggested that lower limb tenotomies followed by bracing are beneficial in prolonging ambulation by 1 or 2 years in patients with DMD. However, these studies are uncontrolled or limited by small sample size. There are currently no randomized, controlled prospective data that confirm the benefit of this widely used approach. Moreover, mild equinus can enhance knee stability by shifting the ground reaction force anterior to the knee axis. Therefore, caution should be exercised because the patient may be at risk of losing the ability to walk following isolated heel-cord surgery. Generally, multi-level tentomies are performed to preserve upright walking posture. Tendon surgery includes the tensor fascia lata, iliotibial band, and gastrocnemius tendon with concomitant release, transfer, or lengthening of the posterior tibial tendon.

Scoliosis will develop in essentially all boys with DMD who have been confined to a wheelchair. Left untreated, this spinal deformity will increase relentlessly at an average rate of 2° per month until the ribs rest on the pelvis. This inevitable progression is associated with a decrease in pulmonary function, although the latter appears to be caused by progression of the muscle disease rather than by mechanical factors related to the spinal deformity. Bracing has not been successful in preventing curve progression but may be used to improve sitting comfort. Segmental spinal instrumentation and fusion has been found to improve sitting balance and quality of life in patients with DMD but has not been shown to alter the decrease in pulmonary function or to increase longevity. Surgery should be performed when the curve approaches 30° and lung function is relatively spared (forced vital capacity greater than 30% to 40% of predicted) to decrease the incidence of pulmonary complications. Typically, posterior instrumentation is performed with segmental fixation from T2 to L5 or to the pelvis if pelvic obliquity is present.

Becker Muscular Dystrophy

BMD is a less common and less severe X-linked recessive muscle disease. BMD results from in-frame mutations in the dystrophin gene and results in a truncated dystrophin protein, in reduced quantities, that retains some structural function. There is a consistent relationship between the quantity of dystrophin present and the clinical severity of the disorder. Although the clinical features of DMD and BMD are similar, patients with BMD have a later age of onset, slower disease progression, and longer life expectancy. Because the same orthopaedic problems occur in both disorders, the orthopaedic treatment of BMD is similar to that outlined for the more severe DMD.

The Sarcoglycanopathies

Defects in the synthesis of sarcoglycan proteins have proven to be responsible for many forms of the autosomal recessive muscular dystrophies known as limb-girdle muscular dystrophies (LGMDs). These diseases, which affect both genders, previously have been indistiguishable based on clinical features and immunohistochemical analysis. Moreover, a similar clinical phenotype results from genetic mutations in any of the four sarcoglycan genes (LGMDs 2C through 2F). Patients with LGMD have progressive proximal muscle weakness in the second or third decade of life that may be a severe, DMD-like disorder or a mild phenotype indistinguishable from BMD. Severely involved pa-

tients may have distal weakness as well. Calf hypertrophy is common, but facial, extraocular, and pharyngeal muscles normally are spared. In contrast to DMD, mentation is spared and cardiomyopathy is less predictable.

Other Limb Girdle Muscular Dystrophies

The remaining LGMDs (1A, 1B, 2A, 2B) do not involve disorders in sarcoglycan proteins; thus, CPK levels are not as elevated. Proximal and distal weakness can be seen as well as childhood, adolescent, or adult onset. Orthopaedic management of all LGMDs is similar to that of DMD and BMD, except that spinal fusion is seldom required because of the relatively late onset of the disease.

Congenital Muscular Dystrophy

Congenital muscular dystrophy (CMD) is characterized by a slowly progressive myopathy that begins in utero or within the first year of life and results in profound motor delay, joint contractures (foot, knee, hip, wrist, fingers, and scoliosis), and inability to walk. Serum CPK usually is elevated moderately. EMGs show a myopathic pattern. Muscle biopsy shows a dystrophic pattern with perimysial and endomysial fibrosis. CMD can be classified at the molecular level into at least two separate autosomal recessive diseases with distinct clinical features and prognoses.

Laminin-α2 deficient CMD is caused by a mutation in the gene encoding the extracellular matrix protein laminin-α2, formerly known as merosin. The deficiency of the laminin-α2 protein disrupts the extracellular anchor of the dystroglycan complex, resulting in membrane instability during muscle contraction. The prognosis is variable, with some patients remaining severely disabled and unable to walk, while others stabilize and remain free of contractures, surviving well into adult life. Most patients have no intellectual impairment.

Fukuyama CMD is caused by a mutation in the gene encoding fukutin, a protein expressed at high levels in skeletal muscle, brain, heart, and pancreas. The exact function of fukutin currently is unknown. Fukuyama CMD occurs predominantly in Japan; it results in profoundly delayed motor and mental development, inability to ambulate, severe mental retardation, and seizures. Eye abnormalities include myopia, retinal pigment mottling, and optic nerve atrophy. Most patients become bedridden by age 10 years, and rarely live beyond age 20 years.

Orthopaedic problems in CMD include congenital hip dislocation, clubfoot, equinus contractures, and scoliosis. Early physical therapy may help prevent soft-tissue contractures. Surgical treatment is standard if the medical condition allows.

Facioscapulohumeral Muscular Dystrophy

Facioscapulohumeral muscular dystrophy (FSHMD) is an autosomal dominant condition with variable clinical phenotypes that have in common slowly progressive weakness of the facial muscles, the shoulder girdle, and the upper arm. Symptoms usually begin in childhood but may be as subtle as inability to whistle or drink from a straw. On physical examination, approximately 90% of patients have some evidence of weakness in the facial or scapular stabilizer muscles by age 20 years. The disease progresses in a descending anatomic fashion, with weakness first affecting the facial muscles followed by the scapular and humeral muscles and finally the pelvic girdle. The deltoid, supraspinatus, and infraspinatus normally are spared.

The etiology of FSHMD is a deletion of a nontranscribed region of DNA at the distal end of chromosome 4 (4q35) that may have a positional effect on the transcription of genes more proximal to the deletion. Although there is a relationship between the size of the deletion and the severity of the disease, the underlying pathogenesis of FSHMD and the genes involved are not understood.

The major orthopaedic problem is scapular winging, which is treated by surgical stabilization of the scapula to the thoracic cage by soft-tissue repair or fusion. The procedure usually is performed only unilaterally, and good deltoid function is a prerequisite.

Myotonic Dystrophy

Myotonic dystrophy is the most common form (frequency of 1:8,000 live births) of adult-onset muscular dystrophy, but it also has a more severe congenital form that is associated with delayed motor development and mental retardation. Despite the autosomal dominant inheritance pattern, the congenital form nearly always is inherited from an affected mother. The disease is caused by a marked expansion in the number of triplet cytosine-thymine-guanine (CTG) repeats in the untranslated region of the gene encoding myotonic dystrophy protein kinase (MDPK), a serine-threonine kinase that appears to be involved in phosphorylation of muscle-specific sodium channels. The disease affects skeletal muscle, smooth muscle, myocardium, the brain, and the eyes.

The age of onset is proportional to the length of the CTG repeat, but the disease usually becomes evident in adolescence. Conditions associated with the adult-onset form include myotonia (inability to relax skeletal muscle), gonadal atrophy, cataracts, frontal baldness, heart disease, diabetes mellitus, and dementia. Wasting of the temporalis and masseter muscles results in the characteristic long, narrow face. In the congenital form, hypotonia, feeding difficulties due to pharyngeal weakness, respiratory failure, and facial weakness are more prominent. Approximately 25% of infants with myotonic dystrophy die because they lack adequate respiratory function. In those who survive, muscle function often improves following the neonatal period. Myotonia is absent at birth but usually develops by age 10 years. Mild or moderate mental retardation affects 75% of children. Muscle biopsy reveals fiber atrophy with central nuclei rather than myopathic changes.

Unlike symptoms of many muscle diseases, weakness of distal muscles of the hands and feet occurs first in myotonic dystrophy. Equinovarus foot deformities may be seen at birth and are difficult to treat, often requiring talectomy. Contractures of the wrist and elbows are common. Hip dislocation is common in young patients. Spinal deformity is more common in patients with positive family histories (and, correspondingly, long CTG repeats).

Emery-Dreifuss Muscular Dystrophy

Emery-Dreifuss muscular dystrophy (EDMD) is an X-linked condition characterized by the triad of early contracture of the elbows, the Achilles tendon, and the posterior cervical muscles. EDMD is the result of a mutation in the gene encoding emerin, a protein that spans the membrane of the cell nucleus. The functional role of emerin may be to stabilize the nuclear membrane against the mechanical stresses generated in muscle cells during contraction.

Children with EDMD have a normal birth and early development but usually experience gait abnormalities and difficulty climbing stairs within the first decade, often before age 5 years. A slowly progressive humeral and peroneal muscle wasting ensues. Fixed equinus contractures of the ankles, flexion contractures of the elbows, and extension contractures of the neck occur in the first and early second decades. The spinal contractures may completely prevent flexion of the head or spine beyond neutral, although forward bending can occur through the hips. Cardiomyopathy and cardiac arrhythmias that may result in sudden death also frequently develop in patients with EDMD.

Orthopaedic treatment is focused on physical therapy and surgical lengthening of ankle equinus contractures. The elbow flexion contractures rarely exceed 35°, and surgical correction rarely is indicated. The paravertebral muscle stiffness may help prevent progression of scoliosis, which often stabilizes in the absence of treatment before surgical correction is needed.

Congenital Myopathy

The congenital myopathies represent a group of disorders with autosomal and X-linked inheritance. Central core myopathy is an autosomal dominant disorder with a gene locus of 19q13.1. There are autosomal dominant (1q42.1 and 1q22-23) and autosomal recessive (2q22, 1q42.1) forms of nemaline myopathy, in which rod-like bodies are seen under electron microscopy of muscle biopsy specimens. Congenital fiber-type disproportion is thought to be autosomal recessive, but the gene locus is not known at this time. Likewise, myotubular myopathy represents a collection of autosomal dominant, autosomal recessive, and X-linked recessive mutations with similar phenotypes.

Infants with congenital myopathies are hypotonic; the muscle weakness is probably static, but function may be lost as the child grows. Weakness is primarily in proximal muscles. Walking may be delayed until age 4 years. In children, Gowers' sign may be positive. Deep tendon reflexes are diminished or absent. Children with nemaline or myotubular myopathy often have long faces with high-arched palates and nasal, high-pitched voices. Those with nemaline myopathy also may have arachnodactyly. Scapular winging may be seen in patients with myotubular myopathy. The CPK often is normal in the congenital myopathies. EMGs are normal or show nonspecific myopathic changes, except in myotubular myopathy, in which the complex repetitive discharges characteristic of fibrillation potentials may be seen. The diagnosis of congenital myopathy is made by examination of muscle biopsy specimens, which often requires electron microscopy. In central core myopathy, muscle biopsy specimens show central round or oval regions without mitochondria and oxidative enzymes in mostly type I fibers. In myotubular myopathy, persistent myotubules of fetal life are seen on biopsy specimens.

There is a notorious association between congenital myopathy, especially central core disease, and malignant hyperthermia. Joint contractures can be severe and may require surgical correction, particularly at the hips or knees.

Charcot-Marie-Tooth Polyneuropathy (Hereditary Motor and Sensory Neuropathy)

In the later part of the 19th century, Charcot, Marie, and Tooth described the features of a polyneuropathy causing weakness and wasting of the legs and feet initially and later wasting of the hands. At the present time, the disorders are collectively referred to as hereditary motor and sensory neuropathies (HMSN), and they are the most common form of polyneuropathy, with a frequency of 1:2,500 individuals. There are at least seven types of HMSN; the most common variety has an autosomal dominant pattern, but recessive and X-linked varieties also exist. Two broad categories of HMSN are recognized, the hypertrophic, demyelinating type I and the rarer, axonal (neuronal) type II. The genetics of these disorders is being established, but it is recognized that they are caused by either DNA duplications or point-mutations in genes controlling myelination (peripheral myelin protein and myelin protein zero). An X-linked dominant disorder has been associated with defects in the gene for connexin, a connecting protein involved with myelination.

Onset of HMSN typically occurs in childhood, but the Dejerine-Sottas variety (HMSN III) is characterized by onset in infancy. Although sensory neuropathy does occur, motor neuropathy characterizes the HMSN. For the demyelinating, hypertrophic form, nerve conduction velocities are uniformly decreased (Table 1). For the neuronal form, the nerve conduction velocities may be slowed only slightly, but the compound muscle action potential is decreased. Nerve biopsy shows the onion bulb hypertrophy of the myelin sheath in the demyelinating, hypertrophic form, and demyelination is seen in the neuronal form. Muscle biopsy shows atrophy of fiber groups.

Common clinical findings include weakness of distal muscles, more in the lower extremity than the upper. The intrinsic muscles of the foot are affected first, then the peroneals. Deep tendon reflexes are diminished or absent in demyelinating forms, especially at the ankles. Sensory functions (eg, vibration sense, light touch position sense) often are impaired distally. In some varieties, patients have tremors, ataxia, spastic paraparesis, deafness, optic atrophy, and retinitis pigmentosa.

Musculoskeletal deformities begin commonly with the foot. Intrinsic muscle weakness results in claw toes, a plantar flexed first metatarsal, and pes cavus. Toe deformities can be treated by flexor to extensor tendon transfers, transfer of the extensor to the metatarsal head, and interphalangeal fusions. Flexible cavus can be treated with plantar release or plantar medial release. In an effort to balance muscle force across the foot, tendon transfers such as centralization of the tibialis anterior or transfer of the tibialis posterior to the dorsum of the foot have been useful. Heel-cord lengthening rarely is required. Usually equinus appears at the forefoot rather than the ankle. Fixed bony varus or cavus deformity can be managed by osteotomy of the os calcis or midtarsal bones. Triple arthrodesis should be reserved as a salvage procedure. The Coleman block test is used to differentiate fixed from flexible deformities by having the patient stand with the lateral border of the foot on a 1-cm block. If the heel tilts out of varus, this is evidence of a flexible deformity that can be treated through soft-tissue surgery.

Hip dysplasia occurs in 6% to 8% of patients with HMSN. Patients usually seek treatment for pain between age 5 and 15 years. Osteotomy of the pelvis or upper femur may be required. Annual hip radiographs might allow earlier intervention, before the patient with hip dysplasia becomes symptomatic. Hand problems are essentially those of the intrinsic minus hand. Transfers such as flexor digitorum sublimis to adductor brevis can be useful. Nerve compression neuropathy can also be improved by surgical releases. Standard operations for the intrinsic minus hand can improve function.

Scoliosis may occur as rarely as in 10% of patients or as commonly as in 50%, depending on the population studied and the criteria used to make the diagnosis. Scoliosis is more common in girls, and most authors agree that the curves behave like those of idiopathic scoliosis. Bracing can be an effective treatment for scoliosis in this disease.

Friedreich's Ataxia

Friedreich's ataxia is a form of spinocerebellar degeneration that occurs at a rate of 1:50,000 live births. It is an autosomal recessive disorder caused by an unstable trinucleotide repeat (GAA) at the 9q21 gene locus. This gene codes for a protein called frataxin. Like myotonic muscular dystrophy, in which there is also an unstable repeat of a trinucleotide group, the severity of the symptoms in Friedreich's ataxia is proportional to the length of the repeat.

In general, symptoms begin before age 20 years. Progressive ataxia and difficulty with gait are the most common symptoms. Dysarthria is common. Physical examination will usually demonstrate absent deep tendon reflexes in both the upper and lower extremities. However, upper motor neuron signs, such as the Babinski sign, are often positive. Decreases in vibration and position sense may be observed. Muscle weakness is usual. The first muscles to weaken are the limb-girdle muscles of the lower extremity, particularly the hip extensors and abductors. Cardiomyopathy is often present and can be identified by electrocardiography. Scoliosis develops in essentially all patients and kyphosis in about two thirds. CPK is normal. EMGs demonstrate loss of motor units in a neurogenic pattern. The nerve conduction velocities are slowed. Less than half the patients will have optic atrophy, nystagmus, distal muscle weakness, deafness, or diabetes mellitus.

Most individuals with Friedreich's ataxia start using a wheelchair at least part-time during the second decade. The ataxia and poor balance cause the patients to stop walking, not muscle weakness. Once wheelchair use begins, disuse atrophy compounds the weakness associated with the disease process, and clinical weakness accelerates. Most patients die in the fourth or fifth decade as a result of cardiomyopathy, pneumonia, or aspiration.

The most common foot deformity in Friedreich's ataxia is pes cavovarus. Nonsurgical treatment is usually ineffective. Tenotomy, lengthening, or transfer of the tibialis anterior and/or posterior have been reported to be successful. Triple arthrodesis is a good salvage procedure.

The scoliosis curve patterns are similar to those observed in idiopathic scoliosis. If the disease onset is early in life, progression is likely. Use of a spinal orthosis may slow the rate of curve progression, but it may make walking more difficult. In some individuals with later onset of symptoms, the curve may never reach 40°, and it may not progress after skeletal maturity. In curves over 40°, posterior spinal fusion is recommended; combined anterior and posterior fusion may be required for particularly large and rigid curves.

Some patients with Friedreich's ataxia report painful muscle cramps, particularly in the hip adductors and quadriceps. Initial treatment should be with massage and heat. Diazepam or baclofen may alleviate symptoms. In some nonambulatory adults with persistent symptoms, tenotomy may be required.

Spinal Muscular Atrophy

The spinal muscular atrophies (SMAs) occur at a rate of 1:20,000 live births. All are autosomal recessive disorders involving a mutation at the 5q13 locus, the site of the survival motor neuron gene. The disease process involves degeneration of anterior horn cells and brain stem motor nuclei. The loss of anterior horn cells is acute and nonprogressive, but progressive weakness occurs as growth progresses beyond muscle reserve. Antenatal diagnosis is available through the survival motor neuron gene deletion test.

The SMAs are generally divided into three types depending on the natural history and severity of symptoms. SMA type I or Werdnig-Hoffmann disease is the most severe type of SMA, with onset at birth to age 6 months. These children are profoundly hypotonic and weak; they never sit without support and generally die before age 2 years.

SMA type II is the intermediate type, with onset before age 18 months. These children achieve sitting but do not stand. Of these individuals, 77% are alive at age 20 years. Life expectancy is into the fourth and fifth decades.

SMA type III is the mild form, known also as Kugelberg-Welander syndrome, with onset after 18 months. Patients achieve both standing and walking and have a normal life expectancy.

Mothers of infants with SMA type I may report decreased intrauterine fetal movement. Infants with

SMA type I have proximal muscle weakness, and the hips assume a frog-leg position of flexion, external rotation, and abduction. Joint contractures are common. Deep tendon reflexes are absent. There may be fasciculations of the tongue.

Children with SMA type II have symmetric muscle weakness in which the proximal muscles are more involved than distal ones. Functional weakness is progressive, and motor milestones are delayed. Fasciculations may be seen not only of the tongue, but also of the trunk and extremity muscles. Joint contractures are common. All patients eventually have scoliosis. EMGs and muscle biopsy show neuropathic changes. CPK and aldolase levels are normal to slightly elevated.

Proximal muscle weakness predominates in SMA type III, although the onset of symptoms is later. Limb-girdle weakness results in a waddling gait. Toe walking is caused by the triceps surae attempting to stabilize the knee to compensate for quadriceps weakness. Gowers' sign may be positive. Deep tendon reflexes are absent. Tongue fasciculations are seen in about half the patients. Scoliosis is less common and less severe.

Intrauterine inactivity can lead to disuse osteoporosis, which may predispose infants with SMA type I to neonatal fractures. These fractures heal with splinting. In children with SMA types II and III, nonsurgical techniques can be used to treat or prevent joint contractures. Orthoses may assist in ambulation. Heel-cord lengthening should be avoided because the strong triceps surae is needed to stabilize the knee.

Hip subluxations and dislocations are not unusual in the face of proximal muscle imbalance. If subluxation is identified early, adductor tenotomy and iliopsoas recession may prevent dislocation. Later, upper femoral varus osteotomy, open reduction, or pelvic osteotomy may be required. Posterior acetabular coverage of the femoral head is poor in SMA, and this fact will affect the selection of pelvic osteotomy.

Patients with SMA who survive into adolescence will eventually have progressive scoliosis as a result of trunk muscle weakness. About one third of patients will have associated kyphosis that is progressive as well. Bracing can help provide sitting balance and slow the rate of curve progression in both ambulatory and nonambulatory patients, but the spinal orthosis can interfere with activities of daily living. If the curve measures more than 40° and the forced vital capacity is more than 30% to 40% of predicted, full-length, posterior spinal fusion with segmental fixation is indicated. Fixation to the pelvis is recommended to address pelvic obliquity. Complications are common and include hemorrhage, pulmonary problems, loss of fixation, infection, pseudarthrosis, and death. Postoperative bracing is not well tolerated. In patients with marginal ambulatory abilities, the ability to walk may be lost following long spinal fusions because the patients can no longer balance by trunk posturing.

Annotated Bibliography

Birch JG: Orthopedic management of neuromuscular disorders in children. *Semin Pediatr Neurol* 1998;5: 78-91.

This is an up-to-date discussion of the principles, rationales, and treatment strategies for orthopaedic problems associated with DMD, SMA, FSHMD, and Charcot-Marie-Tooth disease.

Dietz FR, Mathews KD: Update on the genetic bases of disorders with orthopaedic manifestations. *J Bone Joint Surg Am* 1996;78:1583-1598.

This article is an update on those hereditary conditions that are of interest to the orthopaedist. Included are excellent discussions of the genetics of SMA, muscular dystrophy, and HSMN.

Hart DA, McDonald CM: Spinal deformity in progressive neuromuscular disease: Natural history and management. *Phys Med Rehabil Clin N Am* 1998;9:213-232.

The authors discuss the prevalence, natural history, and treatment of spinal deformity in the muscular dystrophies, SMA, and Friedreich's ataxia. Preoperative evaluation, anesthetic considerations, and outcomes related to the surgical approach are discussed. In SMA type III, surgical spine stabilization may cause the patient to cease ambulation by impairing the patient's ability to compensate for weak muscles.

McDonald CM: Neuromuscular diseases, in Molnar GE, Alexander MA (eds): *Pediatric Rehabilitation.* Philadelphia, PA, Hanley & Belfus, 1999, pp 289-330.

This comprehensive, superbly written description of childhood neuromuscular diseases has an extensive bibliography.

Reitter B, Goebel HH: Dystrophinopathies. *Semin Pediatr Neurol* 1996;3:99-109.

The authors present a comprehensive overview of the dystrophinopathies including pathophysiology, genetics, clinical findings, genotype-phenotype correlation, muscle histomorphology, diagnostic aspects, and therapeutic strategies.

Rideau Y, Duport G, Delaubier A, Guillou C, Renardel-Irani A, Bach JR: Early treatment to preserve quality of locomotion for children with Duchenne muscular dystrophy. *Semin Neurol* 1995;15:9-17.

The authors outline their approach to prolonging ambulation in patients with DMD, which consists of early surgical release of lower extremity contractures, especially the hip flexors, lateral thigh muscles, knee flexors, and Achilles tendon. Their results suggest a positive effect on maintaining muscle strength and ambulation compared to a nonrandomized control group.

Saltzman CL, Fehrle MJ, Cooper RR, Spencer EC, Ponseti IV: Triple arthrodesis: Twenty-five and forty-four-year average follow-up of the same patients. *J Bone Joint Surg Am* 1999;81:1391-1402.

Triple arthrodesis was a mainstay of treatment of foot deformities in neurodegenerative diseases. While this article supports the notion that success of triple arthrodesis diminishes with time, the patients show great satisfaction even at very long follow-up. The authors point out that there has been no control study of the long-term results of untreated foot deformity in these patients.

Tsao CY, Mendell JR: The childhood muscular dystrophies: Making order out of chaos. *Semin Neurol* 1999;19:9-23.

This is an excellent discussion of how the transition from the premolecular to the molecular era of myology has transformed the diagnosis and categorization of childhood muscular dystrophies.

Vignos PJ, Wagner MB, Karlinchak B, Katirji B: Evaluation of a program for long-term treatment of Duchenne muscular dystrophy: Experience at the University Hospitals of Cleveland. *J Bone Joint Surg Am* 1996;78:1844-1852.

This study followed 144 boys with DMD an average of 9 years to document the benefits of a program consisting of physical therapy, Achilles tenotomy, posterior tibial tendon transfer, and knee-ankle-foot orthoses to prolong ambulation.

Voit T: Congenital muscular dystrophies: 1997 update. *Brain Dev* 1998;20:65-74.

The author has compiled a concise and up-to-date review of these rare and heterogeneous muscle disorders, highlighting the molecular features of each disease as well as the sometimes subtle differences in clinical presentation.

Worton R: Muscular dystrophies: Diseases of the dystrophin-glycoprotein complex. *Science* 1995;270:755-756.

This is a very concise, readable summary of the evolution of the present understanding of the structure of the dystroglycan and sarcoglycan complexes, as well as the mutations in the genes encoding these proteins, which are now known to cause many forms of muscular dystrophy. Unfortunately, the information presented already is becoming a little dated in this fast-moving field of research.

Younger DS, Gordon PH: Diagnosis in neuromuscular diseases. *Neurol Clinics* 1996;14:135-168.

This is an excellent review on the clinical and diagnostic features of a variety of muscle diseases.

Classic Bibliography

Beauchamp M, Labelle H, Duhaime M, Joncas J: Natural history of muscle weakness in Friedreich's ataxia and its relation to loss of ambulation. *Clin Orthop* 1995;311:270-275.

Brown RE, Zamboni WA, Zook EG, Russell RC: Evaluation and management of upper extremity neuropathies in Charcot-Marie-Tooth disease. *J Hand Surg Am* 1992;17:523-530.

Bunch WH, Siegel IM: Scapulothoracic arthrodesis in facioscapulohumeral muscular dystrophy: Review of seventeen procedures with three to twenty-one-year follow-up. *J Bone Joint Surg Am* 1993;75:372-376.

Cambridge W, Drennan JC: Scoliosis associated with Duchenne muscular dystrophy. *J Pediatr Orthop* 1987;7:436-440.

Carter GT, Abresch RT, Fowler WM Jr, Johnson ER, Kilmer DD, McDonald CM: Profiles of neuromuscular diseases: Hereditary motor and sensory neuropathy, types I and II. *Am J Phys Med Rehabil* 1995;74(suppl 5):S140-149.

Carter GT, Abresch RT, Fowler WM Jr, Johnson ER, Kilmer DD, McDonald CM: Profiles in neuromuscular diseases: Spinal muscular atrophy. *Am J Phys Med Rehabil* 1995;74(suppl 5):S150-159.

Johnson ER, Abresch RT, Carter GT, et al: Profiles in neuromuscular diseases: Myotonic dystrophy. *Am J Phys Med Rehabil* 1995;74(suppl 5):S104-116.

Kurz LT, Mubarak SJ, Schultz P, Park SM, Leach J: Correlation of scoliosis and pulmonary function in Duchenne muscular dystrophy. *J Pediatr Orthop* 1983;3:347-353.

Miller F, Moseley CF, Koreska J, Levison H: Pulmonary function and scoliosis in Duchenne dystrophy. *J Pediatr Orthop* 1988;8:133-137.

Shapiro F, Specht L: The diagnosis and orthopaedic treatment of childhood spinal muscular atrophy, peripheral neuropathy, Friedreich ataxia, and arthrogryposis. *J Bone Joint Surg Am* 1993;75:1699-1714.

Smith AD, Koreska J, Moseley CF: Progression of scoliosis in Duchenne muscular dystrophy. *J Bone Joint Surg Am* 1989;71:1066-1074.

Sussman MD: Advantage of early spinal stabilization and fusion in patients with Duchenne muscular dystrophy. *J Pediatr Orthop* 1984;4:532-537.

Walker JL, Nelson KR, Stevens DB, Lubicky JP, Ogden JA, VandenBrink KD: Spinal deformity in Charcot-Marie-Tooth disease. *Spine* 1994;19:1044-1047.

Chapter 27

Arthrogryposis Syndromes: Disorders With Congenital Contractures

William J. Shaughnessy, MD

Introduction

The large heterogeneous group of disorders in which congenital joint contractures occur often are referred to as arthrogryposis. The word arthrogryposis literally means "hooked or curved joints." Casual reading of older medical literature might suggest that arthrogryposis is a single disease entity. As individual conditions with multiple joint contractures grew in number, the terms arthrogryposis and arthrogryposis multiplex congenita came to be used in a generic way to group the different conditions. Neither term, however, represents a specific diagnosis. For the purposes of this chapter, arthrogryposis is a term used to describe congenital nonprogressive limitation of movement including, but not limited to, amyoplasia, myelomeningocele, congenital muscular dystrophy, Larsen's syndrome, Möbius' syndrome, and skeletal dysplasias. Whereas these conditions have different etiologies, all are characterized by the presence of joint contractures in different body areas.

Use of the term arthrogryposis to define many different conditions has led to considerable confusion and great difficulty in interpreting the medical literature. From the standpoint of management and treatment, however, the grouping of these very different conditions is useful. Basic principles of treatment usually apply to most congenital contractures. From the perspective of an orthopaedic surgeon, it is therefore reasonable to group these conditions in a single chapter despite the obvious diversity of the pathology.

Etiology and Incidence

The etiology of congenital contractures in a given child is often unknown. Virtually all conditions associated with multiple congenital contractures result from some limitation of intrauterine and early fetal movement. Animal studies have shown that limited intrauterine movement leads to joint contractures at birth. The longer movement is inhibited, the more severe is the contracture. Fetal joint formation in arthrogryposis is usually normal, suggesting that contractures are the result of lack of movement after 8 to 10 weeks of pregnancy when joint formation occurs. Persistent immobility as the result of neuropathic, myopathic, connective tissue, and mechanical processes leads to joint contractures and subsequent abnormal joint development. Several major categories of problems leading to limitation of joint movement are listed in Table 1. The role of environmental factors, teratogens, intrauterine infections, chromosomal abnormalities, and other multifactorial processes in the development of arthrogryposis is unknown. Plasma from mothers of children with arthrogryposis has been shown to inhibit fetal acetylcholine receptor function, suggesting that maternal serum antibodies may play a role in limiting fetal motion and in causing subsequent arthrogryposis. The estimated incidence of arthrogryposis is 1 in 3,000 live births.

Classification

Well over 150 conditions with multiple congenital contractures have been recognized. It is beyond the scope of this chapter to examine each condition. Nonetheless, it is useful to separate and classify individual patients into one of three groups: (1) those with isolated limb involvement, (2) those with limb and other body area involvement (such as craniofacial, vertebral, or cardiac abnormalities), and (3) those with limb involvement and central nervous system dysfunction. Examples of conditions representing these three groups are listed in Table 2. This classification has some utility from the perspective of an orthopaedic surgeon. Patients with more extensive involvement have more limitations and a worse prognosis. Such issues may affect management.

Most orthopaedic surgeons are familiar with amyoplasia, the most common specific arthrogrypotic disorder. Amyoplasia is often referred to as the classic form of arthrogryposis. A significant subset of the arthrogry-

TABLE 1	Causes of Limited Fetal Movement

Cause	Possible Resulting Condition
Myopathic processes	Congenital muscular dystrophy
Neuropathic processes	Myelomeningocele
Connective tissue disorders	Diastrophic dysplasia
Oligohydramnios	Hip dysplasia, knee dislocations
Maternal diabetes	Lumbosacral agenesis

TABLE 2	Classification of Conditions With Congenital Contractures

Type of Disorder	Related Conditions
Limb involvement only	Amyoplasia (classic arthrogryposis)
	Distal arthrogryposis
	Poland anomaly
Limb and other body areas	Diastrophic dysplasia
	Larsen's syndrome
	Nail-patella syndrome
	Osteogenesis imperfecta
	Popliteal pterygium syndrome
	VATER association
Limb and central nervous system	Fetal alcohol syndrome
	Myelomeningocele
	Spinal muscular atrophy
	Congenital muscular dystrophy

posis literature refers to this condition. Approximately 40% of patients with arthrogryposis have amyoplasia. The incidence is estimated to be 1 in 10,000 live births. Although the etiology is unknown, the characteristics of amyoplasia are familiar and include normal intelligence, intact sensation, and relatively symmetric contractures. The contractures are severe and can include clubfoot deformities, fixed extension or occasional flexion contractures of the elbows, volar and ulnar contractures of the wrists, thumb-in-palm deformities, and flexed but relatively rigid interphalangeal joint contractures. Other associated abnormalities include flexed or extended knee contractures, pronation of the forearms, internal rotation of the shoulders, loss of flexion creases, digital hypoplasia, midfacial capillary hemangioma, hip dislocations, and occasional scoliosis. Amyoplasia is considered to be sporadic with a risk to subsequent children estimated to be approximately 5%.

Other less common forms of arthrogryposis that come to the attention of the orthopaedic surgeon include diastrophic dysplasia, distal arthrogryposis, Larsen's syndrome, lumbosacral agenesis, and pterygium syndromes. Although these conditions are quite variable, the basic principles guiding evaluation and management are similar.

Prognosis

Children with arthrogryposis who have significant mental retardation or identifiable chromosomal abnormalities have a much less favorable prognosis, both in terms of longevity and function. Survival during the first year may be compromised by respiratory insufficiency and weakness in those children with central nervous system or trunk involvement. Approximately 20% of children with arthrogryposis do not survive the first year of life. Those that do survive often do well. Among a review of 38 children with amyoplasia, there was an average of 5.7 orthopaedic procedures per child. By age 5 years, 85% were ambulatory, and most were relatively or completely independent in their activities and were in regular classrooms at the appro-

priate grade level. Despite this optimistic outlook, children with arthrogryposis may have various complications as a result of their condition or treatment. These include the development of malignant hyperthermia with general anesthesia or aspiration following surgery because of the lack of normal respiratory function. During growth and development, these individuals also may have spinal abnormalities (scoliosis or kyphosis), osteoarthritis, or pathologic fractures through osteoporotic bone. Obesity is also a potential problem if activities are limited because of joint involvement and immobility.

Evaluation

The initial evaluation of children with arthrogryposis requires obtaining a careful history of the pregnancy and delivery. The newborn examination should document the abnormalities. A multidisciplinary team is essential and should include a pediatrician, neurologist, geneticist, physical therapist, occupational therapist, and social worker.

Management

Management of the child with arthrogryposis often begins before birth if the diagnosis is established by ultrasound. Parental education can be extremely important in preparing the family for what is to follow. A multidisciplinary team is useful because the care of these patients is too complex for one professional to manage without assistance. The primary objective of orthopaedic management for children with arthrogryposis is to obtain maximum function. Function is never sacrificed for the sake of appearance. Improved appearance, facilitating care, control of discomfort, and reducing the risk of pain in adult life are secondary objectives. Because of the large number of disorders with congenital contractures, no single treatment plan can serve as a template for all patients with arthrogryposis.

Despite this, several principles can generally be applied. Long-term goals must be realistic. Independent ambulation or mobility, self-care, and the potential for eventual employment are reasonable goals. Physical and occupational therapy, splinting, and casting are useful and generally should be considered or used before surgical correction of the deformity. Long-term orthotic management is necessary to maintain correction. The risk of developing a recurrent deformity is inversely proportional to age and the use of postoperative orthotics. The earliest orthopaedic treatment is likely to be for birth fractures, which are sustained by 25% of affected children. If a prenatal diagnosis has been made, cesarean section should be considered to avoid these fractures.

Foot and Ankle Deformities
Clubfoot Deformities
Clubfeet represent the most common orthopaedic deformity affecting children with arthrogryposis and are present in up to 90% of children with amyoplasia. The foot deformity is typically stiffer than idiopathic clubfoot. Initial treatment should involve manipulation and serial casting. This may lead to some improvement but is rarely successful in avoiding surgical correction. It is reasonable to continue casting as long as progress is being made. Surgical treatment frequently is done between age 6 months and 1 year and consists of either an extensive posteromedial release or talectomy. The choice remains controversial.

Although recurrence rates of up to 73% have been reported following posteromedial release, most orthopaedic surgeons continue to favor posteromedial release over talectomy. In at least one study, talectomy shows better results, decreased recurrence rates, fewer procedures per foot, and better maintenance of ambulation than with extensive posteromedial release. The obvious advantage of posteromedial release as an initial procedure is that talectomy is available for recurrence or salvage situations. Other treatments for recurrent or severe clubfoot deformities include decancellation of the cuboid and/or talus, triple arthrodesis, or gradual correction with external fixation. Nighttime

and postoperative splinting may lower the recurrence rate and is often used throughout childhood. With treatment, 95% of feet can be made plantigrade, resulting in a satisfactory outcome.

Vertical Talus Deformities
These deformities occur in approximately 5% of children with arthrogryposis. As with other causes of vertical talus, casting rarely is successful and surgical correction usually is necessary between age 6 months and 2 years.

Management of Knee Deformities
Knee joint contractures are common among patients with arthrogryposis. Flexion contractures are present in nearly 50% of children with amyoplasia. Extension contractures occur in 10%. In the absence of motion, the knee joint articular surfaces become deformed. This leads to patellar elongation, flattening of the femoral condyles, and ultimate joint incongruity. Contractures greater than 20° make walking difficult. Conversely, a fixed extended knee allows for standing but makes sitting difficult.

Flexion Contractures
These contractures are treated based on the severity of the contracture. Mild contractures of less than 15° to 20° usually require no treatment except for stretching and physical therapy. For children who have reached an age when standing is possible, typically after 1 year, surgery may be necessary to correct knee flexion contractures of more than 20°. Hamstring lengthening and postoperative splinting are usually sufficient for contractures of 20° to 40°. Moderate contractures of up to 50° may also require a Z-plasty in the popliteal fossa and postoperative serial cast changes to avoid undue tension on the neurovascular structures. More severe contractures of between 60° and 80° require gradual correction with an external fixator or femoral shortening. Postoperative serial casting and chronic bracing are necessary to avoid recurrence. For those unusual, severe contractures of greater than 80° to 90°, correction may only be obtained by a combination of soft-tissue release and application of an external fixator such as in the pterygium syndromes (Fig. 1). Gradual improvement over a period of several weeks is then possible. Rapid recurrence following fixator removal is common if formal soft-tissue procedures and postoperative splinting are not performed.

Severe knee flexion contractures also may be corrected with distal femoral extension producing osteotomies. Internal fixation is necessary to avoid displacement of the osteotomy and injury to the popliteal neurovascular structures. Recurrence of the deformity, at a rate of about 1° per month, often occurs in grow-

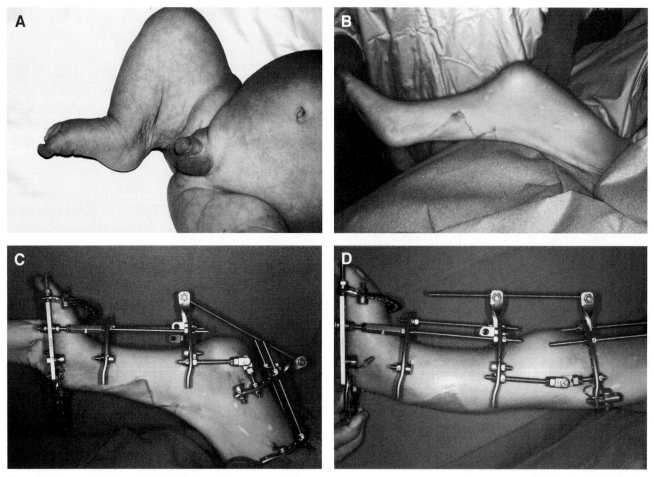

Figure 1 Treatment of severe congenital knee flexion contracture. **A,** A 3-month-old infant with popliteal pterygium syndrome demonstrating 110° knee flexion contracture and popliteal web. **B,** At age 3 years, following daily stretching, serial casting, posterior capsular release, and Z-plasty of the skin has been performed. The residual knee flexion contracture measures 55°. **C,** Treatment involved application of a circular external fixator, distraction at the knee, and slow gradual extension of the knee flexion contracture. **D,** Full extension of the knee has been obtained. Range of motion and splinting were continued until age 6 years.

ing children, so osteotomies are often deferred until near skeletal maturity.

Knee Extension Contractures

These contractures usually are caused by a tight anterior capsule, hypoplasia of the suprapatellar bursa, and replacement of the quadriceps with fibrous tissue. Although knee extension contractures allow for ambulation, sitting, transfers, and shoe tying become difficult. Late degenerative arthritis is common. Quadriceps lengthening with a V-Y plasty allows the passive knee motion to be increased. When combined with correction of clubfeet during the first year of life, the knee flexion aids with rotational control of the foot when casting postoperatively.

Management of the Hip Joint

Flexion contractures are present in 40% of infants with amyoplasia, external rotation contractures in 20%, and abduction contractures in 18%. Flexion contractures of greater than 30° may limit ambulation in those able to walk. Contractures can be corrected with soft-tissue releases if mild or with osteotomies plus soft-tissue surgery if severe.

Unilateral dislocations of the hip are treated to avoid problems related to the associated pelvic obliquity, limb-length discrepancy, and scoliosis. Bracing, traction, or casting are rarely helpful alone. Therefore, surgical treatment involves open reduction through either a medial or anterior incision. Both approaches have been reported to produce satisfactory results in up to 80% of hips. The anterior approach, usually combined with soft-tissue release and proximal femoral shortening, may lead to more stiffness than the medial approach, which is associated with a higher incidence of osteonecrosis.

The management of bilateral hip dislocations in this patient population is controversial. Functional ambulation without pain is possible with bilateral dislocations. Advocates of surgical treatment believe that reduction improves the quality and efficiency of gait.

Management of Scoliosis

Scoliosis can develop in 20% to 35% of patients with arthrogryposis. Scoliosis associated with amyoplasia is usually detected in the first few years of life and leads to the development of a paralytic, C-shaped curve. Curve progression occurs in those with early onset and pelvic obliquity. Brace treatment is recommended for patients with scoliosis of between 25° and 40° but is less successful than in patients with idiopathic scoliosis.

When curve progression to greater than 40° or 50° occurs, spinal fusion with instrumentation usually is recommended. Thoracic and idiopathic-type curve patterns may be treated in the same way as idiopathic scoliosis. Fusion to the pelvis is recommended for patients with paralytic curves and those with lumbosacral obliquity exceeding 15°. The results of surgical treatment are good, but surgical correction is often less than that obtained in patients with idiopathic scoliosis. Several disorders with congenital contractures are associated with spinal segmentation anomalies (congenital scoliosis). The treatment of congenital scoliosis depends on the anomaly and is covered in a separate chapter.

Upper Extremity Management

Management of the upper extremity in children with arthrogryposis is directed at improving function including activities of daily living or ambulation. A few may benefit from surgery, and many will benefit from nonsurgical treatment involving range-of-motion exercises, early splinting, and serial casting. For example, limited shoulder motion ordinarily can be treated with exercises, but internal rotation contractures can be treated with proximal humeral osteotomies and/or soft-tissue releases.

Elbow Extension Contractures

These contractures can be treated with posterior capsulotomy and triceps tendon lengthening. This treatment has been reported to increase elbow flexion from 17° to 67° in one series. Active elbow flexion may be improved using transfer of the triceps, pectoralis, or latissimus dorsi, provided the patient has 90° of passive elbow motion. Transfer of the triceps to the biceps is the most commonly performed procedure, with good results in 80% of patients in two reported series. Shoulder and elbow procedures should be carried out only in children with functional use of the hand and in those who do not require fixed elbow extension for ambulation.

The common volar flexion and ulnar deviation wrist deformities can be improved with splinting shortly after birth. Surgical treatment is indicated for those patients with fixed wrist contractures that interfere with function. This may involve release of the volar wrist capsule, flexor carpi ulnaris tendon transfer to the extensor carpi radialis brevis to maintain position, osteotomy of the distal radius, or intracarpal extension osteotomy. Wrist arthrodesis can be considered when the child is near skeletal maturity. Because recurrent contractures are common, postoperative splinting is essential.

Finger Flexion Contractures

These contractures are best treated with therapy and splinting. Surgical release of proximal interphalangeal joint contractures has not been particularly helpful. Arthrodesis of the interphalangeal joint contractures should be deferred until skeletal maturity.

Thumb-in-Palm Deformities

Treatment usually involves release of the adductor pollicis and Z-plasty of the first webspace. Additional procedures to improve function and decrease occurrence may include sublimis transfer, first metacarpal osteotomy, and first metacarpophalangeal joint arthrodesis. If the brachioradialis is available, it may be transferred to the thumb extensor to balance the first ray.

Conclusion

It is important to emphasize that the child with arthrogryposis often shows surprising dexterity, resourcefulness, and compensatory function so that surgical intervention often is unnecessary. Cure is not possible; therefore, the orthopaedic surgeon must be aware of the rehabilitation, social, and educational needs of these children.

Annotated Bibliography

Akazawa H, Oda K, Mitani S, Yoshitaka T, Asaumi K, Inoue H: Surgical management of hip dislocation in children with arthrogryposis multiplex congenita. *J Bone Joint Surg Br* 1998;80:636-640.

The authors report their results using an extensive anterolateral approach for open reduction of dislocated hips in patients with arthrogryposis. Mean age at surgery was 31 months with 11-year follow-up. All children ultimately walked without gait aids. Eighty percent were believed to have good or excellent results.

Axt MW, Niethard FU, Doderlein L, Weber M: Principles of treatment of the upper extremity in arthrogryposis multiplex congenita type I. *J Pediatr Orthop* 1997;6:179-185.

The authors report their experience treating elbow extension contractures with posterior capsulotomy and triceps tendon transfer in 17 children with arthrogryposis. Marked increased elbow range of motion and functional improvement were noted as a result of the capsular release. Three of five children improved with the triceps tendon transfer.

Brunner R, Hefti F, Tgetgel JD: Arthrogrypotic joint contracture at the knee and the foot: Correction with a circular frame. *J Pediatr Orthop* 1997;6:192-197.

The authors report their treatment of 16 feet and 13 knees in patients with arthrogryposis using a circular external fixator for correction of severe joint contractures. Equinus improved from 30° to 8°. Knee flexion contractures were corrected from 39° to 6°. Partial recurrent knee flexion contractures occurred in most patients following fixator removal.

DelBello DA, Watts HG: Distal femoral extension osteotomy for knee flexion contracture in patients with arthrogryposis. *J Pediatr Orthop* 1996;16:122-126.

The authors report their experience treating knee flexion contractures with distal femoral extension producing osteotomies in 32 knees. Contractures were corrected from 49° to 6°. During follow-up there was loss of 22° of extension at a rate of nearly 1° per month. This study suggests that distal femoral extension osteotomy is effective but should be deferred until near or after skeletal maturity because recurrence occurs in all growing children.

Hall JG: Arthrogryposis multiplex congenita: Etiology, genetics, classification, diagnostic approach, and general aspects. *J Pediatr Orthop* 1997;6:159-166.

This review article is a well-written, easy-to-read summary of arthrogryposis from the perspective of a world-renowned geneticist with an interest in arthrogryposis. The article discusses etiology and an approach to the diagnosis of arthrogryposis.

Jacobson L, Polizzi A, Morriss-Kaye G, Vincent A: Plasma from human mothers of fetuses with severe arthrogryposis multiplex congenita causes deformities in mice. *J Clin Invest* 1999;103:1031-1038.

This study provides evidence that maternal antibodies to fetal acetylcholine receptor might play a role in the development of fetal abnormalities and fixed joint contractures. Injecting pregnant mice with plasma from women whose fetuses had severe arthrogryposis led to abnormalities including joint contractures in the mice fetuses. This suggests a role for the existence of pathologic maternal factors in the development of arthrogryposis.

Murray C, Fixsen JA: Management of knee deformity in classic arthrogryposis multiplex congenita (amyoplasia congenita). *J Pediatr Orthop* 1997;6:186-191.

The management of knee flexion and extension contractures in 44 knees involved with amyoplasia is reported. Ninety percent of those with extension contractures were community ambulators at follow-up. Only 50% of those with initial flexion contractures were community walkers despite aggressive physiotherapy, splinting, and posterior surgical release. The article demonstrates the difficulty in correcting severe knee flexion contractures in this patient population.

Niki H, Staheli LT, Mosca VS: Management of clubfoot deformity in amyoplasia. *J Pediatr Orthop* 1997;17:803-807.

The treatment of clubfoot deformity in 22 children with amyoplasia is reported. Treatment involved stretching, serial casting, surgical posteromedial release, and postoperative splinting. Correction without recurrence was achieved in only 27%. Recurrence was corrected by serial casting and secondary surgery. The authors show that the recurrence of deformity is significantly reduced by nighttime splinting following initial surgical correction.

Sells JM, Jaffe KM, Hall JG: Amyoplasia, the most common type of arthrogryposis: The potential for good outcome. *Pediatrics* 1996;97:225-231.

This retrospective review article describes the birth characteristics, therapeutic interventions, and functional outcomes of 38 children with amyoplasia. After an average of 5.7 orthopaedic procedures per child, multiple casting procedures, splinting, and therapy sessions, 85% of children were ambulatory, and most were relatively or completely independent in their activities of daily living by age 5 years.

Staheli LT, Hall JG, Jaffe KM, Paholke DO (eds): *Arthrogryposis: A Text Atlas.* Cambridge, UK, Cambridge University Press, 1998.

This 178 page multiauthored text is the most up-to-date, authoritative, and complete work available covering arthrogryposis and disorders with congenital contractures. The text provides an overview of arthrogryposis and orthopaedic management principles. Additional chapters on rehabilitation, social and emotional care of the patient, and education make this a required text for anyone involved in the management of patients with congenital contractures.

Szöke G, Staheli LT, Jaffe K, Hall JG: Medial-approach open reduction of hip dislocation in amyoplasia-type arthrogryposis. *J Pediatr Orthop* 1996;16:127-130.

This review reports a high success rate following medial-approach open reduction for hip dislocations in amyoplasia. Eighty percent achieved good results and 12% fair results. Only one of 25 hips redislocated and four had transient evidence of osteonecrosis.

Van Heest A, Waters PM, Simmons BP: Surgical treatment of arthrogryposis of the elbow. *J Hand Surg* 1998;23:1063-1070.

The authors report their treatment of elbow deformities. Eighteen elbows were treated with a variety of triceps, pectoralis, and latissimus tendon transfers to provide elbow flexion. Six extension contractures were treated with elbow capsulotomies and triceps lengthening. Triceps transfers consistently produced better results than latissimus and pectoralis transfers, although the selection for transfer was always based on preoperative muscle strength. The six elbow capsulotomies showed improvement in flexion from 17° to 67°. The authors evaluated range of motion, strength, and function for each child.

Classic Bibliography

Banker BQ: Arthrogryposis multiplex congenita: Spectrum of pathologic changes. *Hum Pathol* 1986;17: 656-672.

Mennen U: Early corrective surgery of the wrist and elbow in arthrogryposis multiplex congenita. *J Hand Surg* 1993;18:304-307.

Sarwark JF, MacEwen GD, Scott CI Jr: Amyoplasia (A common form of arthrogryposis). *J Bone Joint Surg Am* 1990;72:465-469.

Segal LS, Mann DC, Feiwell E, Hoffer MM: Equinovarus deformity in arthrogryposis and myelomeningocele: Evaluation of primary talectomy. *Foot Ankle* 1989;10:12-16.

Sodergard J, Ryoppy S: The knee in arthrogryposis multiplex congenita. *J Pediatr Orthop* 1990;10:177-182.

Solund K, Sonne-Holm S, Kjolbye JE: Talectomy for equinovarus deformity in arthrogryposis: A 13 (2-20) year review of 17 feet. *Acta Orthop Scand* 1991;62: 372-374.

Staheli LT, Chew DE, Elliott JS, Mosca VS: Management of hip dislocations in children with arthrogryposis. *J Pediatr Orthop* 1987;7:681-685.

Thompson GH, Bilenker RM: Comprehensive management of arthrogryposis multiplex congenita. *Clin Orthop* 1985;194:6-14.

Section 5

Spine

Section Editor:
Stephen A. Albanese, MD

Section 5

Spine

Overview

Three chapters in this section review the continuing controversies regarding the value of school screening and nonsurgical management for scoliosis. Since the first edition of this text, much has been learned about curve progression before and after skeletal maturity. Advances in surgical management have focused on improving methods for achieving spine fusion and curve correction. Implant systems have evolved, and the role of anterior surgery, including video-assisted procedures, is explored. The chapter on congenital spine deformities updates information on the incidence, natural history, and importance of imaging intraspinal abnormalities associated with congenital scoliosis. The chapter on Scheuermann's disorder outlines efforts to more conclusively define the normal range of thoracic kyphosis and natural history of the condition. Factors such as chronic pain and deformity progression are important when selecting the most appropriate treatment options. As is true for all the conditions discussed in this section, understanding the etiology and risk of progression are areas of study in spondylolysis and spondylolisthesis, and the chapter describes progress in imaging studies, understanding the natural history of these conditions, and treatment options. The chapter on the pediatric cervical spine abnormalities describes congenital anomalies of the cervical spine, congenital muscular torticollis, trauma, and other syndromes. New developments pertaining to the understanding of natural history and management of these conditions are presented.

Stephen A. Albanese, MD
Section Editor

Chapter 28

Idiopathic Scoliosis: Etiology and Evaluation

Stephen A. Albanese, MD

Epidemiology

Scoliosis is defined as a lateral curvature of the spine. However, this definition is an oversimplification because these deformities generally occur in three dimensions and include alteration of the sagittal plane contour and vertebral rotation. Idiopathic scoliosis, which is the most common type of scoliosis, is a distinct entity with no known etiology. A diagnosis of idiopathic scoliosis should be made only after all other causes of a lateral curve have been excluded.

The study method employed and the minimum Cobb angle used to define true scoliosis influence the reported prevalence of idiopathic scoliosis in the general population. A Cobb angle of 10° currently is widely accepted as the minimum angle necessary to establish the diagnosis of true scoliosis. Over the last 5 years, little new information has been published on the prevalence of idiopathic scoliosis in the general population. Much of the available information was derived from studying patients identified through school screening programs, a method that introduces uncertainty regarding the status of individuals who were not selected for further testing. When a Cobb angle of 10° is used as the minimum angulation to define scoliosis, the prevalence reported in most studies ranges from 1.9% to 3%. The prevalence drops to 0.3% for curves with Cobb angles greater than 20°. There is an overall female predominance, which increases substantially for larger curves. For curves between 11° and 20°, the female-to-male ratio has been reported as 1.4:1. This ratio increases to more than 5:1 for curves that are greater than 20° or those that require treatment.

Patients with idiopathic scoliosis frequently are divided into three groups, based on the age of onset. Infantile-onset scoliosis appears between birth and age 3 years. Juvenile onset occurs between age 4 and 10 years, although some authors define the upper age limit of this group as the beginning of adolescence.

Adolescent onset, the most common type, occurs after age 10 years.

The infantile form affects more boys than girls and includes associated features that distinguish it from other forms of idiopathic scoliosis, such as plagiocephaly and developmental dysplasia of the hip. The clinical course of infantile-onset scoliosis, which usually either resolves spontaneously or progresses significantly, also distinguishes it from other forms (Fig. 1). Infantile-onset scoliosis is uncommon in North America.

The distinction between juvenile-onset scoliosis and the adolescent type is not completely clear. Age demarcation is a somewhat arbitrary distinction between the two because of the difficulty in precisely determining the age of onset in adolescents with already established curves at initial presentation. Recently, more widespread use of MRI has demonstrated that patients with juvenile-onset scoliosis are more likely to have central nervous system abnormalities than those with the adolescent type. Scoliosis cannot be considered idiopathic in patients with identified intraspinal abnormalities. Studies of patients with juvenile-onset scoliosis published prior to the widespread availability of MRI most likely included patients with other conditions, a factor that may account for some of the differences in natural history that were observed in this group. As with patients in the adolescent group, girls with juvenile-onset scoliosis outnumber boys.

Etiology
Genetics

It generally is accepted that genetics plays a role in idiopathic scoliosis. Based on information derived from familial studies, sex-linked dominant, autosomal dominant, and multifactorial inheritance have been postulated. If one parent has idiopathic scoliosis, the risk of scoliosis increases for the children of that individual. The reported magnitude of this risk varies widely; however, girls are at a considerably higher risk than

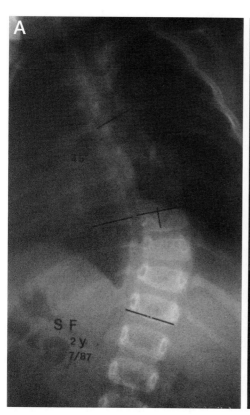

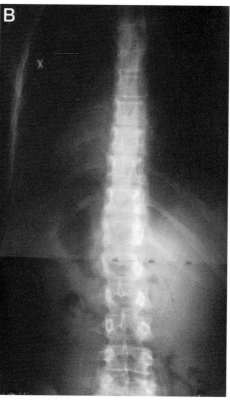

Figure 1 Infantile idiopathic scoliosis is characterized by resolution in some patients. **A,** Radiograph of a 2-year-old girl who had a 42° curve and a rib vertebral angle difference of 25°. MRI was normal. The patient wore a cast for 3 months, followed by a full-time brace for 4 years and a nighttime brace for 2 years. Following treatment, the curve remained minor and bracing treatment was discontinued. **B,** At follow-up at age 14 years, after the patient had been out of the brace for 6 years, the curve is less than 10°.

boys. A family history of scoliosis generally does not help determine the risk of curve progression in patients with idiopathic scoliosis.

Several studies of twins have shown a high concordance for the presence of idiopathic scoliosis in monozygotic twins. In a recent study, DNA fingerprinting used to distinguish between monozygotic and dizygotic twins revealed concordance for the presence of scoliosis in 12 of 13 monozygotic twins (92%) and five of eight dizygotic twins (63%). Because monozygotic twins have all genes in common, the lack of 100% concordance indicates that factors other than genetics can influence the development of idiopathic scoliosis. This and other studies have shown that concordance in dizygotic twins is greater than that observed for siblings in other familial studies. The reason for this disparity is unknown.

Hormones and Growth

The way that hormones and changes in growth pattern affect the etiology of scoliosis is not completely clear. One hypothesis suggests that asymmetrical growth results when the genetically coded developmental program functions incorrectly. Studies that evaluate the role of serum levels of growth-stimulating hormone and other hormones have produced conflicting results. Clinical studies have shown that individuals with idiopathic scoliosis tend to be taller than matched control subjects.

Recently, the role of melatonin in the etiology of idiopathic scoliosis has received much attention. Pinealectomy performed in young chickens has been shown to consistently produce scoliosis with many characteristics that are similar to those observed in humans with idiopathic scoliosis. Replacement of melatonin, which is normally secreted by the pineal gland, has been shown to reverse the effects of pinealectomy in chickens. In another study, however, the excision of the pineal gland in young rats and hamsters did not produce scoliosis. Clinical studies have been unsuccessful in defining the role of melatonin in the production and progression of scoliosis in humans. Studies designed to assess levels of melatonin in patients with idiopathic scoliosis have yielded conflicting results.

Growth, in conjunction with existing short-segment thoracic lordosis or hypokyphosis, has been proposed as a biomechanical explanation for the development and progression of idiopathic scoliosis. An experimental model of scoliosis was created in rabbits by tethering three spinous processes unilaterally to a transverse process below. The scoliosis created by this method resembled idiopathic scoliosis in humans. The authors hypothesized that this method of creating scoliosis combined the lordosis and muscle imbalance theories. The premise of the biomechanical theory, that the apical segment is lordotic in all patients with idiopathic scoliosis, has been questioned. This type of analysis does not account for the anatomic complexity of the spinal column or the role of the multiple dynamic forces acting on the spinal motion segments. Advanced imaging techniques used to reconstruct the three-dimensional anatomic deformity have not successfully predicted curve progression. Biomechanical forces play a role in the progression of large curves; however, their contribution to the etiology and early progression of idiopathic scoliosis remains unresolved.

The role of structural abnormalities of the spine in the etiology of idiopathic scoliosis is not well understood because it is not known whether the observed changes are causes or effects. Convex-concave differences in connective tissue and muscle fiber type as well as the changes observed in disk proteoglycan content generally are considered to be a result, rather than a cause, of scoliosis.

Generalized osteopenia also has been associated with adolescent idiopathic scoliosis. In one study, dual energy x-ray absorptiometry (DEXA) was used to compare bone density of the lumbar spine and proximal femur in girls age 12 to 14 years with scoliosis and a group of age-matched controls. Patients with scoliosis had significantly lower bone density than girls in the control groups. There was a lack of correlation between curve type or magnitude and lower bone mineral density. There is conflicting published information on the existence of left-to-right differences in proximal femoral bone mineral density related to the direction of the curve.

Platelet Function

Elevated platelet calmodulin levels have been demonstrated in patients with progressive idiopathic scoliosis. Calmodulin, a calcium-binding receptor, is involved in the regulation of both skeletal muscle and platelet contractile systems. Observed abnormalities in platelet function are significant, because they may indicate a more general alteration in cellular function, particularly in its relationship to muscle activity. Calmodulin also is of interest because calmodulin antagonists have been shown to inhibit melatonin synthesis in pineal cells in chickens.

Equilibrium System

Abnormal functioning of the equilibrium system has been the focus of numerous studies that have attempted to identify the etiology of idiopathic scoliosis. Some studies have demonstrated variations in vestibular, ocular, and proprioceptive functions. The role of disequilibrium in trunk muscle control was investigated in a recent study in which otolithic vestibular function was tested in 30 patients with idiopathic scoliosis. Twenty patients (67%) with idiopathic scoliosis had greater imbalance of the otolith system than matched control subjects. There was no correlation between the directional preponderance observed and curve magnitude, direction, or rate of progression. No asymmetry was observed in the three patients with congenital scoliosis that were included in the study. Vibratory response, a sensitive indicator of posterior column function, also has been investigated as a possible etiology of idiopathic scoliosis. The role of the brain stem in the equilibrium system is to integrate the afferent input. Anatomic asymmetry in the brain stem in patients with idiopathic scoliosis has been reported in MRI studies.

In summary, the results of research efforts to identify the etiology of idiopathic scoliosis have been inconclusive. Research in this area is continuing in an attempt to improve the clinical management of this condition. Out of necessity, current treatment modalities are directed toward controlling the manifestations of scoliosis. Modalities developed based on an understanding of the etiology are likely to be more effective. In addition, clinical decision making will be further facilitated with better insight into the prediction of curve progression.

Patient Evaluation

History and Physical Examination

Idiopathic scoliosis typically is a diagnosis of exclusion; therefore, obtaining a complete history is an essential component in this process. The severity, duration, and character of any back pain should be noted as well. Radicular pain, abnormal sensation, weakness, incontinence, and balance or coordination problems may indicate neurologic involvement. Predicting remaining growth is critical in determining the probability of curve progression; therefore, determining the patient's level of skeletal maturity is important.

Examination of physical features and body proportions frequently provides clues to conditions that are known to be associated with scoliosis. For example, the position of the trunk and the sagittal plane contours should be noted, and the forward bending test should be done to assess rotational malalignment. The patient is asked to bend forward, placing the palms together and letting the upper extremities hang in a dependent position. The examiner observes the spine from a seated position, checking for any rotation or paraspinal asymmetry. The forward bending test also provides the examiner an opportunity to assess the spine's mobility. The level of the pelvis frequently is an indication of relative limb lengths. Discrepancies in lower extremity circumference and deformities of the feet sometimes are observed in association with intraspinal pathology. The neurologic examination must be thorough. Signif-

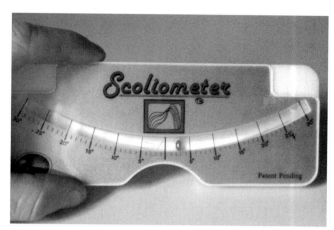

Figure 2 The scoliometer is a fluid-filled inclinometer or level that quantifies rib rotation.

icant intraspinal pathology, such as syringomyelia and spinal cord tumors, can be associated with subtle neurologic abnormalities. The abdominal reflex has received much attention as an early indicator of spinal cord pathology. In one study, four-quadrant abdominal reflex testing was performed on 65 normal individuals. Of these, 39 (60%) had bilaterally equal abdominal reflexes, nine (14%) had an asymmetrical abdominal reflex, and seven (11%) had no abdominal reflex. None of the subjects had an abdominal reflex present on one side and absent on the other. In 16 subjects (25%), the reflex diminished when testing was repeated.

Objective Measurement of Body Shape

Many attempts have been made to quantify the body surface changes observed in patients with idiopathic scoliosis. One of the goals has been to develop a technique without using radiographs that could identify scoliosis, monitor curve progression, and provide information for treatment decisions. These efforts have been hampered by the difficulty in reproducibly measuring body surfaces and the complexity of spinal deformities. In most instances, natural history data and treatment decisions are based on Cobb angles taken from standing AP radiographs. Because the Cobb angle is obtained from a single plane radiographic image, it does not always accurately demonstrate the severity of the three-dimensional spine deformity. In addition, the Cobb angle fails to account for vertebral rotation, a major factor determining the magnitude of body surface changes.

Various methods can be used to measure and document back contours. The most common method includes the use of a scoliometer, a specially designed inclinometer that is used to measure the angle of trunk rotation (Fig. 2). This device provides a simple, effective way to identify patients who need further evaluation and treatment. As the patient bends forward with

hands clasped, the device is gently placed on the surface of the back, perpendicular to the long axis of the body and centered over the apex of the maximum deformity. The angle of trunk rotation is read directly from the device. If the patient has more than one deformity, each curve should be measured independently. In order to identify the maximum rotation for each deformity, it may be necessary to vary the amount of forward flexion.

The first study that evaluated the accuracy of the scoliometer reported data from 1,065 patients referred from screening programs. The angle of trunk rotation measured with the device was correlated with the radiographically determined Cobb angle. Patients with Cobb angles of less than 20° and trunk rotation equal to or greater than 5° were considered to have false-positive results. False-negative results were defined as Cobb angles equal to or greater than 20° and trunk rotation of less than 5°. False-positive results represented 36% of the total results, while false-negative results represented only 1.2%. The mean trunk rotation for patients with a 20° Cobb angle was 7°.

The false-positive results from scoliosis screening programs can result in unnecessary referrals and radiographs. The author of the initial study conducted a follow-up study regarding the use of the scoliometer. In the latter study, further evaluation was recommended for patients with trunk rotation of 7°, resulting in an estimated referral rate of 3% of the individuals screened. The false-negative rate, which is 12% if the goal is to identify curves with a Cobb angle of 20°, drops to 8% for a Cobb angle of 25°. The scoliometer has gained widespread acceptance because it is inexpensive and noninvasive and can be used to obtain objective measurements of large populations.

Diagnostic Imaging
Radiography

AP or posteroanterior (PA) radiographs have been the standard for objective measurement of spine deformities. Use of a 36" cassette allows adequate space to include the entire thoracic and lumbar spine on a single view. For these radiographs, known limb-length discrepancies should be equalized with a lift.

Lateral radiographs should be ordered if the physical findings suggest significant sagittal plane alterations, if the patient is symptomatic or if spondylolisthesis is suspected. Additional views can be obtained when clinical concerns warrant them. Radiographs that are truly lateral to the scoliotic section of the spine frequently demonstrate lordosis of the apical segment.

Bending radiographs are used to assess the flexibility of the deformity. These views are taken preoperatively for the selection of instrumentation levels and when there is a need to determine flexibility for certain types of bracing treatment.

The Cobb technique is considered the standard for measuring scoliosis on radiographs. A recent study evaluating the Cobb technique found interobserver variability averaging 7.2° when the end points were not preselected. The intraobserver variability under similar circumstances averaged 4.9°. When the end points were preselected, observer variability improved, indicating the importance of consistent end point selection when evaluating serial radiographs. Another study found that a 10° measurement difference between radiographs taken at different times was necessary to be 95% confident that a true change in the scoliosis had occurred. A diurnal variation also has been observed. In a study of 19 patients, an average increase of 5° was noted on radiographs obtained in the afternoon compared with those obtained in the morning of the same day. This increase was determined to be statistically significant. Methods of measuring vertebral rotation have not proven to be valuable in the management of most patients with scoliosis. Various measurements have been described to document significant spinal decompensation or trunk shift.

Radiographic ossification of the iliac apophysis begins laterally and extends medially, with eventual fusion to the ilium. The Risser grading system involves dividing this excursion into four segments. Risser grade 1 is ossification of the lateral quarter, Risser grade 2 is ossification of one half of the iliac apophysis, and Risser grade 3 involves excursion into three quarters. Risser grade 4 involves complete excursion of the ossification without fusion, and Risser grade 5 denotes fusion of the ossified apophysis to the ilium. Complete excursion of the ossification requires approximately 1 year. The average time from complete ossification to fusion with the ilium is 2 years.

Published reports have indicated that, for most girls, Risser grade 4 corresponds with the completion of spinal growth. This association was questioned in a study that included a careful statistical analysis of the literature to assess use of the Risser sign as an indication of skeletal age. The authors concluded that chronologic age may be more accurate than the Risser sign for determining skeletal age. The Risser sign is considered a less reliable indicator in boys, because trunk growth frequently is observed after Risser grade 4 is reached. The Risser sign is an easy tool to use because the iliac wings frequently are included on full-length spine radiographs, eliminating the need to obtain separate radiographs of the hand to assess skeletal maturity.

The number of radiographs required to monitor scoliosis until the completion of growth has resulted in concern regarding radiation exposure. Most patients followed on a regular basis are adolescent girls, and there is particular concern about the carcinogenic effects of radiation on breast tissue. In a retrospective study of women previously seen for idiopathic scoliosis between 1935 and 1965, a higher-than-normal rate of breast cancer was reported. The average follow-up was 25.6 years for 973 subjects for whom there was usable information. An average of 41.5 radiographs had been obtained per patient. In this group, breast cancer was identified in 11 patients; six cases are expected in a sample of this size. No breast cancer was detected within 15 years of the initial examination. The ratio of observed cases to expected cases was greater after 30 years for patients with more than 30 years follow-up. This ratio also increased as the estimated dose of radiation and number of radiographs increased. This study involved patients treated before the development of techniques designed to limit the exposure of breast tissue to radiation. The average estimated breast radiation was 12.8 rad. Newer techniques and fewer radiographs taken while following patients have dramatically reduced breast tissue radiation.

A more recent study included a retrospective analysis of radiation exposure for patients seen between 1965 and 1979. The average number of spine radiographs was 12 for women and 10 for men. The theoretic lifetime cancer risk for these patients was calculated to be above the baseline level. The authors advocated the use of PA radiographs of patients with scoliosis because they significantly decreased breast and thyroid exposure to radiation. The risk associated with increased marrow radiation exposure resulting from PA views has been debated. Breast shielding must be employed with AP views. High-speed film, intensifying screens, beam collimation, technique modification, and filters also decrease radiation exposure. Other radiation reduction techniques, such as digital radiography, are being investigated.

Decreasing the number of radiographs can further reduce radiation exposure. Avoiding technical errors reduces the need for repeat studies because of poor quality or incorrect patient positioning. Better objective criteria for obtaining radiographs at the time of initial presentation are needed. Among the important factors to consider are the magnitude of the body surface changes, skeletal maturity, and presence of symptoms. Radiographic views should be limited to those that are likely to yield information pertinent to patient care. The likelihood and influence of curve progression on treatment recommendations should determine the optimal frequency of follow-up radiographs.

Magnetic Resonance Imaging

The role of MRI in the evaluation of patients with scoliosis is evolving. Syringomyelia, Arnold-Chiari malformation, hydromyelia, spinal cord tumor, tethered spinal cord, diastematomyelia, and intraspinal lipoma have been identified in patients with scoliosis that was previously presumed to be idiopathic. Because effective treatment is available in some of these instances, identifying these conditions is important. Treatment not only directly addresses the identified problem, but also may have a beneficial effect on the course of the scoliosis. Arnold-Chiari malformation and hydromyelia are among the more common abnormalities found on MRI of patients with scoliosis. The course of scoliosis following surgical decompression of the Arnold-Chiari malformation was reported in a prospective study of 11 patients younger than age 16 years who had scoliosis and Arnold-Chiari malformations. Follow-up ranged from 20 to 68 months, with a mean of 35 months. Scoliosis improved in eight patients, stabilized in one, and increased in two. Improvement in the curves occurred in all patients younger than age 10 years. Even when no effective treatment is available, the information obtained from MRI studies can be valuable in patient management. Curves with a known etiology should not necessarily be expected to mimic the course of idiopathic scoliosis.

Some authors suggest that all patients with atypical scoliosis be referred for MRI. The problem arises in defining atypical scoliosis. It generally is agreed that the typical patient with scoliosis is, at the time of presentation, an asymptomatic, neurologically normal, adolescent girl, with a right thoracic curve that follows one of several defined typical curve patterns. The proposed indications for ordering an MRI include a neurologic deficit, left thoracic curve, male gender, preadolescent onset, unusually rapid curve progression, lower extremity deformity, and the presence of symptoms. In many reports describing MRI abnormalities in association with these conditions, the patients studied were those selected from a larger population of patients with scoliosis, which makes it difficult to discern the actual incidence of abnormalities associated with these atypical presentations. Cervical, thoracic, and lumbosacral areas of the spine were studied in a prospective and retrospective analysis of MRI evaluations of neurologically normal patients with infantile- and juvenile-onset scoliosis. Of the 34 patients in the prospective group, six (34%) had neural axis abnormalities, which was consistent with the 20% incidence found in the retrospective group. The identified abnormalities included Arnold-Chiari type I malformations and associated cervical or thoracic syrinx, brain stem tumor, diffuse dural ectasia, and low lying conus. The

authors recommended total spine MRIs at presentation for all patients with juvenile-onset scoliosis who had curves greater than 20°.

Currently, cost is the primary disadvantage of routine MRI. Even in selected groups of patients, many of the studies have normal results. Although these studies are noninvasive, many young children require sedation to keep them immobile during the long scanning sequences. MRI is a very sensitive procedure that frequently demonstrates subtle changes. Questions arise as to the relationship between these changes and the scoliosis. As a result, a potential for unnecessary treatment exists. The scoliotic deformity can make MRI technically demanding. Close collaboration with the radiologist and a clear communication of the study goals are essential. It is important that the images extend from the brain stem to the lumbar spine. Proper image sequences and orientation are necessary to limit the occurrence of technically inadequate studies.

Despite some limitations, MRI has made a substantial contribution to the treatment and understanding of scoliosis. The high frequency of abnormal findings on MRIs in preadolescent patients increases skepticism on whether juvenile-onset idiopathic scoliosis really is a distinct diagnosis. Although the precise indications for ordering MRI still are undefined, the examiner must remember that during an evaluation, scoliosis may be the only apparent manifestation of an intraspinal abnormality. Patients with neurologic abnormalities, even stable ones, or features that are believed to be inconsistent with idiopathic scoliosis should be considered for further study.

Computed Tomography/Myelogram

CT is not routinely indicated for patients with scoliosis. When a better definition of the skeletal anatomy is needed, CT combined with two- or three-dimensional reconstruction can be valuable. However, for most indications, myelography and CT myelography have been replaced by MRI. Because stainless steel hardware limits the effectiveness of MRI, myelography combined with CT is preferred for postoperative evaluation of the spinal canal in patients with stainless steel hardware.

Scoliosis Screening

The goal of a screening program is to identify any unrecognized disease or defect. The screening test is not intended to be diagnostic, but rather a method of identifying patients most likely to be affected by the condition in question. Positive results obtained during screening should be referred for diagnosis and, if necessary, treatment of the condition.

School screening for scoliosis has been endorsed by the American Academy of Orthopaedic Surgeons® (AAOS) and the Scoliosis Research Society. The AAOS position statement on school screening recommends screening for girls twice, at ages 10 and 12 years, and once for boys, at age 13 or 14 years.

Results of a 1989 survey dealing with school screening for spine deformity in North America showed that screening was required by law in 15 states, and five states had administrative regulations related to screening. Some form of screening was conducted in all 50 states and the District of Columbia. The tool most commonly used for screening was the inclinometer. During the 1970s, several screening programs were initiated in Canada; however, at the time of the survey, only two provinces were conducting some kind of organized screening.

In a statement published in 1993, the US Preventive Services Task Force concluded that there is insufficient evidence to recommend for or against routine screening for scoliosis.

The World Health Organization has defined principles for a successful screening program. Their guidelines can be used as a framework for exploring in greater depth the controversy that has surrounded these programs.

First, the condition that is being screened should be an important problem. The prevalence of scoliosis has been reported to be in the range of 1.9% to 3% of the population. The prevalence of a spinal curve greater than 30° is 0.3%, which indicates that only a small proportion of curves progress. Although prevalence is low, the reported complications of idiopathic scoliosis have been used to justify the need for school screening. The incidence of back pain and related disability in adult patients with scoliosis is a controversial subject. Although cosmetic and emotional concerns exist, they are difficult to measure. Cardiopulmonary problems are associated with only the most severe cases, which constitute a small fraction of the total number of individuals with scoliosis.

Second, the natural history should be understood. Studies that define the natural history of scoliosis in skeletally immature patients allow the probability of curve progression to be determined based on several factors. The prognosis for curve progression in an individual patient cannot be determined accurately. Inability to precisely predict curve progression may result in management dilemmas once scoliosis is diagnosed. Incomplete knowledge of the natural history has slowed the evolution of nonsurgical treatment.

Third, there should be a suitable screening test that is acceptable to the population being screened. Scoliosis screening tests are based on the identification of body asymmetry. The forward bending test, with or without objective measurement of rotation, is a component of most screening programs. This type of screening generally is well tolerated and easily administered. Its specificity and sensitivity are substantially influenced by the guidelines used to determine a positive test result. The desire to decrease the rate of false-positive results, thereby increasing specificity of the test, has resulted in the recommendation to raise the trunk inclination angle necessary for referral from 5° to 7°. The positive predictive value (ie, the probability that scoliosis exists if the test is abnormal) varies in published reports. Some of the inconsistency is attributed to the minimum Cobb angle used to define true scoliosis. The positive predictive value is lower if a larger minimum angle is used. A potentially harmful effect of screening is an incorrect diagnosis of scoliosis when, in fact, there is either no curve or a curve that is so small that it is inconsequential. Future employment and insurance coverage can be negatively impacted.

Fourth, once the disease is identified, accepted treatment should be available. One goal of scoliosis screening is early identification, which allows the possibility of nonsurgical treatment and limits the number of curves that require surgery, thus improving the outcome. Some authors assume that, unless screening is implemented, many asymptomatic individuals with scoliosis will be unrecognized until very late in the course. The validity of this assumption is questioned, however, because the number of cases and stage of scoliosis identified without screening have not been well documented. A treatment rate of 2.75 per 1,000 individuals screened has been reported.

An improved outcome (a decreased need for surgery) following bracing treatment was noted in one study after screening was implemented. Improvement was attributed to younger skeletal age and smaller curves at the time of the initial diagnosis, a result of the screening program. In another study, a decrease in the number of patients requiring surgery was reported after a comprehensive screening program was initiated. The average curve treated surgically decreased from 60° to 42° over the 8 years of the study. However, an analysis of school screening in Dublin between 1979 and 1990 was unable to demonstrate that the program resulted in a significant change in the number of patients requiring surgery.

Finally, the program should be cost effective. Unfortunately, some program costs are difficult to determine. To establish cost effectiveness, the cost of late diagnosis and related problems must be compared with the cost of the program. Screening itself can be done inexpensively. One study noted that the direct cost of screening was $0.066 for each student. Indirect costs include physician referrals, follow-up visits, treatment, and radiographs. Although the costs associated with follow-up and treatment of patients with positive results have been estimated, these figures are not an accurate indication of the actual costs of screening programs.

The reported referral rate from screening programs has ranged from 3.4% to more than 30%. Much of this variability is a reflection of the screening method employed and the guidelines for referral. When these referral rates are compared to the prevalence of scoliosis, the potentially large expense from false-positive results becomes apparent. In addition, because progression is unpredictable, unnecessary follow-up or treatment of many cases of true scoliosis create another expense that is difficult to evaluate.

In summary, the debate regarding the value of scoliosis screening has not been resolved. The effectiveness of treatment, as it relates to a screening program, assumes that those identified by screening will receive subsequent care. The consistency of this follow-up has been questioned. As more information regarding the natural history and effectiveness of nonsurgical treatment becomes available, a more objective evaluation of the issues will be possible.

Annotated Bibliography

Etiology

Carpintero P, Mesa M, Garcia J, Carpintero A: Scoliosis induced by asymmetric lordosis and rotation: An experimental study. *Spine* 1997;22:2202-2206.

Surgical tethering of the spinal apophysis and transverse apophysis of the three upper vertebrae were performed in 24 4-week old rabbits to create a muscle imbalance of the paravertebral musculature. Surgery was performed on the left side in one half of the rabbits and on the right side in one half. Radiographs were taken at 1 and 3 months following surgery, and the spines were directly measured post mortem using the Cobb technique. Seven rabbits were excluded from the study. Scoliosis developed in the remaining 17 rabbits with convexity facing the opposite side of the surgery. Curve magnitude increased over time in all of the rabbits (range 27° to 42° with a mean of 29°). Rotation of an average of five vertebrae per curve was evident on postmortem radiographs. No statistical difference was found between groups. A significant difference was found between the size of the curve and the rotation of the apex vertebrae. The authors concluded that experimental intrinsic muscle imbalance of a growing rabbit produces results similar to idiopathic scoliosis in humans.

Cheng JC, Guo X: Osteopenia in adolescent idiopathic scoliosis: A primary problem or secondary to the spinal deformity? *Spine* 1997;22:1716-1721.

This study used DEXA to evaluate the bone mineral density of girls between age 12 and 14 years. The bone mineral density of the lumbar spine and proximal femur in subjects with idiopathic scoliosis was compared with age-matched controls. The patients with idiopathic scoliosis had significantly lower bone mineral density. There was a lack of correlation between lower bone mineral density and curve progression.

Fagan A, Kennaway D, Sutherland A: Total 24-hour melatonin secretion in adolescent idiopathic scoliosis: A case-control study. *Spine* 1998;23:41-46.

Radioimmunoassay levels of 6-sulphatoxy melatonin in 24-hour urine samples from patients with adolescent-onset idiopathic scoliosis were measured and compared with matched control adolescents with healed spinal fractures. Even when differences in body weight, body surface area, and body mass index were accounted for, no significant difference was found between groups in diurnal, nocturnal, or total urine 6-sulphatoxy melatonin excretion. In addition, no difference was found in those patients whose curves progressed and those whose curves did not progress.

Goldberg CJ, Fogarty EE, Moore DP, Dowling FE: Scoliosis and developmental theory: Adolescent idiopathic scoliosis. *Spine* 1997;22:2228-2238.

This study explores the relationship between growth and developmental instability in the etiology of idiopathic scoliosis. Subjects were from a school screening program and referrals to a scoliosis clinic. Comparisons were made with control patients. The authors concluded that idiopathic scoliosis can be explained by developmental instability.

Hilibrand AS, Blakemore LC, Loder RT, et al: The role of melatonin in the pathogenesis of adolescent idiopathic scoliosis. *Spine* 1996;21:1140-1146.

In this study, urine samples (nighttime and first morning) were analyzed to compare melatonin levels in a matched case-control study of nine female adolescents with scoliosis (curves of 15° to 40°) and 18 normal adolescents. Melatonin levels were higher in both groups at night. Overall, no significant difference of melatonin levels between the two groups was found even when considering covariant factors (age, weight, hours of sleep, seasonal time outdoors). The authors concluded that melatonin deficiency does not play a role in the pathogenesis of adolescent-onset idiopathic scoliosis in humans.

Inoue M, Minami S, Kitahara H, et al: Idiopathic scoliosis in twins studied by DNA fingerprinting: The incidence and type of scoliosis. *J Bone Joint Surg Br* 1998;80:212-217.

In this study of 21 pairs of twins, DNA fingerprinting was used to determine if the twins were monozygotic or dizygotic. Twelve of the 13 monozygotic pairs (92%) and five of the eight dizygotic pairs (63%) were concordant for the presence of idiopathic scoliosis. This study supports the role of genetics in the etiology of idiopathic scoliosis. The lack of 100% concordance in the monozygotic pairs suggests that other factors also contribute to the development of scoliosis.

Machida M, Dubousset J, Imamura Y, Miyashita Y, Yamada T, Kimura J: Melatonin: A possible role in pathogenesis of adolescent idiopathic scoliosis. *Spine* 1996;21:1147-1152.

Serum melatonin levels were collected and analyzed every 3 hours in a 24-hour time period in five female and five male patients with idiopathic scoliosis and eight female and seven male age-matched controls hospitalized for minor illnesses. Of the 10 patients with idiopathic scoliosis, five had stable curves and five had progressive curves (curves progressing 10° or more in the previous year). Plasma levels of melatonin were determined by radioimmunoassay procedure. Daytime melatonin levels were significantly lower than nighttime levels in all groups. The five patients with progressive curves had significantly lower levels of melatonin in total and nighttime levels than those patients in both the stable and the control group. No difference in levels was established between the groups for daytime melatonin concentration. The authors concluded that the level of melatonin may serve as an indicator for curve progression in patients with idiopathic scoliosis.

O'Kelly C, Xiaoping W, Raso J, et al: The production of scoliosis after pinealectomy in young chickens, rats, and hamsters. *Spine* 1999;24:35-43.

This study was performed to assess the development of scoliosis after pinealectomy in rats and hamsters as compared with chickens. Weekly radiographic examinations of pinealectomized rats, hamsters, and chickens were analyzed for the development of scoliosis. No scoliosis was found in the rats and hamsters. Scoliosis developed in 10 of the 21 chickens. Plasma melatonin levels were 0 for all of the animals. The authors concluded that differences in the physiology and spinal morphology of these animals may be contributing factors to the development of scoliosis.

Wang X, Jiang H, Raso J, et al: Characterization of the scoliosis that develops after pinealectomy in the chicken and comparison with adolescent idiopathic scoliosis in humans. *Spine* 1997;22:2626-2635.

The authors reported that scoliosis developed in 60% of chickens following pinealectomy at age 3 days as compared to a 100% rate reported in other literature. Radiographic characteristics of scoliosis in those chickens with scoliosis were found to be similar to a group of humans with adolescent-onset idiopathic scoliosis. The authors suggested that the few differences may be associated with the biomechanical differences of the two species.

Wiener-Vacher SR, Mazda K: Asymmetric otolith vestibulo-ocular responses in children with idiopathic scoliosis. *J Pediatr* 1998;132:1028-1032.

The role of disequilibrium in trunk muscle control was investigated by testing the otolithic vestibular function in 30 patients with idiopathic scoliosis. Twenty patients (67%) with idiopathic scoliosis had greater otolith system imbalance than matched control subjects. There was no correlation between the directional preponderance observed and the curve magnitude, direction, or rate of progression. There was no asymmetry observed in the three patients with congenital scoliosis who were included in the study.

Patient Evaluation

Gupta P, Lenke LG, Bridwell KH: Incidence of neural axis abnormalities in infantile and juvenile patients with spinal deformity: Is a magnetic resonance image screening necessary? *Spine* 1998;23:206-210.

In this prospective and retrospective study, the authors analyze MRI evaluations of patients with infantile- and juvenile-onset scoliosis. The protocol used included evaluation of the cervical, thoracic, and lumbosacral areas of the spine. The authors recommended a total spine MRI at presentation for all patients with juvenile-onset scoliosis with curves greater than 20°.

Levy AR, Goldberg MS, Mayo NE, Hanley JA, Poitras B: Reducing the lifetime risk of cancer from spinal radiographs among people with adolescent idiopathic scoliosis. *Spine* 1996;21:1540-1547.

This retrospective study included an analysis of radiation exposure for patients seen between 1965 and 1979. The average number of spine radiographs was 12 for women and 10 for men. The theoretic lifetime cancer risk for these patients was calculated to be above the baseline level. The authors advocated the use of the PA view for scoliosis radiographs.

Yngve D: Abdominal reflexes. *J Pediatr Orthop* 1997; 17:105-108.

Abdominal reflexes were tested in 30 adolescent and 35 young adult normal subjects. The abdominal reflex was tested in four quadrants. Bilaterally equal abdominal reflexes were found in 60% of individuals, an asymmetrical abdominal reflex in 14%, and an absent abdominal reflex in 11%. No subjects had an abdominal reflex present on one side and absent on the other. In repeat testing, the reflex diminished in 25% of subjects.

Scoliosis Screening

Goldberg CJ, Dowling FE, Fogarty EE, Moore DP: School scoliosis screening and the United States Preventive Services Task Force: An examination of long-term results. *Spine* 1995;20:1368-1374.

The authors analyzed the school screening program in Dublin between 1979 and 1990. Scoliosis of 40° at or after diagnosis was considered a positive result. A curve of less than 40° at the end of growth generally was not considered a problem. The systematic screening program did not result in a change in the prevalence of mild or significant observed scoliosis.

Morrissy RT: School screening for scoliosis. *Spine* 1999;24:2584-2591.

In this in-depth analysis of the issues related to school screening for scoliosis, the author addresses the pertinent aspects of screening programs and how they apply to school screening for scoliosis.

Classic Bibliography

Asher M, Beringer GB, Orrick J, Halverhout N: The current status of scoliosis screening in North America, 1986: Results of a survey by mailed questionnaire. *Spine* 1989;14:652-662.

Beauchamp M, Labelle H, Grimard G, et al: Diurnal variation of Cobb angle measurement in adolescent idiopathic scoliosis. *Spine* 1993;18:1581-1583.

Bunnell WP: An objective criterion for scoliosis screening. *J Bone Joint Surg Am* 1984;66:1381-1387.

Bunnell WP: Outcome of spinal screening. *Spine* 1993;18:1572-1580.

Carman DL, Browne RH, Birch JG: Measurement of scoliosis and kyphosis radiographs: Intraobserver and interobserver variation. *J Bone Joint Surg Am* 1990;72:328-333.

Carr AJ, Jefferson RJ, Turner-Smith AR: Family stature in idiopathic scoliosis. *Spine* 1993;18:20-23.

Hoffman DA, Lonstein JE, Morin MM, et al: Breast cancer in women with scoliosis exposed to multiple diagnostic x-rays. *J Nat Cancer Inst* 1989;81:1307-1312.

Little DG, Sussman MD: The Risser sign: A critical analysis. *J Pediatr Orthop* 1994;14:569-575.

Lonstein JE, Bjorklund S, Wanninger MH, Nelson RP: Voluntary school screening for scoliosis in Minnesota. *J Bone Joint Surg Am* 1982;64:481-488.

McInnes E, Hill DL, Raso VJ, Chetner B, Greenhill BJ, Moreau MJ: Vibratory response in adolescents who have idiopathic scoliosis. *J Bone Joint Surg Am* 1991;73:1208-1212.

Montgomery F, Willner S: Screening for idiopathic scoliosis: Comparison of 90 cases shows less surgery by early diagnosis. *Acta Orthop Scand* 1993;64:456-458.

Morrissy RT, Goldsmith GS, Hall EC, et al: Measurement of the Cobb angle on radiographs of patients who have scoliosis: Evaluation of intrinsic error. *J Bone Joint Surg Am* 1990;72:320-327.

Muhonen MG, Menezes AH, Sawin PD, et al: Scoliosis in pediatric Chiari malformations without myelodysplasia. *J Neurosurg* 1992;77:69-77.

Position Statement: School Screening Programs for the Early Detection of Scoliosis. Rosemont, IL, American Academy of Orthopaedic Surgeons, 1992.

Rogala EJ, Drummond DS, Gurr J: Scoliosis: Incidence and natural history. A prospective epidemiological study. *J Bone Joint Surg Am* 1978;60:173-176.

Sahlstrand T, Petruson B: A study of labyrinthine function in patients with adolescent idiopathic scoliosis: I. An electro-nystagmographic study. *Acta Orthop Scand* 1979;50:759-769.

Sahlstrand T, Ortengren R, Nachemson A: Postural equilibrium in adolescent idiopathic scoliosis. *Acta Orthop Scand* 1978;49:354-365.

US Preventive Services Task Force: Review article: Screening for adolescent idiopathic scoliosis. *JAMA* 1993;269:2667-2672.

Wilson JMG, Jungner G: *Principles and Practice of Screening for Disease*. Geneva, Switzerland, World Health Organization, 1968.

Chapter **29**

Idiopathic Scoliosis: Natural History and Nonsurgical Management

Stephen A. Albanese, MD

Natural History

Accurate natural history information is essential for determining the most appropriate management of patients with idiopathic scoliosis and evaluating the effectiveness of nonsurgical treatment. Access to large numbers of untreated patients is limited, which makes it difficult to complete long-term natural history studies. The influence of study design on the outcome should be considered when interpreting the results. Retrospective studies of the natural history tend to focus on large curves and underrepresent small to mild curves. Many of the early long-term follow-up studies included patients with scoliosis of mixed etiologies. The minimum curve size used to define scoliosis can influence observed rates of progression in the sample. In addition, the classification of a curve as progressive must take into account the variability of the measurement technique employed.

Idiopathic Scoliosis Prior to Skeletal Maturity

For curves presenting after infancy, the natural history before skeletal maturity differs greatly from that after growth is complete. The natural history of curves prior to skeletal maturity has been evaluated in relatively few studies. The probability of curve progression is the primary consideration in determining treatment indications for this group of patients. Several factors have been examined for their influence on curve progression prior to skeletal maturity.

Progression of scoliosis is known to be associated with growth. The exact mechanism by which this change occurs is still debated. Several studies have shown that curves at greatest risk for progression are those that present at an early age. Late-onset curves, such as those detected after the onset of puberty, are less likely to progress significantly. In one study, patients diagnosed between age 10 and 12 years had an 88% risk of curve progression of at least 5°; for those age 12 to 15 years, the risk was 56%; and for those older than age 15 years, the risk was 29%. In another study, the overall frequency of curve progression at age 10 years was 50%, and at age 13 years, it was 21%. In a study from Scotland, the authors reported on 89 patients with progressive juvenile-onset scoliosis in whom the rate of curve progression increased after age 10 years during the period of accelerated spinal growth.

In a recently published retrospective study analyzing peak height velocity for patients with idiopathic scoliosis, results were compared with data for adolescents who did not have scoliosis. The peak height velocity also was compared with chronologic age, menarchal age, and Risser sign for accuracy in predicting curve progression. Growth ceased in 90% of patients by 3.6 years after peak height velocity. The timing of maximal curve progression was significantly more closely grouped around peak height velocity than chronologic or menarchal age. The authors concluded that the peak height velocity can be used to accurately predict the end of growth. The usefulness of this measurement in the management of patients has not yet been established.

This study also examined the relationship of menarche and the Risser sign to peak height velocity. Progression from a Risser grade 1 to grade 4 occurred over a mean time of 1.4 years. The median time for menarche was 7 months after the peak height velocity. The timing of maximal curve progression was significantly more closely grouped around peak height velocity than chronologic or menarchal age. Curves were more likely to have maximal progression at Risser grade 0 (67% of progressive curves), but 11% of curves had maximal progression at Risser grade 4 or 5. Sixty of the 88 progressive curves were 30° or greater at peak height velocity. Of these, 50 curves (83%) increased to a surgical magnitude. Of the 28 progressive curves that were less than 30° at peak height velocity, only one curve (4%) progressed to a surgical magnitude.

The end of growth in boys is more difficult to predict than in girls. It has been shown that curve progression in boys can occur at an advanced Risser grade. In a recent study, peak height velocity for boys with idiopathic scoliosis was examined. The median height velocity plots were similar to those previously reported by the same institution for girls. Only 61% of the 43 boys in this study had completed growth when they reached Risser grade 5; 90% had completed growth by 3.5 years after peak height velocity. Risser sign was a poor predictor of the time of maximal curve progression. All 13 patients with curves greater than 30° at peak height velocity had curve progression to greater than 45°. Only four of the 29 patients with curves equal to or less than 30° at peak height velocity had curve progression to greater than 45°. The usefulness of peak height velocity as a prospective tool remains unclear.

In a prospective study of 34 patients who underwent anterior spine surgery as part of idiopathic scoliosis correction, superior and inferior vertebral end plates were harvested at the time of surgery and examined histologically for evidence of growth activity. The patient's Risser grade was then correlated with growth activity. There was histologic evidence of significant growth activity in ten of the 14 patients with Risser grade 4.

Although bone age can help identify discrepancies between skeletal and chronologic age, it can be misleading in the prediction of spinal growth. Spinal growth and long bone growth occur at different times. Spinal growth has been observed after skeletal maturity has been documented on wrist and hand radiographs.

Curves that are larger at the time of detection also are at greater risk for progression. In one study, the probability of progression for curves 20° or more was more than twice that for smaller curves. In this study, the average nonprogressive curve was 15°, and the average progressive curve was 20°. In another study, progression of 5° or more occurred in 78% of curves between 40° and 50°, compared with 52% of curves between 20° and 30°. Progression of 10° or more in these two groups was 62% in curves between 40° and 50° and 30% in curves between 20° and 30°.

Although a relationship between curve type and progression is acknowledged, comparison between studies is difficult because of discrepancies in the classification systems used. In general, thoracic curves present earlier and are more likely to progress than lumbar curves. Double curves (thoracic and lumbar) progress more frequently than single curves. In one study, in double curves that worsened, the thoracic curve progressed in 25% of patients, the lumbar curve progressed in 43% of patients, and both curves progressed in 32% of patients.

The female-to-male ratio increases for larger curves, but there is conflicting information regarding the influence of gender on the probability of progression once a curve is identified. Scoliosis in boys can develop later and progress longer than in girls. Follow-up on male adolescents with idiopathic scoliosis is recommended until Risser grade 5 is reached. In a study of patients identified in school screenings, 15% of girls with curves of at least 11° and 4% of boys had at least 5° of progression. Conversely, a greater likelihood of curve progression in boys has been reported in other studies. Finally, in other studies, no difference between genders was reported. This lack of consistency may be a reflection of the small number of boys in most natural history studies. Most studies show no correlation between family history and risk of progression.

Thus, for young patients with scoliosis, the major factors that influence curve progression are skeletal maturity, curve magnitude, and curve type. In the clinical setting, combinations of these factors are useful in assessing the probability of curve progression. For example, curves of 20° to 29° in patients at Risser grade 0 or 1 have a 68% probability of curve progression of 5° or more. For the same curves, the risk of progression in patients at Risser grade 2 to grade 4 is only 23%. Family history, spinal rotation, and gender generally are not helpful in predicting progression.

Idiopathic Scoliosis After Skeletal Maturity

In addition to curve progression, the probability of functional impairment is a concern in adults with idiopathic scoliosis. The effects of scoliosis during adulthood provide much of our rationale for the management of this deformity in adolescence. In an effort to limit future disability, surgery frequently is offered to adolescent patients who are likely to experience curve progression during adulthood. The following information is useful in counseling young patients on the probability of encountering problems related to their scoliosis.

Progression in adults tends to be much slower than that observed in adolescents. Curves of less than 30° at skeletal maturity, regardless of the curve pattern, are unlikely to progress; however, 68% of curves greater than 50° at maturity will very likely progress. Thoracic curves between 50° and 75° progress nearly 1° per year. Lumbar curves greater than 30° are likely to progress and may have translatory shifts. For these curves, a fifth lumbar vertebra seated below the intercrest line seems to provide some protection against translatory shift and progression. The observed progression of right lumbar curves is twice that observed for left lumbar curves.

Most studies indicate that there is little or no relationship between pregnancy and curve progression. In one study, 355 skeletally mature patients with idiopathic scoliosis were reviewed to examine the effects of pregnancy on curve progression. Patients were divided into two groups, based on whether or not they had been pregnant. In both groups, spinal curve progression of at least 10° was noted in 10% of patients. No significant correlation was found between the patient's age at first pregnancy and curve progression. Pregnancy and delivery complications, including cesarean section, have been reported in proportions similar to the average for patients without scoliosis. In general, it is believed that mild to moderate idiopathic scoliosis has no negative effect on pregnancy or delivery.

Cardiopulmonary compromise is uncommon, and symptoms, if they appear, usually are late. Most adolescents with idiopathic scoliosis have normal or near-normal lung volume. Restrictive lung disease is the pulmonary impairment associated with scoliosis. During childhood, even patients with a measured decrease in pulmonary function tend to be asymptomatic. Pulmonary symptoms and decreased vital capacity correlate positively with the severity of the thoracic curve. Marked diminution of pulmonary function in nonsmokers does not occur until the thoracic curve approaches 100°. There is no correlation between lumbar or thoracolumbar curves and pulmonary impairment. In a study of 79 patients with adolescent idiopathic scoliosis with a mean curve of 45°, a reduction in work capacity was found that was unrelated to the nature or extent of spinal deformity. The authors concluded that physical activity should be encouraged for patients with scoliosis to maintain and improve peripheral muscle and cardiovascular conditioning. In a study that sought to identify risk factors for respiratory failure, only patients with less than 45% of predicted vital capacity and a Cobb angle of greater than 110° were at risk for subsequent respiratory failure. Respiratory failure was believed to be the result of age-related diminution of pulmonary function in an already compromised individual. Hypokyphosis further contributes to a decrease in pulmonary function.

Early estimates of mortality rates associated with scoliosis described rates much higher than those predicted for the general population. These studies overestimated the death rate from idiopathic scoliosis because they included patients with scoliosis of other etiologies. A more recent study from Sweden also demonstrated an increase in the mortality rate for a group of patients with scoliosis. However, when the patients with adolescent idiopathic scoliosis were examined separately, it was found that this group was not at increased risk when compared with the expected mortality rates in the general population. Although there are individual exceptions, patients with adolescent idiopathic scoliosis as a group are not at increased risk for early death.

There is conflicting information on the frequency of back pain in patients with scoliosis relative to the general population. Pain along the convexity and concavity of the curve, as well as paraspinal and interscapular pain, has been described. In a long-term follow-up study, chronic back pain was more prevalent in patients with scoliosis than in individuals in the control group. Patients with scoliosis had higher pain scores than individuals in the control group, reflecting greater pain intensity over a longer period of time. No association was noted between the frequency of back pain and the combined factor of curve type and size. There were no significant differences in the prevalence of disabling back pain and activity levels between patients with scoliosis and individuals in the control group. As a group, the daily functioning of adult patients with idiopathic scoliosis is similar to that of the general population.

Cosmetic concerns related to scoliosis frequently are expressed by patients but are difficult to measure objectively. Patients appear to be more self-conscious during their teenage and early adult years than when older. In one study, a positive correlation between the degree of psychological handicap and clinical deformity was shown; however, this finding has been disputed by other authors. In another study, a survey instrument specifically designed to assess the health concerns of adolescents was used to compare adolescents with scoliosis to control subjects without scoliosis. The results indicated that patients with scoliosis were significantly more likely to have suicidal thoughts and concerns about abnormal body development.

Nonsurgical Management

Need for Treatment

Most patients with an established diagnosis of adolescent idiopathic scoliosis do not require treatment. The percentage who do require treatment varies among published reports and is influenced by the composition of the study population, minimum curve size used to define the scoliosis, and the length of time of follow-up. In one study in which patients were identified through school screening, 6.8% of patients with scoliosis required treatment. Nevertheless, periodic observation is necessary to monitor for curve progression.

Multiple factors must be considered when determining the ideal interval between office visits. Progression is not the sole concern; what the progression will mean

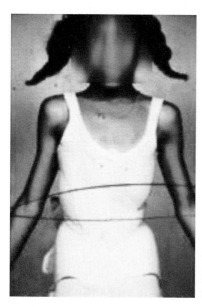

Figure 1 The Boston brace is an underarm brace that is meant to be worn nearly full-time. The brace is made from a preformed module that is customized to the patient, which simplifies brace manufacture.

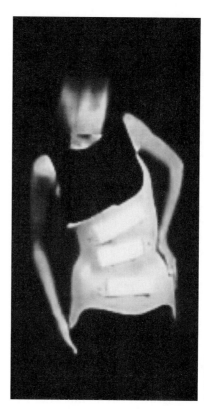

Figure 2 The Charleston brace is a hypercorrective brace that is only used at night and is most appropriate for single curves.

in relation to the management of the patient also must be considered. Skeletal maturity is important, because the potential for further growth has a great influence on the risk of progression. More frequent follow-up visits are required if curve progression will result in a change in treatment. For example, a skeletally immature patient who may need bracing if further progression occurs may need to be reevaluated within 4 months. Conversely, a much longer interval may be suitable for a patient with a small curve for whom more progression could be accepted without changing the management plan. Skeletally mature patients can be allowed a much longer interval between visits because progression, when it occurs, is at a much slower rate. Predetermined guidelines that apply to all patients have not been established. Decisions regarding the follow-up interval must be individualized and the many pertinent factors carefully considered.

The ability to monitor patients according to body surface changes has been limited by the lack of correlation between these changes and the Cobb angle. Natural history data and thresholds for treatment are based on the Cobb angle. If accurate determination of the Cobb angle is critical to patient management, radiographs are a necessity. The number of radiographs ordered should be minimized to limit exposure to radiation. Occasionally, it is possible to monitor body surface changes for smaller curves using a scoliometer. A radiograph should be ordered if a significant change is noted.

Bracing Treatment

The Milwaukee brace was first introduced as a method of postoperative immobilization. Its use was later extended to the nonsurgical management of scoliosis. As

bracing evolved, there was a movement to produce better tolerated and, in some cases, less expensive braces. This resulted in the development of lower profile braces (thoracolumbosacral orthosis) constructed without a superstructure, such as the Boston, Wilmington, and Charleston braces. The Boston brace has a prefabricated design that can be modified to fit the individual patient (Fig. 1). The Wilmington brace is constructed from a thermoplastic material molded to a plaster positive mold from the patient's cast. The Charleston bending brace, designed to conform to a side-bending patient, is for nighttime use (Fig. 2).

Early Milwaukee braces had a mandibular support that caused dental problems and was later replaced by a neck ring. Computer simulations have shown that lateral forces are primarily responsible for correction of scoliosis with use of the Milwaukee brace; longitudinal traction plays a minor role. Some of the correction has been attributed to the role of active muscle forces. In a study using electromyography to assess muscle activity, the difference between braced and unbraced activity was not significant, which suggests that muscle forces were not a major factor contributing to brace correction of scoliosis. The reduction of lumbar lordosis resulting from bracing treatment also is believed to contribute to curve correction.

A study examining the three-dimensional effect of the Boston brace demonstrated significant curve correction in the frontal plane. There also was a significant reduction in the thoracic kyphosis. However, the brace did not significantly change the thoracic apical vertebral rotation or rib hump. In addition, the thoracolumbosacral orthosis strap tension was influenced by the position of the patient, a factor that could change the biomechanical effect of the brace.

The goal of bracing treatment is to control curve progression. Suitable candidates for bracing treatment must fit the profile of the patient at risk for curve progression. Natural history studies and other studies evaluating the effects of bracing have clarified the indications for bracing treatment. Patients should be skeletally immature with a curve in the range of 20° to 40°, have a deformity that they consider cosmetically acceptable, and be willing to accept bracing treatment. Even if progression has not been demonstrated, curves between 30° and 40° in skeletally immature patients should be braced upon presentation. Curves between 20° and 30° can be observed; however, if curve progression of 5° or more occurs in this group, bracing treatment should be initiated. One reason for delaying bracing treatment in this group is to avoid unnecessary treatment of stable curves. The decision to delay treatment must be individualized, especially for patients with curves between 25° and 30°. Because bracing treatment is effective in managing smaller curves, some authors advocate initiating bracing treatment for curves of 25° or greater when the patient is at Risser grade 0. Significant spinal decompensation, even if the curve magnitude is not large enough to meet the usual guidelines, is a relative indication for bracing treatment. Most studies concur that bracing is ineffective in controlling larger curves, especially those greater than 45°. Low-profile braces may be used for curves with the apex at T7 or lower.

Bracing treatment is contraindicated for patients who do not meet the described prerequisites. Thoracic lordosis and hypokyphosis are considered relative contraindications. Adolescents adamantly opposed to bracing treatment, despite counseling on the issues, cannot realistically be expected to comply with bracing treatment requirements.

After the brace is fitted, an in-brace radiograph is compared with the initial radiograph. If adequate correction is not achieved, the brace should be adjusted to maximize correction. Studies have shown that curves that are corrected in the brace by 50% or more are more likely to have a positive response.

The standard recommendation in the past was for the brace to be worn full-time, which was defined as 23 hours per day. However, satisfactory outcomes were observed when patients partially complied with bracing treatment requirements, and this has been interpreted by some authors as an indication that part-time bracing would be as effective as full-time bracing. This issue remains unresolved. Exercise, initially considered an integral component of the bracing regimen, has since been shown to be ineffective. Patients in braces should be monitored periodically to assess for brace-related problems, growth, and clinical changes. A 4- to 6-month interval has been mentioned as a reasonable interval for follow-up visits, but the final determination should be made on an individual basis. Bracing treatment should be continued until skeletal maturity. Weaning the patient from the brace has been advocated, but the value of weaning prior to discontinuing bracing has not been established in the literature.

Numerous reports have examined the efficacy of bracing treatment. Despite evidence supporting this form of treatment, bracing remains quite controversial. Studies often are criticized for the lack of suitable control patients, short follow-up times, and the composition of the study group. To be successful, bracing treatment must positively alter the natural history of scoliosis. As noted, not all patients with scoliosis have curve progression. The sample population must be composed of patients truly at risk for progression, and it must be large enough to demonstrate that, as a group, patients have had a course that differs from the natural history. Differences in sample composition, length of follow-up time, and grouping of curve types are among the factors that make study comparisons difficult. Recent research is summarized in the following discussion.

A long-term follow-up study of 1,020 patients compared the outcome of patients treated with a Milwaukee brace with the natural history as defined in an earlier series from the same institution. Failure was defined as progression of 5° or more. For curves of 20° to 39°, the failure rate was less than that observed in the natural history study. A Risser grade of 0 or 1, or a curve measuring 30° or more at the time bracing treatment was initiated, was a factor that increased the likelihood that surgery would be necessary. As is also true in other series, loss of the correction that was initially achieved in the brace occurred with follow-up.

In contrast, in a study of 102 patients with idiopathic scoliosis treated with a Milwaukee brace, 48% of patients had more than 5° of progression at the time bracing treatment was discontinued. Arthrodesis was performed in 31% of patients. The average in-brace curve correction was better in patients who did not subsequently have curve progression.

In a retrospective review of 76 patients with adolescent idiopathic scoliosis treated with a Wilmington brace for curves ranging from 20° to 39°, curve progression of 5° or more was observed in 28% of patients. This compares favorably with published natural history data. There was a minimum follow-up of 5

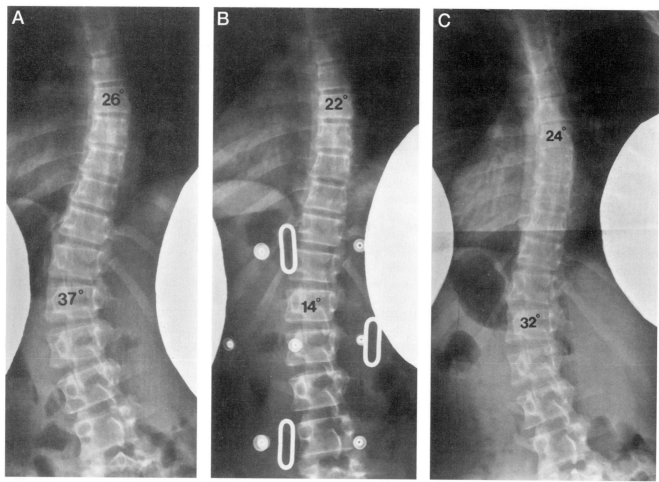

Figure 3 **A,** Prebracing radiograph of a patient with idiopathic scoliosis, with curves measuring 37° and 26°. **B,** An in-brace radiograph of the same patient demonstrating correction of the curves to 22° and 14°. **C,** Radiograph obtained at 5-year follow-up shows some loss of the initial correction achieved in the brace, but the curves remain smaller than those observed on the prebracing radiograph. *(Reproduced from Richards BS: Orthopaedic Knowledge Update: Pediatrics. Rosemont, IL, American Academy of Orthopaedic Surgeons, 1996, pp 101-108.)*

years from the conclusion of bracing treatment for those patients who were not treated surgically. The authors concluded that the Wilmington brace appears to be an acceptable alternative to the Milwaukee brace for the nonsurgical treatment of adolescent scoliosis. The Wilmington brace also was shown to improve pretreatment lateral trunk shift. In a subsequent study from the same institution, the effectiveness of full-time and part-time treatment with a Wilmington brace was compared. Patients treated with electrical stimulation were used as controls. Both full-time and part-time bracing treatments were effective in limiting curve progression. There was no statistically significant difference observed between the effectiveness of bracing in the full-time and part-time groups.

In a study of 295 patients treated with a Boston brace, young age and larger pretreatment curves were found to increase the probability of the need for surgery. Bracing treatment of curves greater than 40° had a high failure rate. A strong correlation between the best in-brace correction and follow-up correction was observed (Fig. 3).

The results suggested that the Boston brace is beneficial. In another study, 32 patients treated with a Boston brace were compared with 32 paired untreated patients from a separate institution. All patients were at Risser grade 0. Follow-up was terminated when patients were weaned from the brace. No statistically significant difference in curve progression was noted between the two groups. The small number of patients and the short follow-up time are weaknesses of this study.

One prospective study compared curve progression in two groups of adolescent patients with idiopathic scoliosis. A total of 111 patients underwent bracing treatment and 129 were observed. Electrical surface stimulation was used to treat 46 patients. The method of management was determined by the preference of the 10 centers involved in the study. Follow-up was incomplete for 14% of patients. Failure was defined as curve progression of 6° or more as observed on two consecutive radiographs. Bracing treatment was found to have a significant beneficial effect on curve progression, even if all patients with incomplete follow-up were considered failures. There was no difference in curve progression between patients who were observed and those who received electrical stimulation. This study did not address the effect of nonsurgical treatment on the probability of the need for surgery.

The Charleston brace is designed to bend the trunk toward the convexity of the curve being treated, thus correcting the deformity. It is intended for nighttime use, which makes it less of a burden for patients. However, double major curves are a special concern, because the side bending that corrects one curve could accentuate the curve in the opposite direction. One study of 139 patients who were Risser grade 0, 1, or 2 with curves between 25° and 49° showed that bracing treatment was associated with curve progressions of less than 5° in 83% of patients. In a follow-up study of 98 patients from this group, the authors reported that 66% of patients showed improvement or less than 5° of curve progression. Treatment failure was reported in 20 patients (20%); fifteen of these patients had surgery and two others were offered surgery but declined. Six patients with single lumbar curves had excellent results following bracing treatment. Those with double curves had the poorest results. The authors concluded that nighttime bracing was effective in managing adolescent idiopathic scoliosis. Another study showed effectiveness of this brace only in single curves of less than 35°.

New braces that incorporate dynamic correction of scoliosis currently are being investigated. The tendency is to be more aggressive when treating small curves to prevent development of large structural deformities. The results of these methods are still preliminary.

Compliance

Compliance with bracing often is difficult to assess. One study that evaluated compliance found that only 15% of the patients wore the brace for the recommended hours of brace wear. Average wear for the entire group was 65% of the recommended time. Compliance was better in grade school children than in adolescents. In a study of the Boston brace, compliance was compared in patients whose brace had a superstructure and those that did not. Contrary to expectations, compliance was similar between the two groups.

Function and Social Impact

In a study designed to determine the long-term impact that bracing had on patients' lives, an assessment of Milwaukee brace treatment indicated that treatment and control groups were similar. Low back pain, however, was less frequent in the treatment group. In a study examining pulmonary function in patients wearing a thoracolumbosacral orthosis, patients were examined three times over a 2-year period. Results showed a significant reduction in vital capacity, forced vital capacity, func-

tional residual capacity, and residual volume with in-brace measurements compared with out-of-brace measurements. The authors concluded that brace wear did not result in permanent harm in pulmonary function during the 2-year observation period. However, adaptive changes in breathing pattern were observed in patients after several months of bracing treatment. Reduction in glomerular filtration rate, effective renal plasma flow, and urinary sodium secretion also have been noted shortly after application of the Boston brace. These changes are believed to be the result of reduction in the transverse area of the body caused by the brace. It is unlikely that the observed changes in renal function have long-term clinical significance. Other complications related to bracing treatment include skin ulceration or hypersensitivity, exacerbation of lordosis, and alteration of the normal fat distribution in the hip area.

Electrical Stimulation

Lateral electrical surface stimulation (LESS), which was introduced in 1977, is another type of nonsurgical treatment. The goal of LESS is to achieve active curve correction through intermittent transcutaneous muscle stimulation on the convex side. This alternative to bracing treatment was designed for nighttime use. Although early reports on the results were encouraging, numerous subsequent studies have shown that treatment with LESS results in a course that parallels the disease's natural history. This discrepancy in results has been attributed to the selection of patients at low risk for progression and short follow-up time in the early studies. Surface stimulation is no longer considered an effective method for the management of scoliosis.

Implantable electrical stimulation also has been attempted. Here, too, the early studies reported successful results. A subsequent study of the same patients by investigators who were not involved in the design of the device failed to demonstrate effectiveness. Physical therapy and manipulation have not been shown to alter the natural history of idiopathic scoliosis.

Annotated Bibliography

Natural History

Little DG, Song KM, Katz D, Herring JA: Relationship of peak height velocity to other maturity indicators in idiopathic scoliosis in girls. *J Bone Joint Surg Am* 2000;82:685-693.

In this retrospective study, peak height velocity for 120 patients with idiopathic scoliosis was analyzed. The results were compared with data for adolescents who did not have scoliosis. The peak height velocity also was compared with chronologic age, menarchal age, and Risser sign for accuracy in predicting curve progression. The authors concluded that peak height velocity can be used to accurately predict the end of growth. The usefulness of this measurement in the management of patients has not yet been established.

Noordeen MH, Haddad FS, Edgar MA, Pringle J: Spinal growth and a histologic evaluation of the Risser grade in idiopathic scoliosis. *Spine* 1999;24:535-538.

In this prospective study, 34 patients underwent anterior spine surgery as part of the correction of idiopathic scoliosis. Superior and inferior vertebral end plates were harvested at the time of surgery and examined histologically for evidence of growth activity. The patients' Risser grade was then correlated with the growth activity.

Payne WK, Ogilvie JW, Resnick MD, Kane RL, Transfeldt EE, Blum RW: Does scoliosis have a psychological impact and does gender make a difference? *Spine* 1997;22:1380-1384.

A health survey instrument designed to assess the health concerns of adolescents was completed by 34,706 adolescents. From this group, 685 adolescents with scoliosis were identified and compared with a control group. The results indicated that the patients with scoliosis were significantly more likely to have suicidal thoughts and concerns about abnormal body development. The analysis also showed that the adolescents' concerns were influenced by gender. The author concluded that scoliosis is a risk factor for psychological issues and health-compromising behavior.

Robinson CM, McMaster MJ: Juvenile idiopathic scoliosis: Curve patterns and prognosis in one hundred and nine patients. *J Bone Joint Surg Am* 1996;78:1140-1148.

The authors reviewed the medical records and radiographs of 109 (67 girls and 42 boys) consecutive juvenile patients with scoliosis (presentation between age 3 and 10 years). Curve progression was observed in 104 patients. Eighty-nine patients with progressive curves were followed to skeletal maturity. The rate of curve progression increased after age 10 years. Sixty-seven of the 89 patients who were followed to skeletal maturity were treated with arthrodesis. The authors reported that the prevalence of patients with juvenile onset idiopathic scoliosis at their institution was 8% of the total of patients with idiopathic scoliosis.

Song KM, Little DG: Peak height velocity as a maturity indicator for males with idiopathic scoliosis. *J Pediatr Orthop* 2000;20:286-288.

In this retrospective analysis, 43 male patients met the inclusion criteria of a diagnosis of idiopathic scoliosis, visits to the institution for at least 2 years with recorded height measurements through the adolescent growth spurt, and progression from at least Risser grade 0 to grade 4 during the follow-up period. The purpose of the study was to assess the usefulness of the peak height velocity in predicting curve progression and compare it to commonly used factors such as the Risser sign, closure of the triradiate cartilage, and chronologic age. The usefulness of peak height velocity as a prospective tool remains unclear.

Weinstein SL: Long-term follow-up of pediatric orthopaedic conditions: Natural history and outcomes of treatment. *J Bone Joint Surg Am* 2000;82:980-990.

The author summarized the natural history and outcomes of treatment of several conditions that involve pediatric patients. The long-term follow-up of scoliosis was addressed, as well as curve progression, pulmonary function, and back pain.

Nonsurgical Management

Allington NJ, Bowen JR: Adolescent idiopathic scoliosis: Treatment with the Wilmington brace. A comparison of full-time and part-time use. *J Bone Joint Surg Am* 1996;78:1056-1062.

In this retrospective analysis of patients with idiopathic scoliosis treated with a Wilmington brace, the effectiveness of full-time and part-time bracing treatment was compared. Ninety-eight patients were treated with full-time bracing, and 49 were treated with part-time bracing. Forty-one patients treated with electrical stimulation were used as controls to assess the effectiveness of the brace treatment. There was no statistically significant difference observed between the effectiveness of full-time and part-time bracing.

Korovessis P, Filos KS, Georgopoulos D: Long-term alterations of respiratory function in adolescents wearing a brace for idiopathic scoliosis. *Spine* 1996;21:1979-1984.

The pulmonary function was evaluated in 30 adolescents who were treated for idiopathic scoliosis with a Boston brace. The patients were evaluated at the beginning of treatment and at 12 and 24 months. At each interval, pulmonary function was measured both in and out of the brace. Values for vital capacity, forced vital capacity, functional residual capacity, and residual volume were statistically significantly less while the patients were wearing the brace. The authors concluded that wearing the brace resulted in a significant but reversible impairment of pulmonary function.

Labelle H, Dansereau J, Bellefleur C, Poitras B: Three-dimensional effect of the Boston brace on the thoracic spine and rib cage. *Spine* 1996;21:59-64.

A stereoradiographic technique was used to obtain three-dimensional reconstructions of the spine and rib cage in patients with adolescent idiopathic scoliosis who were treated with the Boston brace. Patients were evaluated in and out of their braces. Significant curve correction in the frontal plane was demonstrated as well as a significant reduction in the thoracic kyphosis. The brace did not significantly change the thoracic apical vertebral rotation or rib hump. The patient's position influenced the brace strap tension.

Nachemson AL, Peterson LE: Effectiveness of treatment with a brace in girls who have adolescent idiopathic scoliosis: A prospective, controlled study based on data from the Brace Study of the Scoliosis Research Society. *J Bone Joint Surg Am* 1995;77:815-822.

This prospective study involved 10 centers in which treated and untreated patients with adolescent idiopathic scoliosis were compared. There were 129 observed and 111 braced patients. Forty-six patients were treated with electrical stimulation. The method of management was determined by the center's preference. There was no difference in curve progression between the electrical stimulation and observation groups.

Noonan KJ, Weinstein SL, Jacobson WC, Dolan LA: Use of the Milwaukee brace for progressive idiopathic scoliosis. *J Bone Joint Surg Am* 1996;78:557-567.

The results of Milwaukee brace treatment for 102 patients with idiopathic scoliosis was retrospectively reviewed. The statistical analysis included 88 patients. More than 5° of curve progression was observed at the end of bracing treatment in 42 patients (48%). In 37 patients (42%), either the patient's curve was large enough to warrant surgery, or surgery was actually performed. The average in brace correction was better in the group of patients who did not have curve progression. The authors questioned the effectiveness of Milwaukee brace treatment for altering the natural history of idiopathic scoliosis.

Price CT, Scott DS, Reed FR Jr, Sproul JT, Riddick MF: Nighttime bracing for adolescent idiopathic scoliosis with the Charleston Bending Brace: Long-term follow-up. *J Pediatr Orthop* 1997;17:703-707.

The authors reported on a long-term follow-up study of patients treated with a Charleston bending brace for adolescent idiopathic scoliosis. All patients in this study were in the preliminary study. A diagnosis of idiopathic scoliosis, skeletal immaturity (Risser grade 0, 1, or 2), age of 10 years or older, and a curve in the range 25° to 49° were requirements for inclusion in the study. Of 98 patients, 65 showed improvement or less than 5° change in curvature. Curve progression in 17 patients resulted in the need for surgery; 15 patients underwent surgery, two were offered surgery but declined. All six single lumbar curves had excellent results; however, the response to bracing treatment was poor in patients with double curves. The risk of curve progression was greater for more skeletally immature patients than for patients with larger initial curves. The authors concluded that the Charleston bending brace was as effective as other types of orthotic management of adolescent idiopathic scoliosis.

Classic Bibliography

Axelgaard J, Brown JC: Lateral electrical surface stimulation for the treatment of progressive idiopathic scoliosis. *Spine* 1983;8:242-260.

Bassett GS, Bunnell WP, MacEwen GD: Treatment of idiopathic scoliosis with the Wilmington brace: Results in patients with a twenty to thirty-nine-degree curve. *J Bone Joint Surg Am* 1986;68:602-605.

Bassett GS, Bunnell WP: Effect of a thoracolumbosacral orthosis on lateral trunk shift in idiopathic scoliosis. *J Pediatr Orthop* 1986;6:182-185.

Betz RR, Bunnell WP, Lambrecht-Mulier E, MacEwen GD: Scoliosis and pregnancy. *J Bone Joint Surg Am* 1987;69:90-96.

Bjure J, Nachemson A: Non-treated scoliosis. *Clin Orthop* 1973;98:44-52.

Bunnell WP: The natural history of idiopathic scoliosis before skeletal maturity. *Spine* 1986;11:773-776.

Cochran T, Nachemson A: Long-term anatomic and functional changes in patients with adolescent idiopathic scoliosis treated with the Milwaukee brace. *Spine* 1985;10:127-133.

Dhar S, Dangerfield PH, Dorgan JC, et al: Correlation between bone age and Risser's sign in adolescent idiopathic scoliosis. *Spine* 1993;18:14-19.

DiRaimondo CV, Green NE: Brace-wear compliance in patients with adolescent idiopathic scoliosis. *J Pediatr Orthop* 1988;8:143-146.

Emans JB, Kaelin A, Bancel P, et al: The Boston bracing system for idiopathic scoliosis: Follow-up results in 295 patients. *Spine* 1986;11:792-801.

Goldberg CJ, Dowling FE, Hall JE, et al: A statistical comparison between natural history of idiopathic scoliosis and brace treatment in skeletally immature adolescent girls. *Spine* 1993;18:902-908.

Karol LA, Johnston CE II, Browne RH, et al: Progression of the curve in boys who have idiopathic scoliosis. *J Bone Joint Surg Am* 1993;75:1804-1810.

Kearon C, Viviani GR, Killian KJ: Factors influencing work capacity in adolescent idiopathic thoracic scoliosis. *Am Rev Respir Dis* 1993;148:295-303.

Lonstein JE, Carlson JM: The prediction of curve progression in untreated idiopathic scoliosis during growth. *J Bone Joint Surg Am* 1984;66:1061-1071.

Lonstein JE, Winter RB: The Milwaukee brace for the treatment of adolescent idiopathic scoliosis: A review of one thousand and twenty patients. *J Bone Joint Surg Am* 1994;76:1207-1221.

Nachemson AL, Peterson LE: Effectiveness of treatment with a brace in girls who have adolescent idiopathic scoliosis: A prospective, controlled study based on data from the Brace Study of the Scoliosis Research Society. *J Bone Joint Surg Am* 1995;77:815-822.

O'Donnell CS, Bunnell WP, Betz RR, et al: Electrical stimulation in the treatment of idiopathic scoliosis. *Clin Orthop* 1988;229:107-113.

Pehrsson K, Bake B, Larsson S, et al: Lung function in adult idiopathic scoliosis: A 20-year follow-up. *Thorax* 1991;46:474-478.

Pehrsson K, Larsson S, Oden A, et al: Long term follow-up of patients with untreated scoliosis: A study of mortality, causes of death, and symptoms. *Spine* 1992; 17:1091-1096.

Piazza MR, Bassett GS: Curve progression after treatment with the Wilmington brace for idiopathic scoliosis. *J Pediatr Orthop* 1990;10:39-43.

Rogala EJ, Drummond DS, Gurr J: Scoliosis: Incidence and natural history. A prospective epidemiological study. *J Bone Joint Surg Am* 1978;60:173-176.

Weinstein SL, Ponseti IV: Curve progression in idiopathic scoliosis. *J Bone Joint Surg Am* 1983;65:447-455.

Wynarsky GT, Schultz AB: Trunk muscle activities in braced scoliosis patients. *Spine* 1989;14:1283-1286.

Chapter 30

Idiopathic Scoliosis: Surgical Management

John J. Grayhack, MD

Introduction

Surgical management of idiopathic scoliosis is continually evolving given our greater understanding of the pathophysiology and natural history of the disorder. Modifications to the surgical treatment have been driven by assessment of these factors and the successes and failures of different techniques.

Although the indications for surgical treatment of idiopathic scoliosis remain largely unchanged, the extent or type of surgical intervention continues to evolve. Considerations regarding both the patient and curve must be addressed. The patient's physiologic, skeletal, and chronologic age, pain and pulmonary function, cosmetic satisfaction, and social concerns must be considered, and indicators of skeletal maturity must be assessed because of their association with the risk of curve progression. Most natural history and treatment studies are based on the Risser grade and age at menarche. The curve's magnitude, location, balance, rotation, and evidence of progression are important factors in determining both the need for and extent of surgery. Studies also indicate the relative importance of cosmetic concerns to patients and their families.

A decision to perform surgery that is based on any single parameter, such as curve magnitude, is inappropriate. General indications for surgery can be derived from natural history studies that predict the risk of progression and subsequent clinical outcome. In most cases, a premenarchal patient who is Risser grade 0 to 2 (skeletally immature) with a curve greater than 40° or curve progression despite appropriate bracing can be considered for surgery.

Prolonged bracing may be indicated in preadolescents despite a curve greater than 40° or curve progression in the brace. A pediatric patient may benefit from further growth to gain height or skeletal maturity to avoid postoperative "crankshaft" changes. Interim curve progression from 40° to 55° would have little effect on the type of surgery performed and its long-term outcome.

A skeletally mature patient with a thoracic curve of more than 50°, a thoracolumbar/lumbar curve of more than 40° with marked apical rotation or translation, a double major curve of more than 50°, or significant imbalance may be considered a candidate for surgery. Natural history studies have documented progression of these curves, despite skeletal maturity.

Preoperative Evaluation

The initial preoperative assessment must include a thorough history, physical examination, and imaging studies. Other causes of the curvature and any atypical characteristics must be investigated as well. The patient's birth and developmental history and a thorough history of trauma, infection and medical conditions, and treatments must be evaluated. A review of systems to identify potential etiologies, such as neurologic or muscular disease or inflammatory or neoplastic causes, is necessary. Although an accompanying backache is more common than previously believed, significant pain, functional difficulties, or neurologic symptoms should prompt further investigation. A history of cardiovascular or respiratory involvement is an important consideration in assessing the risk of surgery.

History, clinical examination, and imaging studies are used to assess the patient's physiologic and skeletal maturity. Clarification of menstrual history, assessment of the Risser grade and height velocity, and skeletal age based on radiographs of the hand, elbow, and/or pelvis can help predict remaining growth. In turn, the planned surgical procedure may be modified to avoid risks of postoperative curve deformation such as "add-on" or crankshaft phenomena.

The physical examination is an essential component in assessment and treatment of idiopathic scoliosis. Possible alternative etiologies must be identified. Clinical assessment of balance and alignment plays a sig-

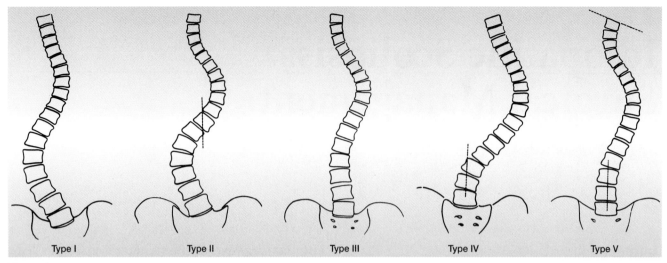

Figure 1 Diagrammatic representation of the King-Moe classification of idiopathic scoliosis. *(Adapted with permission from King HA, Moe JH, Bradford DS, et al: The selection of fusion levels in thoracic idiopathic scoliosis. J Bone Joint Surg Am 1983;65:1302-1313.)*

nificant role in the selection of surgical procedures, particularly in patients with double thoracic and double major curve patterns (King-Moe type I, II, and V classifications) (Fig. 1). Assessment of the deformity, especially at the rib cage, remains the most critical factor for most patients and their families. As more limited fusions are performed, flexibility of the remaining curves becomes more important.

A full-length standing coronal and sagittal plane radiograph on a single 14" × 36" cassette is the standard view for judging curve magnitude, balance, and rotation. Although supine side-bending coronal views are widely used for assessing flexibility, balance, and disk space mobility, some surgeons prefer variations such as "push-prone" and fulcrum-bending views. Supine AP side-bending views to maximum bend should be obtained on 36" cassettes. Fulcrum-bending views are obtained with the patient in a side-lying position over a bolster at the apex. In some studies, this view appears to be more reproducible; however, ascertaining which of the views is most helpful in determining appropriate surgical levels has been questioned.

The use of preoperative MRI in idiopathic scoliosis is limited. The specific indications for MRI include presence of a neurologic deficit, left lower thoracic curve or juvenile idiopathic curvature, with relative indications that include neck pain, headache, significant or disproportionate back pain, and characteristics that are beyond the expected parameters, such as significant imbalance or exceedingly rapid curve progression.

Preoperative assessments of pulmonary or neurologic function, such as pulmonary function test or somato-sensory-evoked potential (SSEP) monitoring, are of limited value unless the history and physical examination disclose specific abnormalities.

Curve Patterns

Classification of idiopathic scoliosis has assumed greater significance, with increased emphasis on using the most limited extent of fusion possible with more powerful instrumentation. The emphasis on three-dimensional assessment that focuses on correction of balance in both the sagittal and coronal planes and correction of rotational deformity makes a greater understanding and consideration of the multiplanar deformity necessary. The King-Moe classification remains the most widely used standard; however, several studies have questioned its inter- and intraobserver reliability. In recent studies, a new classification system by Lenke and associates has proven to be more reproducible and has important clinical implications in the selection of appropriate surgical treatment. This new classification has been particularly helpful in assessing double major curves with larger and less flexible thoracic curves (King-Moe type II curves) and double thoracic curves (King-Moe type V curves).

The presence of sagittal plane deformities such as thoracic hypokyphosis or lordosis has influenced the choice of surgical technique.

Techniques and Instrumentation

The goal of surgical intervention is to favorably alter the natural history of the disorder. This can be best achieved by realigning the spine within normal anatomic limits in all three planes while avoiding adverse effects and maintaining the alignment until fusion occurs. The goal is a well-balanced spine with a limited extent of fusion that can stand the test of time. Surgical techniques and instrumentation are evolving so that these goals can be attained.

TABLE 1 | Selection of Posterior Fusion Levels for Idiopathic Scoliosis

Upper End Vertebra	Lower End Vertebra
End Cobb vertebra	End Cobb vertebra or lower
Stable, neutrally rotated vertebra	Neutral or nearly neutral rotation
No significant proximal kyphosis on lateral view	No caudal kyphosis on lateral view
Include any upper curve that is greater than approximately 40° or causes clavicle tilt	Rarely below L4 in idiopathic scoliosis
	Disk below opens both ways during bending
	Vertebra becomes stable and horizontal during bending

The upper and lower extent of fusion should satisfy as many of these criteria as possible

Anterior Approaches

The role of anterior spinal fusion, with and without instrumentation, is expanding as the indications for fusion are more widely recognized and techniques and instrumentation become more advanced. Anterior fusion and instrumentation alone has been used widely for lumbar or thoracolumbar curves of sufficient flexibility and balance. This approach allows for greater correction while using a more limited extent of fusion. Allowing lower lumbar segments to remain unfused has been associated with a decreased incidence of low back pain in long-term studies. Similarly, success has been reported in achieving better sagittal and coronal plane correction when using isolated thoracic anterior instrumentation with limited extent of fusion, compared to posterior instrumentation and fusion. The long-term value of limiting the extent of fusion in such cases has not been established, and there is a risk that prominent hardware will irritate or perforate viscera and neurovascular structures.

Anterior release and fusion has been advocated in patients with significant sagittal plane deformity, such as apical lordosis in a thoracic curvature, and in curvatures that demonstrate significant rigidity. Residual curvatures of more than 45° or less than 50% correction, as assessed on side-bending radiographs, may benefit from the addition of anterior surgery to more traditional posterior spinal instrumentation and fusion.

Supplemental anterior fusion in skeletally immature patients has been advocated to avoid the crankshaft phenomenon. This tendency for the growing spine to demonstrate progressive deformity after solid posterior fusion has been well documented. The risk is most significant in patients who are younger than age 10 years or who are premenarchal and at Risser grade 0, particularly in the presence of open triradiate cartilage.

Anterior spinal instrumentation has evolved significantly so that optimal correction of the coronal curva-

ture is achieved while sagittal alignment is restored or maintained. Previous anterior instrumentation systems, such as the Dwyer cable, lacked the intrinsic stability to maintain or recreate the sagittal contour. Recently developed systems with solid rods have been supplemented with anterior interbody structural grafts or cages to alleviate this problem. Studies have shown the advantages of the newer systems, which include greater correction, derotation, and the ability to limit the extent of the fusion. However, irritation and perforation of viscera and neurovascular structures by indwelling instrumentation are continuing possibilities. Although adequate soft-tissue coverage of prominent hardware may be achieved with muscle and pleural rotation flaps, this risk represents a potential significant disadvantage of these approaches, particularly with anterior thoracic instrumentation.

Video-Assisted Surgery

Video-assisted thoracoscopic surgery has demonstrated results that are equivalent to those of open thoracotomy techniques. With the use of multiple intercostal portals, excellent visualization and more direct approaches at each level allow for resection of the disk, anterior longitudinal ligament, and vertebral end plates, as well as osteotomy and bone grafting. Anterior instrumentation of the thoracic spine using thoracoscopy has been tried in a few select centers. The advantages of this approach have been examined in preliminary reports, but long-term benefits have yet to be established.

Segmental Posterior Spinal Instrumentation

Recent studies have confirmed the superior restoration and maintenance of sagittal and coronal correction with segmental posterior spinal instrumentation compared with previously used systems such as Harrington

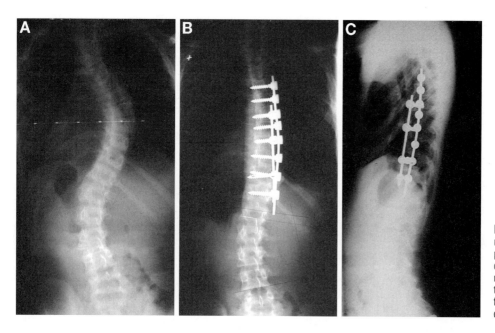

Figure 2 King-Moe type II (false double major) scoliosis in a 14-year-old boy. **A,** The patient's Risser sign was 0. The thoracic curve measured 65° and the lumbar curve measured 51°. **B** and **C,** Anterior instrumentation and fusion of T5 through T12 was performed to minimize the extent of fusion, decompensation, and curve progression.

rods. However, the long-term clinical outcome is not yet proven to be positively affected. Guidelines for selection of fusion levels with posterior instrumentation are provided in Table 1. Placement of pedicle screws at the caudal level or even more proximally has been demonstrated to improve vertebral alignment and, in certain patients, allows for a more limited fusion while maintaining balance. Again, the long-term outcome has not been assessed. The orthopaedic surgeon's experience and judgment should determine whether this approach should be used.

Bone Grafts

With the advent of the newer generation of instrumentation, the rate of successful bony fusion with appropriate bone grafting techniques is increasing. Although instrumentation techniques have continued to evolve, the success of spinal fusion still relies on meticulous technique. Facetectomy is essential. The standard for bone grafting is an autogenous graft, harvested from the rib, iliac crest, or spinous processes. Allograft and bone substitutes have been tested in animal models and in limited clinical settings. Results have been encouraging, resulting in their increased usage as osteoconductive bone graft extenders (to increase volume). Materials with greater osteoinductive and osteogenic properties currently are being investigated.

Monitoring

Electronic intraoperative neurologic monitoring has become widely accepted because it allows a level of confidence in the safety of surgical spinal manipulation. The use of SSEP with or without motor-evoked potential (MEP) monitoring during surgery for idiopathic

TABLE 2	Ideal Criteria for Selective Thoracic Fusion of False Double Major (King-Moe Type II) Curves

Description

Thoracic:lumbar curve Cobb ratio greater than 1:2

Thoracic rotation greater than lumbar rotation

Thoracic apical vertebral translation greater than lumbar translation

Lumbar curve magnitude less than or equal to 50°

No thoracolumbar kyphosis

Risser sign equal to or greater than 1

scoliosis has proved to be both sensitive and specific. On rare occasions, the use of SSEP alone may cause motor deficits to be missed. If monitoring is not available, a wake-up test is indicated.

Classification and Treatment of Curves

Specific surgical recommendations by curve type have been modified by changes in classification systems and wider acceptance of specific techniques such as anterior spinal release, anterior spinal instrumentation, and use of pedicle screws. Reports of anterior fusion and instrumentation or the use of thoracic pedicle screws in thoracic curves have been restricted to short-term follow-up studies at major centers. Advocates of these techniques cite as advantages the decreased number of segments fused and improved immediate correction in both the sagittal and coronal planes.

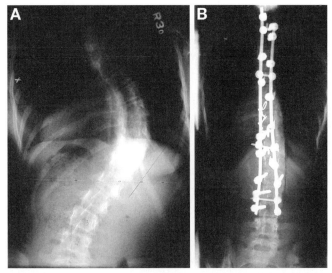

Figure 3 **A,** King-Moe type III thoracic curve measuring 73° was treated with posterior fusion and instrumentation. Bending radiographs (not shown) taken before surgery showed that the curve was corrected to 40°. **B,** L3 was selected as the distal fusion level, and bending radiographs showed that after surgery, L3 became stable and horizontal and the disk below L3 opened in both directions.

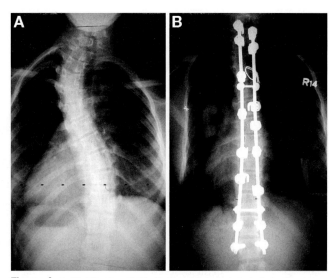

Figure 4 **A,** King-Moe type V (double thoracic) scoliosis typically involves an upper left, lower right thoracic curve. **B,** Both curves were fused because they were structurally similar.

King-Moe type I curves (those with a predominant lumbar curve and secondary thoracic curve) have been assessed by the relative flexibility of the two curves on side-bending films. If the thoracic curve is sufficiently rigid (greater than approximately 30° on the bending films) to affect skeletal balance, posterior instrumentation and fusion of both curves is the norm. Because of long-term sequelae of loss of lumbar lordosis, ie, "flatback," maintenance of lumbar lordosis is emphasized. Often, the thoracic curve is less significant, so selective anterior lumbar spinal instrumentation and fusion will suffice. Systems with rigid rods and anterior spacers (structural grafts or cages) have resulted in better correction of sagittal plane deformity with maintenance of lordosis. King-Moe type II curves (those with a predominant thoracic curve and secondary lumbar curve) have been further classified by deviation from the midline (apical vertebral translation) and flexibility. Guidelines for identification of King-Moe type II curves in which the thoracic curve can be selectively fused are shown in Table 2. These more specific criteria have been developed to assist surgeons in determining the appropriateness of selective thoracic fusion (Fig. 2). The more extensive correction of rotation that can be achieved during selective thoracic fusion with newer segmental instrumentation has resulted in decompensation of the lumbar curve. This overcorrection leaves the curve without instrumentation unable to compensate. Several authors have recommended only limited rotational correction, preferring translation and distraction and varied caudal hook and screw patterns instead.

Posterior fusion that is required for both curves in patients with type II curves may result in fusion of low lumbar segments. However, this has been associated with an increased incidence of lower back pain, most often in patients with loss of sagittal alignment. Attempts to prevent this problem have been made by maintaining or restoring lumbar lordosis or using pedicle screw patterns that allow satisfactory correction with less extensive fusion. The long-term outcomes of these modifications remain unproven.

Type III curves are thoracic curves with no lumbar curve deviation past the midline. These curves traditionally have been treated with posterior instrumentation and fusion (Fig. 3). Recent attention has been focused on the accompanying hypokyphosis or apical lordosis and the limited extent of the fusion. Anterior release and more powerful correction with posterior instrumentation has addressed sagittal plane deformity. Instrumentation to T12 has been associated with decompensation; therefore, fusion to L1 or L2 has been advocated. In selected centers, use of thoracic pedicle screws has achieved significant sagittal and coronal plane correction. With this procedure, one or two fewer caudal levels have been fused than traditionally indicated. However, the risks of thoracic pedicle screw placement have not been documented. Extensive training is required before this approach can be used, and the long-term benefit has yet to be established.

Type IV curves have been treated with posterior fusion alone. In recent studies, the caudal extent of fusion has been limited to L3 using lumbar pedicle screws, particularly if L3 demonstrates neutral rotation and the L3-4 disk space reverses its wedging on side-bending films. The rod bend must be reversed to maintain lumbar lordosis.

In patients with a type V curve, the upper thoracic curve must be carefully evaluated. Radiographs must be carefully reviewed to identify the presence of this curve and whether inclusion in instrumentation is necessary. Upper thoracic curves that are greater than 25°, an elevated left shoulder, limited flexibility on radiographic side bending, and apical rotation should be considered for inclusion (Fig. 4).

Complications

The rate of short-term surgical complications for idiopathic scoliosis is relatively low. Surgical complexity continues to increase; however, studies have demonstrated the relative safety of techniques such as insertion of lumbar and thoracic pedicle screws and placement of sublaminar wire when performed by experienced surgeons.

Although late complications have been reviewed, sufficiently long terms of follow-up are scarce. In one study, late infections appeared in 1.7% of patients at a mean of 3.1 years after surgery. All patients were readily treated with implant removal, débridement, primary closure, and 1 week of antibiotic therapy.

A 2-year follow-up of 87 patients with iliac crest bone grafts demonstrated that 21 patients (24%) reported pain; daily activities were affected in 13 (15%) of these patients and eight (9%) were treated with nonsteroidal anti-inflammatory drugs.

Annotated Bibliography

Introduction

Bridwell KH, Shufflebarger HL, Lenke LG, Lowe TG, Betz RR, Bassett GS: Parents' and patients' preferences and concerns in idiopathic adolescent scoliosis: A cross-sectional preoperative analysis. *Spine* 2000;25:2392-2399.

This article reported on a multicenter prospective study of 91 parents and patients, each of whom completed a preoperative questionnaire regarding a planned surgery for adolescent idiopathic scoliosis. Of greatest concern to both parents and patients was neurologic deficit, of least concern was scar location and appearance. The primary reason for surgery was to reduce future pain and disability.

Preoperative Evaluation

Cheung KM, Luk KD: Prediction of correction of scoliosis with use of the fulcrum bending radiograph. *J Bone Joint Surg Am* 1997;79:1144-1150.

The use of side-bending radiographs over a fulcrum in the decubitus position was compared to preoperative assessments from weight-bearing and supine side-bending radiographs. The fulcrum-bending studies better predicted the flexibility and final correction obtained by segmental spinal instrumentation.

Do T, Fras C, Burke S, Widmann RF, Rawlins B, Boachie-Adjei O: Clinical value of routine preoperative magnetic resonance imaging in adolescent idiopathic scoliosis: A prospective study of three hundred and twenty-seven patients. *J Bone Joint Surg Am* 2001;83: 577-579.

In this prospective study of MRI findings obtained for 327 patients with typical adolescent idiopathic scoliosis with a neurologically unremarkable history and physical examination, four patients had Arnold-Chiari type I malformation, two had spinal cord syrinx, and one had abnormal fatty infiltrate of the tenth thoracic vertebral body. None of the patients required neurosurgical intervention. All underwent spinal instrumentation and fusion without neurologic sequelae.

Little DG, Song KM, Katz D, Herring JA: Relationship of peak height velocity to other maturity indicators in idiopathic scoliosis in girls. *J Bone Joint Surg Am* 2000;82:685-693.

Peak height velocity in girls with adolescent idiopathic scoliosis was studied retrospectively. When compared with the general population, patients in the study showed a similar growth curve. In 90% of the patients, growth ceased 3.6 years after peak height velocity. Peak height velocity more sharply defined growth patterns and maximal progression of curves than chronologic age, menarche, and Risser sign. At the time of peak height velocity, 60 patients had curves of greater than 30°; curves progressed to greater than 45° in 50 of these patients. Curves progressed to greater than 45° in only one of 30 girls with curves of less than 30°.

Curve Patterns

Cummings RJ, Loveless EA, Campbell J, Samelson S, Mazur JM: Interobserver reliability and intraobserver reproducibility of the system of King et al. for the classification of adolescent idiopathic scoliosis. *J Bone Joint Surg Am* 1998;80:1107-1111.

The interobserver and intraobserver reliability of the King-Moe classification of adolescent idiopathic scoliosis was studied. Preoperative radiographs of 63 patients were assessed by five observers, with a median interobserver reliability Kappa coefficient of 0.44 and median intraobserver coefficient of 0.64, demonstrating "fair" reproducibility and "poor" reliability.

Lenke LG, Betz RR, Harms J, et al: Adolescent idiopathic scoliosis: A new classification to determine extent of spinal arthrodesis. *J Bone Joint Surg Am* 2001;83:1169-1181.

The authors report on a new classification system for adolescent idiopathic scoliosis. The five developers of the system and seven independent surgeons who tested the system found that it was reproducible and reliable. The system is meant to assist the surgeon in selecting fusion levels and approaches.

Techniques and Instrumentation

Betz RR, Harms J, Clements DH III, et al: Comparison of anterior and posterior instrumentation for correction of adolescent thoracic idiopathic scoliosis. *Spine* 1999; 24:225-239.

This prospective study compared results of anterior spine fusion in 78 patients with posterior spine fusion in 100 patients. All patients had King-Moe type II to V curves and were followed for a minimum of 2 years. In the anterior spine fusion group, hyperkyphosis was seen in 40% of patients with preoperative kyphosis of 20°. In addition, a high incidence of pseudarthrosis, loss of correction, and rod breakage occurred in this group. The coronal correction was similar in both groups, and sagittal correction was better in the anterior spine fusion group. Most patients (97%) with anterior spine fusion had fusion limited to L1 or above; in the posterior spine fusion group, fusion limited to L1 or above was possible in only 18% of patients.

Liljenqvist UR, Halm HF, Link TM: Pedicle screw instrumentation of the thoracic spine in idiopathic scoliosis. *Spine* 1997;22:2239-2245.

The authors of this prospective study of 32 consecutive patients with adolescent idiopathic scoliosis who were treated with thoracic pedicle screws reported that 22% of the screws penetrated the pedicle cortex and 3% penetrated the vertebral cortex. There were no neurologic or vascular complications, although one screw was replaced because of proximity to the aorta. Pedicle screws achieved slightly better coronal correction when compared to hook constructs; however, the difference was not statistically significant.

Padberg AM, Wilson-Holden TJ, Lenke LG, Bridwell KH: Somatosensory- and motor-evoked potential monitoring without a wake-up test during idiopathic scoliosis surgery: An accepted standard of care. *Spine* 1998;23:1392-1400.

This is a retrospective study of 500 patients who underwent surgery for idiopathic scoliosis. All patients were monitored with SSEP and neurogenic MEP techniques. There were no false-negative results; however, there were seven false-positive results. Two true-positive results were noted. Normal neurologic results were predicted 100% of the time using a combination of normal SSEP and MEP techniques.

Regan JJ, Mack MJ, Picetti GD III: A technical report on video-assisted thoracoscopy in thoracic spinal surgery: Preliminary description. *Spine* 1995;20:831-837.

This is a preliminary report of 12 patients who underwent anterior thoracic spinal fusion with video-assisted thoracoscopy. The authors reported little postoperative pain with this procedure, short hospital stays, and little or no morbidity. They determined that with consistently improving surgical skills, a number of thoracic spine procedures using video-assisted thoracoscopy can safely be performed.

Sanders JO, Little DG, Richards BS: Prediction of the crankshaft phenomenon by peak height velocity. *Spine* 1997;22:1352-1356.

In this retrospective review, 43 patients with idiopathic scoliosis who were at Risser grade 0 at the time of surgery were evaluated for timing of peak height velocity. All patients with closed triradiate cartilage were found to be beyond peak height velocity. All patients who had fusion before or during the peak height velocity had postoperative curve progression. In patients with open triradiate cartilage, surgery during or before peak height velocity was found to be a strong predictor of the crankshaft phenomenon.

Suk SI, Kim WJ, Kim JH, Lee SM: Restoration of thoracic kyphosis in the hypokyphotic spine: A comparison between multiple-hook and segmental pedicle screw fixation in adolescent idiopathic scoliosis. *J Spinal Disord* 1999;12:489-495.

This is a retrospective study of correction of thoracic hypokyphosis in patients with adolescent idiopathic scoliosis using multiple hook constructs and pedicle screw fixation. At a minimum 2-year follow-up, patients in the segmental screw fixation group demonstrated significantly better restoration of kyphosis than those in the multiple hooks group, creating kyphosis that was similar to that in patients who did not have preoperative hypokyphosis.

Sweet FA, Lenke LG, Bridwell KH, Blanke KM: Maintaining lumbar lordosis with anterior single solid-rod instrumentation in thoracolumbar and lumbar adolescent idiopathic scoliosis. *Spine* 1999;24:1655-1662.

This was a prospective study of 20 consecutive patients with lumbar/thoracolumbar curves treated with anterior single rod and intervertebral cage instrumentation. Follow-up at 2 years after surgery showed maintenance of coronal plane correction and sagittal plane lordosis.

Classification and Treatment of Curves

Suk SI, Kim WJ, Lee CS, Lee SM, Kim JH, Chung ER, Lee JH: Indications of proximal thoracic curve fusion in thoracic adolescent idiopathic scoliosis: Recognition and treatment of double thoracic curve pattern in adolescent idiopathic scoliosis treated with segmental instrumentation. *Spine* 2000;25:2342-2349.

In this retrospective study of 40 patients with double thoracic curves with a left upper thoracic curve of greater than 25°, fusion of the upper thoracic curve was successful in achieving a level postoperative shoulder height in patients with preoperative level shoulders or an elevated left shoulder.

Complications

Clark CE, Shufflebarger HL: Late-developing infection in instrumented idiopathic scoliosis. *Spine* 1999;24: 1909-1912.

The authors reported on a retrospective review of 1,247 patients who underwent posterior instrumentation for adolescent idiopathic scoliosis. At a 5- to 14-year follow-up, late infection developed in 22 patients (1.7%) at a mean of 3.1 years postoperatively. Most cultures were positive after 10 days, with low-virulence skin organisms. Treatment consisted of removal of hardware, primary closure, and antibiotic therapy for 7 days, administered intravenously for the first 48 hours.

Skaggs DL, Samuelson MA, Hale JM, Kay RM, Tolo VT: Complications of posterior iliac crest bone grafting in spine surgery in children. *Spine* 2000;25:2400-2402.

In this review of perioperative and postoperative complications of harvesting posterior iliac crest bone grafts in children, 214 patients' charts were retrospectively reviewed and 87 patients were interviewed at least 2 years postoperatively. Perioperatively, there were two infections and one arterial injury. Of the patients participating in the 2-year follow-up, 21 (24%) had pain; pain affected daily activities in 13 of these patients (15%) and eight (9%) required nonsteroidal anti-inflammatory drugs.

Classic Bibliography

Bridwell KH, McAllister JW, Betz RR, Huss G, Clancy M, Schoenecker PL: Coronal decompensation produced by Cotrel-Dubousset "derotation" maneuver for idiopathic right thoracic scoliosis. *Spine* 1991;16: 769-777.

Harrington PR: Treatment of scoliosis correction and internal fixation by spine instrumentation. *J Bone Joint Surg Am* 1962;44:591-610.

King HA, Moe JH, Bradford DS, Winter RB: The selection of fusion levels in thoracic idiopathic scoliosis. *J Bone Joint Surg Am* 1983;65:1302-1313.

Lenke LG, Bridwell KH, Baldus C, Blanke K: Preventing decompensation in King type II curves treated with Cotrel-Dubousset instrumentation: Strict guidelines for selective thoracic fusion. *Spine* 1992;17: S274-S281.

Lenke LG, Bridwell KH, O'Brien MF, Baldus C, Blanke K: Recognition and treatment of the proximal thoracic curve in adolescent idiopathic scoliosis treated with Cotrel-Dubousset instrumentation. *Spine* 1994;19: 1589-1597.

Richards BS: Lumbar curve response in type II idiopathic scoliosis after posterior instrumentation of the thoracic curve. *Spine* 1992;17:S282-S286.

Sanders JO, Little DG, Richards BS: Prediction of the crankshaft phenomenon by peak height velocity. *Spine* 1997;22:1352-1357.

Steel HH: Rib resection and spine fusion in correction of convex deformity in scoliosis. *J Bone Joint Surg Am* 1983;65:920-925.

Suk SI, Lee CK, Kim WJ, Chung YJ, Park YB: Segmental pedicle screw fixation in the treatment of thoracic idiopathic scoliosis. *Spine* 1995;20:1399-1405.

Chapter 31

Congenital Spine Deformities

Steven E. Koop, MD

Introduction

Congenital malformations of vertebrae may result in deformity of the spine. For some patients the spinal deformity causes few, if any, problems. For others the vertebral malformations lead to severe deformities that result in pain, cardiopulmonary dysfunction, or neurologic deficit. Moreover, congenital vertebral malformations frequently are associated with malformations of other organs or structures. The orthopaedist will need to assess the whole patient while calculating the risk for spinal deformity and treating that deformity when needed.

Etiology and Associated Anomalies

By definition, congenital vertebral anomalies are the result of anomalous embryonic vertebral development. Most anomalies occur in the first 8 weeks after conception, when the neural tube completes closure and individual vertebrae are formed. The precise cause of vertebral malformation remains unknown. Reports of twins with similar congenital vertebral anomalies are very rare, and one center demonstrated that less than 1% of patients with congenital spine deformities have a known relative with the problem. Certain syndromes that include anomalous vertebral formation, such as myelomeningocele, are known to occur more frequently in some families. Genome studies have identified candidate human gene sites for congenital vertebral malformation based on known mouse mutations with phenotypes similar to those of human syndromes. It also is possible that environmental factors such as chemical toxins or radiation play a role in these malformations, but that is not clearly understood.

The embryologic development of the spinal column coincides with the development of numerous other organs and systems, and it is not unusual for patients with congenital vertebral anomalies to have congenital anomalies elsewhere. The type of vertebral anomaly that occurs does not predict the type or location of any associated anomalies. Malformations may occur in other organ systems, within the spinal canal and the neural tissue, or in musculoskeletal sites remote from the spine.

Structural abnormalities of the urinary tract occur in 18% to 37% of individuals with congenital vertebral anomalies. Renal agenesis, duplication, ectopia, and fusion are the most common abnormalities, followed by ureteral anomalies and reflux. Renal agenesis and ectopia also are frequently associated with genital anomalies. All urinary tract anomalies occur more often in patients with congenital scoliosis than in the general population. The great majority of renal tract anomalies are asymptomatic in childhood, but some of these asymptomatic anomalies may have serious consequences. Hydronephrosis that is caused by reflux or ureteral obstruction can silently destroy renal function.

The group of associated anomalies includes lesions of the spinal column and its content. Intraspinal anomalies are found in 18% to 41% of individuals with congenital spine deformities. They are most common in children with congenital scoliosis and distinctly less common in the presence of congenital kyphosis. Diastematomyelia, the most common and troublesome intraspinal anomaly, is present in 5% to 16% of patients. Diastematomyelia may be defined as a complete or partial osseous or fibrocartilaginous septum within the spinal canal that invaginates or splits the neural tissue. When results of several studies are combined, 9% of diastematomyelias occur between T1 and T6, 27% between T7 and T12, and 64% in the lumbar spine. The female to male ratio for diastematomyelia is 8:1, compared to 2.5:1 for congenital scoliosis. Although the overall prevalence of diastematomyelia in congenital vertebral anomalies is 5% to 16%, one author reported that 46% of those patients who had a hemivertebra and same-level unsegmented bar also had a diastematomyelia. Other intraspinal anomalies are tethered cord, low conus, diplomyelia, syrinx, and lipoma. The detection of these anomalies has increased with wider use of MRI.

The list of possible musculoskeletal anomalies is extensive. It has been noted in reviews that 2% to 5% of individuals with diverse upper limb anomalies will also have congenital vertebral anomalies. In 1972, the acronym VATER was created to group together vertebral anomalies, anal anomalies, tracheoesophageal fistula, and partial or complete radial limb dysplasias. Since that time, the term VATER association has been used to describe the nonrandom association of multiple malformations of the vertebrae, lower gastrointestinal tract, trachea and esophagus, renal tract, lungs, heart, and radius. Vertebral anomalies also have been associated with malformations of the ear, lip, and palate (Goldenhar's syndrome), scapula and clavicle (Sprengel's malformation), and pectoral muscles and hand (Poland's syndrome). These conditions have no clear embryologic explanation and no clear pattern of inheritance.

A disconcerting finding among children with congenital scoliosis and kyphosis is the high incidence of congenital cervical vertebral anomalies, often referred to as Klippel-Feil syndrome (first reported in 1912, when an individual with anomalous cervical vertebrae, short neck, low posterior hairline, and restricted cervical motion was described). Cervical vertebral anomalies have been reported in 298 of 1,215 patients who had congenital scoliosis and kyphosis. These anomalies may occur at single or multiple sites, have no clear correlation with particular forms of congenital scoliosis, and are usually asymptomatic in early childhood. Congenital cervical vertebral anomalies represent sites of potential instability and may necessitate restrictions in athletic activities.

Classification

There are two basic types of vertebral malformation: failure of a portion of a vertebra to form and failure of adjacent vertebrae to fully separate from each other. The deformity that results from either of these malformations depends on the location of the malformation within the vertebra. Complete failure of separation of two adjacent vertebrae would result in a loss of growth in height but no angular deformity because the vertebrae are normal in shape and growth potential is balanced. Failure of formation of one side of a vertebra (right or left, or the vertebral body) would result in angular deformity from the shape of the vertebra and the unbalanced growth that occurs over many years. A hemivertebra is an example of a failure of formation. The combination of failure of formation on one side of a vertebra and failure of separation of the adjacent vertebrae represents the most extreme example of

unbalanced growth: active growth on one side and no growth on the opposite side of the spine. Failures of formation and segmentation can occur at single or multiple sites in the spine (adjacent to or remote from each other) and can occur together as a mixed pattern of anomalies.

Vertebral anomalies that result in hyperkyphosis, typically in the region of the spine between T10 and L2, have a specific classification system. Type I deformities are the result of anterior failure of formation. Type II deformities are the result of anterior failure of separation. Type III deformities are those resulting from mixed malformations.

Evaluation

The presence of a congenital vertebral anomaly should prompt a careful history and physical examination. The association of congenital vertebral anomalies with other anomalies confirms the importance of a thorough physical examination of children who have such anomalies, although the examiner need not expect to discover multiple additional anomalies. A special emphasis must be placed on the neurologic examination, which can be difficult to perform in young children. Inquiries should be made about pain, sensory changes, weakness, and changes in bowel or bladder function. The examination should include assessment of strength, sensation, and deep tendon reflexes in the upper and lower extremities. Abdominal reflex changes may be a subtle sign of spinal cord or canal pathology.

Radiographs remain the best method to characterize the vertebral anomalies and detect change in the deformity. In children younger than age 2 years, radiographs may be done supine and include AP and lateral views. When children are able to stand in a reliable manner the radiographs may be done upright. The interval between radiographs depends on the type of congenital anomaly, the age of the child, and if known, the previous behavior of the deformity. The rapid growth that occurs from birth to age 3 years may require radiographs every 3 months, particularly in the presence of unilateral hemivertebrae and a segmentation failure on the opposite side. The slower growth of the juvenile years may allow follow-up every 6 to 12 months. The onset of adolescent growth will shorten the time between visits to 4 to 6 months. Careful analysis of sequential radiographs is required to detect emerging deformity. Anomalous vertebral anatomy can make it very difficult to reliably and reproducibly measure deformity. It is best to view radiographs from several points in time side by side and then to measure the Cobb angle using the same landmarks in each film. Coned-down radiographs will enhance bone detail. Severe deformities may necessitate a Stagnara view

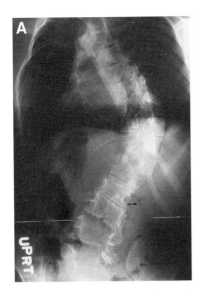

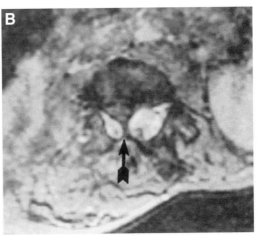

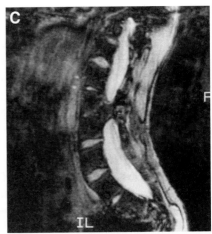

Figure 1 Congenital scoliosis in a teenage girl. **A,** Diastematomyelia is noted at the L2-3 region. **B** and **C,** MRI studies demonstrate a split in the neural elements in the transverse plane and sagittal plane. *(Reproduced from Richards BS (ed): Orthopaedic Knowledge Update: Pediatrics. Rosemont, IL, American Academy of Orthopaedic Surgeons, 1996.)*

(oblique view taken with the patient sufficiently turned to fully display the scoliosis) to see the vertebral structural anomalies.

Until recently, intravenous pyelography (IVP) has been the most common imaging technique used to identify abnormalities in the renal tract. Recent studies suggest that ultrasonography has 95% of the accuracy of an IVP and also may be used as an acceptable screening tool.

Clinical findings associated with diastematomyelia have been consistent. Cutaneous lesions (especially hair patches) are found in 55% to 79% of patients, anisomelia (usually calf or thigh circumference asymmetry) is found in 52% to 58% of patients, and foot deformity (most commonly cavus and almost always unilateral) is found in 32% to 52% of patients. Neurologic deficits, such as reflex changes, weakness, and sensory deficits are found in 58% to 88% of patients with diastematomyelia. Important radiographic findings consistent with diastematomyelia include spina bifida occulta, which occurs in 76% to 94% of patients, and widened interpedicular distance at the level of diastematomyelia, which occurs in 94% to 100% of patients (Fig. 1). Neurologic deficits also may occur in the presence of other intraspinal anomalies (hindbrain malformation, hydromyelia, distal cord tethering, lipomas), severe scoliosis caused by the combination of hemivertebrae and a bar, and congenital kyphosis caused by failure of formation of one or more vertebral bodies.

It is unnecessary to use MRI or myelography to study the spinal canal of every child with a congenitally anomalous vertebral column. In young children sedation or general anesthesia is required for MRI, and the process of obtaining these images must be weighed against the need to have information about the spinal canal and its contents. Diagnostic studies should be obtained when significant back or leg pain,

neurologic deficit, foot deformity, radiologically evident diastematomyelia or interpedicular widening, or combined unsegmented bar and hemivertebrae are present. Studies also should be obtained for all spinal fusion candidates. In these situations an understanding of spinal canal and cord pathology is essential for planning treatment. Myelography is now reserved for severe deformities for which the planar images of MRI are less effective.

Natural History

Deformity of the spine may be the result of local vertebral architecture, unbalanced growth potential, or compensatory curves. Results of two studies of congenital scoliosis, one with 251 patients and one with 234 patients, showed that approximately 75% of the patients required treatment before they reached maturity. The rate of deformity change and its final severity depended on the type and site of the deformity. Block or wedged vertebrae had the least deformity and the slowest rate of change (curve increase of 0 to 2° per year). Scoliosis due to a single hemivertebra was less severe than if two or more consecutive hemivertebrae were present, with rates of change between 0 and 5° per year. Fully segmented hemivertebrae with a contralateral bar (failure of separation), particularly at the thoracolumbar junction, always resulted in severe scoliosis. The rate of progression was 5° per year in the upper thoracic area, 6° to 8° per year in the lower thoracic area, and 10° or more per year in the thoracolumbar area.

A study of 112 individuals with congenital kyphosis demonstrated that deformity progression was most rapid and severe in two circumstances: Type III combined failure of formation and failure of separation and type I failure of formation (especially when two consecutive vertebral bodies failed to form). Neurologic deficits occurred in 7 of 68 patients with type I deformities, 0 of 24 with type II deformities, 0 of 12 with type III deformities, and 4 of 8 patients with deformities so severe that the exact vertebral malformations could not be determined. The apex of the kyphosis in patients with neurologic deficits was usually located between T6 and T11.

By comparison, the long-term evaluation of individuals with Klippel-Feil syndrome and congenital scoliosis is much less gloomy. A study of 32 individuals over the span of at least 10 years found that only seven (22%) had symptoms and only two required cervical surgery. Twenty-seven of the 32 did have surgery for congenital scoliosis in the thoracic or lumbar spine. Pain was associated with the presence of congenital cervical stenosis or a fusion in the thoracic spine that had extended to or above the cervicothoracic junction.

Treatment

Treatment begins with detection of changes in spinal deformity associated with vertebral anomalies. Severe deformities may require immediate treatment, but milder deformities may be monitored with radiographs obtained over a period of months or years. The interval between observations depends on the risk of progression associated with particular vertebral anomalies, the age of the child, and the prior behavior of the deformity. The radiographs must be of high quality and carefully measured, as described above.

Braces have a limited role in the management of congenital scoliosis. For infants, an open-frame brace that carefully applies pressure to the soft thorax may help control compensatory scoliosis. In older children, braces may be useful to help control long flexible curves or compensatory curves. Braces cannot be expected to halt growth-related deformity resulting from marked growth imbalance (such as hemivertebrae with opposing failure of segmentation, or type I kyphosis resulting from failure of vertebral body formation). Continued use of a brace in the face of relentless deformity progression should be avoided.

There are many surgical options for treating congenital scoliosis, including posterior spinal fusion, anterior spinal fusion, combined anterior and posterior spinal fusion, vertebral excision, and convex posterior hemiarthrodesis with anterior hemiepiphyseodesis (by partial disk and end-plate excision). Instrumentation may be used as a part of fusion or as a temporary means of curve control while delaying fusion. The surgeon chooses the best surgical procedure according to the vertebral pathology, the behavior of the deformity, and evaluation of the child with the deformity.

Posterior fusion is the benchmark against which to compare all other methods. It is the oldest surgical technique and the simplest and safest. Indications for posterior spinal fusion for congenital scoliosis include moderate size curves and curves with slow progression. Lordotic scoliosis is a relative contraindication to posterior fusion alone. Indications for posterior fusion for congenital kyphosis include patients who have anterior bar formation and wedged vertebrae (type II deformities) and less than 50° of angulation. The fusion should include the entire kyphotic area, plus one level above and one below when feasible. This may result in some spontaneous correction of the kyphosis and lead to a very satisfactory cosmetic appearance. The posterior fusion technique should include facetectomy and copious bone graft so that the result is a thick, wide fusion mass that will resist later growth deformity. The iliac crest is the most common source for autogenous bone graft, and it can be supplemented with local bone from decortication and facet removal or with rib if an anterior procedure is performed simultaneously. When iliac graft is impractical (very young children) or insufficient (long fusions), allograft bone may be used successfully.

Anterior spinal fusion as a single surgical solution outside the cervical spine is applicable for progressive congenital lordosis caused by posterior segmentation defects. Anterior spinal fusion is commonly used in combination with posterior spinal fusion. Anterior spinal fusion is more complex surgically, but it may improve deformity correction, reduce the incidence of pseudarthrosis, and prevent the bending of the posterior fusion caused by future growth (crankshaft phenomenon). Combined anterior and posterior spinal fusion for congenital scoliosis is indicated for children with substantial growth potential; deformities with marked growth imbalance, such as both hemivertebrae and a bar; large rigid curves; and excessive kyphosis. Indications for a combined anterior and posterior spinal fusion for congenital kyphosis include failure of anterior vertebral formation (type I deformities) or other deformities that occur with severe kyphosis.

Instrumentation reduces dependence on postsurgical casts and braces and may enhance deformity correction. Fusion rates may be improved by providing stability to the vertebrae during bone healing. Instrumentation also is associated with a higher risk of neurologic deficit that includes paralysis, particularly in patients with significant kyphosis. Instrumentation should never be used without presurgical imaging of the spinal canal, and it must be done with spinal cord monitoring or an intraoperative wake-up test. In carefully selected patients, instrumentation without fusion may be a prelude to the definitive spinal fusion.

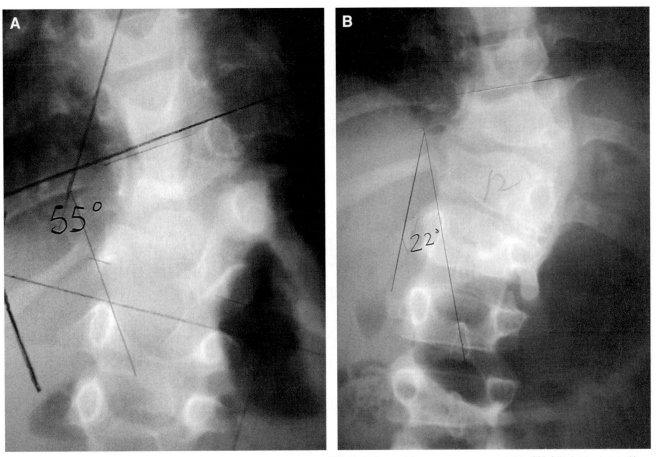

Figure 2 **A,** Hemivertebra in a 5-year-old patient caused progressive curvature to 55°. **B,** At 4-years follow-up, curve was corrected to 22° following treatment with an anterior and posterior convex hemiepiphyseodesis.

In patients with congenital scoliosis without spinal canal lesions, instrumentation without fusion may be used to control long curves with mixed anomalies or compensatory curves. However, there are significant risks associated with this method, and repeated surgeries to modify rod length may be needed. Possible complications associated with the use of this instrumentation method include hook dislodgment, rod fracture, junctional kyphosis at the upper end of the instrumentation, and soft-tissue fibrosis from repetitive incisions and dissection. Repeated surgery for rod length modification or replacement is necessary every 6 to 9 months. Use of a brace is mandatory.

Convex hemiarthrodesis and hemiepiphyseodesis is a procedure designed to prevent deformity progression and allow deformity improvement by surgically creating an anterior and posterior bar on the convexity of the scoliosis. This procedure is best performed on curves of limited length (five or fewer vertebrae), limited magnitude (less than 70°) with little or no kyphosis, and real concave growth potential. The entire curve segment must be included when performing this procedure, and it may be appropriate to also include one level above and one level below the curve.

Although curve stabilization is the most common outcome after this procedure, curve correction after surgery may occur in children younger than age 5 years (Fig. 2). The procedure generally consists of partial diskectomy and bone grafting, with convex posterior facetectomy and fusion included. Some authors report success in achieving anterior growth arrest by a transpedicular vertebral body decancellation.

One of the most controversial surgical procedures for congenital scoliosis is hemivertebra excision. Excision of a hemivertebra may be considered the equivalent of an apical wedge excision and may be used when that type of curve correction is needed (Fig. 3). The best indication for the procedure is a lumbosacral hemivertebra that causes an oblique angulation of the lumbar spine and significant trunk decompensation. The entire hemivertebra must be removed and the entire curve fused for the procedure to be successful. Failure to remove all of the hemivertebra increases the risk of nerve root impingement, and failure to fuse the whole curve may result in progressive deformity. Complications include neurologic deficits, pseudarthrosis, and progression of deformity above or below the resection site, necessitating secondary procedures to

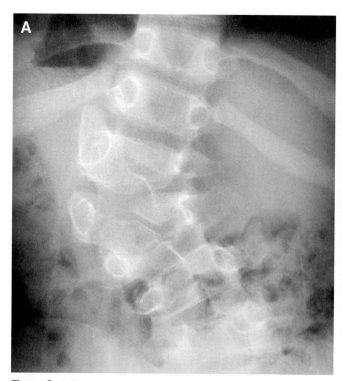
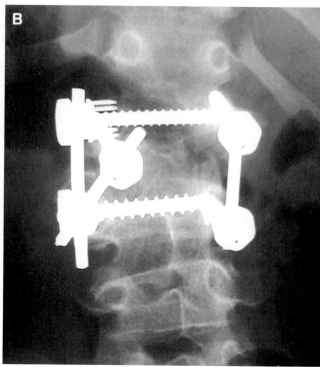

Figure 3 **A,** Progressive hemivertebra in a 9-year-old boy that caused significant deformity throughout his lumbar spine. **B,** An instrumented hemivertebra excision was performed to correct the deformity with minimal limitation of lumbar mobility.

extend the original surgical fusion. Multilevel vertebrectomy is a rare procedure performed as an attempt to create correction through instability, making internal fixation essential. This procedure carries with it the highest risk of neurologic deficit.

Although traction rarely is used in congenital scoliosis, it may be appropriate at times. Traction may be a means to gain slow, gradual deformity correction in a patient who is awake and whose neurologic function can be closely monitored. Indications for the use of traction include severe complex deformities, some compensatory curves with marked decompensation (between anterior and posterior procedures), and also following osteotomies and unilateral bars before final fusion. A thorough evaluation of the spinal canal is essential before traction is used.

An unsegmented bar usually results in a progressive and rigid deformity. Fusion in situ stops deformity progression but does not improve the deformity. Osteotomy of the bar may create some flexibility and allow deformity reduction before definitive fusion.

Common MRI findings include malformations of the hindbrain with neural elements in the upper cervical spinal canal, syrinx formation in the cervical and thoracic spinal cord, diastematomyelia, tethering of the distal cord caused by fibrous bands, and lipomas of the cauda equina in the lumbar spinal canal. Syrinx management may include decompression of the foramen magnum and the floor of the fourth ventricle if hind-

brain neural tissue is present in the upper cervical canal. This decompression may change the mechanics of cerebrospinal fluid flow and indirectly reduce syrinx size. Some neurosurgeons will insert a shunt directly into the syrinx. Division of fibrotic cord tethers is done in the presence of persistent back or leg pain, neurologic deterioration, or deformity progression that requires fusion with instrumentation. Commonly cited reasons to excise a diastematomyelia include progressive neurologic deficit and impending spinal fusion surgery with instrumentation. Most authors do not recommend excision of a diastematomyelia in the absence of a neurologic deficit or with a stable neurologic deficit, although one investigator recommends excision in all children in whom it is predicted that growth will create a spinal deformity that will require spinal fusion.

Summary

The care of children with congenital vertebral anomalies begins with a careful patient evaluation that includes physical examination and spine deformity assessment. Treatment solutions are selected based on what is best for the particular deformity and on results of the patient evaluation. The physician must be open-minded and able to offer the patient a number of treatment options. Finally, children with congenital spine deformities must be followed to maturity. Often, patients with congenital spine deformities may need two or more episodes of treatment to achieve the best possible results for correction of the deformity.

Annotated Bibliography

Etiology and Associated Anomalies

Giampetro PF, Raggio CL, Blank RD: Synteny-defined candidate genes for congenital and idiopathic scoliosis. *Am J Med Genet* 1999;83:164-177.

The authors attempt to identify candidate genes for human congenital scoliosis by reviewing mouse mutations with phenotypes affecting the spine.

Loder RT, Hernandez MJ, Lerner AL, et al: The induction of congenital spinal deformities in mice by maternal carbon monoxide exposure. *J Pediatr Orthop* 2000;20:662-666.

In this study of pregnant mice exposed to varying levels of carbon monoxide, there were no deformities in the controls and a 77% incidence of congenital vertebral anomalies in mice exposed to 600 parts per million of carbon monoxide in the first 10 days of gestation.

Evaluation

Prahinski JR, Polly DW Jr, McHale KA, Ellenbogen RG: Occult intraspinal anomalies in congenital scoliosis. *J Pediatr Orthop* 2000;20:59-63.

This study reports the results of MRI in 30 consecutive patients with congenital spine deformities. Nine (30%) had intraspinal anomalies, including tethered cord, syringomyelia, lipoma, and diastematomyelia. The authors point out the poor correlation between physical examination, plain radiographs, and MRI findings.

Natural History

McMaster MJ: Congenital scoliosis caused by unilateral failure of vertebral segmentation with contralateral hemivertebrae. *Spine* 1998;23:998-1005.

This article examines the behavior of congenital scoliosis caused by this particular anomaly. The combination of growth on one side of the spine and complete absence of longitudinal growth on the opposite side inevitably results in severe deformity. The author also reports the presence of intraspinal and neurologic anomalies, as well as anomalies in other organ systems.

McMaster MJ, Singh H: Natural history of congenital kyphosis and kyphoscoliosis: A study of one hundred and twelve patients. *J Bone Joint Surg Am* 1999;81:1367-1383.

This study examines congenital vertebral anomalies that result in deformity in the sagittal plane. The authors expand the existing classification system and emphasize that this pattern of congenital vertebral malformation has the highest risk of neurologic defect, including paraplegia.

Theiss SM, Smith MD, Winter RB: The long-term follow-up of patients with Klippel-Feil syndrome and congenital scoliosis. *Spine* 1997;22:1219-1222.

In this study of 32 individuals with congenital malformations of cervical vertebrae, most patients also had congenital scoliosis or kyphosis. The authors found few complaints of pain in those individuals who did not undergo cervical fusion. Complaints of pain were most common in those individuals who had undergone fusion for thoracic congenital scoliosis if the fusion extended into the cervical spine.

Treatment

Holte DC, Winter RB, Lonstein JE, Denis F: Excision of hemivertebrae and wedge resection in the treatment of congenital scoliosis. *J Bone Joint Surg Am* 1995;77:159-171.

This article reports the results of this procedure in 37 consecutive patients. The authors state that the primary indication for hemivertebra excision is rigid decompensation of the spine. Thirteen patients required additional surgery: six to extend the original arthrodesis and three to repair a pseudarthrosis. Neurologic deficits occurred in eight patients, although only one was permanent.

Classic Bibliography

Beals RK, Robbins JR, Rolfe B: Anomalies associated with vertebral malformations. *Spine* 1993;18:1329-1332.

Day GA, Upadhyay SS, Ho EK, Leong JC, Ip M: Pulmonary functions in congenital scoliosis. *Spine* 1994;19:1027-1031.

Drvaric DM, Ruderman RJ, Conrad RW, Grossman H, Webster GD, Schmitt EW: Congenital scoliosis and urinary tract abnormalities: Are intravenous pyelograms necessary? *J Pediatr Orthop* 1987;7:441-443.

McMaster MJ: Occult intraspinal anomalies and congenital scoliosis. *J Bone Joint Surg Am* 1984;66:588-601.

McMaster MJ, Ohtsuka K: The natural history of congenital scoliosis: A study of two hundred and fifty-one patients. *J Bone Joint Surg Am* 1982;64:1128-1147.

Miller A, Guille JT, Bowen JR: Evaluation and treatment of diastematomyelia. *J Bone Joint Surg Am* 1993;75:1308-1317.

Winter RB, Moe JH, Lonstein JE: The incidence of Klippel-Feil syndrome in patients with congenital scoliosis and kyphosis. *Spine* 1984;9:363-366.

Winter RB, Lonstein JE, Denis F, Sta-Ana de la Rosa H: Convex growth arrest for progressive congenital scoliosis due to hemivertebrae. *J Pediatr Orthop* 1988;8:633-638.

Winter RB, Moe JH: The results of spinal arthrodesis for congenital spinal deformity in patients younger than five years old. *J Bone Joint Surg Am* 1982;64:419-432.

Winter RB, Moe JH, Eilers VE: Congenital scoliosis: A study of 234 patients treated and untreated. Part I: Natural history. *J Bone Joint Surg Am* 1968;50:1-15.

Winter RB, Moe JH, Eilers VE: Congenital scoliosis: A study of 234 patients treated and untreated. Part II: Treatment. *J Bone Joint Surg Am* 1968;50:15-47.

Winter RB, Moe JH, Lonstein JE: Posterior spinal arthrodesis for congenital scoliosis: An analysis of the cases of two hundred and ninety patients, five to nineteen years old. *J Bone Joint Surg Am* 1984;66: 1188-1197.

Chapter 32

Scheuermann's Disorder

Steven E. Koop, MD

Introduction

In 1921, Holger Scheuermann, a Danish physician, described a type of increased rounding or hyperkyphosis of the thoracic spine that he believed to be distinct from the increased rounding of poor posture. Whereas postural thoracic hyperkyphosis is a flexible curvature with normal vertebral structures and intervertebral disks, Scheuermann's observations included increased thoracic kyphosis in adolescence, wedging of vertebral bodies, and irregularity of vertebral end plates. In 1964, Sorenson proposed a criterion by which the term Scheuermann's kyphosis could be applied: three adjacent vertebrae with wedging of at least 5°. Despite this strict criterion, the definition of Scheuermann's disorder is not clear; it may include radiographic findings of inflexible hyperkyphosis, vertebral wedging, disk narrowing, end-plate irregularities, and Schmorl's nodes.

Prevalence and Cause

Because the diagnosis of Scheuermann's disorder is based on angular measurement of kyphosis and abnormal end-plate and disk appearance, it is important to define normal thoracic kyphosis and the usual appearance of disks and end plates. A single measurement of the Cobb angle cannot describe normal thoracic kyphosis. Instead, normal is defined by a range of measurements obtained from the standardized standing lateral radiographs of a large number of individuals. In a recent study of 121 children and adolescents, researchers calculating two standard deviations above or below the mean determined a range of thoracic kyphosis between 20° and 50° to be normal. Others state that average thoracic kyphosis increases with age. Results of an MRI study of the thoracic spine in 90 asymptomatic individuals indicated that 38% had end-plate changes consistent with Scheuermann's disorder and as many as 58% had evidence of disk bulges, herniations, and annular tears. In another MRI study of 12 children with Scheuermann's disorder, typical findings included

Schmorl's nodes, loss of disk height, altered disk hydration, and variable herniation of nuclear material. Despite the prevalence of findings in imaging studies, it appears that approximately 1% of adolescents have the outward appearance or the symptoms of Scheuermann's disorder.

The cause of Scheuermann's disorder is unknown. Speculation centers on two possibilities: biologic predisposition to abnormal vertebral column growth (caused by familial predisposition, hormonal abnormalities, and vitamin deficiencies) and application of stress to the immature spine resulting in aberrant spinal growth. Studies of the substance of vertebral end plates and disks demonstrate disordered collagen and proteoglycans and abnormal chondrocytes, but researchers have been unable to determine whether these changes are the cause of abnormal growth or the consequence of stress-altered growth. The mechanical theory rests on the knowledge that growth cartilage subjected to abnormal application of force will change its pattern of growth. Abnormal compressive loads might inhibit growth in vertebral body height, causing a wedge shape and may cause the intervertebral disk to form abnormally or deteriorate. Studies of brace treatment that include evidence of restoration of anterior vertebral height support this theory, but little is known about the type of stress application that leads to abnormal vertebral growth. A similar radiographic appearance in family members of individuals with Scheuermann's disorder suggests a biologic predisposition in some people. Results of a recent study of 12 individuals supported the belief that predisposition to Scheuermann's disorder may be transmitted by an autosomal dominant pattern of inheritance with variable expression. The bone density of individuals with Scheuermann's disorder appears to be similar to that of other adolescents.

Uncertainty about the etiology of Scheuermann's kyphosis has allowed the use of terms such as disease, disorder, or condition. A single term, Scheuermann's disorder, could be used to represent a spectrum of clinical presentations. At one end of the spectrum would be those individuals with spinal deformity caused by focal wedging of vertebral bodies. At the other end of the spectrum would be those individuals who have normal sagittal contours, but who also experience disk narrowing, end-plate irregularities, and Schmorl's nodes. Such a spectrum may be artificial and bring together unrelated conditions, but, because definitive explanations for these findings are lacking, it would provide a reasonable framework to organize patients and their problems.

Presentation and Evaluation

Most young people with Scheuermann's disorder are evaluated because of excessive rounding of the back, which appears after the onset of accelerated adolescent growth. Often this rounding is a bigger concern for parents than for the adolescent. When pain does exist, it usually is associated with rapid growth, activities that emphasize forward flexion or lifting, or athletic activities. Symptoms may be present for weeks or months and often are described as dull, aching, annoying, or nonradiating pain. The pain is usually at the apex of deformity or in the lumbar region. Neural defects are rare in this age group. The condition is slightly more common in girls (1.4 to 2.0:1 girl:boy ratio).

Increased thoracic kyphosis generally is evident at physical examination. It may be accompanied by increased lumbar lordosis and a forward thrust of the head. Forward bending accentuates the kyphosis and helps characterize its location in the spine. Stiffness of the deformity, which is atypical for postural kyphosis or roundback, may be demonstrated by its persistence when the patient is lying supine on a bolster positioned at or just below the apex of the kyphosis. Reduced straight leg raising as a result of hamstring tightness is common.

Radiographs must be done in a consistent manner to allow comparisons across time and between patients. A standing lateral 2-m view taken with the arms supported parallel to the floor, including the entire spine from the lower cervical to the upper lumbar area, will permit measurement of kyphosis and characterization of disk and end-plate changes. A similar AP view will quantify scoliosis, if present. A lateral view that emphasizes bone detail will facilitate more precise measurement of vertebral wedging, and a supine lateral view with hyperextension over a bolster at the apex of the kyphosis will help quantify the rigidity of the deformity (Fig. 1).

MRI is not routine. It is indicated when neural deficits are found or when the description of pain seems

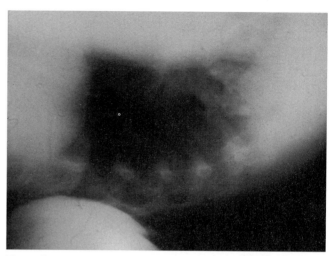

Figure 1 Curve flexibility can best be evaluated with a radiograph of supine hyperextension with a bolster at the apex of the curve.

inconsistent with radiographic assessment or clinical appearance. Worrisome pain reports might include extreme pain, pain remote from the kyphosis, radicular pain, night pain, or pain that fails to respond to rest, anti-inflammatory medications, or brace support.

Natural History

Natural history studies are inconsistent in their descriptions of the consequences of Scheuermann's disorder. A study from Iowa compared a group with Scheuermann's disorder to a control group. All of the participants were between age 25 and 82 years. Patients with Scheuermann's disorder had pain that was more intense and in a different location than that in individuals in the control group. Individuals with severe kyphosis experienced the most intense pain, especially if the apex of the deformity was above T8. Overall, the effect of this pain was not remarkably different than that experienced by the control group. Individuals in the group with Scheuermann's disorder demonstrated less trunk flexibility and usually held less physically demanding jobs. Otherwise, their education, total amount of time absent from work, recreational activities, pain medication use, and self-esteem were similar to those of the control group. Restrictive lung disease was found only in those individuals with kyphosis greater than 100°, with a deformity apex above T8. Other studies state that Scheuermann's disorder can cause severe and debilitating pain as a result of degenerative changes.

Neural deficits resulting from Scheuermann's disorder are rare during adolescence but somewhat more frequent in adulthood. Some studies have demonstrated that neural deficits may be the result of thoracic disk herniation, epidural cysts, or severe focal kyphosis.

While most studies emphasize pain or neural deficits, altered appearance is an important issue. There are few features of a child that concern parents as much as increased rounding of the back, or thoracic kyphosis. Most parents consider it unsightly and believe it is the result of poor posture. They seek to have thoracic kyphosis corrected during childhood because they fear it will become a stigma for their child during adulthood. The Iowa study examined self-image but the study population was exclusively adults, with 62 out of 67 older than 35 years. The authors reported that the Scheuermann's group was more likely to be single. They also found a correlation between increased concerns about appearance and more severe kyphosis, but they noted that increased age correlated with decreased concern about appearance. The opinions of adolescents and young adults may be quite different. The importance of body image at this age should not be underestimated.

Other studies have been focused on individuals with normal sagittal curves who have disk narrowing, end-plate irregularities, and Schmorl's nodes, particularly in the lower thoracic and upper lumbar regions. Diagnostic imaging centers, where many individuals with back pain are evaluated with MRI and CT, have reported a possible relationship between Scheuermann's disorder, radiographic findings, and early adult degenerative disk disease, particularly in the lumbar spine. Many of the individuals who undergo diagnostic imaging have already undergone surgical procedures and show degenerative changes in disks above the fusion in the mid and lower lumbar spine. A prospective study of Danish adolescents failed to find a correlation between radiographic changes in the spine and adult pain unless pain was already significant during adolescence or a family history of low back pain existed.

Treatment

Nonsurgical Treatment

Treatment of Scheuermann's disorder is generally directed at reducing pain or improving appearance. The only nonsurgical methods available for these problems are stretching and strengthening exercises and brace treatment. Stretching and strengthening, combined with modification of activities that incite pain, are likely to improve pain symptoms but will not reduce hyperkyphosis.

The goals of brace treatment include pain reduction and improvement of the hyperkyphosis. Studies of brace treatment of Scheuermann's disorder have widely variable results. Bracing will reduce pain and may improve deformity. The effect of brace treatment depends on the age of the child and the severity of the hyperkyphosis at the start of brace wearing. A younger child (before reaching adolescent growth velocity) has

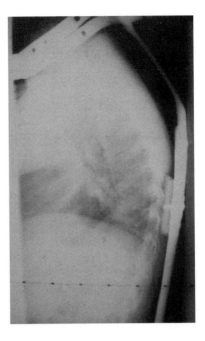

Figure 2 The Milwaukee brace provides the best three-point correction of kyphosis.

sufficient remaining growth to respond to bracing by restoring anterior vertebral body height. A moderate deformity (thoracic kyphosis less than 70° or diffuse thoracic hyperkyphosis rather than focally angulated deformity, especially thoracolumbar or lumbar) represents a smaller growth-restoration challenge.

The outcome of brace treatment is closely correlated to phases in the response of the kyphosis to the brace. Reduction in the kyphotic angular measurement is a necessary first response to the brace. If the kyphosis does not improve, then the curve is very rigid, the brace is not being worn sufficiently, or the brace is not mechanically effective. The Milwaukee brace provides the best three-point correction forces for kyphosis reduction (Fig. 2) but is much more visible than a thoracolumbosacral orthosis (TLSO), a major concern for image-conscious adolescents. A TLSO may be acceptable for deformities in the low thoracic or thoracolumbar area. A skilled orthotist and patience are required to achieve initial correction slowly over several weeks. If the Milwaukee brace vigorously corrects the hyperkyphosis, the brace will create excessive pressure under the posterior pads or under the neck ring and will not be worn. Therefore, the brace should be built with the idea of gradual kyphosis reduction resulting from brace modifications that progressively increase correction forces. Older studies of brace treatment suggested an alternative method of kyphosis reduction before a brace was constructed: serial casts were used to reduce kyphosis and the brace was built to hold the correction. Once the kyphosis is reduced, the correction must be maintained until growth stops. This maintenance may necessitate wearing the brace as much as 20 out of 24 hours. Premature reduction in brace-wearing time may inhibit restoration of anterior vertebral height, resulting in loss of correction.

The best candidate for brace treatment is a child with visible but moderate deformity that concerns him or her, pain, and accelerating growth. Such a child is motivated by self-interest to wear a brace. The worst candidate for brace treatment is an adolescent in the later stages of growth who has no pain and is unconcerned about the appearance of hyperkyphosis. That young person sees no merit in wearing a brace.

Surgical Treatment

Surgical treatment of Scheuermann's disorder during adolescence and young adulthood means spinal fusion. Indications for spinal fusion in that age group include pain that is unresponsive to nonsurgical treatment or deformity that is worsening or has become unacceptable in appearance. Indications for spine surgery later in adulthood include pain or neural deficit.

Studies have suggested that a Cobb angle of 70° of kyphosis is an indication for spinal fusion, but this seems an inadequate criterion. Kyphosis of that magnitude spread over the entire thoracic spine may not be obvious compared to 70° of kyphosis in the upper thoracic spine or 30° of kyphosis at the thoracolumbar junction or in the upper lumbar spine. Choosing exact deformity parameters to justify spinal fusion is, therefore, very difficult. Parameters include deformity size, location, and behavior as well as appearance and pain symptoms. Natural history studies suggest the curves most likely to be troublesome later in life. Severe hyperkyphosis with an apex above T8 is the deformity most likely to be painful, progressive, and associated with pulmonary dysfunction. Severe hyperkyphosis with an apex in the middle or lower thoracic spine is associated with reports of disk herniation and pain or neural deficit during adulthood.

The goal of spinal fusion is to improve deformity. Improvement of the deformity means reducing the hyperkyphosis to an amount that is cosmetically acceptable while preserving trunk balance and alignment. Depending on the nature of the deformity, this goal may be achieved by a posterior fusion with dual-rod, multiple-hook segmental instrumentation. In some cases, the posterior procedure may need to be combined with division of the anterior longitudinal ligament, multilevel disk excision, and interbody bone grafting. The indications for this additional anterior procedure include large, stiff deformities, especially those with very focal kyphosis. Depending on the site of the deformity, the anterior procedure may be done using thoracotomy (particularly if the diaphragm must be mobilized), or thoracoscopy (by surgeons experienced in that technique). Postoperative support with a brace or even a cast may be appropriate to protect the

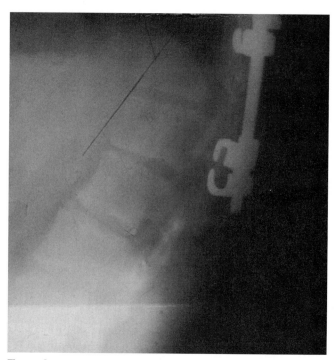

Figure 3 Junctional kyphosis at the upper or lower (shown here) ends of the fusion is a possible complication of surgery.

fusion, particularly if the deformity was severe or if the adolescent's activity is likely to result in significant application of stress to the instrumentation.

Complications of posterior spinal fusion during adolescence and young adulthood include infection, blood loss sufficient to require transfusion, neural deficit, failure of the instrumentation, pseudarthrosis, and sagittal malalignment resulting from deformity above or below the fusion segment. Short segment kyphosis immediately above or below the fusion region is a troublesome complication of spinal fusion in Scheuermann's disorder (Fig. 3). Failure to include all vertebrae in the kyphotic segment during a spinal fusion is a common cause of progressive kyphosis above or below the fusion segment. Excessive deformity correction, to a magnitude less than 50% of the original measurement, appears to be associated with increased risk of kyphosis just above the rods, with a compensatory and unsightly cervical hyperlordosis. Failure to include the first lordotic disk space and nonwedged vertebra below the kyphotic segment appears to be associated with an increased risk of short segment kyphosis below the fusion.

Some older adults with characteristic radiographic changes of Scheuermann's disorder may experience pain that is refractory to all nonsurgical treatment, and a few may have neural deficits. MRI in such cases may demonstrate thoracic disk herniations, intraspinal cysts, and anterior cord compression. Diskography may help identify which of several disks with similar appearance on imaging studies is the source of pain. Surgery tailored to the specific pathology, such as disk excision and spinal fusion, can relieve neural deficits and pain.

Annotated Bibliography

Prevalence and Cause

Boseker EH, Moe JH, Winter RB, Koop SE: Determination of "normal" thoracic kyphosis: A roentgenographic study of 121 "normal" children. *J Pediatr Orthop* 2000;20:796-798.

The purpose of this retrospective study was to determine the range of "normalcy" in the radiographic measurement of thoracic kyphosis in 121 children. A range of 20° to 50° described the mean plus or minus two standard deviations.

Wood KB, Garvey TA, Gundry C, Heithoff KB: Magnetic resonance imaging of the thoracic spine: Evaluation of asymptomatic individuals. *J Bone Joint Surg Am* 1995;77:1631-1638.

An MRI examination was carried out on 60 individuals who had never experienced any significant back pain and 30 currently asymptomatic individuals who had experienced low back pain only. Sixty-six of the 90 had positive anatomic findings at one or more thoracic level, including disk herniation (37%), bulging disk (53%), annular tear (58%), deformation of the spinal cord (29%), and Scheuermann-like endplate changes (38%). These findings document the high prevalence of anatomic irregularities in the MRI studies of the thoracic spine in asymptomatic adults.

Presentation and Evaluation

Swischuk LE, John SD, Allbery S: Disk degenerative disease in childhood: Scheuermann's disease, Schmorl's nodes, and the limbus vertebra. MRI findings in 12 patients. *Pediatr Radiol* 1998;28:334-338.

The authors report a study of the MRI findings of 12 children with clinical and radiographic manifestations of Scheuermann's disorder. Findings included loss of disk height, altered disk hydration, and herniation of nuclear material.

Natural History

Harreby M, Neergaard K, Hesselsoe G, Kjer J: Are radiologic changes in the thoracic and lumbar spine of adolescents risk factors for low back pain in adults? A 25-year prospective cohort study of 640 school children. *Spine* 1995;20:2298-2302.

This long-term prospective study of Danish adolescents did not find a strong correlation between radiographic changes in the spine and back pain during adulthood. Of greater importance were back pain during adolescence and a family history of low back pain.

Treatment

Chiu KY, Luk KD: Cord compression caused by multiple disc herniations and intraspinal cyst in Scheuermann's disease. *Spine* 1995;20:1075-1079.

Anterior cord compression caused by intraspinal cysts and disk herniation was improved by disk excision, cyst drainage, and spinal fusion.

Winter RB, Schellhas KP: Painful adult thoracic Scheuermann's disease: Diagnosis by discography and treatment by combined arthrodesis. *Am J Orthop* 1996;25:783-786.

This is a case report of an adult with refractory thoracic back pain and characteristic radiographic and MRI findings of Scheuermann's disease. Diskography at two apical disks reproduced the pain symptoms, which were relieved by combined anterior and posterior fusion.

Classic Bibliography

Gilsanz V, Gibbens DT, Carlson M, King J: Vertebral bone density in Scheuermann disease. *J Bone Joint Surg Am* 1989;71:894-897.

Heithoff KB, Gundry CR, Burton CV, Winter RB: Juvenile discogenic disease. *Spine* 1994;19:335-340.

Ippolito E, Bellocci M, Montanaro A, Ascani E, Ponseti IV: Juvenile kyphosis: An ultrastructural study. *J Pediatr Orthop* 1985;5:315-322.

Lowe TG, Kasten MD: An analysis of sagittal curves and balance after Cotrel-Dubousset instrumentation for kyphosis secondary to Scheuermann's disease: A review of 32 patients. *Spine* 1994;19:1680-1685.

McKenzie L, Sillence D: Familial Scheuermann disease: A genetic and linkage study. *J Med Genet* 1992;29:41-45.

Murray PM, Weinstein SL, Spratt KF: The natural history and long-term follow-up of Scheuermann's kyphosis. *J Bone Joint Surg Am* 1993;75:236-248.

Sachs B, Bradford D, Winter R, Lonstein J, Moe J, Willson S: Scheuermann kyphosis: Follow-up of Milwaukee-brace treatment. *J Bone Joint Surg Am* 1987;69:50-57.

Sturm PF, Dobson JC, Armstrong GW: The surgical management of Scheuermann's disease. *Spine* 1993;18:685-691.

Chapter 33

Spondylolysis and Spondylolisthesis

Erik C. King, MD

John F. Sarwark, MD

Introduction

The words spondylolysis and spondylolisthesis are derived from the Greek words spondylos (vertebra), lysis (break or defect), and olisthesis (movement or slipping). Spondylolysis is a unilateral or bilateral defect in the pars interarticularis of the vertebra. In the pediatric and adolescent populations, spondylolysis is most common at L5. Spondylolysis has been reported at other levels in the lumbar spine, but this is rare in the pediatric population. Cervical and thoracic spondylolysis also are rare.

Spondylolisthesis is a forward slippage of a vertebra relative to the vertebra caudal to it. The most common site for spondylolisthesis is L5 on S1, but slippage of L4 on L5 does occur in rare cases. Spondylolisthesis is classified into five subtypes: dysplastic, isthmic, degenerative, traumatic, and pathologic. Dysplastic (type I) and isthmic (type II) are the most common types of spondylolistheses in the pediatric population. These two types are discussed exclusively in this chapter.

Prevalence and Etiology

Spondylolysis is believed to be virtually nonexistent at birth. Spondylolysis in a newborn has never been reported, and the earliest cases of spondylolysis reported have been in infants age 6 weeks and 10 months. The prevalence of spondylolysis rises to between 4% and 5% at age 5 years, and increases with age until 20 years, at which time it remains constant. In a longitudinal study by Fredrickson and associates, the prevalence of L5 spondylolysis, with or without spondylolisthesis, was 4.4% in 6-year-old children and 5.8% in adults. Spondylolysis is twice as common in boys as in girls. The incidence of spondylolysis is increased in individuals who participate in athletic activities that require repetitive forceful hyperextension of the spine, such as gymnastics, diving, wrestling, and weight lifting (Fig. 1).

In dysplastic spondylolisthesis, forward slippage of a vertebra results from congenital anomalies of the lumbosacral articulation, most commonly a deficiency of a component of the L5-S1 facet joint. Such anomalies are present at birth and may be discovered incidentally in younger age groups. The incidence of dysplastic spondylolisthesis is not known. It is twice as common in girls as in boys.

In isthmic spondylolisthesis, forward slippage of a vertebra results from a defect in the pars interarticularis. The incidence of isthmic spondylolisthesis also is not well known; however, it commonly is believed that this disorder is virtually nonexistent at birth. Reported rates of spondylolisthesis among patients who have spondylolysis range from 50% to 81%. As is the case with spondylolysis, the incidence of isthmic spondylolisthesis increases after age 5 years. High-grade slippage is four times more common in girls, and girls are more likely to be symptomatic.

Inheritance plays a role in the development of spondylolysis and spondylolisthesis. Incidence rates ranging from 27% to 69% have been reported among first-degree relatives of children with these disorders. Familial predisposition is greater for dysplastic spondylolisthesis than for the isthmic type. Racial differences in incidence rates also have been documented. In the United States, the prevalence of spondylolysis among Caucasians (6.4% in males and 2.3% in females) is more than twice that among African-Americans (2.8% in males and 1.1% in females). The highest prevalence of any ethnic group is 26% in Alaskan Eskimos.

Wiltse and associates proposed that isthmic spondylolysis is the result of a fatigue fracture through a congenitally weak pars interarticularis. Researchers are attempting to identify such a predisposing anatomic abnormality. In a recent study, histologic examination of lumbar spines of human fetuses age 8 to 20 weeks of gestation was used to correlate the histologic development of the pars interarticularis with isthmic spon-

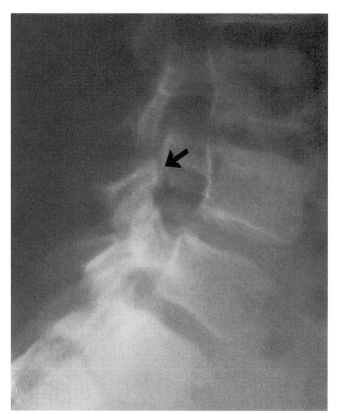

Figure 1 Spondylolysis at L4 in a 10-year-old boy injured while high jumping.

dylolysis. An uneven distribution of ossification was found within the pars of the lower lumbar spine (L4 and L5). This finding was in contrast to the uniform ossification in the pars of the upper lumbar spine and in the pedicles of all levels of the lumbar spine. The researchers concluded that areas of uneven ossification might form stress risers on which repetitive loading forces act to produce fatigue fractures.

Whether the congenitally weak area is larger or weaker in affected individuals than in unaffected individuals is not known. However, it is commonly agreed that isthmic defects ultimately result from stress fractures. Biomechanical studies have shown that repetitive microtrauma to the pars occurs when the inferior facet of one vertebra is driven repetitively into the pars interarticularis of the next caudal vertebra. Any activity that entails frequent extension or hyperextension of the lumbar spine exacerbates this trauma, and individuals who participate in such activities are predisposed to pars stress fractures.

The pars of young children are particularly susceptible to stress injury because they are thinner and weaker than are those of adults. Furthermore, mechanical stress on the pars is greater in children because of the increased lumbar lordosis in their posture and gait. Increased lordosis also explains the 50% incidence of spondylolysis that occurs in Scheuermann's disease. Individuals who have Scheuermann's disease typically

have increased lumbar lordosis that compensates for the increased kyphosis in the thoracic or thoracolumbar regions of their spines. This hyperlordosis causes increased stress forces across the pars, leading to an increased predisposition for spondylolysis. Finally, the fact that spondylolysis and spondylolisthesis have never been found in nonhuman species, including semi-erect primates, supports the theory that upright posture plays a role in the etiology. Thus, the etiology of spondylolysis and spondylolisthesis is multifactorial and involves congenital, traumatic, and developmental factors.

Natural History

Clinically, it usually is difficult to predict whether a spondylolytic defect will heal in a specific patient. Most complete pars defects do not heal radiographically, even in cases where clinical symptoms resolve. A few authors have reported radiographic healing in children and adolescents following immobilization in a cast or brace, but these typically are individuals who had an acute onset of symptoms following a specific injury.

A recent study of the skeletons of prehistoric and early historic Canadian Eskimos adds to the understanding of healing in spondylolysis and supports clinical experience. In this study, spondylolysis was not found in the vertebrae of the skeletons of infants or children. The youngest individuals whose spines showed evidence of spondylolysis were young adults who had either incomplete or complete spondylolysis. As the age of the individuals increased, incomplete defects were less common, and complete defects were more common. Based on the relative frequency of defects, the authors concluded that in the study population, most incomplete defects progressed to complete defects. Furthermore, they theorized that osseous healing of pars defects, incomplete or complete, rarely occurred.

Despite a few exceptions, most spondylolytic defects do not heal; they become pseudarthroses. In an attempt to explain this propensity for pseudarthrosis formation, a group of surgeons conducted a study in which they injected methylene blue dye into the facet joint immediately proximal to the pars defect in patients undergoing surgery for bilateral spondylolysis. They found a high frequency of dye in the pars defect and in the facet joint distal to the pars defect. Based on these findings, the authors suggested that leakage of synovial fluid from a facet joint into a pars defect may play a role in the pathogenesis of spondylolytic pseudarthroses.

Slip progression occurs in approximately 5% of patients with spondylolisthesis. Progression is more common in girls, in patients with dysplastic spon-

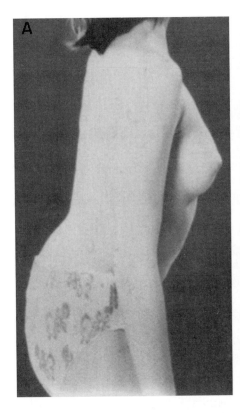
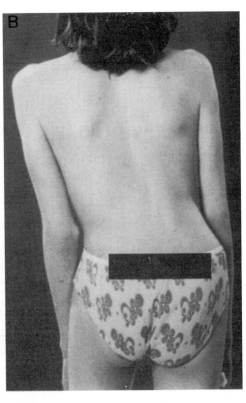

Figure 2 A, Patient with severe grade IV spondylolisthesis at L5-S1. **B,** Note list from sciatic scoliosis.

dylolisthesis, and when the slippage at initial presentation is greater than 50%. Slip progression is rare after skeletal maturity. Other risk factors for progression are greater slip angle, vertically oriented sacrum, dome shaped sacrum, skeletal immaturity, and dysplastic type.

When progression does occur, it usually occurs during the adolescent growth spurt and is most likely the result of intervertebral disk degeneration. Using diskography and MRI, abnormalities have been demonstrated both in the intervertebral disk at the level of the slip and in the disk at the level above. Disk herniation in adolescents with spondylolisthesis has been reported but is rare.

Clinical Findings

Spondylolysis and spondylolisthesis seldom are symptomatic in young children. Symptoms develop before age 18 years in 13% of the children known to have spondylolysis. Typically, symptoms develop during the adolescent growth spurt. Even then, the pain is rarely severe enough for the patient to seek medical attention. Radiographic features that correlate with pain are slippage greater than 25%, L4 spondylolysis or spondylolisthesis, and early disk degeneration.

Back pain is the most common initial complaint. Clinically, the pain is localized to the low back, and to a lesser extent, the posterior aspects of the buttocks and thighs. The pain is believed to be caused by motion at the pars defect and derangement of normal lumbosacral biomechanics. Recent studies suggest that the pain signals originate from mechanoreceptors located in fibrocartilage masses within spondylolytic sites. These mechanoreceptors may sense instability and transmit this information as pain. Nociceptive free nerve endings also have been found within tissue obtained from pars defects at the time of corrective surgery on patients with symptomatic spondylolysis and spondylolisthesis.

Many children who do not have pain are diagnosed because of postural deformity (Fig. 2) or abnormal gait. Typical findings during physical examination include restricted spine motion, a step-off in the lower lumbar area, tenderness to palpation, lumbar lordosis, lumbosacral kyphosis, flattening of the buttocks, and hamstring tightness. Patients with tight hamstrings demonstrate a pelvic waddle gait characterized by stiff legs, short stride, and pelvic rotation. The etiology of hamstring tightness is not known, although several unproven theories have been proposed, including nerve root irritation and microinstability of the lumbosacral spine. In general, hamstring tightness resolves after surgical arthrodesis.

Radicular pain in the lower extremities is unusual, but may occur in cases of severe slippage. Neurologic testing usually is normal. In severe isthmic spondylolisthesis, occasional abnormal findings include diminished or absent deep tendon reflexes in the ankle and weakness of the extensor hallucis longus. Tight hamstrings or radicular symptoms in themselves are not indicators of neurologic deficit.

Scoliosis occurs in 13% of patients with spondylolysis and in 23% to 48% of patients who have symptomatic spondylolisthesis. Three patterns of scoliosis occur: sciatic, olisthetic, and idiopathic. Sciatic scoliosis, also known as spasm scoliosis, is a lumbar curve resulting from muscle spasm. This pattern is not structural and resolves after resolution of symptoms related to the underlying spine pathology. Olisthetic scoliosis is a rotational deformity caused by an asymmetric slip at the spondylolisthetic level. Approximately two thirds of olisthetic curves resolve with surgical stabilization of the spondylolisthesis. Idiopathic scoliosis is structural and does not correct with lumbosacral arthrodesis. Approximately one fourth of these patients require surgical stabilization for the scoliotic deformity. The incidence of spondylolysis and spondylolisthesis in patients who have adolescent idiopathic scoliosis is 6.2%.

Radiologic Evaluation

The mainstay of initial diagnostic imaging remains standing posteroanterior and lateral lumbosacral radiographs. The central x-ray beam should be centered over the lumbosacral joint when obtaining the lateral view. Oblique views may provide a better picture of the pars area and often increase the yield of positive results. Up to 20% of cases of spondylolysis will be missed in young children if oblique views are not obtained. In addition, flexion and extension lateral radiographs may be helpful in assessing the magnitude of instability. The classic finding of a pars defect on an oblique radiograph is a break in the collar of the scottie dog (Fig. 3). The intact but elongated pars seen in dysplastic spondylolisthesis also has been described as the greyhound sign.

Bone scintigraphy is more sensitive than radiography in detecting acute pars defects. Two types of scintigraphy, planar bone scintigraphy (PBS) and single-photon emission computed tomography (SPECT), are commonly performed. SPECT has been shown to be more sensitive and specific than PBS. In addition, quantitative SPECT may have a use in the determination of healing of a pars injury following treatment. Normalization of the SPECT ratio correlates with clinical improvement (Fig. 4).

CT sometimes is useful, particularly in patients in whom a pars defect is strongly suspected but not seen on lateral or oblique radiographs. Failure to see a pars defect on an oblique radiograph may be caused by an incomplete defect or because the plane of the defect is not adequately aligned with the x-ray beam. When

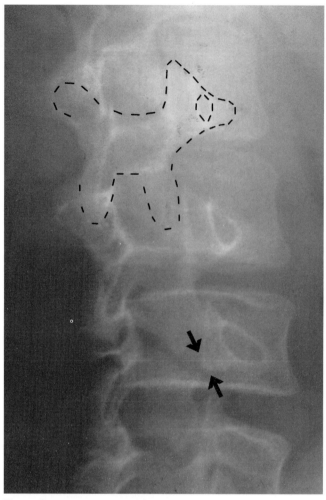

Figure 3 The posterior elements of the spine form a figure resembling a "scottie dog" on the oblique radiograph (dotted lines). A spondylolysis is apparent as a break in the neck of the dog (arrows).

CT is used, thin sections of 1.5 mm or less should be performed.

The utility of MRI in the evaluation of spondylolysis and spondylolisthesis is limited. It is associated with a high false-positive rate when used to diagnose pars defects. In the diagnosis of pars defects, MRI is reported to have a sensitivity of 57% to 86%, specificity of 81% to 82%, positive predictive value of 14% to 18%, and negative predictive value of 97% to 99%. However, in cases of neurologic deficit, either MRI or CT-myelography is highly recommended.

Grading

Systems for classification of spondylolisthesis are based on the amount of translation, lumbosacral kyphosis, and sacral inclination seen on spot standing lateral radiographs of the lumbosacral spine (Fig. 5). In addition to these measured parameters, morphologic changes in the shape of L5 and S1 are noted.

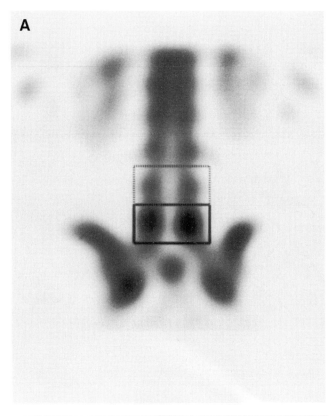

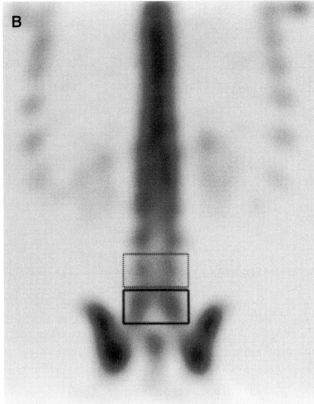

Figure 4 A, SPECT image of the lumbar spine in a patient with spondylolysis demonstrating localization at L5 (solid rectangle) as compared with activity at L4 (dotted rectangle). The pars activity ratio of L5 to L4 was 1.65. **B,** SPECT image of the same patient after treatment with a thoracolumbosacral orthosis. The pars activity ratio of L5 to L4 was 1.29, 21% reduced from that seen in Fig. 4B.

The Meyerding grading system is the one most commonly used. This classification system is based on the amount of anterior translation of the superior vertebra (L5) relative to the inferior vertebra (S1): grade I, 1% to 25%; grade II, 26% to 50%; grade III, 51% to 75%; grade IV, 76% to 100%; grade V, greater than 100% (spondyloptosis). Alternatively, slip percentage as described by Taillard may be used. Lumbosacral kyphosis is most commonly graded by measuring the slip angle. In the normal individual, the slip angle measures 0° or a negative value; slip angles greater than 45° are associated with a higher risk of progression. Sacral inclination is the angle formed by the intersection of a line along the posterior edge of the sacrum and a line parallel to the vertical axis of the body. Other grading systems include the modified Newman classification and the displacement index.

Dubousset classifies spondylolisthesis into two types based on the magnitude of the lumbosacral angle. The lumbosacral angle measures the degree of kyphosis between L5 and the posterior wall of the sacrum and is thus the complement angle to the slip angle. Spondylolisthesis with a horizontal sacrum (lumbosacral angle more than 100°) often does not progress, unless there is a concomitant increase in translational slippage, which can occur in a small number of patients. In the presence of a horizontal sacrum, nonsurgical treatment with rest, orthotic management, and an exercise program often will resolve symptoms (pain, radiculopathy, and gait disturbance). Spondylolisthesis with a vertical sacrum (lumbosacral angle less than 100°) is progressive and can produce neurologic impairment, cosmetic deformity, and functional disability. This latter type requires surgical intervention.

Treatment

Spondylolysis

Asymptomatic spondylolysis discovered incidentally can be managed with observation. Treatment of symptomatic patients consists initially of rest, nonsteroidal anti-inflammatory drugs (NSAIDs), activity modification, physical therapy, bracing, or cast application. Reports of recent studies indicate that early bracing of acute symptomatic spondylolysis is more likely to resolve symptoms than is activity restriction alone. Similarly, radiographic osseous union is more likely to occur if the immobilization is implemented during the early stages of the lytic process rather than the terminal stages.

Activity modification consists of limiting those physical activities in which hyperextension of the spine occurs. If the symptoms resolve, the patient may then resume all previous activities. Spine immobilization with a modified lumbosacral orthosis that reduces lum-

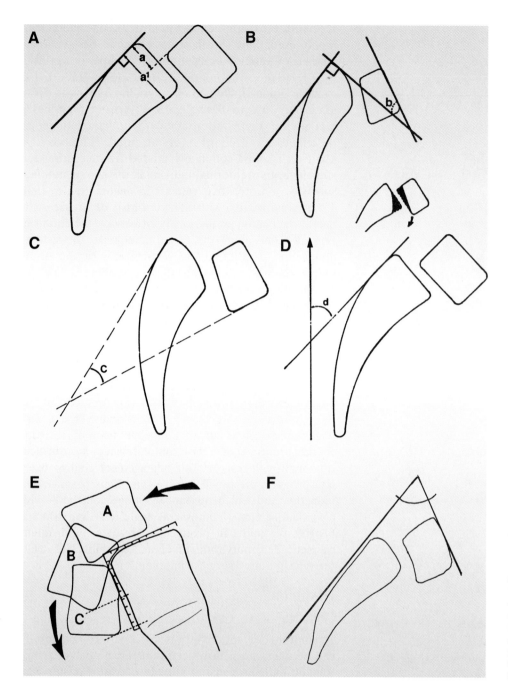

Figure 5 Measurement of spondylolisthesis. **A,** Measurement of the amount of forward displacement (a) and the sagittal diameter of S1 (a^1) allows calculation of the percent slip. **B,** Measurement of the slip angle (b), which is the kyphosis at the area of the slip (the L5-S1 kyphosis). As the slip increases, growth is inhibited at the anterior lip of S1 and the posterior lip of L5, causing the vertebra to become trapezoidal so that using the bottom of L5 does not accurately measure the angular deformity. **C,** Measurement of the sagittal rotation angle (c), which also represents the L5-S1 kyphosis and equals the slip angle. **D,** Measurement of the sacral inclination (d). *(Reproduced with permission from Lonstein JE: Spondylolysis and Spondylolisthesis, in Morissey R, Weinstein S (eds): Lovell and Winter's Pediatric Orthopaedics, ed 5. Philadelphia, PA, Lippincott Williams and Wilkins, 2001, p 782.)* **E,** Modified Newman spondylolisthesis grading system. Two numbers are used to measure the degree of the slip; one is along the sacral end plate and the second is along the anterior portion of the sacrum so that A = 3 + 0; B = 8 + 6, and C = 10 + 10. *(Reproduced with permission from DeWald RL: Spondylolisthesis, in Bridwell KH, DeWald RL (eds): The Textbook of Spinal Surgery, ed 2. Philadelphia, PA, Lippincott-Raven, 1997, p 1207.)* **F,** The lumbosacral angle, measured between the posterior border of the sacrum and the superior end plate of L5.

bar lordosis generally is recommended for patients who remain symptomatic after treatment with rest and activity modification.

Physical therapy often is prescribed after acute pain episodes and generally is more effective when focused specifically on training muscles that are the dynamic stabilizers of the spine, ie, the deep abdominal and paraspinal muscles. Strengthening of the quadriceps and hamstrings further strengthens the pelvic girdle and thus should be included in the program as well. The indications for surgical intervention in spondylolysis are persistent or increasing pain of more than 6 months duration, hamstring spasm, and/or radiculopathy.

Spondylolisthesis

Indications for treatment of spondylolisthesis are pain, radiculopathy, gait disturbance, hamstring contracture, and cosmetic dissatisfaction. Treatment selection is based on severity, skeletal maturity, duration of symptoms, magnitude of slip, and morphologic features of the slip.

Guidelines suggested by Wiltse and Jackson remain useful for most patients. Any child in whom spondylolisthesis is discovered early, especially if younger than age 10 years, requires radiographic follow-up every 6 months initially. If the condition remains stable, follow-up every 6 to 12 months until skeletal maturity is advised. In spondylolisthesis of less than 25% in an asymptomatic child, observation only is recommended. Activities are not limited. In spondylolisthesis of 25% to 50% in an asymptomatic child, Wiltse and Jackson recommended limiting participation in contact sports and sports necessitating hyperextension of the lumbar spine such as football, gymnastics, and diving. This last recommendation has been questioned recently because no study has ever proven that restriction from competitive or contact sports decreases progression in low severity (grade I and II) spondylolisthesis.

Symptomatic spondylolisthesis of less than 50% translation initially should be treated nonsurgically, including NSAIDs, rest, activity modification, lumbosacral orthosis, and physical therapy (as described for spondylolysis). Treatment of symptomatic grade I and II spondylolisthesis using antilordotic braces generally has been shown to eliminate symptoms. If symptoms do not resolve after an adequate trial of nonsurgical management, fusion in situ should be offered. In spondylolisthesis of greater than 50% in a growing child, with or without symptoms, surgery should be recommended.

Surgical Treatment

The selection of surgical procedures depends on the amount of slippage, degree of lumbosacral kyphosis, and patient and surgeon preference. Options include direct repair, posterolateral arthrodesis, anterior arthrodesis, decompression, reduction, and instrumentation.

Direct Repair

Direct repair is best suited for spondylolysis between L1 and L4 not associated with spondylolisthesis. Successful repair at L5 is less predictable. A prognostic technique used by some surgeons is the injection of a local anesthetic agent into the pars defect before recommending surgical repair. Proponents of this technique suggest that patients who report pain relief following injection will be more likely to benefit from surgical repair.

Several techniques of direct repair have been described. The four most common are described here. Each includes débridement of the spondylolytic pseudarthrosis and application of autologous bone graft harvested from the spinous process or the iliac crest. In the Scott wiring technique, a wire is passed around the transverse processes at the spondylolytic level and then tightened around the spinous process at the same level. In a modification of the Scott technique, a wire is looped around cortical screws placed into each pedicle and then tightened around the spi-

nous process. Buck's technique uses a lag screw placed across the defect. In a newer technique, the construct on each side of the spine consists of a pedicle screw, rod, and laminar hook. This construct is believed to provide more rigid fixation than the previous three techniques. It has been used successfully on patients with spondylolysis, predominantly adults, with and without grade I or II spondylolisthesis.

Clinically, 80% of properly selected patients heal after direct repair techniques. Resolution of symptoms has been reported in patients in whom the isthmic defect is still visible on CT. In animal cadaveric studies, each of the four fixation techniques adequately restores intervertebral stiffness comparable to that of the intact condition. However, the pedicle screw-rod-hook construct allows the least amount of motion across the spondylolytic defect during flexion. Compared to arthrodesis, direct repair also has the advantage of preserving motion segments.

Another direct repair technique recently has been described. In this technique, pedicle screws are placed into the involved vertebra and then the loose posterior arch is stabilized with a solid V-shaped rod that rests against the inferior aspect of the spinous processes and laminae. The pars interarticularis spondylolytic defect is then bone grafted. This technique has several theoretical advantages. First, it is mechanically stronger than wiring techniques. Second, it avoids placement of wires or hooks into the spinal canal. Finally, more surface area remains for bone grafting because no screws are passed directly through the pars defect as in Buck's technique. Experience with this technique is limited, however, and no long-term results are available.

Posterolateral Arthrodesis

Bilateral posterolateral arthrodesis in situ remains the standard for the surgical stabilization of spondylolysis and spondylolisthesis. Results with this technique have been consistently good to excellent, with 83% to 95% rates of fusion. With lower grade L5-S1 slips, single-level fusion from L5 to S1 is adequate. However, with slips of greater than 50%, the fusion should extend from L4 to S1. In severe slips, a pantaloon cast is recommended for 3 to 4 months postoperatively to enhance fusion rates. A cast is unnecessary if internal fixation is used. In some children with high-grade slips, progression has been noted after arthrodesis in situ despite solid fusion apparent on radiographs. Therefore, close radiographic follow-up should be continued until skeletal maturity.

Anterior Arthrodesis

For severe spondylolisthesis, combined anterior and posterior procedures sometimes are performed. Ante-

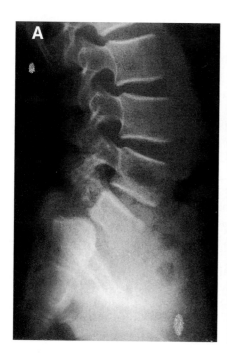

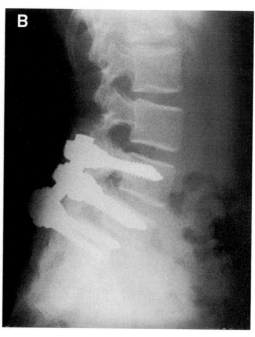

Figure 6 A, Twelve-year-old patient with back pain and Meyerding grade IV spondylolisthesis. Slip angle is 32°. **B,** The patient underwent surgical reduction with pedicle screws from L4 to S1 and arthrodesis. Postoperatively, pain was completely resolved, with a Meyerding grade 2 and a slip angle of less than 5°.

rior arthrodesis is attractive for two reasons. First, anterior diskectomy facilitates partial or complete reduction of spondylolisthesis. Second, anterior bone graft in conjunction with posterior surgery increases the rate of fusion. Anterior arthrodesis of the vertebral bodies also can be achieved through a single posterior surgical approach using the transsacral fibular bone grafting technique. However, this technique is performed predominantly for spondyloptosis and for salvage after failed posterolateral arthrodesis.

Decompression

Neurologic deficit is the most commonly cited reason for neural decompression. However, this indication is controversial because many surgeons have found that neurologic deficits usually resolve after solid fusion without decompression. If decompression is performed, arthrodesis must be done concurrently. An unacceptably high rate of progression has been shown to occur following the Gill decompression procedure in children; therefore, this technique is not recommended.

Spondylolisthesis Reduction

As described earlier, posterolateral arthrodesis in situ has been performed with reproducible success for low- and high-grade spondylolisthesis. In the past, reduction was indicated exclusively for patients in whom significant sagittal imbalance existed or to accompany neural decompression. Proposed advantages of reduction of slips greater than 50% include lower risk of pseudarthrosis, lower risk of slippage progression, elimination of the need to extend fusion to L4, decreased traction on the cauda equina, and deformity correction.

Both closed and open reduction techniques currently are used. Closed reduction techniques include pelvic suspension, halo-femoral traction, and postoperative hyperextension casting. The goal is to stretch the soft tissue holding the displaced vertebra and then pull the vertebra back into normal alignment. Open reduction techniques include: (1) anterior release and arthrodesis followed by postoperative reduction casting; (2) anterior release followed by intraoperative reduction and fusion with or without instrumentation; (3) posterior decompression and arthrodesis followed by slow reduction in extension and then anterior arthrodesis with internal fixation; and (4) posterior pedicle screw instrumentation techniques (Fig. 6). Injury of L5 nerve roots and the cauda equina have been reported with each of these techniques. The primary goal of reduction is to reduce lumbosacral sagittal kyphosis, and in most cases, no attempt is made to reduce the translational displacement. Attempts to reduce translation significantly increase the risk of traction injury to L5 nerve roots.

Vertebrectomy

The Gaines procedure is a two-stage vertebrectomy for spondyloptosis. The goal of this procedure is to correct the deformity and neurologic compromise accompanying these severe slips. In the first stage, the anterior lumbosacral spine is approached transperitoneally or retroperitoneally. The body of L5, the L4-5 disk, and the L5-S1 disk are removed. The second stage is performed either the same day or up to 2 weeks later. In this stage, the posterior spine is approached through a posterior midline incision. The loose neural arch and the pedicles of L5 are excised after distraction with a Harrington outrigger. The body of L4 is then reduced onto S1 and stabilized with pedicle screw instrumentation.

The rate of neurologic injury associated with the Gaines procedure may be higher than with in-situ fusion. However, many of these patients have preexisting neurologic dysfunction. Reportedly, patient satisfaction following this procedure is high.

Annotated Bibliography

Prevalence and Etiology

Jones DM, Tearse DS, el-Khoury GY, Kathol MH, Brandser EA: Radiographic abnormalities of the lumbar spine in college football players: A comparative analysis. *Am J Sports Med* 1999;27:335-338.

The purpose of this study was to determine whether there is a higher prevalence of lumbar spine abnormalities in football players before competing at the Division I level. Lumbar spine radiographs of 104 freshman college football players were compared with those of 83 age-matched individuals participating in preemployment physical examinations at a local factory. The rate of spondylolysis was not significantly different: 4.8% in the athletes and 6.0% in the control group.

Merbs CF: Incomplete spondylolysis and healing: A study of ancient Canadian Eskimo skeletons. *Spine* 1995;20:2328-2334.

Four hundred prehistoric and early historic skeletons from the Northwest Territories of Canada were examined for evidence of spondylolysis. Spondylolysis was found in 51 individuals, with 110 separate sites (sides) affected. The lysis was incomplete at 34 of these sites.

Natural History

Morita T, Ikata T, Katoh S, Miyake R: Lumbar spondylolysis in children and adolescents. *J Bone Joint Surg Br* 1995;77:620-625.

These authors investigated 185 adolescents younger than age 19 years with spondylolysis. The pars defects were classified into early, progressive, and terminal stages. Of the 346 pars defects in 185 patients, 39.6% were early, 29.5% progressive, and 30.9% in the terminal stages. Nonsurgical management produced healing in 73.0% of the early, 38.5% of the progressive, and none of the terminal defects. These results suggest that spondylolysis is caused by repetitive microtrauma during growth and can be successfully treated nonsurgically if treatment is started in the early stage.

Sagi HC, Jarvis JG, Uhthoff HK: Histomorphic analysis of the development of the pars interarticularis and its association with isthmic spondylolysis. *Spine* 1998;23: 1635-1639.

This study analyzes the histologic development of human fetal lumbar spine pars interarticularis to draw inference regarding the development of spondylolysis. Lumbar spines of human fetuses age 8 to 20 weeks gestation were examined

microscopically. The pars begins to ossify at 12 to 13 weeks gestation by endochondral ossification. The ossification center originates in the region of the pars in lower lumbar vertebrae, resulting in uneven distribution of trabeculation and cortication in this region. Uneven distribution of isthmic ossification results in formation of a potential stress riser in the region of the pars in lower lumbar vertebrae, which could be susceptible to fatigue fracture.

Clinical Findings

Congeni J, McCulloch J, Swanson K: Lumbar spondylolysis: A study of natural progression in athletes. *Am J Sports Med* 1997;25:248-253.

Forty athletically active young people with back pain, a diagnosis of spondylolysis, normal radiographs, and positive bone scans were studied. CT was used to further characterize the spondylolytic lesion and to determine healing of the lesion. Eighteen patients (45%) demonstrated chronic non-healing fractures, 16 (40%) demonstrated acute fractures in various stages of healing, and six (15%) demonstrated no obvious fractures.

Hasegawa S, Yamamoto H, Morisawa Y, Michinaka Y: A study of mechanoreceptors in fibrocartilage masses in the defect of pars interarticularis. *J Orthop Sci* 1999;4: 413-420.

The authors investigated the origin of low back pain associated with lumbar spondylolysis and spondylolytic spondylolisthesis by removing fibrocartilage masses from the lytic sites in symptomatic patients and staining the masses to examine mechanoreceptors. Comparison with mechanoreceptors in normal lumbar facet joint capsules showed that there were more mechanoreceptors in the fibrocartilage masses and a greater proportion of atypical structures at lytic sites. The authors theorize that these masses play a protective role by sensing instability via mechanoreceptors and transmitting this information as pain, while acting as ligament-like tissue that connects and stabilizes the separated vertebral arches.

Schneiderman GA, McLain RF, Hambly MJ, Nielsen SL: The pars defect as a pain source: A histologic study. *Spine* 1995;20:1761-1764.

Tissue from the pars defects of six adult patients with symptomatic spondylolysis and spondylolisthesis was obtained at surgery, and a histologic study was conducted to identify and characterize neural elements in this tissue. Neural elements, including free nerve endings believed to have nociceptive function, were identified in all specimens, although the density varied between specimens. These findings suggest that the pars defect may be a source of back pain in some patients with symptomatic spondylolysis.

Radiologic Evaluation

Anderson K, Sarwark JF, Conway JJ, Logue ES, Schafer MF: Quantitative assessment with SPECT imaging of stress injuries of the pars interarticularis and response to bracing. *J Pediatr Orthop* 2000;20:28-33.

Thirty-four patients were observed clinically between 1987 and 1996 and were studied with an initial and at least one follow-up SPECT scintigram. Initial radiographs and planar bone scans failed to demonstrate the pars lesion in 53% and 19% of the patients, respectively. The average SPECT ratio before brace treatment was 1.45. After treatment, this ratio significantly decreased to 1.27. The reduction in SPECT ratio of patients who remained symptomatic at follow-up averaged only 2.8% as compared with 13% for the remainder of the patients.

Saifuddin A, White J, Tucker S, Taylor BA: Orientation of lumbar pars defects: Implications for radiological detection and surgical management. *J Bone Joint Surg Br* 1998;80:208-211.

The authors studied the variation in orientation of spondylolytic lesions on CT scans of 34 patients with 69 defects. Only 32% of defects were orientated within 15° of the 45° lateral oblique plane. These authors believe that lateral oblique radiographs should not be considered as the definitive investigation for spondylolysis. They suggest that CT scans with reverse gantry angle are more appropriate than oblique radiography for the assessment of spondylolysis.

Treatment

Gillet P, Petit M: Direct repair of spondylolysis without spondylolisthesis, using a rod-screw construct and bone grafting of the pars defect. *Spine* 1999;24:1252-1256.

The authors report the results of an original technique of pars repair for spondylolysis without spondylolisthesis. Their surgical technique uses bone grafting and internal fixation consisting of pedicle screws and a V-shaped rod resting against the inferior aspect on the spinous process and the posterior aspects of the laminae. The first 10 patients who underwent this technique had an average follow-up of 35 months. The mean age at surgery was 26 years (range, 16 to 48 years). Six patients had an excellent result, one good, one fair, and two poor. No complications related to the specific design of the construct were encountered.

Kakiuchi M: Repair of the defect in spondylolysis: Durable fixation with pedicle screws and laminar hooks. *J Bone Joint Surg Am* 1997;79:818-825.

Direct repair of a defect in the pars interarticularis was performed using bone-grafting and internal fixation with a pedicle screw, rod, and laminar hook. The procedure was performed in 16 patients who had a bilateral defect of the pars interarticularis with or without grade I or II spondylolisthesis in whom nonsurgical treatment failed. Only patients who noted temporary relief of pain after the area of the defect had been infiltrated with lidocaine were included in the study. After an average 25-month follow-up, oblique radiographs showed osseous union in the previous defect bilaterally in all 16 patients. Thirteen patients were free of symptoms, three had major improvement with occasional low-back pain, and none had complications.

Muschik M, Hahnel H, Robinson PN, Perka C, Muschik C: Competitive sports and the progression of spondylolisthesis. *J Pediatr Orthop* 1996;16:364-369.

The authors investigated the effects of several years of competitive sports training on children and adolescents with spondylolisthesis. They performed a retrospective radiologic and clinical study of 86 young athletes with spondylolysis or spondylolisthesis drawn from a special school in Germany for competitive athletes. The mean degree of displacement was 10.1% at the beginning of the observation. Displacement increased in 33 athletes, did not progress in 36 athletes, and decreased in 7 athletes. The authors conclude that there is no justification for generally advising children and adolescents with limited spondylolytic spondylolisthesis not to take part in competitive sports.

O'Sullivan PB, Phyty GD, Twomey LT, Allison GT: Evaluation of specific stabilizing exercise in the treatment of chronic low back pain with radiologic diagnosis of spondylolysis or spondylolisthesis. *Spine* 1997;22: 2959-2967.

The authors studied the effectiveness of physiotherapy, specifically training of muscles surrounding the lumbar spine in the treatment of patients with chronic low back pain and a radiologic diagnosis of spondylolysis or spondylolisthesis. Forty-four patients were assigned randomly to two treatment groups. The first group underwent a 10-week program involving the specific training of the deep abdominal muscles, with coactivation of the lumbar multifidus proximal to the pars defects. The control group underwent a 10-week program as directed by their treating practitioner. After treatment, the specific exercise group showed a statistically significant reduction in pain intensity and functional disability levels that was maintained at a 30-month follow-up. The control group showed no significant change in these parameters.

Pellise F, Toribio J, Rivas A, Garcia-Gontecha C, Bago J, Villanueva C: Clinical and CT scan evaluation after direct defect repair in spondylolysis using segmental pedicular screw hook fixation. *J Spinal Disord* 1999;12:363-367.

Direct defect repair using segmental pedicular screw hook fixation was carried out in nine patients with spondylolysis (mean age, 24.2 years). One patient was fused 3 years after isthmic reconstruction. In the remaining eight patients, after a mean follow-up of 41 months, three self-evaluation scales revealed a significant improvement in clinical status. CT scans performed on seven patients showed bilateral bony union in two, unilateral union in three, and no healing in two. No correlation was observed between the radiographic appearance of the pars and the clinical status.

Tokuhashi Y, Matsuzaki H: Repair of defects in spondylolysis by segmental pedicular screw hook fixation: A preliminary report. *Spine* 1996;21:2041-2045.

Direct repair of pars defects was performed on six patients with lumbar spondylolysis using segmental pedicle screw-rod-hook fixation in conjunction with bone grafting. Postoperatively, all patients with low back pain or radicular pain experienced significant relief. Radiographs showed five patients to have a bilateral union and one a unilateral union. There were no instrumentation failures.

Classic Bibliography

Bell DF, Ehrlich MG, Zaleske DJ: Brace treatment for symptomatic spondylolisthesis. *Clin Orthop* 1988;236; 192-198.

Boxall D, Bradford DS, Winter RB, Moe JH: Management of severe spondylolisthesis in children and adolescents. *J Bone Joint Surg Am* 1979;61:479-495.

Bradford DS, Boachie-Adjei O: Treatment of severe spondylolisthesis by anterior and posterior reduction and stabilization: A long-term follow-up study. *J Bone Joint Surg Am* 1990;72:1060-1066.

Burkus JK, Lonstein JE, Winter RB, Denis F: Long-term evaluation of adolescents treated operatively for spondylolisthesis: A comparison of in situ arthrodesis only with in situ arthrodesis and reduction followed by immobilization in a cast. *J Bone Joint Surg Am* 1992; 74:693-704.

Fredrickson BE, Baker D, McHolick WF, Yuan HA, Lubicky JP: The natural history of spondylolysis and spondylolisthesis. *J Bone Joint Surg Am* 1984;66: 699-707.

Frennered AK, Danielson BI, Nachemson AL: Natural history of symptomatic isthmic low-grade spondylolisthesis in children and adolescents: A seven-year follow-up study. *J Pediatr Orthop* 1991;11:209-213.

Harada T, Ebara S, Anwar MM, et al: The lumbar spine in spastic diplegia: A radiographic study. *J Bone Joint Surg Br* 1993;75:534-537.

Lehmer SM, Steffee AD, Gaines RW Jr: Treatment of L5-S1 spondyloptosis by staged L5 resection with reduction and fusion of L4 onto S1 (Gaines procedure). *Spine* 1994;19:1916-1925.

Pizzutillo PD, Hummer CD III: Nonoperative treatment for painful adolescent spondylolysis or spondylolisthesis. *J Pediatr Orthop* 1989;9:538-540.

Saraste H: Long-term clinical and radiological follow-up of spondylolysis and spondylolisthesis. *J Pediatr Orthop* 1987;7:631-638.

Seitsalo S, Osterman K, Hyvarinen H, Tallroth K, Schlenzka D, Poussa M: Progression of spondylolisthesis in children and adolescents: A long-term follow-up of 272 patients. *Spine* 1991;16:417-421.

Stanitski CL, Stanitski DF, LaMont RL: Spondylolisthesis in myelomeningocele. *J Pediatr Orthop* 1994;14: 586-591.

Wiltse LL, Jackson DW: Treatment of spondylolisthesis and spondylolysis in children. *Clin Orthop* 1976;117: 92-100.

Chapter 34

Pediatric Cervical Spine

Brian G. Smith, MD

Introduction

Cervical spine disorders in children encompass the spectrum of pathologies, including congenital, developmental, traumatic, inflammatory, and connective tissue abnormalities. Careful diagnostic assessment and appropriate early management remain the cornerstones of treatment and avoiding potentially devastating complications.

Understanding differences between the developing pediatric cervical spine and the adult spine is critical. The developmental anatomy of the pediatric spine is unique and influences diagnostic and management considerations. The more horizontal orientation of the upper cervical facets and increased ligamentous laxity in children combine to permit greater cervical mobility, especially in children younger than age 8 years. This contributes to some of the differences observed between children and adults when comparing the nature and type of cervical spine injuries they sustain. The pediatric cervical spine is more flexible than that of the adult as exemplified by pseudosubluxation of C2 and C3 and an increased normal atlanto-dens interval in children (4 to 5 mm). Radiographic variability is common in children because of hypermobility, incomplete vertebral ossification, and the presence of synchondroses.

Klippel-Feil Syndrome

Klippel-Feil syndrome (KFS) is defined as a cervical anomaly that includes a congenital fusion. It comprises the entire range of osseous anomalies of the cervical spine associated with limited motion and frequently (one third of cases) includes genitourinary anomalies. The classic triad of low posterior hairline, short neck, and limited range of motion is found to occur in less than half of patients with KFS. Associated conditions frequently identified in these patients include congenital scoliosis, Sprengel's deformity, hearing impairment, synkinesis, and congenital heart disease. Presenting symptoms often include neck pain or limited motion.

When radiographs of the cervical spine confirm the diagnosis of KFS, further evaluation and assessment of possible associated conditions, especially those involving the renal system, is warranted.

The incidence of neurologic symptoms requiring surgery and the associated predisposing cervical abnormalities recently has been evaluated. In a study of 57 patients, 21 (37%) had neurologic symptoms requiring surgery, whereas in another study of 32 patients, only seven (22%) had neurologic symptoms, with two having surgery. In both studies, degenerative changes at an unfused segment and cervical stenosis were correlated with the development of neurologic problems. In yet another study of 19 children and adolescents with KFS, five patients (26%) had neurologic symptoms, with four requiring surgery. An increased risk of neurologic symptoms was related to the severity of occipitocervical abnormalities and cervical instability, findings that have been identified in previous studies. Neither age nor number of mobile segments was found to correlate with the development of neurologic symptoms.

The possible genetic cause of KFS recently has been studied extensively using cytogenic banding studies in three families with KFS. In one family with a dominant mode of KFS transmission, all affected individuals had a chromosome 8 inversion. A new four-type classification system recently has been proposed, which is based on the time of development of the radiographic appearance and morphology of vertebral fusions. This classification scheme distinguishes KFS classes by differences in the location of the vertebral fusion and modes of inheritance and is clinically relevant in the identification of the different additional anomalies associated with each class.

Congenital Muscular Torticollis

Torticollis is a term describing a characteristic head tilt and rotation that in young infants may cause adverse molding of the head and generate plagiocephaly. A variety of conditions may produce torticollis, but congenital muscular torticollis (CMT) is now considered possibly to be secondary to a compartment-like syndrome in the sternocleidomastoid muscle (SCM) produced by a stretch injury during delivery. The healing process results in SCM contracture, manifesting at age 6 or 8 weeks as a firm mass within the body of the muscle, a so-called pseudotumor. The contracture of the SCM restricts range of motion of the head and neck, producing deformation of the skull and face in the first year of life. Differential diagnosis of wry neck in an infant would include visual/ocular abnormalities, inflammation or infection of the pharynx, neoplasms of the spinal cord, trauma, and atlantoaxial rotatory displacement.

Microscopic analysis in 16 children undergoing surgery for torticollis of the pseudotumor permitted determination of the ratio of myoblasts to fibroblasts. Based on this ratio, the potential development of torticollis from pseudotumor was postulated.

CMT has been theorized to represent one aspect of the molded baby syndrome in which crowding of the infant in a small uterus during the last trimester contributes to stretching of the SCM. Associated with the concept has been the co-incidence of hip dysplasia in infants with CMT, which has been reported as high 15% to 20% in the past. Hip dysplasia was diagnosed in only 2.4% of 624 patients with torticollis in one study and nearly 7% of 510 patients in another. Yet another study, in which patients with CMT were evaluated specifically for dysplasia, identified six of 77 patients (8%) with dysplasia, all of whom required treatment.

Prompt diagnosis and early treatment with a stretching program generally result in a correction of the contracture and reduction of the plagiocephaly. More than 1,000 infants with torticollis were evaluated in two recent studies, with manual stretching yielding good to excellent results in more than 90% of patients in one study and 97% in the other. In one report, the success of stretching and nonsurgical treatment was correlated directly with the patient's age at diagnosis and initiation of treatment. Symptoms completely resolved in all 28 patients with CMT who started treatment by age 3 months.

Surgical release or lengthening of the contracted SCM is done in those children who are seen late or who do not respond to nonsurgical treatment. Excellent results in more than 96% of patients undergoing surgery recently were reported.

Rotatory Subluxation

Rotatory subluxation or atlantoaxial rotatory subluxation (AARS) is a common cause of acquired torticollis in children. A child may come to the orthopaedist with a head tilt and rotation following an upper respiratory or pharyngeal infection (Grisel's syndrome). Inflammation-induced laxity of the alar and transverse ligaments and capsular structures is considered the etiology of the disorder, and the ligamentous laxity may also be secondary to juvenile rheumatoid arthritis or present in children with Down or Morquio's syndromes. Other causes of AARS include trauma and surgical procedures of the head and neck. If an early diagnosis is made, prompt treatment with nonsteroidal anti-inflammatory drugs (NSAIDs), a collar, physical therapy, or traction with a halter often is successful.

Dynamic CT of the upper cervical spine in maximal right and left rotation is the diagnostic study of choice, with 40° rotation to the right and left considered normal. However, even in normal children, uncovering the facet joints may be misinterpreted as subluxation. It is the lack of reducibility that characterizes AARS. A recent study using dynamic CT in 10 normal healthy children demonstrated wide contact loss between the facets of C1 and C2 of 74% to 85% of the articular surface in right and left rotation and was interpreted by three blinded radiologists as AARS. The authors concluded that the diagnostic concepts of rotatory subluxation should be reevaluated, because the normal C1-C2 rotation on CT assessment has not been reported previously.

Twenty patients with AARS and an average age of 6 years underwent treatment at an average of 11 days after onset of symptoms. Seven patients had a history of pharyngitis, four had recently had head or neck surgery, four had sustained some type of trauma, and in five patients no obvious cause was identified. Most patients responded to nonsurgical care that initially in all patients was either cervical collar immobilization and NSAIDs or cervical traction for a mean of 4 days with an average of 4 lb of weight. Six patients (30%) either did not respond to these measures or had a recurrence of AARS and required posterior atlantoaxial fusion. The delay of diagnosis or treatment correlated with the failure of nonsurgical treatment.

Cervical Disk Calcification

Cervical disk calcification is a rare phenomenon that occurs in the cervical and thoracic spines of children. It is characterized by calcification of the nucleus pulposus. In a series of nine children with an average age of 8.5 years at the time of diagnosis and a 5-year average follow-up, the presenting symptoms included neck pain and stiffness; laboratory work-up was unrevealing. This study confirmed the self-limited nature of the disorder; symptomatic treatment lead to pain reduction within

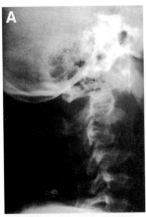 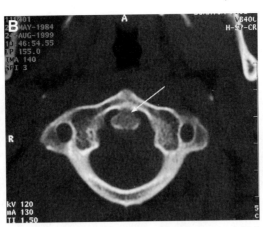 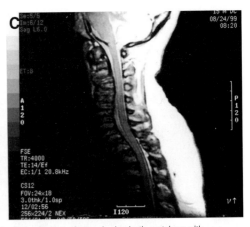

Figure 1 **A,** Lateral radiograph of the spine of a 15-year-old boy with spondyloepiphyseal-type skeletal dysplasia. Radiograph reveals dysplastic vertebrae with platyspondyly and an apparent increased subluxation of the ring of C1 on a dysplastic and shortened odontoid process, with an apparent os odontoideum. **B,** CT scan shows an apparent fusion between the posterior arch of C1 and the cephalad portion of the odontoid process (*arrow*). **C,** MRI scan of the sagittal plane shows no cervical spinal cord impingement. Flexion MRIs demonstrated slight atlantoaxial subluxation with an increase of the predental space but no evidence of cord compression.

weeks. The radiographs returned to normal within 6 months.

Osteochondrodysplasias

The osteochondrodysplasias are a varied group of heritable abnormalities of bone or cartilage formation and remodeling. Patients with these disorders generally are characterized as having short stature and ligamentous laxity; they often have significant cervical spine abnormalities as well. Precise diagnosis of a short-statured child requires radiographic evaluation supplemented with genetics consultation and appropriate laboratory analysis; often, these tests may not be accomplished until early childhood. Cervical instability may develop in these patients, often with few clinical signs or symptoms, and must be considered and evaluated with periodic radiographs. Cervical spine involvement may occur at the atlanto-occipital area (basilar invagination), atlantoaxial, or mid cervical spine levels (Fig. 1).

Basilar invagination may occur in patients with osteogenesis imperfecta, Morquio's syndrome, or more rarely with achondroplasia or spondyloepiphyseal dysplasia. Patients may remain asymptomatic for several decades and then may also experience headache, neck pain, and subtle neurologic symptoms for years prior to diagnosis. Lateral cervical radiography and MRI remain the best means of diagnosis (Fig. 2).

Twenty-five patients with basilar invagination secondary to osteochondrodysplasias recently were evaluated. The most common presenting symptom was headache, and the average age at presentation was 12 years. All patients had posterior occipitocervical fusion. Those with reducible invagination underwent posterior fossa decompression while those with irreducible ventral compression underwent transoral-transpharyngeal decompression. Fusion eventually was successful

in all patients, although 80% had progressive invagination requiring prolonged external immobilization.

Cervical kyphosis may be present in patients with Larsen's syndrome or diastrophic dysplasia. It is more often progressive with growth in patients with Larsen's syndrome and may cause neurologic compromise. A total of 11 patients with cervical kyphosis, four with Larsen's syndrome and seven with diastrophic dwarfism, recently were reviewed in two separate studies. Common radiographic findings included posterior element hypoplasia, dysraphism, and apical vertebral body retrocession causing narrowing of the spinal canal. In one study, cervical kyphosis of greater than 40° in four patients with Larsen's syndrome was treated with posterior fusion at an average age of 14 months. Anterior growth continued in three patients, resulting in stabilization or improvement of the kyphosis. Pseudarthrosis in the fourth patient resulted in progressive kyphosis with neurologic compromise, requiring anterior decompression. Neurologically normal patients with Larsen's syndrome or diastrophic dysplasia may be seen, but evidence of spinal cord compression on MRI or neurologic symptoms warrant surgical stabilization.

Trisomy 21

Patients with Down syndrome may have upper cervical instability secondary to generalized ligamentous laxity. Approximately one in five patients with trisomy 21 have at least a mild degree of C1-C2 instability. Atlanto-occipital instability is documented to occur in these children as well. A study of 90 children with Down syndrome identified atlantoaxial instability in seven patients, none of whom were symptomatic. Of the 67 patients available for reevaluation, no new cases

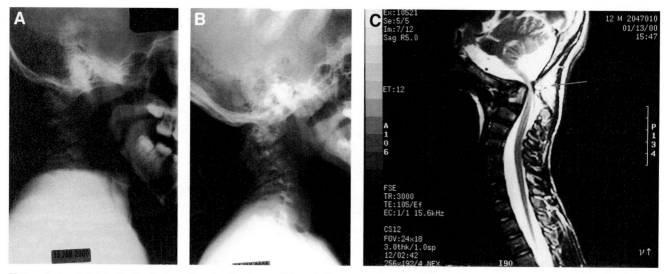

Figure 2 **A** and **B,** Lateral and extension radiographs of a 12-year-old boy who is blind and mentally retarded whose care providers have reported increasing dysfunction in his right arm. Radiographs reveal severe congenital dysplasia of the craniocervical junction and severe occipitocervical kyphosis with basilar invagination. **C,** MRI depicts the severe congenital anomaly of C1 with a deficient posterior arch. The arrow indicates subluxation of C2 into the foramen magnum with severe spinal cord compression and kinking. A mass effect within the spinal cord is consistent with edema.

of instability were identified and two of the original seven actually improved.

Atlanto-occipital translation (AOT) and instability recently have been evaluated in patients with Down syndrome. The method of Wiesel and Rothman for sagittal AOT was used to evaluate 38 children with Down syndrome and 34 control children. The average translation was 2.3 mm in the Down group, 0.61 mm in the control group, with 1.0 mm the normal adult standard. Because only one of 38 patients had any neurologic symptoms or signs, the authors concluded that less than 3 mm AOT should be considered clinically insignificant in these patients. Clinical assessment and dynamic MRI findings were more reliable in confirming AOT instability in patients with trisomy 21.

The precise indications for cervical spine fusion in patients with Down syndrome remain uncertain. Flexion-extension radiography in 84 patients identified an atlanto-dens interval of greater than 4 mm in 17 (20%). Positive neurologic findings were also found in five (29%) of these patients, but similar findings were present in 18 (27%) of the normal patients with Down syndrome, indicating that the presence of either of these findings alone is not sufficient to warrant surgery.

Upper cervical spinal fusion in children with Down syndrome is a potentially risky and challenging surgical endeavor. Fifteen patients with Down syndrome undergoing upper cervical spine arthrodesis had a major complication rate (73%) at an average follow-up of 74.6 months. Neurologic improvement occurred in three, but two had neurologic deterioration. Twelve of 15 patients (80%) had achieved solid arthrodesis by

follow-up. Neurologic signs and significant radiographic findings must be present to warrant surgery in this patient population.

Postlaminectomy Kyphosis

Postoperative cervical spine deformity has been documented following decompression surgery in growing children. Surgical decompression in 32 children with Chiari malformations produced kyphosis requiring fusion in one patient and mild kyphosis in two patients at a follow-up of 3.7 years. This low (9%) incidence of postsurgical deformity is a testimony to the value of minimizing bone resection in growing patients, especially avoiding violation of the facet joint during cervical laminectomy.

Trauma

Because the developing spine of a child tends to be more cartilaginous, especially at younger ages, than the mature spine of an adult, the pattern and nature of cervical spine injuries (CSI) in children often is different than that occurring in adults. Because an accepted protocol for cervical spine clearance in comatose children does not exist, a protocol was proposed during a recent pilot study. Fifteen obtunded children were evaluated by three-view standard radiography and CT scans as necessary. In order not to miss the unique spinal cord injuries without radiographic abnormality (SCIWORA) of children, patients who 5 days postinjury still had an altered mental status and unreliable physical examinations with normal radiographic studies underwent flexion-extension cervical spine fluoroscopy with monitoring of somatosensory-evoked potentials

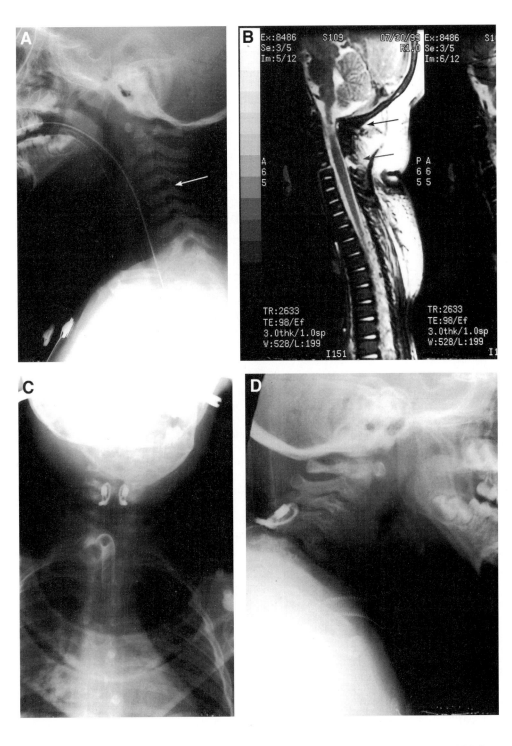

Figure 3 **A,** Lateral radiograph of the cervical spine of a 24-month-old boy who was ejected from a car. Arrow indicates the widened space between C4 and C5. **B,** MRI scan obtained after the patient was stabilized. Traumatic changes are noted at the C4-C5 level, particularly in the posterior elements secondary to flexion-distraction injury through the cephalad portion of C5 (*solid arrow*). Open arrow indicates edema and obvious trauma in the cord at the craniocervical junction. Clinically, the patient had quadriplegia at C2 even though the radiographic injury was at C4-C5. **C** and **D,** AP and lateral views obtained 8 weeks postoperatively following posterior fusion at C4-C5 and stabilization with sublaminar cables. Although solid fusion was achieved, the patient has a tracheostomy and is ventilator dependent.

(SSEPs). Median nerve SSEPs, which correlate with compromise of the cervical cord, were monitored unless an injury below C5 was suspected, in which case the ulnar nerve also was assessed. Those with abnormal SSEPs underwent MRI studies. Based on this protocol, it was possible to render management decisions for all patients. The improved efficacy of this management protocol in obtunded children currently is being evaluated by the authors in a multicenter randomized study.

The value of MRI in evaluating CSI was confirmed in another recent study of 52 children with CSI and negative radiographs and CT scans who had persistent findings or symptoms of instability or injury. Sixteen of the 52 patients (31%) had abnormal findings present on MRI, with posterior ligamenatous injury the most common finding.

A recent review documented the relatively high incidence of SCIWORA in children with CSI. Of 72 children with CSI on the basis of their discharge diagnosis from a children's medical center over a 5-year period, 40 had radiographic evidence of CSI and 32 had SCIWORA. Lateral radiographs had a sensitivity of 94% and three-view radiographs had the same sensitivity in children with radiographically evident CSI. Younger children tended to have higher, more proximal cervical spine lesions (fractures or dislocations) than older children (Fig. 3).

In a study of 32 children with CSI sustained over a 7-year period, 53% had abnormal neurologic findings. Children older than age 10 years tended to have adult pattern type injuries, usually below C4. Of 17 patients with neurologic injury, two died, six had permanent sequelae, and nine recovered fully. The high morbidity of CSI in children coupled with the tendency for these injuries to be caused in motor vehicle accidents underscores the importance of properly restraining children in motor vehicles.

Surgical Techniques and Results

Traditional techniques continue to evolve, and new procedures are being developed for the surgical management of pediatric cervical spine disorders. In a retrospective review of 23 patients undergoing occipitocervical fusion with occipitocervical wiring, arthrodesis was successful in all but one patient. Fifteen of the patients had fusion using a technique in which a threaded Kirschner wire (K-wire) was passed through the spinous process of the distal instrumented cervical vertebra, usually C2. Anchoring the occipital wire to the percutaneously placed spinous process K-wire produced no significant increase in risk of complications. In another study, 16 children with atlantoaxial instability (AAI) underwent either odontoid screw fixation for odontoid fractures or transarticular screw fixation of C1-C2. A halo was not used postoperatively; only a Miami J collar was used. Fusion was successful in all patients 3 months postoperatively without major complications or neurologic problems.

Improvement of cervical alignment following fusion for cervical kyphosis in children also has been documented recently. Four of 12 patients with immediate postoperative malalignment and cervical kyphosis following C1-C2 fusions were found over a follow-up of more than 6 years to have increased bone formation on the anterior vertebral cortex, resulting in remodeling of the deformity over time. Problems with the use of multistranded sublaminar cables were identified in one study of 25 children undergoing fusion. In two of six instances in which the cable was used, erosion of the intact arch of C1 was identified. The authors concluded that sublaminar multistranded cables should not be used to provide internal fixation of the cervical spine for fusions in children.

Summary

The pediatric cervical spine remains a challenge for the physician managing the potentially complex disorders that may affect it. The differences in mobility and types of injuries of the pediatric cervical spine compared with those of the adult are important in treatment considerations. Accurate early diagnosis of pediatric cervical spine disorders will enable prompt appropriate care and help to avoid potential future deformity and disability.

Annotated Bibliography

Klippel-Feil Syndrome

Baba H, Maezawa Y, Furusawa N, Chen Q, Imura S, Tomita K: The cervical spine in the Klippel-Feil syndrome: A report of 57 cases. *Int Orthop* 1995;19:204-208.

In a review of 57 patients with KFS, progressive neurologic symptoms developed in 21 patients (37%) and 19 required surgery. Neurologic compromise was associated with cervical stenosis and degenerative changes at an unfused segment.

Clarke RA, Catalan G, Diwan AD, Kearsley JH: Heterogeneity in Klippel-Feil syndrome: A new classification. *Pediatr Radiol* 1998;28:967-974.

Three families with KFS were studied extensively with cervical and thoracic spinal radiographs and chromosomal analysis using cytogenic banding studies. A new four-type classification system is proposed that distinguishes classes of KFS by differences in patterns of vertebral fusion, associated anomalies, and modes of inheritance.

Rouvreau P, Glorion C, Langlais J, Noury H, Pouliquen JC: Assessment and neurologic involvement of patients with cervical spine congenital synostosis as in Klippel-Feil syndrome. *J Pediatr Orthop B* 1998;7:179-185.

Of 19 children and adolescents with KFS followed for an average of more than 12 years, five patients had neurologic complications leading to surgery in four, and three patients had radiographic evidence of hypermobility. Neurologic symptoms occurred at an average age of 16.5 years and were related to age or the number of mobile vertebral segments. The severity of occipitocervical abnormalities and cervical instability were associated with an increased risk of neurologic problems.

Theiss SM, Smith MD, Winter RB: The long-term follow-up of patients with Klippel-Feil syndrome and congenital scoliosis. *Spine* 1997;22:1219-1222.

Data are presented on 32 patients with KFS followed longitudinally for more than 10 years who presented originally with congenital scoliosis. Cervical symptoms developed in only seven patients (22%), with two requiring surgery. Fusion to the cervicothoracic junction and cervical stenosis were two factors found to be associated with the development of cervical symptoms.

Thomsen MN, Schneider U, Weber M, Johannisson R, Niethard FU: Scoliosis and congenital anomalies associated with Klippel-Feil syndrome types I-III. *Spine* 1997;22:396-401.

The authors reviewed data on 57 patients with KFS treated for more than 25 years at their center. A wide variety of associated anomalies were identified, with more than 70% of the patients demonstrating scoliosis. Patients with type II KFS (fusion isolated to the cervical spine) had the lowest incidence of scoliosis.

Congenital Muscular Torticollis

Cheng JC, Tang SP: Outcome of surgical treatment of congenital muscular torticollis. *Clin Orthop* 1999;362:190-200.

Data on 84 patients undergoing surgical treatment over a 10-year period for CMT are presented. Surgery was performed before age 1 year in 26%, between 1 and 3 years in 23%, and between 3 and 10 years in 38%. More than 96% of the patients had good or excellent results, while 1.2% required a second operation.

Cheng JC, Tang SP, Chen TM: Sternocleidomastoid pseudotumor and congenital muscular torticollis in infants: A prospective study of 510 cases. *J Pediatr* 1999;134:712-716.

These authors evaluated 510 infants with sternomastoid pseudotumor prospectively over 10 years, with an average follow-up of 3.5 years. Nearly 93% were seen by age 3 months, with a mean age of 24 days. Breech presentation and assisted delivery were highly correlated with pseudotumor, and almost 7% of patients had hip dysplasia, which correlated with the severity of the clinical rotational deficit. More than 90% of the patients had good or excellent results with early intervention with a manual stretching program performed by physical therapists, while 34 patients (6.7%) required surgery.

Demirbilek S, Atayurt HF: Congenital muscular torticollis and sternomastoid tumor: Results of nonoperative treatment. *J Pediatr Surg* 1999;34:549-551.

In this study, 57 infants and children were followed over a 5-year period to evaluate the effectiveness of active and passive stretching exercises. A regular standardized exercise program was used by the parents. Avoidance of surgery was considered successful treatment, and all 28 patients who started treatment at age 3 months or earlier had resolution of their symptoms. The success rate of nonsurgical treatment declined with increasing age at presentation.

Tang S, Liu Z, Quan X, Qin J, Zhang D: Sternocleidomastoid pseudotumor of infants and congenital muscular torticollis: Fine-structure research. *J Pediatr Orthop* 1998;18:214-218.

Light and electron microscopy were used to investigate the tissue of 16 children undergoing surgery for sternocleidomastoid pseudotumor at infancy and 34 children with CMT. Myoblasts were found in the pseudotumors, and their degree of degeneration and their ratio to fibroblasts were theorized to have a significant impact on the outcome of the pseudotumors and the potential development of torticollis.

Walsh JJ, Morrissy RT: Torticollis and hip dislocation. *J Pediatr Orthop* 1998;18:219-221.

Seventy-seven patients with torticollis were seen over a 7-year period and were evaluated radiographically for hip dysplasia. Six patients (8%) were diagnosed with hip dysplasia; all required treatment. Four of these six were known at the time of referral to have hip dysplasia.

Rotatory Subluxation

Subach BR, McLaughlin MR, Albright AL, Pollack IF: Current management of pediatric atlantoaxial rotatory subluxation. *Spine* 1998;23:2174-2179.

Twenty patients with a mean age of 6 years and an average of 11 days of symptoms were treated for AARS. Five patients were treated with a rigid cervical collar and anti-inflammatory agents, and four had spontaneous reduction while the fifth patient required fusion because a course of traction failed. In 15 of 16 patients treated with cervical traction, normal alignment was restored at an average of 4 days. Six of the 20 patients (30%) ultimately required posterior fusion for either failure or recurrence of reduction. The length of delay of diagnosis or treatment correlated with the likelihood of failure of nonsurgical treatment.

Villas C, Arriagada C, Zubieta JL: Preliminary CT study of C1-C2 rotational mobility in normal subjects. *Eur Spine J* 1999;8:223-228.

Radiographic and clinical evaluation of 10 normal, healthy, asymptomatic children (average age 9 years) was performed to determine the normal rotatory mobility at C1-C2. Radiographic evaluation included lateral radiographs in neutral and maximal flexion and CT in maximal left and right rotation at the C1-C2 articular processes joint. A wide contact loss of 74% to 85% of the total articular surface was found on images at the C1-C2 facet in all 10 children. Three independent and blinded radiologists concluded that all patients had rotatory subluxation. The authors conclude that a real potential for overdiagnosis of upper cervical spine rotational problems in children exists, and they suggest that the diagnostic concepts of C1-C2 rotatory fixation and subluxation be revisited.

Cervical Disk Calcification

Ventura N, Huguet R, Salvador A, Terricabras L, Cabrera AM: Intervertebral disc calcification in childhood. *Int Orthop* 1995;19:291-294.

Calcified intervertebral disks were followed in nine children (average age 8.5 years) for an average of 5 years, with a minimum follow-up of 2 years. A total of 12 disks were involved, with most in the cervical spine. Presenting symptoms included pain and limited motion; laboratory work-up was unremarkable. Treatment was symptomatic, and pain resolved within a few weeks. The disk calcification disappeared within 2 to 6 months.

Osteochondrodysplasias

Forese LL, Berdon WE, Harcke HT, et al: Severe mid-cervical kyphosis with cord compression in Larsen's syndrome and diastrophic dysplasia: Unrelated syndromes with similar radiologic findings and neurosurgical implications. *Pediatr Radiol* 1995;25:136-139.

Seven patients with diastrophic dwarfism and four patients with Larsen's syndrome, all with midcervical kyphosis, were reviewed. Posterior element hypoplasia and dysraphism and retrocession of the apical vertebral bodies were common.

Johnston CE II, Birch JG, Daniels JL: Cervical kyphosis in patients who have Larsen syndrome. *J Bone Joint Surg Am* 1996;78:538-545.

Cervical kyphosis averaging more than 40° in four patients with Larsen's syndrome was treated with posterior fusion at an average age of 14 months. In three patients, the kyphosis either stabilized or improved by continued anterior growth. Pseudarthrosis in the fourth patient resulted in progessive kyphosis and ultimately required anterior decompression and fusion for an acute neurologic deficit.

Sawin PD, Menezes AH: Basilar invagination in osteogenesis imperfecta and related osteochondrodysplasias: Medical and surgical management. *J Neurosurg* 1997;86:950-960.

Twenty-five patients with symptomatic basilar invagination secondary to congenital osteochondrodysplasias, including 18 patients with osteogenesis imperfecta, were evaluated. The average age at presentation was 12 years. Headache was the most common symptom, but 12 patients presented with quadriparesis. Treatment included posterior occipitocervical fusion in all patients, with those having a reducible invagination undergoing posterior fossa decompression and those with irreducible ventral compression having transoral-transpharyngeal decompression. Fusion was successful in all patients, but progressive invagination developed in 80% of patients, which was treated with prolonged external orthotic immobilization.

Trisomy 21

Doyle JS, Lauerman WC, Wood KB, Krause DR: Complications and long-term outcome of upper cervical spine arthrodesis in patients with Down syndrome. *Spine* 1996;21:1223-1231.

Fifteen patients with Down syndrome and a history of upper cervical spine arthrodesis for instability were reviewed at an average of 74.6 months. Major complications including nonunion, loss of reduction, neurologic deterioration, and infection developed after surgery in 11 of the 15 patients (73%). A second procedure was required in six patients, and 12 patients (80%) achieved solid arthrodesis. Improvement was noted in only three patients, however, and neurologic status deteriorated in two postoperatively.

Ferguson RL, Putney ME, Allen BL Jr: Comparison of neurologic deficits with atlanto-dens intervals in patients with Down syndrome. *J Spinal Disord* 1997;10:246-252.

Flexion-extension radiographs were obtained in 84 patients with Down syndrome to identify those with subluxation of the atlanto-dens interval (ADI) of greater than 4 mm. Subluxation was found in 17 patients (20%). Positive neurologic findings were found in five patients (29%) with subluxation, but similar findings were identified in 18 patients (27%) without subluxation. The authors conclude that an abnormal ADI and positive neurologic findings alone are not sufficient criteria to recommend spinal fusion in patients with Down syndrome.

Karol LA, Sheffield EG, Crawford K, Moody MK, Browne RH: Reproducibility in the measurement of atlanto-occipital instability in children with Down syndrome. *Spine* 1996;21:2463-2468.

Sixty pairs of lateral cervical spine radiographs in 34 children with Down syndrome were reviewed twice by four different observers. Using the technique of Wiesel and Rothman and the basion-axial interval, translational motion between the occiput and C1 was recorded and intra- and interobserver variability was calculated. Measurement of these intervals was not statistically reproducible. The authors concluded that clinical symptoms and MRI assessment also are necessary to confirm instability in these patients.

Matsuda Y, Sano N, Watanabe S, Oki S, Shibata T: Atlanto-occipital hypermobility in subjects with Down's syndrome. *Spine* 1995;20:2283-2286.

AOT was evaluated using the method of Wiesel and Rothman on lateral flexion-extension radiographs in 38 children with Down syndrome and then compared with those of 34 control children. Whereas more than 1 mm of translation indicates instability in adults, the average translation in the patients with Down syndrome was 2.3 mm compared to 0.61 mm in the control group. Only one of these 38 patients was found to have neurologic signs or symptoms suggestive of instability, leading the authors to suggest that AOT of less than 3 mm in patients with Down syndrome is likely to be clinically insignificant.

Morton RE, Khan MA, Murray-Leslie C, Elliott S: Atlanto-axial instability in Down's syndrome: A five year follow-up study. *Arch Dis Child* 1995;72:115-119.

Ninety school children with Down syndrome were evaluated radiographically for AAI. AAI was identified in seven children, none of whom had signs or symptoms. Five years later, 67 patients (74%) were reviewed. No new cases of AAI were found, and two of the original seven with AAI actually improved while the other five remained symptom free. Three radiographs taken on the same day in these patients showed a maximal variation of 1.0 mm.

Postlaminectomy Kyphosis

McLaughlin MR, Wahlig JB, Pollack IF: Incidence of post laminectomy kyphosis after Chiari decompression. *Spine* 1997;22:613-617.

The results of surgical decompression of Chiari malformations in 32 children (average age, 4.9 years) were reviewed to determine the incidence of cervical kyphosis and instability after surgery at a mean of 3.7 years. One patient had clinical and radiographic evidence of kyphosis requiring fusion, and two patients had mild kyphosis radiographically. The low (9%) incidence of kyphosis in this report suggests that overaggressive laminectomy be avoided to minimize postoperative kyphosis in these patients.

Trauma

Baker C, Kadish H, Schunk JE: Evaluation of pediatric cervical spine injuries. *Am J Emerg Med* 1999;17:230-234.

Seventy-two children with CSI were reviewed. Radiographically evident CSI was present in 40 patients, while 32 had SCIWORA. Abnormal physical examination findings of the neck were present in 80% of patients, and six patients (16%) with SCI had abnormal neurologic findings. Lateral radiographs alone had a sensitivity of 79% for SCI and three-view radiographs had a sensitivity of 94%, indicating that this is the minimum radiographic assessment required for children with CSI. Younger children tended to have more CSI than older children.

Finch GD, Barnes MJ: Major cervical spine injuries in children and adolescents. *J Pediatr Orthop* 1998;18: 811-814.

The incidence of CSI in 32 children younger than age 15 years over a 7-year period was reviewed. Motor vehicle accidents caused most of the injuries in younger children, whereas recreational sports caused those in older children. Associated injuries were present in 31%, and 53% had abnormal neurologic findings. Children younger than age 10 years were more likely to have upper CSI, whereas those patients older than age 10 years tended to have adult pattern injuries. Of 17 patients with neurologic injury, two died, nine had a full recovery, and six had permanent sequelae. All 10 patients treated with reduction or surgery had satisfactory outcomes.

Givens TG, Polley KA, Smith GF, Hardin WD Jr: Pediatric cervical spine injury: A three-year experience. *J Trauma* 1996;41:310-314.

Over a 3-year period, 34 children were treated for CSI, most sustained in motor vehicle accidents. Head injuries were associated with CSI in 53% of patients, and overall mortality was 41% (14 patients). CSI below C4 occurred in 50% of patients age 8 years or younger, tending to discount the theory that young children sustain CSI primarily above C4.

Keiper MD, Zimmerman RA, Bilaniuk LT: MRI in the assessment of supportive soft tissues of the cervical spine in acute trauma in children. *Neuroradiology* 1998;40:359-363.

Fifty-two children with cervical spine trauma were evaluated with MRI despite negative radiographs and CT scans when symptoms persisted or unexplained findings of instability or injury were seen. Positive MRI findings were present in 16 patients (31%), with posterior ligamentous injury the most common finding. MRI influenced the surgical management of all four patients requiring posterior stabilization and was superior to CT for assessment of spinal cord hemorrhage and injury.

Scarrow AM, Levy EI, Resnick DK, Adelson PD, Sclabassi RJ: Cervical spine evaluation in obtunded or comatose pediatric trauma patients: A pilot study. *Pediatr Neurosurg* 1999;30:169-175.

Because an accepted protocol for evaluation of CSI in obtunded pediatric trauma patients does not exist, 15 patients were evaluated using a new cervical spine clearance protocol. Evaluation included three-view standard radiography and CT as necessary. Patients with altered mental status and normal radiographs underwent flexion-extension cervical spine fluoroscopy with monitoring of SSEP. Patients with SSEP changes or abnormal movement by fluoroscopy had MRI. This protocol is recommended as a safe method to evaluate CSI in children.

Surgical Techniques and Results

Lowry DW, Pollack IF, Clyde B, Albright AL, Adelson PD: Upper cervical spine fusion in the pediatric population. *J Neurosurg* 1997;87:671-676.

Upper cervical spine arthrodesis for spinal instability was performed in 25 children with an average age of 9 years. After surgery, nine of 10 children showed improvement or resolution of abnormal preoperative neurologic findings. Arthrodesis occurred in 21 of 25 patients after the initial operation and in all but one patient by final follow-up. Erosion of a multistranded sublaminar cable through the intact arch of C2 occurred in two of six patients in whom it was used, prompting the authors to stop using this as a means of fixation in children.

Rodgers WB, Coran DL, Emans JB, Hresko MT, Hall JE: Occipitocervical fusions in children: Retrospective analysis and technical considerations. *Clin Orthop* 1999;364:125-133.

The results of occipitocervical fusion in 23 patients were reviewed. Fifteen had a technique incorporating a threaded K-wire passed transversely through the spinous process to anchor an occipital wire. At an average follow-up of 5.8 years, successful arthrodesis had been achieved in all but one patient, and overall results and incidence of complications compared very favorably to prior studies in the literature.

Wang J, Vokshoor A, Kim S, Elton S, Kosnik E, Bartkowski H: Pediatric atlantoaxial instability: Management with screw fixation. *Pediatr Neurosurg* 1999;30:70-78.

AAI was treated surgically with screw fixation and fusion in 16 children (average age, 9.4 years). Three patients with type II fractures underwent odontoid screw fixation, while the 13 remaining patients had posterior C1-C2 transarticular screw fixation. A Miami J collar only was used postoperatively in all children. All patients had achieved arthrodesis by 3 months after surgery with no major complications or neurologic deterioration.

Classic Bibliography

Cheng JC, Au AW: Infantile torticollis: A review of 624 cases. *J Pediatr Orthop* 1994;14:802-808.

Toyama Y, Matsumoto M, Chiba K, et al: Realignment of post operative cervical kyphosis in children by vertebral remodeling. *Spine* 1994;19:2565-2570.

Wiesel SW, Rothman RH: Occipitoatlantal hypermobility. *Spine* 1979;4:187-191.

Index

f indicates figure
t indicates table